W9-BII-864

Orthopaedic Management of
Metastatic Bone Disease

Orthopaedic Management of Metastatic Bone Disease

KEVIN D. HARRINGTON, M.D.

Clinical Associate Professor of Orthopaedic Surgery,
University of California, San Francisco,
School of Medicine, San Francisco, California

with 486 *illustrations and* 2 *four-color plates*
illustrations by Susan Taft

THE C. V. MOSBY COMPANY

ST. LOUIS • WASHINGTON, D.C. • TORONTO 1988

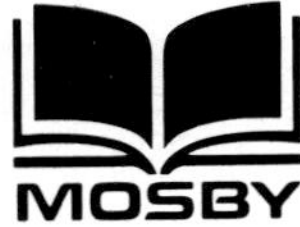

A TRADITION OF PUBLISHING EXCELLENCE

Editor: *Eugenia A. Klein*
Assistant editor: *Lynn Gerdemann Hughes*
Manuscript editor: *George B. Stericker, Jr.*
Design: *Liz Fett*
Production: *Ginny Douglas*

Printed in the United States of America

The C.V. Mosby Company
11830 Westline Industrial Drive, St. Louis, Missouri 63146

Library of Congress Cataloging-in-Publication Data

Harrington, Kevin D.
Orthopaedic management of metastatic bone disease.

Includes bibliographies and index.
1. Bones—Cancer—Surgery. 2. Metastasis—Surgery.
I. Title. [DNLM: 1. Bone Neoplasms—surgery. 2. Neoplasm Metastasis. WE 258 H299o]
RD675. H37 1988 619.99'471 87-15266
ISBN 0-8016-2102-X

AC/MV/MV 9 8 7 6 5 4 3 2 1 03/A/372

CONTRIBUTORS

STEPHEN R. BUNKER, M.D.
Nuclear Medicine Service,
Children's Hospital of San Francisco;
Assistant Clinical Professor of Radiology,
University of California,
San Francisco, California;
Assistant Clinical Professor of Radiology,
George Washington University,
Washington, D.C.

KATHLEEN M. FOLEY, M.D.
Associate Professor of Neurology and Pharmacology,
Cornell University Medical College;
Chief, Pain Service,
Department of Neurology,
Memorial Sloan-Kettering Cancer Center,
New York, New York

KEVIN D. HARRINGTON, M.D.
Clinical Associate Professor of Orthopaedic Surgery,
University of California, San Francisco,
School of Medicine,
San Francisco, California

BETH C. KLEINER, M.D.
Magnetic Resonance Fellow,
Diagnostic Networks, Incorporated,
San Francisco, California

ALEXANDER MAUSKOP, M.D.
Pain Fellow,
Department of Neurology,
Memorial Sloan-Kettering Cancer Center,
New York, New York

TILLMAN M. MOORE, M.D.
Professor of Clinical Orthopaedics,
University of Southern California School of Medicine;
Chief, Orthopaedic Surgery,
Kenneth J. Norris Cancer Hospital;
Director, Oncology Service,
Orthopaedic Hospital,
Los Angeles, California

STEVEN B. NEWMAN, M.D.
Assistant Clinical Professor of Medicine,
Section of Neurology-Oncology,
University of California–Los Angeles Center for Health Sciences,
Los Angeles, California

To *Roger Murphy*
John Bond
Mary Gordon

young and old,
who suffered this disease
with courage and tenacity, and even humor,
and rose above their debility to gain strength
in living even as life ebbed away.

Yield not to misfortunes, but go all the more boldly to face them.

Happy is he who knows how to bear the estate of slave or king, and who can match his countenance with either lot. For he who bears his ills with even soul has robbed misfortune of its power.

Seneca, 61AD

Calamity is man's true touchstone.

Francis Beaumont, 1608

PREFACE

The last 15 years have witnessed dramatic advances in the palliative management of patients with metastatic bone disease. Cancer chemotherapy has improved both in predictability and in efficacy, and the means of minimizing the side effects of that treatment have progressed apace. Improved techniques for the assessment of hormonal sensitivity of tumors, particularly carcinomas of the breast, have greatly enhanced the oncologist's ability to surpress the activity of metastases often for a long time. Radiotherapy protocols now reflect an expanded flexibility in tailoring both the time and the dosage fractionation to the individual requirements of any one patient.

Ironically, as patients have survived longer with metastatic bone disease and as the quality of their lives has improved, distribution and extent of their bone metastases and the incidence of pathological fractures have increased as well. Whereas 20 years ago a pathological long bone fracture was a preterminal event, today most patients can expect to live almost 2 years after their first fracture. Complicated reconstructive procedures of the hip, knee, pelvis, and upper extremities now must be considered for selected patients with prolonged anticipated survival. Pathological fractures of the spine, not infrequently resulting in progressive neurological compromise, now warrant operative decompression and stabilization. Prophylactic fixation of impending fractures is required with increasing frequency.

As the demand has risen, techniques for the assessment of pathological fractures or impending fractures have improved markedly as have the means for operative stabilization or reconstruction of affected bones and joints. The orthopaedic surgeon has become an integral part of the cancer treatment team and plays a major role in affording pain relief, resumption of ambulation, and enhancement of survival. He must understand the limitations as well as the advantages of the various diagnostic modalities available to him. He must also understand, at least in a general sense, hormonal and chemotherapeutic measures available to his patient and how each may enhance or may interfere with the efficacy of his reconstruction.

This book is designed as a practical primer for the surgeon interested in the management of metastatic bone disease. It is subdivided into three sections covering diagnostic modalities, medical therapy, and orthopaedic reconstruction. Each chapter is authored by an individual with great expertise and experience in his or her field and with an interest in presenting concise and practical recommendations with direct clinical application.

It is hoped that the reader will find here the information required to realistically assess any patient with metastatic bone disease and to proceed confidently with an organized approach to the overall management of that patient including the complications which may result from such management.

CONTENTS

Orthopaedic Management of
Metastatic Bone Disease

CHAPTER 1

INTRODUCTION

Cancer has been known and feared since antiquity, and malignant growths of the extremities, either primary or metastatic, were among the earliest excuses for attempts at surgical extirpation (Fig. 1-1). The concept of metastatic disease was only vaguely understood, and the sudden occurrence of a pathological fracture, dramatically rendering a person paralyzed or with a spontaneous but agonizing deformity, typically was considered re-

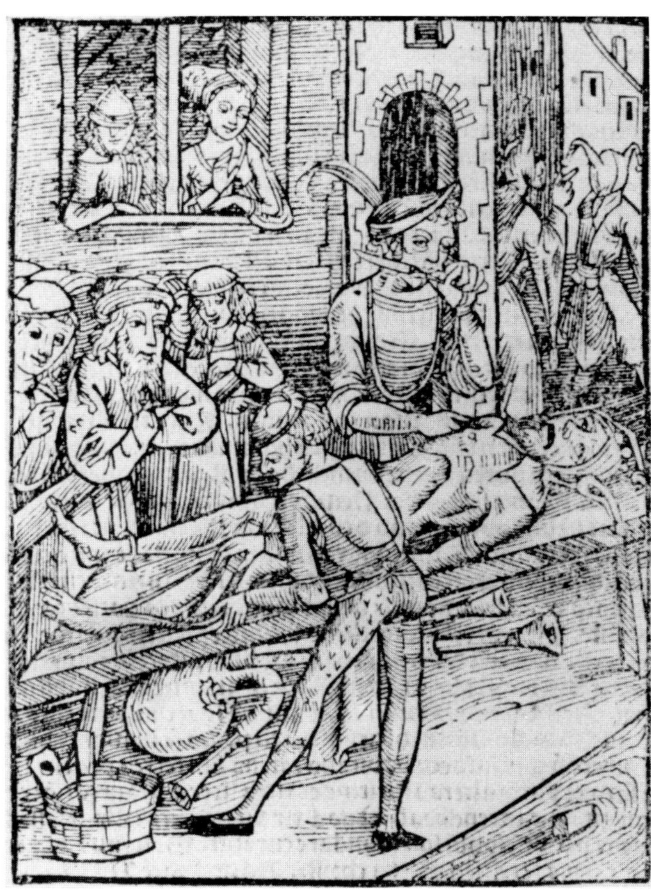

FIGURE 1-1 Medieval surgical technique for removal of an extremity tumor, in this case considered the result of inordinate pride and inadequate religious zeal (note that the patient wears a foolscap). (From Brant, S.: Das Narrenschiff [The Ship of Fools], 1494; woodcut by Albrecht Dürer, 1511.)

flective of some divine or satanic intervention (Fig. 1-2).

Perhaps the most dramatic misunderstanding of the evolution of skeletal metastases occurred during the reign of Elizabeth I of England. Elizabeth, never married but perpetually the focus of intriguing suitors, was herself enamored of Lord Robert Dudley. Unfortunately, Dudley's suit was twice encumbered. To begin with, he was already married to one of Elizabeth's ladies in waiting, Amy Robsart (Fig. 1-3). Moreover, because he was English and could offer no prospect of international alliances through marriage, the possibility of his marrying the Queen was considered a diplomatic disaster by most of her ministers. When an obvious breast malignancy developed in Amy Robsart and it became apparent that she would not long survive, her husband's neglect appeared the more callous and Elizabeth's complete monopoly of his company the more cruelly selfish. His detractors were not slow to find advantage in this and began to circulate rumors that Dudley might attempt to hasten his wife's demise. Sure enough, within a week, Amy Robsart was found at home dead with a broken neck but without evidence of foul play. A storm of protest erupted. Eighteen months of malicious gossip had put Dudley and even Elizabeth under a high degree of suspicion. A revolution was predicted by some, there was talk that the Queen would join her inamorato in the Tower, and a court of inquiry was in fact con-

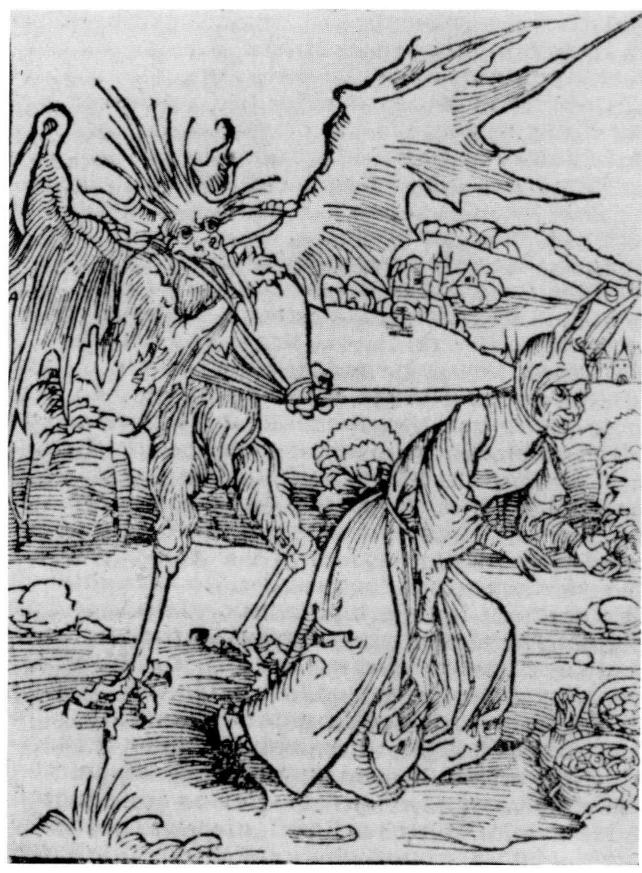

FIGURE 1-2 Woman struck down by Satan in the guise of a stork-like creature. In the Middle Ages spontaneous fractures, paralyses, and the like often were considered a manifestation of either divine or satanic intervention depending on the life-style of the afflicted. (From Brant, S.: Das Narrenschiff [The Ship of Fools], 1494; woodcut by Albrecht Dürer, 1511.)

vened. Eventually the jury brought in a verdict of accidental death, and the government was saved. Although the coroner was unable to link the malady in her breast with her broken neck, it was established that she had suffered an apparently spontaneous fracture and consequent paralysis. It was not until almost three centuries later that her death could be attributed to a metastatic pathological fracture of the upper cervical spine, probably at the second or third cervical level.[37]

Although the relationship between primary and metastatic cancers gradually came to be understood, even into the nineteenth century, virtually the only definitive treatment for extremity malignancies was physical and chemical cauterizations, excision of superficial masses, or amputation. Benjamin Rush, a signer of the Declaration of Independence, founder of the first American medical school, and one of America's earliest and most distinguished physicians, with an interest in extremity cancer, described his technique for the management of a fungating metastatic malignancy in the thigh (Figs. 1-4 and 1-5):

> Dress the bone with Lint dip't in a Tincture of Myrrh and Aloes . . . and keep up a Discharge of Matter by injecting Barley Water with honey . . . . Recommend above all things Fresh air and Gentle Exercise . . . if she cannot do the latter, have recourse to the Flesh brush.

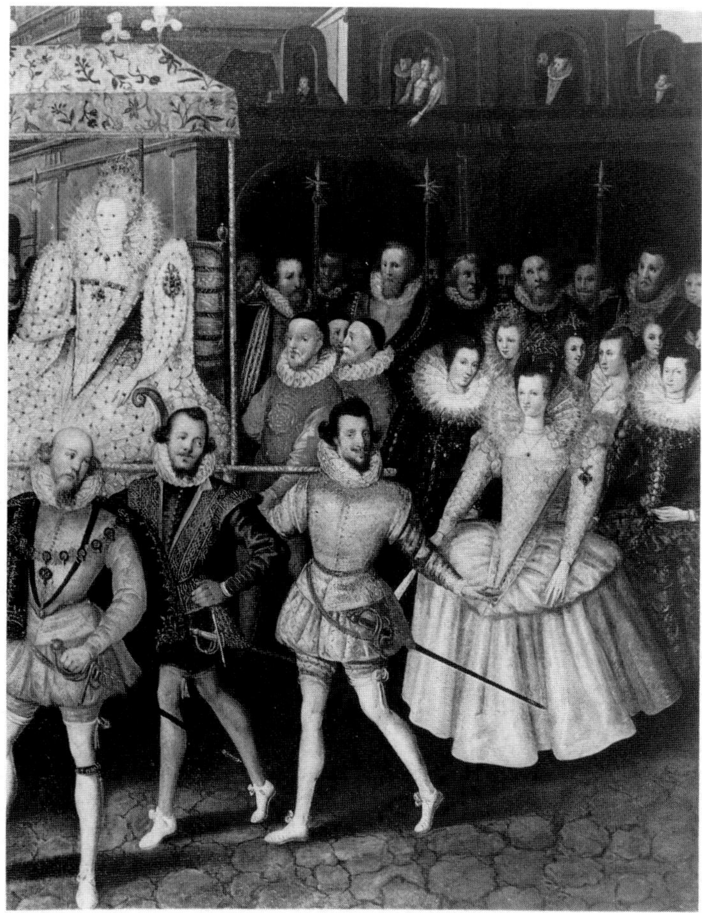

FIGURE 1-3 Queen Elizabeth being carried by her courtiers. Painting attributed to Robert Peake, the Elder, c. 1600. The Garter Knights depicted here include *(second from the left)* Robert Dudley, long the Queen's favorite. His wife, Amy Robsart, probably is at the extreme right in the black dress.

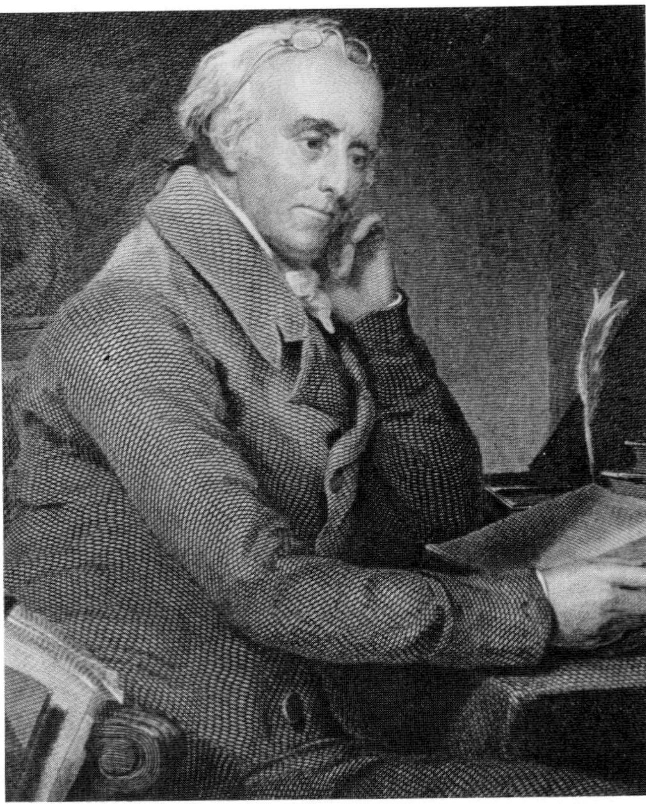

FIGURE 1-4 Benjamin Rush (1745-1813) was the most influential American physician and one of the first with an interest in the treatment of bone cancer. Although his techniques of tissue debridement and cauterization were advanced for his day, he was also an advocate of bloodletting and of purging with calomel.

Such homeopathic and largely ineffective measures (Fig. 1-6) promoted a certain apathy with regard to the management of metastatic bone disease, even while John Hunter, Ashley Cooper, and other innovative surgeons were making great advances in developing the techniques for preserving limbs affected by other disease processes. External immobilization of tumor fractures was on occasion effective in relieving pain and enhancing mobility, but it was not until the early twentieth century, when techniques began to be developed for internal fracture splintage, that patients with advanced bony metastases could be helped significantly. As those techniques have improved, particularly since World War II, so have the surgeon's ability to enhance the quality of life for advanced cancer sufferers.

Since accurate records concerning cancer first were recorded, the incidence of the disease has increased. Although much of this statistical increase may represent an artifact of early diagnostic inaccuracy, there is no doubt that cancer has become a progressively more common disease as the population ages. For example, the overall incidence of cancer in the United States in 1975 was 75% higher than in 1933 while the average life expectancy was increasing by only 10 years. During the past five decades the population of the United States has indeed increased dramatically, as both men and women are living longer and infant mortality rates have decreased. Heart disease still is the single most common cause of death, accounting for 38% of all mortality in the United States in 1981,[32] but recent advances in the management of coronary artery disease have led to a significant reduction in that percentage and give promise of an even greater improvement during the next decade.

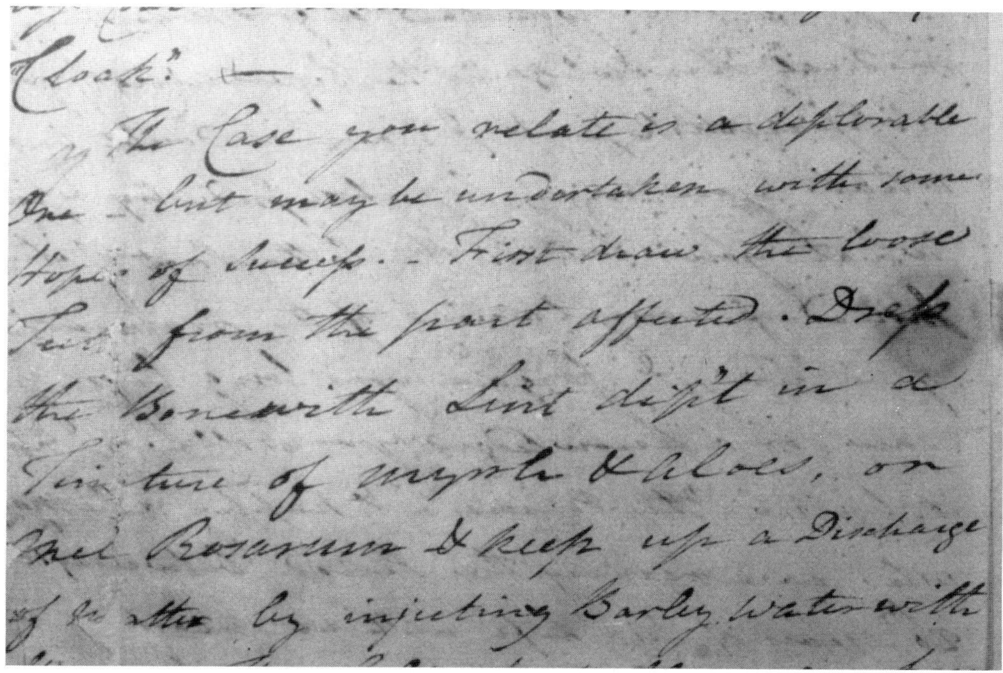

Cloak: —
The Case you relate is a deplorable
One but may be undertaken with some
Hope of Success. - First draw the loose
Teeth from the part affected. Dress
the Bone with Lint dipt in a
Tincture of myrrh & Aloes, or
Mel Rosarum & keep up a Discharge
of Matter by injecting Barley water with

FIGURE 1-5 Portion of a letter from Rush to one of his former students, Dr. Elisha Hall, dated July 13, 1773. His technique of tumor tissue debridement is discussed in the text.

Cancer is the second leading cause of death in the United States, accounting for 21% of all deaths in 1981 and 24% in 1984. In 1981, 432,000 Americans died of cancer. In 1985 there were 482,000 deaths and 910,000 new cancers cases reported.[32] A statistical analysis of these trends reveals that a child born in the United States in 1985 has a better than one-in-three chance of eventually contracting invasive cancer (excluding epidermal skin cancer and carcinoma in situ). For males born in 1985, the chances of dying from metastatic cancer are almost one in four, and for females almost one in five.[31] Breast cancer alone strikes between 1 in 10 and 1 in 14 women worldwide. Incidence and mortality parallel each other and have changed little in the past half-century.

Although these statistics seem discouraging at first glance, they must be balanced against the fact that more aggressive palliative treatment of patients with established metastases, using sophisticated combinations of hormonal manipulation, chemotherapy, and radiotherapy, have been successful in prolonging these patients' lives and improving their general well-being. Almost half of all newly diagnosed cancer patients are alive 5 years later. Of women with breast carcinoma diagnosed between 1977 and 1979, 81% were alive 5 years later and 34% of these were alive with metastases. Those percentages had increased from 63% and 18% respectively in 1960.[32] When one correlates these figures with the fact that an estimated 120,000 new cases of breast cancer will be diagnosed in the United States in 1985, it can be projected that there will be well over a half million women in this country living with metastatic carcinoma of the breast during the next 5 years. The number of patients alive with metastases from other cancers will be in excess of 2 million. For many of these patients, living with a metastatic malignancy becomes akin to living with any other chronic disease process, requiring periodic medical evaluations and strict adherence to a drug or hormonal therapy protocol with minimal side effects.

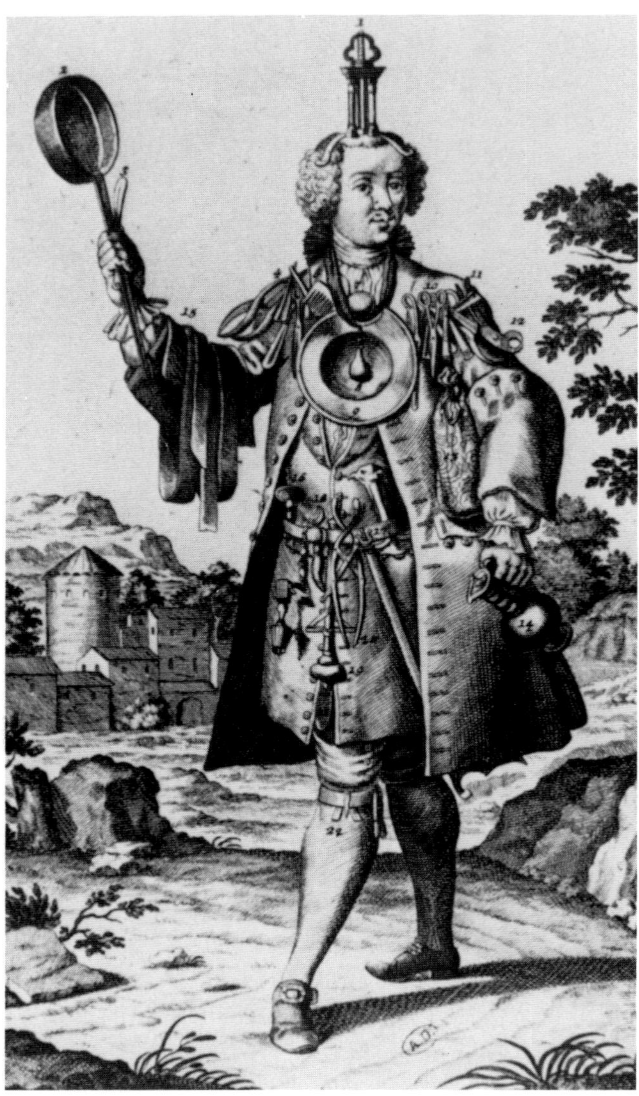

FIGURE 1-6 Engraving by Martin Engelbrecht (c. 1761) entitled "Cancer Surgeon/ Barber" showing some of his varied equipment, which included an amputation saw, a trepan, extraction forceps, and clamps.

INCIDENCE OF PATHOLOGICAL FRACTURE

It is unfortunate that coincident with the improvements in overall cancer palliation has come an increase in clinically apparent bone metastases and from these an increase in subsequent pathological long bone fractures. Simply stated, as patients survive for progressively longer periods after cancer metastases develop, the incidence of metastatic involvement of bone increases apace. Not surprisingly patients with tumors such as breast and prostatic carcinomas, which have a prognosis for the longest survival after development of bone metastases, are the ones who have the highest likelihood of eventually sustaining a complicating pathological fracture. As seen in Table 1-1, 61% of all metastatic pathological fractures occur in patients with disseminated breast carcinoma and the majority of other fractures also occur in patients with cancers having the longest anticipated survival.

Metastatic carcinoma is the most common malignancy of bone, affecting more than 40 times as many patients as are affected by all other types of bone cancer combined.[2,20] In fact, it has been estimated that over 60% of women with disseminated breast cancer have radiographic evidence of bone metastases, and the incidence is much higher when measured by bone scanning techniques[17,18,25] (Table 1-2). Jaffe[21] has stated that if careful postmortem examinations were performed on all patients dying of malignancies over 90% would show evidence of skeletal metastases.

The time of appearance of bone metastases varies depending on the tumor of origin. Staley,[33] in a study of skeletal metastases from breast carcinoma, found that when a metastasis developed it did so in more than half of his patients within 18 months of mastectomy. Enis et al.,[12] reporting on a smaller series of patients with primary malignancies of various origins, found that the mean duration of disease prior to the development of the first metastatic pathological fracture in patients with breast cancer was 72 months whereas the mean duration in patients with other primary malignancies was only 5.6 months.

Statistics on the occurrence of pathological fractures in patients with recognized skeletal metastases are more difficult to find. Higinbotham and Marcove[20] reported that of 1800 patients treated for skeletal metastases at Memorial Sloan-Kettering Cancer Center in New York between 1931 and 1964, 9.5% sustained pathological fractures. Their figures, from a cancer referral center where patients at high risk of such fractures are more concentrated, undoubtedly do not accurately reflect the overall national incidence. Staley[33] has estimated that the true incidence of pathological fractures in patients with skeletal metastases is closer to 5%. Even accepting this lower figure, it becomes obvious that the challenge of anticipating and managing these difficult problems will have to be faced more and more commonly in the future.

Advances in cancer palliation allow longer survival for patients who may feel relatively well and essentially pain free until their skel-

TABLE 1-1 Types and Distribution of Primary Cancers

	Number	Percent
Breast	162	41
Kidney	38	43 (Kidney through Undifferentiated)
Lung	36	
Prostate	24	
Bowel	21	
Thyroid	6	
Undifferentiated (origin unknown)	20	
Other	24	16 (Other through Lymphoma)
Myeloma	36	
Lymphoma	26	
TOTAL	393	

TABLE 1-2 Incidence of Bone Metastases at Autopsy in Selected Malignant Diseases

Primary site	Involvement (%)
Breast	50-85
Lung	30-50
Prostate	50-70
Hodgkin's	50-70
Kidney	30-50
Bladder	12-25
Thyroid	40
Melanoma	30-40

etal disease reaches the point of incipient or actual fracture. The question of how aggressive the orthopaedic surgeon should be in recommending operative treatment for patients with metastases and impending or actual fractures straddles the boundary between medical science and philosophy. The surgeon must avoid allowing his compassion for a patient in pain to push him toward performing an operation from which that patient, because of the advanced nature of his disease, cannot readily benefit. On the other hand, there is no way that any physician, be he oncologist or surgeon, can predict the survival of a given patient with metastatic malignancy. In my experience many oncologists tend to overestimate rather than underestimate the prognosis for survival of a patient with a pathological fracture, perhaps subconsciously hoping that the surgeon, by stabilizing the patient's fracture and relieving his pain, may also somehow stimulate an immunological reserve previously untapped.

In general, if a patient's basic disease will allow him at least 4 to 6 weeks of life and if fixation of his fracture will enhance that remaining life then the hope for relief of pain, ease of nursing care, and release from the financial grip of hospitalization makes surgical stabilization of that fracture the treatment of choice. Among the most optimistic and motivated patients I have treated are those with the most dismal overall prognosis. The fact that many of these individuals do indeed survive following effective stabilization of their fractures, often for periods in excess of what had been projected initially, perhaps lends credence to the seemingly unscientific optimism so often expressed by the referring oncologist.

Improvement in survival statistics undoubtedly is a reflection of advances in many parameters of cancer therapy—including chemotherapy, hormonal manipulation, radiotherapy, and nutrition. Among these advances, however, must also be numbered the many improvements in techniques for secure and lasting internal fixation of pathological fractures.

PAIN RELIEF

One important therapeutic advance has been the use of methylmethacrylate as an adjunct to internal fixation by conventional devices or as a material for partial reconstruction of bone defects also managed by prosthetic replacement. Because most patients have received local irradiation prior to the occurrence of a pathological fracture, the likelihood of that fracture's healing spontaneously is slim. (The radiobiological factors predisposing to nonunion are discussed in Chapter 11.) Consequently, operative fixation of a pathological fracture offers, with few exceptions, the only opportunity for relief of pain and restoration of the ability to walk again.

More than 50% of patients with lytic long bone metastases do not enjoy lasting relief of pain following irradiation alone, even if a fracture does not occur.[7,36] Once a pathological fracture has occurred, neither radiation nor chemotherapy alone offers any chance for pain relief. Prior to the use of methylmethacrylate to augment conventional internal fixation of long bone fractures, such fixation was borderline at best and statistics for pain relief after fixation were discouraging. Since methylmethacrylate has been used to ensure rigid fixation of most fractures, the overwhelming majority of patients enjoy relief of pain postoperatively[19] (Table 1-3). Analyzing pain relief after operative fixation of more than 450 pathological fractures or impending long bone fractures, Habermann et al.[17] found that 97% of their patients had good or excellent relief of pain when methylmethacrylate was utilized along with internal fixation or prosthetic replacement but that only 78% had such relief when acrylic cement was not utilized to augment fixation.

TABLE 1-3 **Pain Relief After Internal Fixation of Pathological Fractures (augmented by PMMA), 186 Patients**

	Number	Percent
Excellent (no regular analgesics after the initial postoperative period)	86	46
Good (occasional analgesics)	74	40
Fair (regular analgesics)	21	11
Poor (no improvement)	5	3

RESUMPTION OF AMBULATION

The achievement of rigid fixation also has been responsible for a dramatic improvement in statistics concerning the resumption of ambulation postoperatively. For example, Takita and Watne[35] attempted conventional internal fixation without adjunctive methylmethacrylate in 16 of 29 pathological fractures of the lower extremities, considering the remaining 13 to be unsuitable even for attempts at fixation. Of the 16 patients operated on, none were able to walk independently postoperatively and just 8 were able to walk with the aid of crutches or a walker. Thus, only 27% of their patients regained even a partially ambulatory status after suffering a fracture. Similarly, Parrish and Murray[27] excluded approximately one third of the patients in their series from consideration for internal fixation because they felt that the extent of bone destruction about the fracture site precluded prosthetic replacement or internal fixation by conventional means. The remaining 96 patients were treated either by prosthetic replacement or by internal fixation, but in no instance was methylmethacrylate used as an adjunct to conventional fixation techniques. Only 49 patients (52%) regained the ability to walk and 29 of those required the assistance of crutches or a walker. Thus only 36% of their total patient group were able to walk, even with external aids.

These discouraging results should be compared with present-day statistics showing that the use of acrylic cement to augment conventional fixation methods has greatly improved the solidarity of such fixation and thus the likelihood of any given patient's walking again (Table 1-4). In our experience,[18,19] of the 366 patients so managed 94.6% became ambulatory postoperatively, 50% of them without requiring the assistance of a cane, crutches, or any other such device. Habermann[16] and Habermann et al.[17] have reported similarly impressive improvement in the rate of resuming ambulation for patients whose pathological fracture fixations were augmented by polymethylmethacrylate. More than 95% of their patients regained the ability to walk whereas only 75% of those treated without methylmethacrylate resumed walking.

ENHANCED SURVIVAL

In addition to the relief of pain and the resumption of walking, a third important factor to consider in assessing the adequacy of fracture fixation is how long these patients survive after a pathological fracture occurs. As already noted, advances in overall cancer palliation have played an important role in improving survival statistics. However, none of these advances has been more important than the orthopaedic surgeon's ability to achieve freedom from local pain and to restore independent walking.

Prior to the development of modern techniques for fixation of these fractures, the mean survival of all patients after their first pathological fracture was only 7.8 months.* Parrish and Murray[27] and Perez et al.[28] found that patients with fractures secondary to metastatic breast cancer enjoyed a better prognosis but the mean survival still was only 11.6 months. Takita and Watne[35] found a significantly better prognosis for patients with peritrochanteric fractures (mean 11.6 mo) than

*References 5, 6, 20, 23, 27, 28, 33, 35.

***TABLE 1-4* Postoperative Ambulatory Status of 366 Patients With Pathological Fractures Who Were Able to Walk Before Operation**

	Breast Primary	Other Primary	Total	Percent
Bedridden	2	7	9	5.4
Wheelchair-bound	4	7	11	
Weight-bearing with support	61	105	166	94.6
Full weight-bearing	89	91	180	

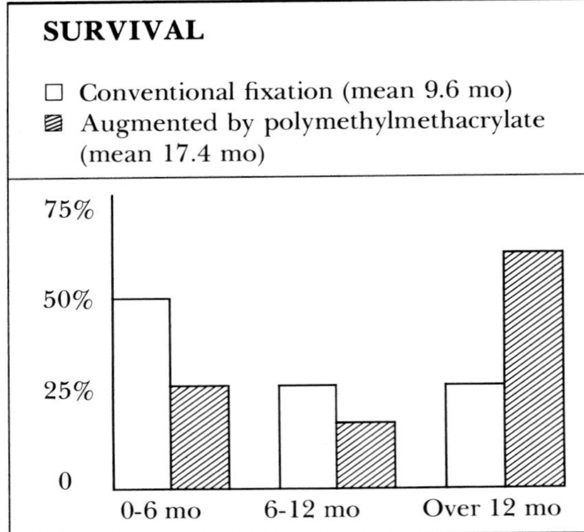

for those with pathological fractures of other long bones (7.1 mo). However, the number of patients in each group was small and a large percentage in the former group had primary malignancies with a more favorable survival prognosis. Patients suffering pathological fractures of the spine resulting in neurological impairment or intractable pain from spinal instability faced an even more dismal prognosis. Before the development of effective techniques for spinal decompression and stabilization, the average survival of such patients at the University of California, San Francisco, was 3.3 months.

Since methylmethacrylate has been used to augment fixation, survival rates have improved dramatically (box). Habermann[16,17] has reported a mean survival of 12 months for all his patients whose long bone fractures or impending fractures were so managed, which represents an improvement of almost 20% in 1-year survival statistics when compared to the statistics for patients with similar fractures managed by internal fixation but without acrylic cement augmentation. Perhaps the most striking example of this improvement in prognosis was for patients with metastatic breast cancer, of whom 75% survived more than 1 year after fracture fixation (mean 21 mo).[16] Our own experience is similar to Habermann's and is summarized in Table 1-5. Of our 289 patients, 61% sustained pathological fractures secondary to metastatic breast cancer and their mean postoperative survival was 24.6 months, with 28% still alive more than 3 years postoperative.

***TABLE 1-5* Postfracture Survival (by tumor), 289 Patients**

	Mean Time (mo)
Breast	24.6
Myeloma	25.6
Lymphoma	25.8
Bladder, prostate	32.9
Kidney	14.6
Lung	4.1

There is also no question that the survival of patients with metastatic breast cancer has been enhanced greatly by improved chemotherapy and hormonal manipulation. A decade ago the unpredictable response rate to hormone manipulation in such patients prompted the use of chemotherapeutic regimens as the initial means of controlling widespread disease. More recently, however, the introduction of hormonal receptor assays has allowed for patients with a poor chance of response to be excluded from hormone treatment. Sixty percent of breast cancer patients with a positive test for cytoplasmic estrogen receptors (ER+) will respond to hormonal manipulation despite widespread metastatic bone disease.[24] The introduction of antiestrogen compounds has simplified hormonal treatment, since these drugs are as effective as major endocrine ablation or additive hormonal treatment and yet are without many of the side effects of those therapies.[1] Most oncologists now employ hormonal manipulation as the initial course of management for ER+ breast cancer with bone metastases, reserving chemotherapy for when hormonal manipulation becomes ineffective.

Unfortunately, such dramatic improvements in the nonoperative management of metastatic bone disease have not been reported for other tumor types. Medical management of most malignancies other than breast cancer has changed relatively little in the past decade. However, even patients with these other malignancies enjoy a much better prognosis for survival after a pathological fracture because of the greatly improved success in effective stabilization of that fracture. For example, patients with fractures secondary to myeloma, the second largest group, now enjoy a mean survival of 26 months;

those with hypernephroma, a mean survival of 14.6 months. In fact, only patients with fractures secondary to metastatic lung malignancies have anywhere near as dismal a prognosis for survival (4.1 mo) today as they did a decade ago[13,18] (Table 1-5).

FRACTURE HEALING

The encouraging improvements in relief of fracture pain, restoration of walking ability, and, ultimately, prolongation of survival with an acceptable quality of life all are attributable primarily to markedly improved fracture stabilization. Even as patients live for longer periods after such surgery, however, a new concern arises about how many of these fractures ultimately will progress to true bony union in the face of preoperative or postoperative irradiation. As a corollary to this question the concern also arises about how long even the most rigid stabilization can be expected to withstand the daily stresses of walking if true bony union does not occur. Pugh et al.[29] demonstrated experimentally that pathological fractures whose fixation has been augmented by methylmethacrylate require a much higher load to fail than do those fixed without cement. Moreover, when failure does occur the fixation assembly of a metal splint augmented by acrylic cement can continue to bear a surprisingly large load with only minimal deformation. However, if true bony union does not supervene, complete loss of stability will eventually occur even in the face of such stabilization.

The overall reported incidence of bony union of pathological fracture secondary to metastatic malignancy varies between 7.5% and 45%, with a mean of 30%,[13,18,27,28] even after effective internal fixation of the fracture. Although preoperative irradiation has been implicated repeatedly as the principal deterrent to bony union, there is some evidence to suggest that other factors may play a part as well. For example, the prognosis for union of a pathological fracture is determined to some extent by the cell type of the primary tumor responsible. Fractures secondary to myeloma, lymphoma, or metastatic prostate carcinoma have a significantly higher union rate than do those from metastatic hypernephroma or lung carcinoma. Gainor and Buchert[13] found an incidence of 67% union in fractures occurring with myeloma, 44% with hypernephroma, 37% with breast cancer, and no instances with lung cancer metastases. However, they also noted that if patients survived their fracture fixation by more than 6 months, no matter the primary, over three fourths of those fractures ultimately healed. In fact, of those breast cancer patients who survived more than 6 months, 82% showed fracture union. Our experience confirms this.

The presence of viable tumor cells at the fracture site may also interfere with healing. Bonarigo and Rubin[4] demonstrated that lymphosarcoma cells experimentally injected into a long bone fracture site in a rat resulted invariably in a nonunion even in the absence of radiation. Galasko[14] has reviewed additional evidence to suggest that a variety of tumor cell–mediated factors could interfere with fracture healing, at least under experimental conditions. There is also evidence, again primarily of an experimental nature, to suggest that certain chemotherapeutic agents may interfere with pathological fracture healing, at least in children.[13,34] However, neither the presence of tumor cells nor the use of adjunctive chemotherapy appears to be of any real clinical significance in affecting the incidence of bony union of metastatic fractures in adults.

Similarly there is no evidence that the presence of intramedullary methylmethacrylate in combination with an internal fixation device materially affects the rate of healing of such fractures, unless a large amount of acrylic is allowed to become interposed between the fracture surfaces. Several authors have reported uncomplicated healing of such fractures where large defects have been filled by cement as long as rigid fixation has been achieved and postoperative radiation has been limited to 3000 cGy.*

There is overwhelming evidence, both clinical and experimental, however, that fracture healing is adversely affected by local irradiation. Clinically the incidence of pathological fracture nonunion following conventional-dose radiotherapy (4000 to 5000 cGy) approaches 70%, even in areas such as the intertrochanteric region of the femur, which ordi-

*A centigray (cGy), the currently accepted designation, is the same as a rad.

narily have an excellent prognosis for bony union.[14,18] In contrast, the majority of lesions (85%) irradiated and internally fixed before a fracture occurs show evidence of healing with restitution of bony architecture.[4] Not only is this fact a strong argument for prophylactic internal fixation of impending fractures whenever possible (see Chapter 11), it also suggests that different mechanisms exist for the healing of a fracture and for the filling in of a lytic defect.

Cooley and Goss[8] studied the effect of irradiation on fracture repair in normal animal bones. One thousand rads (centigrays) delayed callus formation for 1 week, 2000 retarded it for 3 weeks, and 3000 completely prevented bone repair. Similarly Bonarigo and Rubin[4] demonstrated experimentally that 2000 cGy prevents both tumor progression and bony union at the site of a pathological fracture unless that fracture previously has been rigidly internally fixed. The interference with bony union occurs because, in the absence of rigid fixation, chondrogenesis is a necessary precursor of osteogenesis and ultimate fracture union. Chondrogenesis is far more radiosensitive than is osteogenesis. Consequently, when rigid internal fixation of a pathological fracture cannot be achieved by conventional means, healing cannot be expected if the fracture is irradiated. Chondrogenesis is not necessary for healing of lytic lesions prior to a fracture, a fact that explains the high rate of such lesions' filling in with bone after prophylactic fixation. Bone grafting of fractures that have been or will be subjected to local irradiation usually is ineffective in promoting bony union unless more than 6 months has elapsed since the completion of such local radiation. By that time in the majority of instances, unless extremely high doses of irradiation were employed, the bone will have regained its osteoblastic and chondroblastic capabilities and bone grafting may stimulate union as with any conventional fracture nonunion.

Clinically Blake,[3] Coran et al.,[9] Gainor and Buchert,[13] and Harrington[18] have demonstrated that the incidence of fracture healing improves markedly in humans if no more than 2500 to 3000 cGy is administered locally preoperatively or within the first 6 months postoperatively. By concentrating local irradiation in a brief interval, it is possible to get the same tumoricidal effect from a relatively small total irradiation dose as from a much larger dose administered over several weeks. For example, 1700 cGy given over 2 to 3 days is equivalent to 3200 cGy given over 3 weeks. Twenty-two hundred centigrays administered over 6 days is equivalent to 4400 in 4 weeks.[22] With modern methods of radiotherapy administration, the skin desquamation and other deleterious effects of these concentrated doses can be made equivalent to those of the prolonged fractionated treatment method.

It has been demonstrated experimentally[15] that just 300 cGy of local irradiation to a metastatic focus in bone results in the death of 90% of the oxygenated tumor cells, 600 cGy causes the death of 99% of oxygenated cells, 900 cGy the death of 99.9%, and 2000 cGy the death of more than 99.999%.

By concentrating the radiation dose to 2200-2500 cGy administered in 6 to 7 days, one can expect the following results for pathological fractures from bone metastases secondary to carcinomas of the breast, prostate, and thyroid and from sarcomas of the lymphoma and myeloma type:

- A 96% incidence of remission, of which 26% will be permanent[15]
- Healing of 94% of major lytic lesions (internally fixed when necessary before the complication of a fracture)[4]
- Healing of 86% of adequately fixed pathological fractures[18]
- A major financial saving to the patient

At present, radiotherapy is billed on a unit-treatment basis. Thus 2200 cGy administered in 4 to 6 days costs less than one third as much as 4400 cGy administered in 4 weeks.[10,15]

There is no evidence that the presence of internal fixation devices, prostheses, or methylmethacrylate interferes with the efficacy of radiation therapy. Moreover, irradiation of methylmethacrylate does not significantly alter its physical properties with regard to shear or compressibility even with doses far exceeding those normally used.[11,26] Scullin et al.[30] have shown that up to 20,000 cGy does not compromise the strength of either the cement itself or its interface with bone.

In summary, the incidence of metastatic bone disease has increased geometrically in the past 20 years as patients are generally living longer, more are contracting malignancies, and more are surviving longer with their malignancies. The complication of bone metastases, including pathological fractures of the long bones, spine, and pelvis, presents added demands to the orthopaedic surgeon. He or she must employ specialized techniques because of the difficulty of achieving rigid and lasting fracture stabilization and because gaining bony union in the face of tumor lysis, chemotherapy, and radiation also is more difficult. The techniques of fixation just outlined will be expanded on greatly in later chapters dealing with the specific management of fractures and impending fractures of particular regions. Suffice it to say that as the prospect for prolonged survival after fracture fixation improves so too do the indications for aggressive management of these problems. Similarly, the excellent likelihood of achieving pain relief and restoring a patient's ability to resume walking offers a very positive outlook to these unfortunate individuals, who in the recent past were often considered unmanageable except by progressively increasing doses of narcotic analgesics. Finally, as radiation protocols are altered to encourage true bony union of these fractures, the approximately 35% of patients who enjoy prolonged survival need not face the ultimate failure of artificial stabilization alone.

One final point is worth emphasizing. In focusing on the variety of technical challenges that each of these patients presents, the physician must never lose sight of the individual personality of the patient himself. Every cancer patient needs a realistic appraisal of his chances for survival and of the ratio of risks to benefits for any proposed procedure. However, once a decision has been made to proceed with reconstruction through a metastatic lesion, it is exceedingly important that all physicians involved maintain a spirit of enthusiasm and optimism through the end of postoperative rehabilitation. The cancer patient requires a longer time and more effort than a healthy individual to realize the potential benefits of any operation. The cancer patient is sensitive to every nuance of disinterest or frustration manifested by his physicians and often may subconsciously be looking for an excuse to give up struggling against his disease. As the reader will learn from the following chapters, there is much that can be done to enrich the quality of these patients' remaining months or years. It is the responsibility of the physician to educate them to that potential and to find a balance between ensuring a reasonable degree of comfort during their struggle, on the one hand, and inspiring them to push ahead with recovery, on the other.

— REFERENCES

1. Bezwoda, W.R., et al.: Treatment of metastatic breast cancer in estrogen receptor positive patients, Cancer **50:**2747, 1982.
2. Bickel, W.H., and Barber, J.R.: Pathologic or spontaneous fractures, G.P. **3:**41, 1951.
3. Blake, D.D.: Radiation treatment of metastatic bone disease, Clin. Orthop. **73:**89, 1970.
4. Bonarigo, B.C., and Rubin, P.: Non-union of pathologic fracture after radiation therapy, Radiology **88:** 889, 1967.
5. Bremner, R.A., and Jellifee, A.M.: The management of pathological fracture of the major long bones from metastatic cancer, J. Bone Joint Surg. **40B:**652, 1958.
6. Campbell, C.J.: Palliation of metastatic bone disease. In Hickey, R.C., editor: Palliative care of the cancer patient, Boston, 1967, Little, Brown & Co.
7. Cheng, D.S., et al.: Non-operative management of femoral, humeral, and acetabular metastases in patients with breast carcinoma, Cancer **45:**1533, 1980.
8. Cooley, L.N., and Goss, R.J.: The effects of transplantation and x-irradiation on the repair of fractured bones, Am. J. Anat. **102:**167, 1958.
9. Coran, A.G., et al.: The management of pathologic fractures in patients with metastatic carcinoma of the breast, Surg. Gynecol. Obstet. **127:**1225, 1968.
10. Dutreix, J., et al.: Concentrated irradiation palliative radiotherapy for tumors affecting the oesophagus, brain, bones, and mediastinum, Ann. Clin. Res. **3:**9, 1971.
11. Eftekhar, N.S., and Thurston, C.W.: Effect of irradiation on acrylic cement with special reference to fixation of pathologic fractures, J. Biomech. **8:**53, 1975.
12. Enis, J.E., et al.: Methylmethacrylate in neoplastic bone destruction. In The hip. Proceedings of the Hip Society, St. Louis, 1973, The C.V. Mosby Co.
13. Gainor, B.J., and Buchert, P.: Fracture healing in metastatic bone disease, Clin. Orthop. **178:**297, 1983.
14. Galasko, C.S.B.: Pathological fractures secondary to metastatic cancer, J. R. Coll. Surg. Edinb. **19:**351, 1974.
15. Garmatis, J.: Concentrated irradiation for metastatic bone disease, Radiology **126:**235, 1978.
16. Habermann, E.T.: Evaluation and management of malignant pathological fractures of the long bones, spine, and pelvis. In Instructional Course 305. Presented at the A.A.O.S. meeting, New Orleans, February, 1986.
17. Habermann, E.T., et al.: The pathology and treatment of metastatic disease of the femur, Clin. Orthop. **169:**70, 1982.
18. Harrington, K.D.: New trends in the management of lower extremity metastases, Clin. Orthop. **169:**53, 1982.
19. Harrington, K.D., et al.: Methylmethacrylate as an

adjunct in internal fixation of pathological fractures, J. Bone Joint Surg. **58A:**1047, 1976.

20. Higinbotham, N.L., and Marcove, R.C.: The management of pathological fractures, J. Trauma **5:**792, 1965.
21. Jaffe, H.L.: Tumors and tumorous conditions of the bones and joints, Philadelphia, 1958, Lea & Febiger.
22. Koskinen, E.V.S., and Nieminen, R.A.: Surgical treatment of metastatic pathological fracture of major long bones, Acta Orthop. Scand. **44:**539, 1973.
23. Marcove, R.C., and Yang, D.J.: Survival times after treatment of pathologic fractures, Cancer **20:**2154, 1967.
24. McGuire, W.L., et al.: The current status of oestrogen and progesterone receptors in breast cancer, Cancer **39:**2934, 1977.
25. McNeil, B.J.: Rationale for the use of bone scans in selected metastatic and primary bone tumors, Semin. Nucl. Med. **8:**336, 1978.
26. Murray, J.A., et al.: Irradiation of polymethylmethacrylate. In vitro gamma radiation effect, J. Bone Joint Surg. **58A:**1067, 1976.
27. Parrish, F.F., and Murray, J.A.: Surgical treatment for secondary neoplastic fractures. A retrospective study of ninety-six patients, J. Bone Joint Surg. **52A:**665, 1970.
28. Perez, C.A., et al.: Management of pathologic fractures, Cancer **29:**684, 1972.
29. Pugh, J., et al.: Biomechanics of pathologic fractures, Clin. Orthop. **169:**109, 1982.
30. Scullin, J.P., et al.: The effect of radiation on the shear strength of acrylic bone cement, Clin. Orthop. **129:** 201, 1977.
31. Seidman, H., et al.: Probabilities of eventually developing or dying of cancer—United States 1985, CA **35**(1):36, 1985.
32. Silverberg, E.: Cancer statistics, 1985, CA **35**(1):19, 1985.
33. Staley, C.J.: Skeletal metastases in cancer of the breast, Surg. Gynecol. Obstet. **68:**683, 1956.
34. Stanisavljevic, S., and Babcock, A.L.: Fractures in children treated with methotrexate for leukemia, Clin. Orthop. **125:**139, 1977.
35. Takita, H., and Watne, A.L.: Operative treatment of pathologic fractures, Surg. Gynecol. Obstet. **116:** 683, 1963.
36. Tong, D., et al.: The palliation of symptomatic osseus metastases, Cancer **50:**893, 1982.
37. Williams, N.: All the Queen's men, London, 1972, Sphere Books, Ltd.

CHAPTER 2

MECHANISMS OF METASTASES

Perhaps it is redundant to emphasize that although the primary tumor focus establishes the clinical behavior of any given cancer it is the distant metastasis that almost invariably produces progressive disability and eventual death. In fact, it is the ability of a tumor cell to be transported from its primary location to a distant site and to establish a viable metastatic focus in that site that qualifies it as a malignancy. Consequently, although control of the primary tumor is important and in fact determines whether a patient can be cured, it is the control of metastases that determines the duration and quality of survival.

Most metastases probably do not develop after removal of a primary tumor but rather were present before the ablation of that primary (surgical excision or radiation). Occasionally metastases will be solitary and curable by secondary resection. Such an event is uncommon with any malignancy but should be considered a possibility particularly after diagnosed cancers of the kidney and thyroid. Far more typically, patients have multiple but clinically undetectable metastases at the time of primary tumor ablation and it is only under the influence of further stimuli—hormonal in a positive sense or immunological insufficiency in a negative one—that these foci grow and become clinically apparent. The concept that these so-called micrometastases often exist at the time of the original tumor diagnosis has led oncologists to attempt to prognosticate which patients with primary cancers are likely to have late clinical evidence of metastatic disease and how such disease may be prevented or at least minimized. For example, on the simplest plane, it has long been recognized that women with large breast cancers, those with skin invasion, or those with a multiplicity of nodes have the greatest likelihood of developing distant metastases. More subtly, the histological grading of a given malignancy correlates with the likelihood of metastases[30] and, debatably, that tumor's hormonal responsiveness may also determine its likelihood of spreading.[7]

In recent years many patients at high risk of metastatic disease on a statistical basis have been started on a protocol of prophylactic hormonal manipulation or chemotherapy. The early results of such intervention do not clearly show an increased overall percentage of survivors, although in most studies the duration of survival has been prolonged.

As knowledge in this field expands, there has followed an increased interest in the mechanisms of metastatic spread of tumor cells. That process has been found much more complex than initially imagined and includes a host of interrelationships, which can best be subdivided into two groups:

1. The systemic factors that influence where cancers tend to metastasize and how they will behave as metastatic foci
2. The mechanical factors influencing the actual release of cancer cells into the circulation and how those cell reach and ultimately become established in their host organs

SYSTEMIC FACTORS INFLUENCING METASTASES

Although numerous tumor cells gain access to the circulation, principally through the capillary system but also through lymphatic channels, few are capable of establishing a metastatic focus. The tumor cell must complete a long series of steps initially enabling it to become detached from the primary tumor site and finally enabling it to establish sufficient growth at a distant site to become clinically significant.

Some cancers have a distinct predisposition to involve bone (Tables 2-1 and 2-2). Based on large postmortem studies, lung cancer has been noted to metastasize to bone between 24% and 55% of the time, breast cancer between 47% and 85% of the time, prostatic carcinoma between 33% and 85%, and renal carcinoma approximately 35% of the time. Conversely, carcinomas of the pancreas, uterus, and gastrointestinal tract metastasize to bone in less than 10% of cases despite the abundant hematogenous routes affording skeletal access from these sites. Paget[49] in 1889 first emphasized this disparity with his comment that whereas thyroid cancer, for example, produces "bone deposits with astonishing frequency, the bones are remarkable in their freedom from disease" from gastric cancer. When cancers do metastasize to bone, at least 85% of the time multiple foci can be appreciated by nuclear scanning or roentgenographic techniques once a single focus has become symptomatic.

Although nineteenth century physicians generally subscribed to the fact that cancers typically spread by direct extension from an original tumor mass, the fact that certain tumors spread distantly and to preferential tissues (such as bone) did not go altogether unrecognized. Hodgkin[38] in 1848 felt that such preferential recipient sites possessed "some power which arrests certain molecules already in the circulation, and that so arrested they become fresh starting points for the production of the morbid growth." He and others cited examples of metastatic foci that appeared to flourish at the ends of ribs (near the vertebrae or at the costochondral junctions) rather than in the rib midsections. In 1888 Targett[60] postulated that this phenomenon in some way might be related to the development of rickets, but Paget more generally concluded that "it is not such a matter of chance what bone shall be attacked by a secondary growth."

In modern times this concept of "organ selectivity" has been described fully by Onguibo,[47,48] who pointed out that certain tumors seem to select a particular metastatic location and that this preference can be demonstrated by experimental observation. Kinsey,[40] for example, injected malignant cells with an observed preference for establishing foci within the lungs into animals in whom lung tissue had

***TABLE 2-1* Incidence of Skeletal Metastases**

Tumor Site	Author	Year	Percent
Breasts	Kaufman	1929	52
	Abrams et al.	1950	73
	Jaffe	1958	85
	Drury et al.	1964	74
	Galasko	1972	84
	Willis	1973	47
Prostate	Kaufman	1902	70
	Bumpus	1921	33
	Pürckhauer	1929	54
	Abrams et al.	1950	84
	Jaffe	1958	85
	Drury et al.	1964	65
	Roy et al.	1971	70
Thyroid	Ehrhardt	1902	28
	Kaufman	1929	34
	Abrams et al.	1950	50
	Drury et al.	1971	60
Kidneys	Symmers	1917	33
	Copeland	1931	35
	Willis	1973	40
Bronchus	Abrams et al.	1950	32
	Drury et al. (all tumors)	1964	40
	Drury et al. (oat cell)	1964	55
	Willis	1973	30
	Oyamada et al.	1978	60
Esophagus	Clayton	1928	5
	Kaufman	1929	7
	Willis	1973	6
Gastrointestine	Poscharissky	1930	3
	Kaufman	1929	3
	Abrams et al.	1950	11
	Willis	1973	7
Rectum	Kaufman	1929	11
	Abrams et al.	1950	13
	Drury et al.	1964	8
Bladder	Drury et al.	1964	42
Uterine cervix	Drury et al.	1964	50
Ovaries	Abrams et al.	1950	9

TABLE 2-2 **Distribution of Skeletal Metastases**

Author, year	Lenz and Freid, 1931	Kaufman, 1902	Pürckhauer, 1929	Simpson, 1926	Aufses, 1930	Willis, 1973
Tumor	Mammary	Prostatic	Prostatic	Thyroid	Rectal	Miscellaneous
Site (%)	Pelvis (63)	Lumbar vertebrae (79)	Vertebrae (90)	Skull (39)	Vertebrae (33)	Vertebrae (62)
	Vertebrae (59)	Femur (68)	Femur (37)	Vertebrae (32)	Femur (25)	Ribs (57)
					Ribs (25)	
	Femur (54)	Ilium (62)	Pelvis (23)	Pelvis (14)	Skull (13)	Skull (35)
					Sternum (13)	
	Ribs (40)	Thoracic vertebrae (56)	Skull (16)		Humerus (8)	Femur (22)
		Ribs (56)			Pelvis (8)	
					Sacrum (8)	
	Skull (36)	Sternum (35)	Ribs (13)			Pelvis (19)
	Humerus (27)	Skull (32)	Sternum (10)			Humerus (10)
						Sternum (10)
Patients	81	34	30	77	24	68

been transplanted subcutaneously. Metastases developed within the subcutaneous implanted lung despite its separate anatomical location and generally poor access to the systemic circulation. In a similar experiment Fidler et al.[28] injected cultured cancer cells into mice. The cells from lung metastases that the animals developed were then recultured and injected into a second set of mice. The process was repeated ten times, and the number of lung metastases was observed to increase with each sequence.

In 1860 Virchow[66] postulated the existence of "an ichorous juice" emitted by a cancer that somehow allowed its cells to pass through certain organs without clinical evidence of implantation only to become multiply established in a different type of tissue. Eve[26] in 1883 found metastatic tumors "not uncommonly in the liver and bones while the lungs remain perfectly free, although the cancer elements must have passed through the pulmonary circulation in order to reach the organs first named." Modern research suggests that it is the host tissues as well as the tumor cells themselves that produce materials enhancing the establishment of metastases.

Hayashi et al.,[36] Mundy and Spro,[45] and Ushijima et al.[62] have demonstrated that certain host tissues can produce a chemotactic substance attractive to tumor cells. Bone-derived chemotactic factors appear to be particularly active. Experimentally, metastatic deposits have been shown to occur preferentially at the sites of bone trauma[29] because of the accelerated release of chemotactic factors from traumatized bone. It also has been demonstrated[45] that such a factor or factors are released, albeit at a slower rate, during the normal process of bone turnover. Normal bone is continually being remodeled by the coupled process of resorption and reformation. The chemotactic factor probably is a breakdown product of bone collagen released during this process. In vitro bone collagen has exhibited a chemotactic influence on tumor cells under certain circumstances.

Within any primary tumor are innumerable cells that may metastasize, but these cells are not a homogeneous population. Fidler et al.,[28] Springfield,[57] and Weiss[67] have emphasized that all cells in a given tumor presumably originated from a single cell, which then lost its normal growth-controlling mechanism.

Nevertheless, the resulting tumor consists of a heterogeneous population of cells and, in fact, colonies of different cell types exist within a single clinical tumor. The behavior of these subcell types is not identical, and a metastasis that originates from one subcell type usually demonstrates some subtle characteristic differences from the primary tumor. Although typically the metastases can be recognized by a pathologist as originating from a primary tumor, because of the microscopic similarities between them, more sophisticated histopathological analysis demonstrates as many significant dissimilarities as similarities between a metastatic lesion and its parent tumor. For example, a thyroid carcinoma, whether anaplastic or well differentiated, typically presents as histologically well differentiated when metastasizing. This tendency was first recognized by Coats[18] in 1888 and had been described for other tumors well before the beginning of the twentieth century.

The fact that metastatic foci behave much more aggressively than the parent primary tu-

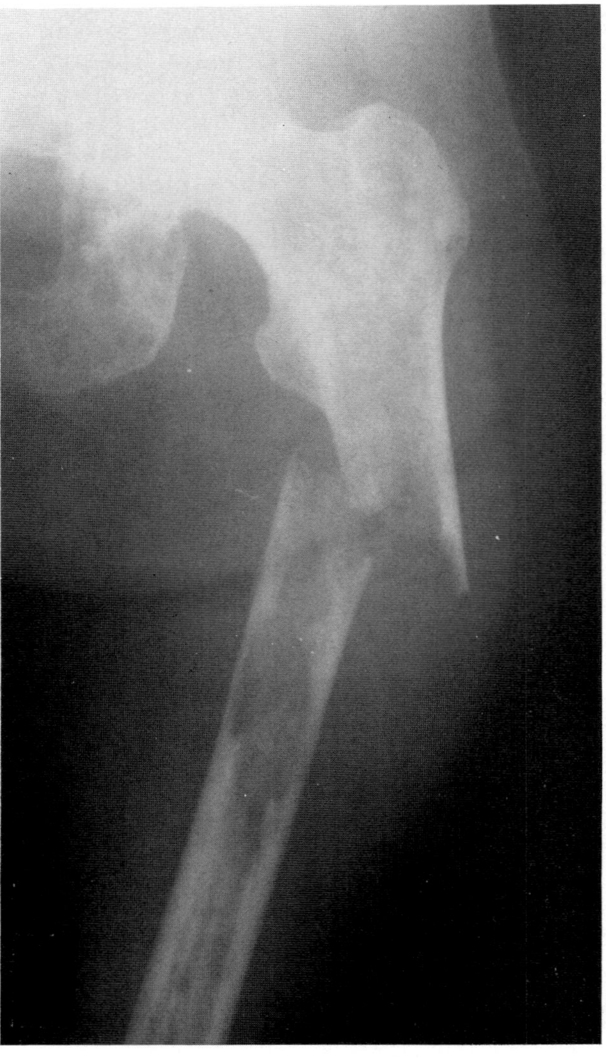

FIGURE 2-1 Pathological fracture of the femur through extensive lytic metastases from breast cancer. The patient had undergone a mastectomy 16 years earlier and had been free of apparent disease until this fracture occurred. Prophylactic mastectomy of the opposite breast revealed no evidence of malignancy. This kind of long quiescent cancer suddenly remanifesting itself in the form of an aggressive bony metastasis is not rare.

mor, and in fact may be the first manifestation of an occult primary malignancy, also is well recognized. Again this phenomenon was described more than a century ago, first being emphasized by Morgan[44] in 1879 when he noted that an enlarging lump on a baby's shoulder, which had been ascribed to "some rough handling on the part of the nurse," had actually been proved to be the initial manifestation of a renal malignancy.

There also appear to be systemic influences that may encourage clinical dormancy or at least latency in an already established metastatic focus. This phenomenon appears to be particularly common in bone metastases. Greenhow[33] noted in 1874 that it was not uncommon for cancers to reappear "after long intervals of latency in situations at a distance from the original site" and he cited a case in which a breast cancer "declared itself in the spine after an interval of fifteen years of good health." In our own experience, similarly long and unpredictable periods of latency followed by a sudden and aggressive reactivation of the tumor are not at all uncommon (Fig. 2-1).

The question of regression of cancer deposits is also noteworthy. Laurence[41] first described in 1855 a malignancy of the "right upper jaw" that "after the fourth operation grew again, and at the same time, some new growths made their appearance—one on the left upper jaw and two on the cranium. However, after it was removed for the fifth time, strange to say, the three others disappeared spontaneously." Again such a phenomenon is not uncommon in our experience, even with metastatic foci that have behaved in a most aggressive manner. A particularly impressive example is a 52-year-old woman with breast cancer metastatic to the thoracic spine who became completely paraplegic from spinal cord compression (Fig. 12-20, *A* to *C*). At the time of anterior decompression and stabilization of her midthoracic spine, numerous malignant implants were observed throughout the pleura and a moderately sized malignant pleural effusion existed. Despite receiving only local radiation to the spine and no chemotherapy, she is now more than 10 years postoperative and has no evidence of residual neurological deficit or active malignancy anywhere.

It is probable that late recurrence of metastatic cancer after a prolonged latency reflects changes in cell-mediated immune responses, as have been shown repeatedly in preterminal cancer patients.[39] Such immunological suppression is demonstrated by a significant delay in skin homograft rejection by terminal cancer patients.[10] Since this immune mechanism is largely mediated by lymphocytes, it was also not surprising that autotransplantations of tumor cells admixed with autogenous leukocytes were temporarily rejected in only half of preterminal cancer patients compared to a rejection rate of 100% in noncancer patients with appropriately controlled transplants.[10] These experiments furnish support for the hypothesis that the suppression of cell-mediated immunity favors implantion of tumor metastases. Such a mechanism might also be invoked to explain the accelerated dissemination of tumor cells in the terminal stages of cancer.

Factors that may favor spontaneous regression of tumor metastases are less easily understood. Among specific allegedly inhibitory factors described have been the by-products of bacterial infection (the so-called Coley's toxins),[46] hormonal suppression,[39] and viral oncolysis.[55] An example of the viral phenomenon was reported by Southam[55] and concerned a case of what he called Hodgkin's disease in an 11-year-old child who was almost clinically moribund and had contracted measles. The child promptly exhibited a dramatic remission, and there was no evident relapse during a follow-up of more than 18 years. Southam subsequently confirmed an at least temporary and predictable remission using the West Nile virus in the therapy of human reticulum cell sarcoma, and from this he postulated that subclinical viral infection might account for some of the apparently spontaneous cancer remissions that have been seen. Cassel and Garrett[14] have also described experimental work aimed at identifying common characteristics of such oncological viruses. They reported an apparent association between neurotropism and viral oncolysis and thus demonstrated at least the theoretical feasibility of inducing the oncolytic property in viruses by neurotropic adaptation.

MECHANISMS OF METASTASIS

The metastatic process is conventionally described as a five-step event: (1) release of cells from the primary tumor, (2) invasion of efferent lymphatic or vascular channels, (3) dissemination of these cells to tissues distant from their source, (4) endothelial attachment and invasion of the new host, and (5) growth of the original colony into a metastatic tumor focus.

Separation of Cells From the Primary Tumor

The first stage, separation of tumor cells from the primary malignancy, appears to be due to a combination of loss of intercellular cohesiveness and subsequent transport within the original tumor interstitial tissue enhanced by local collagen hydrolysis. Springfield[57] has summarized this initial phase, in which the cohesiveness normally encountered between cells is lacking in malignancies. Usually any cell is influenced by surrounding similar cells, such that its growth characteristics are determined to a great degree by its immediately adjacent neighbors. Control is apparently mediated via the cell membrane and is referred to as contact inhibition.[2,28] This contact inhibition prevents overgrowth of the normal cell population. The cell membrane also provides a cohesiveness between normal cells to prevent their separation from each other. Benign tumors appear to lack contact inhibition but are cohesive, whereas malignant tumors lack both contact inhibition and cohesiveness. This dual lack allows isolated cells to exit the main body of a malignant tumor and metastasize to a distant location. There is some evidence[15,52] that the lack of both contact inhibition and cohesiveness is the result of abnormal electrical charges within the cell wall of malignant tumor cells.

Once separated from adjacent cells within the primary tumor, the malignant cells are capable of traversing the tumor interstitial tissue by means of two mechanisms. First, they take advantage of hemoconcentration and consequent strong convective currents forcing fluid out of the primary malignancy.[45] Second, the cells are capable of producing degradative enzymes that destroy connective tissue within and adjacent to the tumor.

With regard to the first mechanism, invasion of the tissue surrounding a primary tumor by neoplastic cells and dissemination of these cells through lymphatic vessels have long been recognized as the principal means of local tumor spread. Gullino[34] and Gullino et al.[35] have demonstrated experimentally that significant hemoconcentration of efferent tumor blood can be measured and that between 5% and 10% of the fluid entering a tumor does not exit by way of venous drainage. Since the total water content of the tissues is constant, the excess fluid oozes out of the tumor surface into the interstitial spaces and into the lymphatics of surrounding tissues. Indirect evidence of this phenomenon[34] is the presence of edematous halos around large tumors and the rapid transfer to the tumor periphery of dyes injected into its center. In fact, it has been demonstrated[35] that the hydrostatic pressure of the tumor interstitial fluid is severalfold higher than in the subcutaneous area surrounding the tumor.

Although such convection currents would encourage cancer cells to escape their host environment, the interstitial environment of a solid tumor contains collagen and glycosaminoglycans in amounts that make the passive movement of the cell impossible unless the cell itself is able to modify its environment. Thus it has long been postulated that for tumor cells to escape into the surrounding tissues and invade local vessels as a route to distant spread, they also must have the secondary capability of producing hydrolases and proteolytic enzymes. Such enzymes have been isolated experimentally.[27,34,52] Specific collagenases and their activators are measurable in fluid surrounding neoplastic cells, although the conditions that control their interactions still are somewhat obscure. The importance of collagenese secretion in the formation of metastases, however, was emphasized by the observation that tumor cells with the highest metastasizing capability also showed the highest collagenese-secreting activity. Specifically, Liotta et al.[42] demonstrated that the degradation of type IV collagen (basement membrane) in vitro was highest in tissue culture lines producing the highest rate of metastases in experimental animals.

Vascular Invasion

There is good evidence that once tumor cells have escaped their parent they must invade local vessels to spread to distant sites as tumor emboli. Venous penetration appears to play a much more important role than does lymphatic infiltration in the development of distant metastases. Spread by the lymphatic system probably is important only as far as the regional lymph nodes are concerned; from there the venous system is the carrier.

Unfortunately, the exact mechanism by which tumor cells cross a tumor wall is not yet clearly established. It appears that the proteolytic enzymes secreted by the tumor cells, and already shown to be so important in enhancing the release of those cells from the parent tumor, also are critical to peripheral vessel invasion. Poste and Fidler[51] and Roos and Dingemais[52] have demonstrated defects in both the endothelial wall and the basement membrane of capillaries within tissue adjacent to tumor masses. It is probable that these defects are created by tumor-secreted enzymes and allow the tumor cells to gain access to the systemic circulation by the same method (diapedesis) as is used by inflammatory cells to enter or exit the circulation. Cameron[13] has postulated that hyaluronidase may be the most important vessel invasion–promoting factor, both in enhancing the egress of cells from the parent tumor into the general circulation and in allowing these cells to invade the tissues of organs in which they ultimately establish metastatic foci.

Transport

Once free in the circulation, cancer cells are able to migrate further depending on the local organ blood flow, general patterns of systemic circulation, and perhaps a particular vulnerability of peripheral tissue (such as bone marrow) due to peculiarities of sinusoidal permeability. The primary factor affecting migration, however, appears to be the ability of those cells to survive within the circulation during transport. Nineteenth century investigators concluded that cancer cells "carried with them to distant parts independent powers of life and nourishment."[11] In 1878 Coats[18] believed that "the elements of certain tumors are in a peculiarly active state, and when transported by blood vessels refuse to be subjected to the destructive powers of the part."

In point of fact, fewer than 0.1% of the circulating cells appear to survive within the circulation.[28] The cause of cell death during transport is not clear. The immune surveillance system, whereby host T-lymphocytes attack tumor cells, undoubtedly plays a role although the exact interactions involved still are unclear.[51,52] A macrophage response has been recorded[15,28,51] that may represent a tumor antigen–stimulated response or a nonspecific immunological reaction to "foreign" tumor protein. Clark[15] also has demonstrated a nonimmunogenic response of macrophages to some tumor cells whose surfaces lack contact inhibitors.

Circulating tumor cells appear to be protected in part by a fibrin-platelet coagulum that surrounds the cells.[28,29,40] This coagulum isolates the circulating malignant cells from the hostile environmental factors of the host just described, allowing them to multiply in some safety and to produce a small and protected colony.[39,56,69,70] The exact pathogenesis of fibrin deposition by circulating cancer cells, however, is unclear. The phenomenon may be attributable to a coagulant factor secreted by healthy circulating tumor cells[61] or to a coagulant released by damaged tumor cells. Experimental evidence[53] does demonstrate that the lethally damaged tumor cells somehow exert a stimulating influence on the growth of their viable neighbors. Finally, it has been shown[61] that the plasmin-antiplasmin system is defective in human cancer patients and the normal mechanisms that inhibit intravascular fibrin formation are either deficient or lacking.

Fibrinogen antibodies labeled with ^{131}I have been employed in clinical detection and even in radioisotope therapy of human tumors.[56] It is not surprising that anticoagulants have successfully reduced the growth rate of cancer transplants in animal experiments. In the series of Agostino et al.,[1] the rate in warfarin-treated animals decreased from 86% of control to as little as 10%. Conversely, since fibrinolytic enzymes exert an anticoagulant effect of sorts, inhibitors of such enzymes have been shown[16] to increase the percentage of successful tumor implants in experimental animals. Unfortunately, the use of anticoagulants in humans prone to metastatic disease, although logical, has not proved to be of any predictable effectiveness in reducing metastatic implants.[43,59]

Circulatory Factors Affecting Metastases

As already noted, it can be assumed that cancer cells metastasize to bone almost exclusively by the hematogenous route. The distribution of those metastases, however, is not uniformly dispersed within the skeleton, the axial skeleton being involved much more commonly than the appendicular skeleton. (See Table 2-2.) This has been shown by radiographic, scintigraphic, and autopsy studies.

Relative to other organs, skeletal metastases are much more common than would be predicted from the low (11 ml/kg/min) overall perfusion rate of bone[39] or from the fact that skeletal blood flow accounts for only 4% to 10% of cardiac output.[20,21] Were the distribution of metastases dependent on blood flow alone, the kidney, with its perfusion rate of 4600 ml/kg/min, would be expected to have the highest incidence of metastases. In fact, the frequency of renal metastases is disproportionately low when considered on the basis of organ perfusion alone.

True, if different portions of bone circulation are examined individually it can be perceived, at least experimentally, that the perfusion rate of the red marrow portion of the axial skeleton is as high as 510 ml/kg/min.[20,21] Moreover, Weiss[66] and others have demonstrated that the microstructure of hematopoietic marrow renders it particularly vulnerable to tumor cell concentration and ultimate invasion. Nutrient arteries to bone with abundant red marrow spaces tend to subdivide into capillaries as they near the endosteal margin of the bone. These capillaries, in turn, become continuous with a rich venous sinusoidal system, which has a capacity six to eight times that of the osseous arterial system and where the circulation of blood and tumor cells effectively comes to a standstill. The walls of these sinusoids are intermittently discontinuous, apparently allowing free exchange of

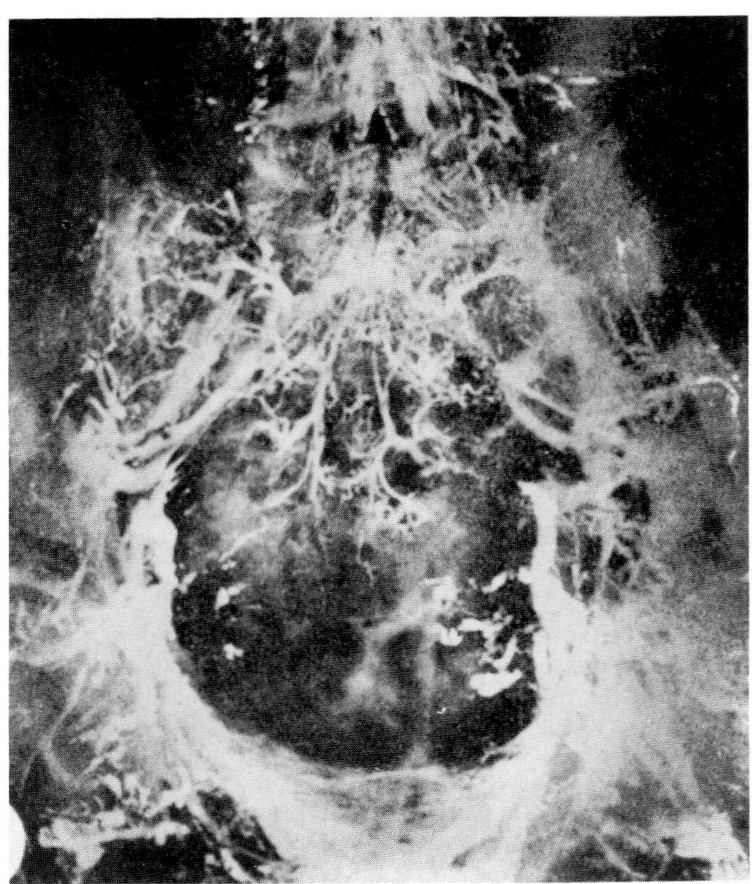

FIGURE 2-2 Illustration from Batson's first publication[3] on the vertebral venous plexus showing the extensive spread of contrast material into the vertebral system from an injection in the deep dorsal vein of the penis. (From Batson, O.V.: AJR **78:**195, 1957.)

circulating blood cells with the intersinusoidal cords of hematopoietic tissue. This anatomical arrangement, encouraging ready access of circulation to the red marrow, unfortunately also carries with it the penalty of vulnerability to metastases.

The high predilection of metastases for becoming established in axial bone marrow, however, in preference to equally rich hematopoietic tissues in the appendicular skeleton argues for specific circulatory factors outside the general arterial circulation. The spine is by far the most common site of metastatic disease, irrespective of the primary tumor responsible. Within the spine the vertebral body usually is affected first, although the initial roentgenographic finding may be the destruction of a pedicle. The usual order of spinal involvement is lumbar, thoracic, cervical, and finally sacral. Most authors agree that this high incidence of vertebral, and in particular lumbar vertebral, metastases is because of a peculiar two-way circulation in the vertebral venous plexus described by Batson in 1940 and bearing his name.[3-5,37] Batson demonstrated both in cadavers and in experimental animals that when dye is injected into the deep dorsal veins of the penis it spreads initially into the prostatic venous plexus and subsequently into the veins about the sacrum, ilium, and lumbar spine, thus mimicking the typical spread of prostatic carcinoma (Fig. 2-2). Although the dye spread up the spine, this spread did not involve the caval system of veins. When the volume of dye was increased, the material reached the base of the skull and even entered the cranial cavity without ever passing through the lungs.

This vertebral system of veins had been recognized as early as the sixteenth century. Vesalius[64] appears to have been the first to observe veins leaving the spinal canal (Fig. 2-3, *A*). In 1611 Vedus-Vedius[65] demonstrated the longitudinal cervical venous sinuses and postulated at least some degree of interconnection (Fig. 2-3, *B*). It was Willis,[68] however, in 1664 who first described the longitudinal and intercommunicating transverse sinuses throughout the entire length of the spinal cavity (Fig. 2-3, *C*), and his concept of vertebral plexus anatomy was further refined by Vieusseus in 1685 (Batson[5]) (Fig. 2-4, *A*). Thereafter no further work was done, and apparently no interest was expressed, in this system until the work of Breschet[9] in the early nineteenth century.

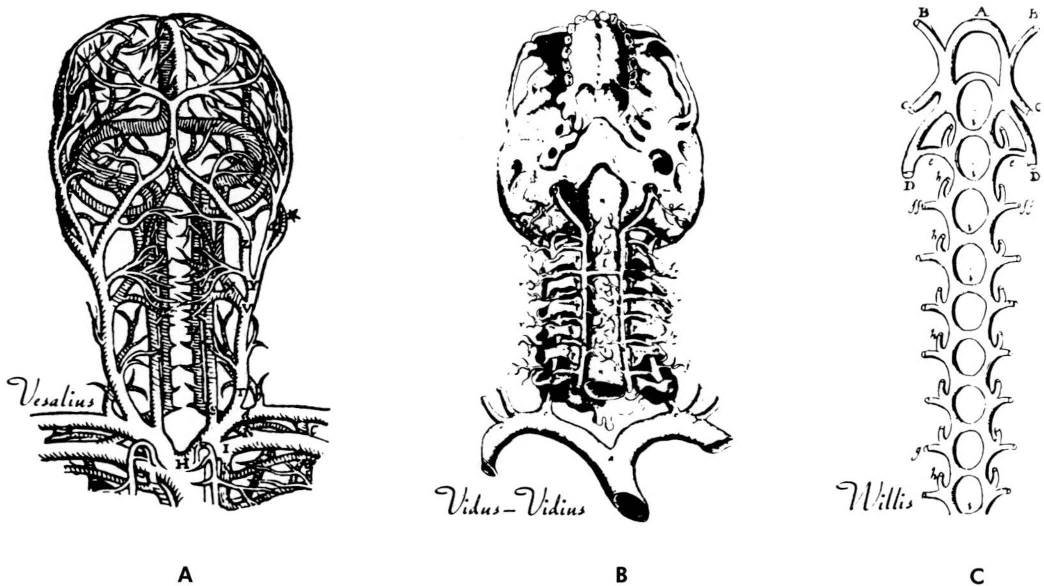

FIGURE 2-3 **A,** Vesalius was the first to illustrate veins leaving the spinal canal. **B,** Vidus-Vidius first illustrated the longitudinal sinus. He showed only one cross-connection. **C,** Willis showed the cross-connections of the entire canal. (From Batson, O.V.: AJR **78:**195, 1957.)

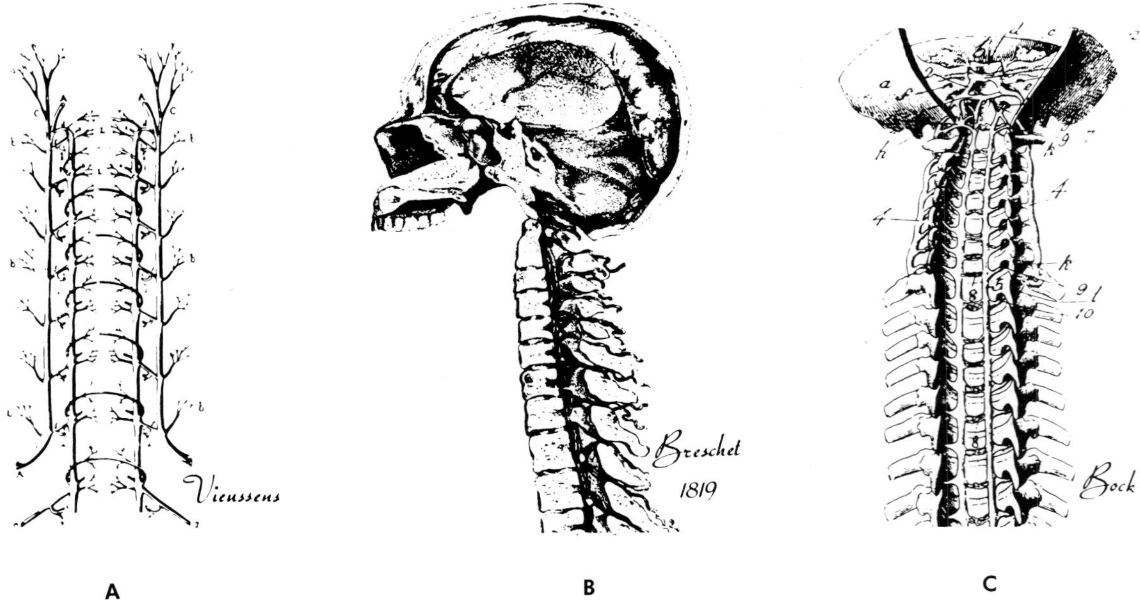

FIGURE 2-4 **A,** Vieussens' illustration and description of the vertebral plexus in the spinal canal showed it to be more complicated than had Willis'. **B,** Breschet gave an excellent description and the best illustrations of the vertebral vein system up to that time (1819). **C,** Bock in 1823 showed the cross connections as a simple tube. (From Batson, O.V.: AJR **78:**195, 1957.)

Breschet was the first to demonstrate that the vertebral venous system was not simply an orderly arrangement of intercommunicating "tubes" lying on the surface of the vertebral bodies, as had been illustrated by Willis (Fig. 2-3, *C*) and Bock (Fig. 2-4, *C*), but instead consisted of the primary longitudinal basilar veins, which branch through an extensive network of sinusoids within the vertebral bodies themselves and in fact communicate with similar venous channels along the anterior longitudinal networks (Figs. 2-4, *B,* and 2-5). He showed that, although the blood in these sinusoids eventually reaches the heart, the veins do not themselves converge toward the heart. Instead, the general arrangement is longitudinal (Figs. 2-5 and 2-6). In his depictions, however, there was an absence of valves and it appeared that the blood could flow freely in either direction without impedance. The network also appeared to function as a large reservoir whose volume capacity was much larger than would have been required simply to return the blood brought in by the arteries.

As represented in Breschet's drawings, this network could be divided into three intercommunicating systems (Figs. 2-5 and 2-6): (1) the central system within the spinal canal and consisting of vessels surrounding the spinal dura, (2) the system of venous sinusoids within the vertebral bone, and (3) the plexus external to the vertebral column and surrounding it. Batson demonstrated that each of these networks was much larger than had previously been suspected. He also showed that the paradural network, being the largest of the three, forms an almost continuous meshwork around the dura lining the spinal canal (Fig. 2-7).

After his initial demonstration that retrograde venous circulation from the prostatic plexus into the vertebral venous network closely mimicked the observed patterns of spread of prostatic carcinoma (Fig. 2-2), Batson began to investigate the ramifications of his proposal to see whether tumor spread from other organs could be explained similarly. He showed that dye injected into a small venule in the breast traveled by way of the

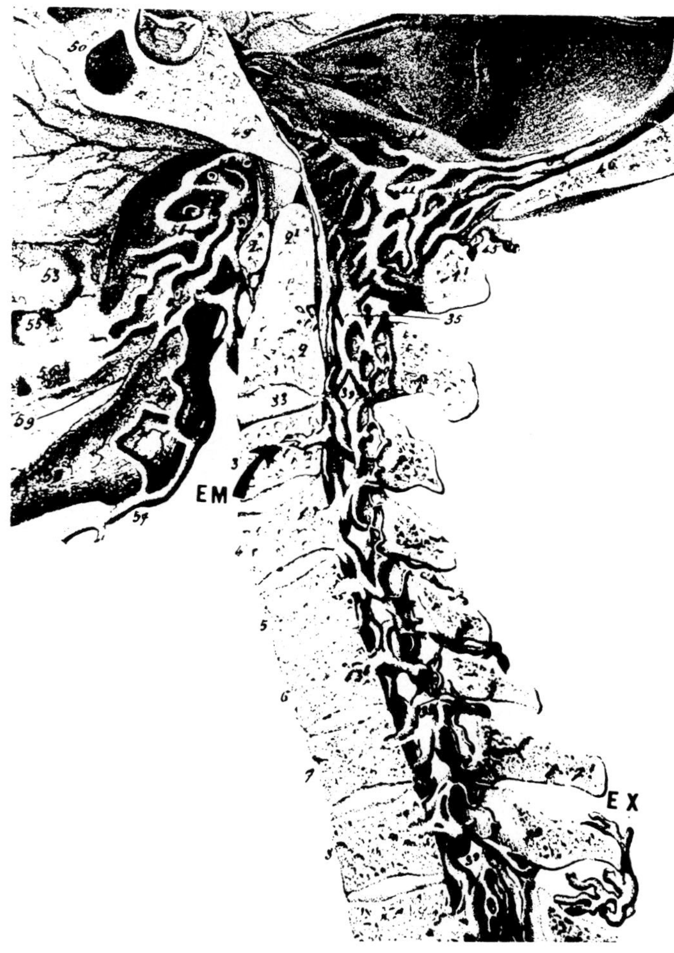

FIGURE 2-5 The longitudinal venous sinuses with both cross and circle connections. *EM,* Emissary channels into the vertebral bodies; *EX,* posterior external plexus. (Reproduced by Batson from Breschet's life-sized lithograph, 1828.) (From Batson, O.V.: AJR **78:**195, 1957.)

superficial breast veins to enter not only into the intravertebral sinusoids and eventually the sinuses of the cranium but also into the venous anastomoses about the clavicle, intercostal veins, and humeral head.[5] Thus it was shown that the venous system of the skin and breast communicates both with the deep vertebral plexus and with the apparently valveless plexuses well outside the axillary skeleton.

This and other experiments eventually led Batson[3-5] to classify the veins of the human body into two principal groups: those within the pressure chamber of the thoracoabdominal cavity and those outside this cavity (Fig. 2-8). Within the cavity are the caval, pulmonary, portal, and azygos systems. The veins of the extremities that possess valves are part of the caval system. By contrast, outside the cavity are the veins of the head and neck, veins of the body wall (including the intercostal vessels), and valveless veins of the extremities. These outside vessels, Batson[5] wrote,

> mutually continuous with the veins of the vertebral column (the true vertebral veins), form a separate and distinct group of vessels . . . called the vertebral vein system. This system parallels, joins, and at the same time bypasses the cavity veins. It unites the superior vena cava to the inferior vena cava, like the azygos veins but outside the pressure cavity.

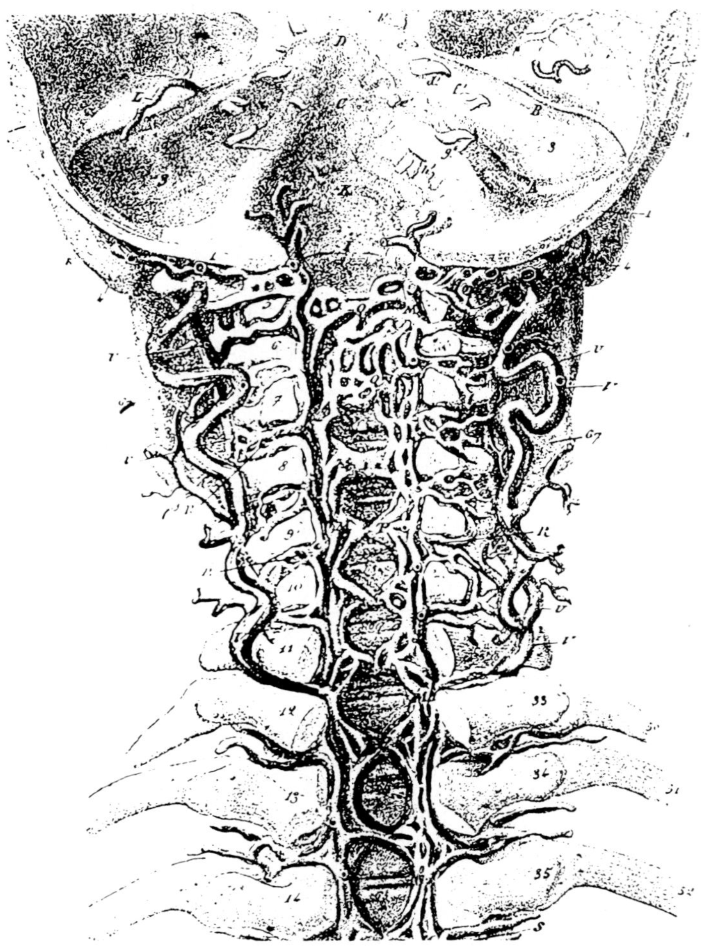

FIGURE 2-6 The extradural anterior sinuses are paired and plexiform in this view from Breschet. The cross connections unite with the large bone emissaries in the middle of the vertebral bodies. The paired sinuses become a network near the skull. (From Batson, O.V.: AJR **78:**195, 1957.)

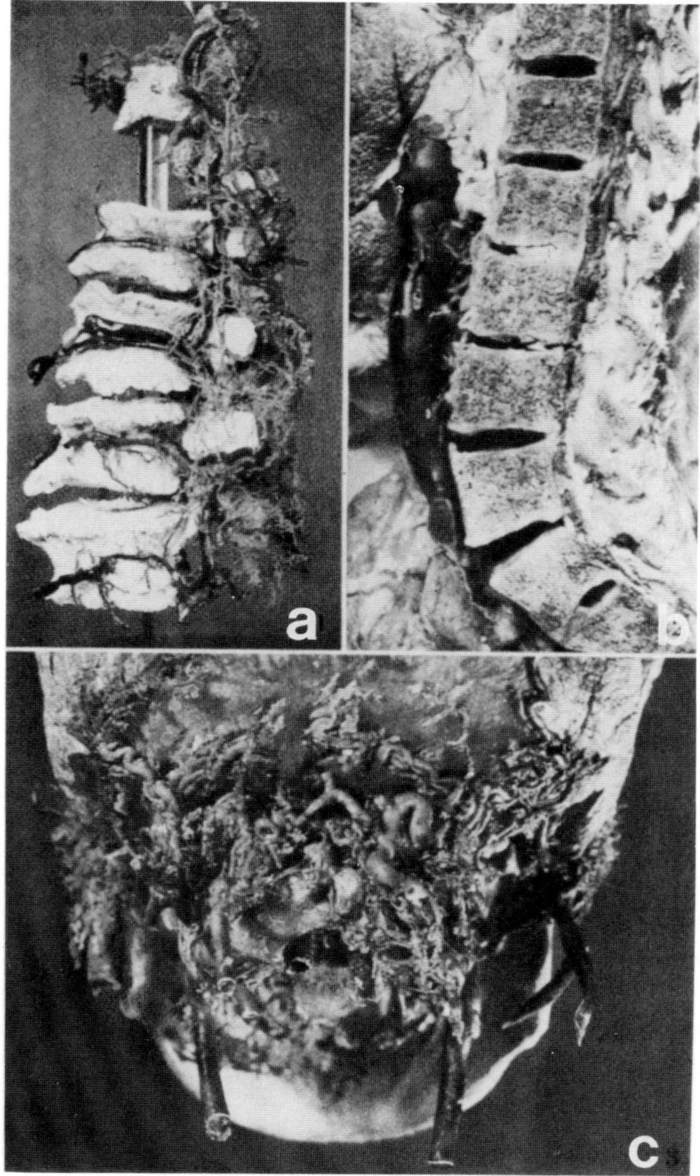

FIGURE 2-7 Batson's preparations of vertebral veins. **A,** Corrosion specimen, human, showing the rich network around the vertebral column. **B,** The extradural vertical network and extensive intraosseus net. An emissary joins the inferior vena cava. **C,** The base of the skull from behind. Note the posterior extravertebral plexus, with two vertical channels contained within the spinal canal. (From Batson, O.V.: AJR **78:**195, 1957.)

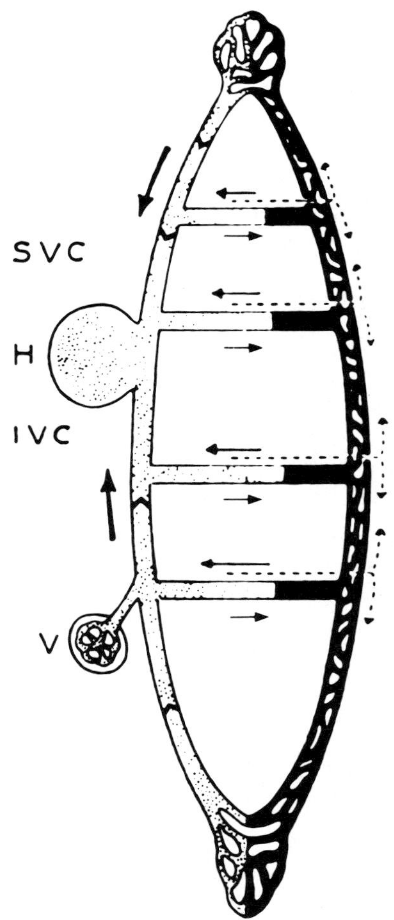

FIGURE 2-8 Herlihy's concept of the venous network as modified by Batson. The valveless vertebral vein system is on the right in black; all the other body veins are on the left. The middle communications flow in either direction depending on extravenous pressures. *SVC,* Superior vena cava; *H,* heart; *IVC,* inferior vena cava; *V,* venous plexuses of the peripheral musculature. (From Batson, O.V.: AJR **78:**195, 1957.)

In every act of straining, coughing, or lifting, blood not only is prevented from entering the thoracoabdominal system but actually is squeezed out into this outside system described by Batson. Similarly, tumor cells from cancers of the breast, lungs, thyroid, pelvic organs, and retroperitoneal tissues, which have direct access to the vertebral venous system, can be distributed anywhere along the network without entering the portal, pulmonary, or caval systems. The distribution of metastases from such cancers is easily explainable by this hypothesis. For example, in the living human, the normal direction of flow is from the prostatic plexus to the inferior vena cava. When intraabdominal pressure is increased, blood flows into the vertebral venous plexuses and from there spreads into the intercostal vessels, avoiding the vena cava. Cells from the breast and thyroid enter the system through intercostal and cervical veins respectively. (See p. 309.)

Numerous workers[17,31,63] have investigated and verified Batson's hypothesis. Tumor cells injected into the femoral veins of experimental mammals while the intraabdominal pressure was elevated briefly were diverted from the caval plexus into the vertebral venous plexus. In the majority of these animals pulmonary lesions developed, indicating that some of the tumor cell suspension also entered the caval system. However, these direct tumor emboli in the lungs did not extend through the pulmonary arterioles or capillaries, thus disproving the nineteenth century concept that vertebral metastases arose by seeding from secondary tumors in the lungs.[23]

Host Endothelial Attachment

Once tumor cells have reached a peripheral site suitable for the development of a metastatic focus, direct attachment of these cells to vessel endothelium must occur before the tissues of the host organ can be invaded. The tendency of cancer cells to adhere to vascular endothelium, as distinct from the mere formation of tumor emboli, provides the basis for establishing "beachheads" prior to interstitial invasion.

Nineteenth century investigators[22,54] felt that cancer cells simply became lodged in peripheral vessels small enough to allow those cells to become wedged as emboli. Modern investigators,[69,70] however, have demonstrated that cancer cells (as visualized microscopically in the rabbit's ear, for example) have an ability to cling to the endothelium even when the capillary diameter is two to three times the size of the cancer cell and the blood is flowing quite briskly. This stickiness is not dependent on or related to endothelial damage but appears rather to be due to the production by the tumor cells of the fibrin-like substance already described. This substance not only protects the cells from host defense mechanisms but also enhances their fixation to the vessel endothelium.[28,40,70] Wood et al.[70] observed the formation of a fibrin thrombus that surrounded the tumor cells within 30 minutes of their fixation to the capillary endothelium. Although the thrombus disappeared within 12 to 24 hours, the cancer cells remained attached to the endothelium and after 24 hours began to undergo mitotic division. Cell invasion of the entothelium began 48 hours after adherence to the capillary wall. At 72 hours the incipient metastasis was established.[69,70]

Penetration of the endothelium and movement of the cancer cell into the host interstitium appear to be enhanced both by the secretion of a "spreading factor" by the cells[31] and by a remarkable ameboid motility of the cells in vivo. This spreading factor, variable from one tumor type to another, appears to be some type of hyaluronidase[13] that can promote the exfoliation of mesothelial cells of the vessel wall before there is any actual contact with the tumor cells themselves.[8] The tumor cells then replace the mesothelial cells on the denuded surface and breach the basement membrane by ameboid motion.

The ameboid motility of cancer cells in vitro is not impressive.[25] However, in vivo these cells have been observed to move at speeds up to 7.68 μm/min as compared to adjacent fibroblasts and tissue macrophages, which are virtually nonmotile.[70] Interestingly, in experimental animals that had widespread metastases but were not preterminal the lymphocytes adjacent to small metastatic foci also demonstrated enhanced motility whereas the more moribund the animals became the less active were the lymphocytes.

Final Establishment of a Metastatic Focus

In clinical observations of cancer patients, as in the study of experimental animals, the acceptance of a metastatic tumor deposit appears to depend on the suppression of lyphocyte-mediated immunological responses. This has been demonstrated indirectly in terminal cancer patients by the much less rapid rejection of skin homografts than occurs in other cancer patients.[10]

Once a colony of tumor cells has become established within a peripheral site, it may be termed a micrometastasis. However, it will not become a clinically significant tumor focus unless it obtains its own vascular supply.[15] Secretion of "a tumor angiogenesis factor" was demonstrated first by Folkman (Springfield[57]). The factor attracts vessels to a small tumor colony that would otherwise remain viable only through local tissue diffusion of nutrients and be incapable of subsequent invasion itself. Again, the production of this angiogenesis factor appears to be blocked in part by postimmune responses, presumably mediated through lymphocytes. This phenomenon explains, perhaps, the late appearance of metastases long after resection of the original tumor focus. In such instances (Fig. 2-1) it can be postulated that a micrometastasis established years earlier only much later attracts the vasculature required for growth. It is against such viable but as yet poorly vascularized peripheral tumor colonies that adjuvant chemotherapy probably is most effective.

In addition to a vascularizing factor produced by all tumors that metastasize successfully, some tumors also appear to be able to secrete specific factors that enhance the establishment of their colonies in particular organs. As described in Chapter 7, breast, prostatic, lung, renal, and thyroid tumors all secrete osteoclast-activating factors that enhance their successful establishment in bone.[31]

In summary, for cancer cells to form viable metastatic foci, an exceedingly complex series of interactions must occur between those cells and the host environment. On the one hand, it seems amazing that any cancer cells are able to survive their escape from the parent malignancy, much less become established as independent colonies capable of fostering further metastases. On the other hand, considering the multiplicity of apparent defenses that each cancer cell possesses to avoid its own annihilation and enhance colonization of distant vital organs, it seems surprising that any primary tumor ever can be removed before distant metastases have become established. Obviously, in any given individual, a delicate balance exists that can be tipped in favor of either side. The major determinant in this equation, as yet poorly defined experimentally and minimally influenceable clinically, probably is the complex of immune defenses normally active in the human body. In the healthy individual, this stands as an impenetrable bastion; in the cancer patient it has been breached to varying degrees. Only when we have learned to exert some influence on this immune system will there be cause for optimism that any or all of the complex steps in tumor growth and metastasis can be controlled.

REFERENCES

1. Agostino, D., et al.: Effect of prolonged coumadin treatment on the production of pulmonary metastases in the rat, Cancer **19:**284, 1966.
2. Ambrose, E.J.: The surface properties of mamalian cells in culture. In The proliferation and spread of neoplastic cells. Twenty-first Symposium on fundamental cancer research, Baltimore, 1967, The Williams & Wilkins Co.
3. Batson, O.V.: The function of the vertebral veins and their role in spread of metastases, Ann. Surg. **112:**138, 1940.
4. Batson, O.V.: Vertebral vein system as mechanism for spread of metastases, A.J.R. **48:**715, 1942.
5. Batson, O.V.: The vertebral vein system. Caldwell lecture, 1956, A.J.R. **78:**195, 1957.
6. Beale, L.: The microscope and its application to clinical medicine, London, 1854, Highly.
7. Bezwoda, W.R., et al.: Treatment of metastatic breast cancer in estrogen receptor positive patients, Cancer **50:**2747, 1982.
8. Birbeck, M.S.C., and Whatley, D.N.: An electron microscopic study of the invasion of ascites tumor cells into the abdominal wall, Cancer Res. **25:**490, 1965.
9. Breschet, G.: Recherches anatomiques, physiologiques et pathologiques sur le système veineux et spécialement sur les cavaux veineux des os, Paris, 1828-1832, Villaret & Cie.
10. Brunschwig, A., et al.: Host resistance to cancer: clinical experiments by homotransplants, autotransplants, and admixture of autologous leukocytes, Ann. Surg. **162:**416, 1965.
11. Budd, W.: Remarks on the pathology of cancer, Lancet **2:**266, 1841-1842.
12. Butler, T.P., et al.: Bulk transfer of fluid in the interstitial compartment of mammary tumors, Cancer Res. **133:**3084, 1975.
13. Cameron, E.: Hyaluronidase and cancer, Long Island City, N.Y., 1966, Pergamon Press, Inc.
14. Cassel W.A., and Garrett, R.E.: Relationship between viral neurotropism and oncolysis. I, Study of vaccinia virus. II, Study of influenza virus, Cancer **20:**433, 440, 1967.
15. Clark, R.L.: Systemic cancer and the metastatic process, Cancer **43:**790, 1979.
16. Clifton, E.E., and Agostino, D.: Effect of inhibitors of fibrinolytic enzymes on development of pulmonary metastases, J. Natl. Cancer Inst. **33:**753, 1964.
17. Coman, D.R., et al.: Studies on the mechanisms of metastasis. The distribution of tumors in various organs in relation to the distribution of arterial emboli, Cancer Res. **11:**648, 1951.
18. Coats, J.: A case of simple diffuse goitre, with secondary tumours of the same structure in the bones of the skull, Trans. Pathol. Soc. Lond. **38:**399, 1887.
19. Coats, J.: Case of multiple cancerous tumours, many of them cystic, in the lungs, brain, bones &c., the primary tumour probably in the lung, Trans. Pathol. Soc. Lond. **39:**326, 1888.
20. Cumming, J.D.: A study of blood flow through bone marrow by a method of venous effluent collection, J. Physiol. **162:**13, 1962.
21. Cumming, J.D., and Nutt, M.E.: Bone marrow blood flow and cardiac output in the rabbit, J. Physiol. [Lond.] **162:**30, 1962.
22. De Morgan, C.: Discussion on cancer, Trans. Pathol. Soc. Lond. **25:**287, 387, 1874.
23. Drury, A.B., et al.: Carcinomatous metastasis to the vertebral bodies, J. Clin. Pathol. **17:**448, 1964.
24. Ecoffier, J., et al.: Étude de réseau veineux dans les os longs du lapin, Rev. Chir. Orthop. **43:**29, 1957.
25. Enterline, H.T., and Coman, D.R.: The ameboid motility of human and animal neoplastic cells, Cancer **3:**1033, 1950.
26. Eve, F.S.: Lectures on cystic tumours of the jaws, and on the etiology, general characters, and the relations of tumours, Br. Med. J. **1:**241, 1883.
27. Fidler, I.J.: Tumor heterogeneity and the biology of cancer invasion and metastasis, Cancer Res. **38:** 2651, 1978.

28. Fidler, I.J., et al.: The biology of cancer invasion and metastasis, Adv. Cancer Res. **28:**149, 1978.
29. Fisher, B., et al.: Trauma and the localization of tumor cells, Cancer **20:**23, 1967.
30. Fisher, E.R., et al.: Pathologic findings from the National Surgical Adjuvant Breast Project. VIII. Relationship of chemotherapeutic responsiveness to tumor differentiation, Cancer **51:**181, 1983.
31. Galasko, C.S.B.: Skeletal metastases and mammary cancer, Ann. R. Col. Surg. Engl. **50:**3, 1972.
32. Grantham, F.H., et al.: Primary mammary tumors connected to the host by a single artery and vein, J. Natl. Cancer Inst. **50:**1381, 1973.
33. Greenhow, E.H.: Discussion on cancer, Trans. Pathol. Soc. Lond. **25:**362, 1874.
34. Gullino, P.M.: Techniques for the study of tumor physiopathology, Methods Cancer Res. **5:**45, 1970.
35. Gullino, P.M., et al.: The interstitial fluid of solid tumor, Cancer Res. **24:**780, 1964.
36. Hayaski, H., et al.: Chemotactic factors associated with the invasion of cancer cells, Nature [Lond.] **226:**174, 1970.
37. Henriques, C.Q.: The veins of the vertebral column and their role in the spread of cancer, Ann. R. Coll. Surg. Engl. **31:**1, 1962.
38. Hodgkin, T.: Cases illustrative of some consequences of local injury, Med. Chir. Trans. **31:**253, 1848.
39. Johnston, A.D.: Pathology of metastatic tumors in bone, Clin. Orthop. **73:**8, 1970.
40. Kinsey, D.L.: An experimental study of preferential metastasis, Cancer **13:**674, 1960.
41. Laurence, J.Z.: The diagnosis of surgical cancer, London, 1855, Churchill.
42. Liotta, L.A., et al.: Metastatic potential correlates with enzymatic degradation of basement membrane collagen, Nature **284:**67, 1980.
43. Michaels, L.: Cancer incidence and mortality in patients having anticoagulant therapy, Lancet **2:**832, 1964.
44. Morgan, J.H.: Sarcoma of the scapula in infant, followed by multiple sarcoma in various organs and tissues, Trans. Pathol. Soc. Lond. **30:**399, 1879.
45. Mundy, G.R., and Spro, T.P.: The mechanisms of bone metastasis and bone destruction by tumor cells. In Weiss, L., and Gilbert, H.A., editors: Bone metastasis, Boston, 1981, G.K. Hall & Co.
46. Nauts, H.C., et al.: A review of the influence of bacterial infection and of bacterial products (Coley's toxins) on malignant tumors in man, Acta Med. Scand. (suppl.) **276:**5, 1953.
47. Onguigbo, W.I.B.: Recognition and treatment of pathologic fractures in the nineteenth century, Surgery **77:**553, 1975.
48. Onguigbo, W.I.B.: Sensitivity and rejectivity in cancer metastasis, Med. Hypoth. **5:**185, 1979.
49. Paget, S.: The distribution of secondary growths in cancer of the breast, Lancet **1:**571, 1889.
50. Pitts, B.: Columnar carcinoma of humerus secondary to tumour of upper part of rectum, Trans. Pathol. Soc. Lond. **42:**267, 1891.
51. Poste, G., and Fidler, I.J.: The pathogenesis of cancer metastasis, Nature **283:**139, 1980.
52. Roos, E., and Dingemais, K.P.: Mechanism of metastasis, Biochim. Biophys. Acta **560:**135, 1979.
53. Seelig, K.F., and Revesy, L.: Effect of lethally damaged tumor cells upon the growth of admixed viable cells in diffusion chambers, Br. J. Cancer **14:**126, 1960.
54. Simon, J.: Some points of science and practice concerning cancer, Br. Med. J. **1:**219, 1878.
55. Southam, C.M.: Tumor resistance in cancer patient. In Wissler, R.W., et al., editors: Endogenous factors influencing host-tumor balance, Chicago, 1967, University of Chicago Press.
56. Spar, I.L., et al.: I^{131}-labeled antibodies to human fibrinogen. Diagnostic studies and therapeutic trial, Cancer **20:**865, 1967.
57. Springfield, D.S.: Mechanisms of metastasis, Clin. Orthop. **169:**15, 1982.
58. Steinbach, H.L., et al.: Osseous phlebography, Surg. Gynecol. Obstet. **104:**215, 1957.
59. Suzman, M.M.: In Pickering, G., editor: Symposium on anticoagulant therapy, London, 1961, Harvey & Blythe, Ltd.
60. Targett, J.H.: Multiple sarcomata of skull, ribs, and glands, Trans. Pathol. Soc. Lond. **39:**306, 1888.
61. Thornes, R.D.: Fibrinogen and the interstitial behaviour of cancer. In Wissler, R.W., et al., editors: Endogenous factors influencing host-tumor balance, Chicago, 1967, University of Chicago Press.
62. Ushijima, K., et al.: Characterization of two different factors chemotactic for cancer cells from tumor tissues, Virchows Arch. [Cell Pathol.] **21:**119, 1976.
63. Van den Brenk, H.A.S., et al.: Venous diversion trappings and growth of blood-borne cancer cells en route to the lungs, Br. J. Cancer **31:**46, 1975.
64. Vesalius, A.: De humani corporis fabrica, Basel, 1543, Andreas Oporinus..
65. Vidus-Vidius (Guido Guidi): De anatomia corporis humani, Venice, 1611, Iuntas, Fig. 2.
66. Virchow, R.: Cellular pathology, London, 1860, Churchill.
67. Weiss, L.: Dynamic aspects of cancer cell populations in metastasis, Am. J. Pathol. **97:**601, 1979.
68. Willis, T.: Cerebri anatomia, London, 1664, Martyn & Allestry.
69. Wood, S., Jr.: Experimental studies of the intravascular dissemination of ascites V_2 carcinoma cells in the rabbit with special reference to fibrogen and fibrinolytic agents, Bull. Swiss Acad. Med. Sci. **20:**92, 1964.
70. Wood, S., Jr., et al.: Factors influencing the spread of cancer—locomotion of normal and malignant cells in vivo. In Wissler, R.W., et al., editors: Endogenous factors influencing host-tumor balance, Chicago, 1967, University of Chicago Press.

PART I

DIAGNOSTIC MODALITIES

CHAPTER 3

BONE IMAGING

Stephen R. Bunker   Beth C. Kleiner

Diagnostic imaging provides the cost-effective and noninvasive means to accurately evaluate the skeleton for possible metastases. The highly sensitive radionuclide survey is performed initially, allowing the entire skeleton to be evaluated. Since initial investigations of ^{99m}Tc-labeled bone imaging compounds in the early 1970s, several improvements in both imaging instrumentation and radiopharmaceutical properties have taken place. Skeletal scintigraphy in the 1980s represents a noninvasive diagnostic procedure with extreme sensitivity and the ability to image the entire skeleton with a minimum of exposure to ionizing radiation. It is the imaging modality of choice to initially search for osseous metastases.

Comparative studies assessing the relative accuracies of scintigraphy and roentgenographic surveys of the skeleton have demonstrated that from 30% to 50% of lesions identified by scan are not detected by conventional roentgenograms. Skeletal scintigraphy was falsely negative in only about 2% of lesions, and a false-positive rate of similar magnitude was estimated.* The shortcomings of roentgenograms in detecting trabecular bone lesions have been known for some time. Lesional size of at least 1.5 cm and a 50% loss of bone mineral content were initially recognized as requirements for x-ray detection.[1] Furthermore, an estimated 10% of metastatic bone deposits occur in the extremities,[20] whose distal portions are frequently not included in roentgenographic surveys.

Most tumor sites become manifest as focal or regional areas of increased radiotracer accumulation compared to "normal" distribution of activity in the contralateral or adjacent bones (Fig. 3-1). This focal increase in tracer deposition is related to the extent and magnitude of bone repair that occurs in response to tumor osteolysis. The regional hyperemia that is associated with this osteoblastic reparative process is felt to be a major associated factor in "overexposing" the affected bone region to the circulating tracer. Finally, tumor cells or their elaborated metabolites may cause an osteoblastic response by direct stimulation.[3]

Much less commonly, tumor sites will produce focally reduced or absent tracer deposition compared to the adjacent bone (Fig. 3-2). These photopenic lesions are most often associated with roentgenographically lytic, destructive processes that elicit little or no osteoblastic repair by virtue of either extensive or rapid destructive osteolysis (or both) with or without compromise of the nutrient vascular supply to the affected area.

In general, then, skeletal scintigraphy is used to screen for bone metastases from a wide variety of primary neoplasms, with roentgenographic evaluation of suspicious or nonspecific areas of abnormality utilized as a correlative modality. As with all such strategies or algorithms (Fig. 3-9), however, major exceptions exist and interaction of the nuclear physician or radiologist with the referring or

Text continued on p. 41.

*References 3, 6, 7, 9, 17, 19, 21-23, 27.

A

B

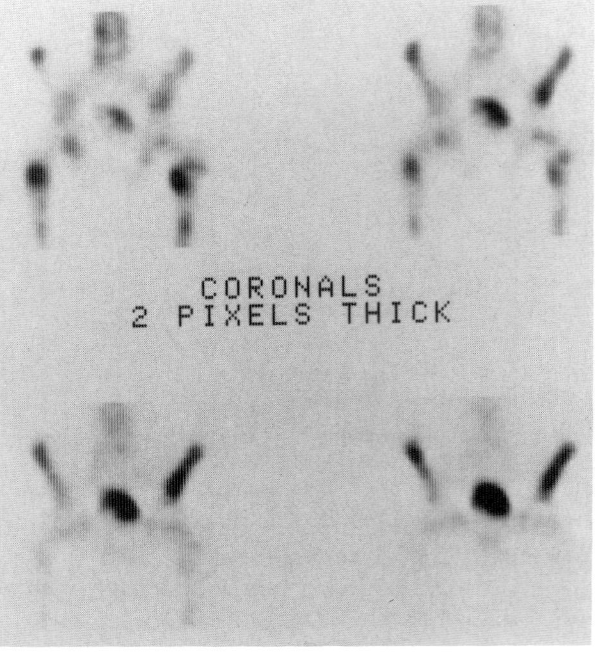

FIGURE 3-1 Prostatic carcinoma. **A,** An anterior whole body radionuclide image is used to evaluate the entire skeleton. Multiple focal areas of increased tracer deposition can be seen in the shoulders, ribs, lumbar spine, pelvis, and proximal femora. **B,** Contiguous coronal single photon emission computed tomographic (SPECT) images, posterior-to-anterior, demonstrate superior contrast resolution. Focal abnormalities in both femoral heads are more clearly delineated than on the anterior whole body image.

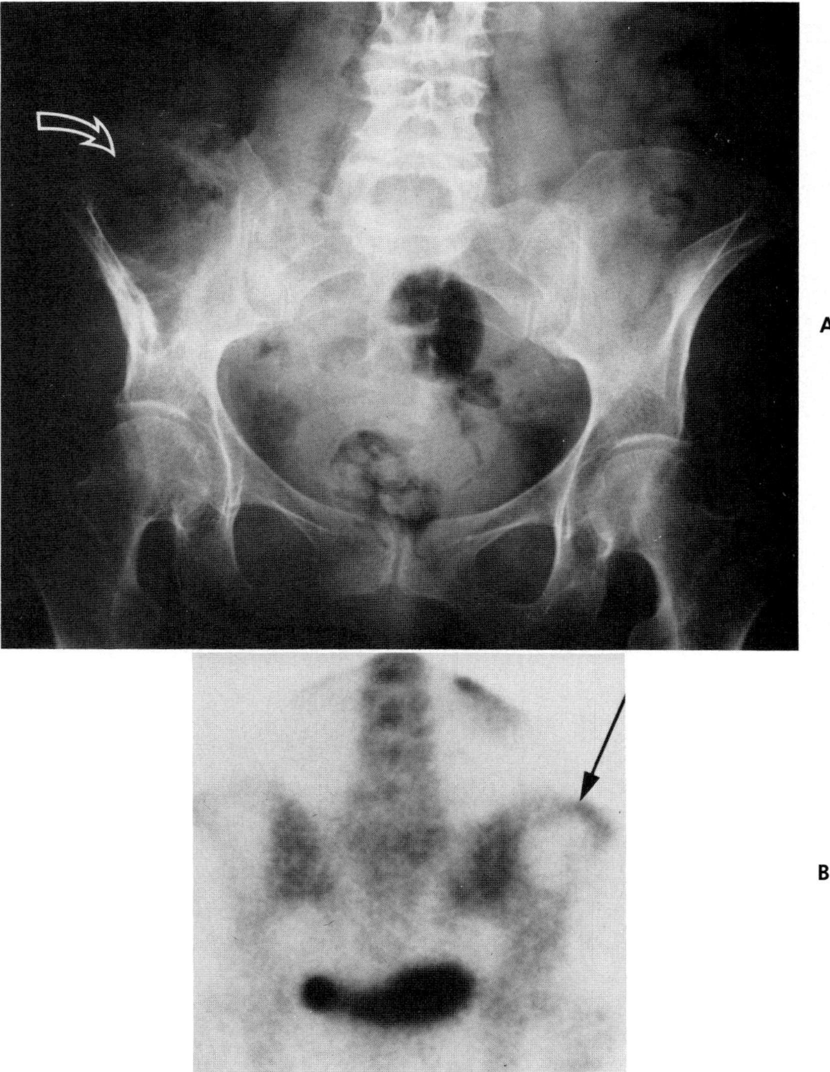

FIGURE 3-2 Multiple myeloma. **A,** An AP roentgenogram of the pelvis demonstrates a lytic expansile lesion involving the right superolateral iliac wing *(arrow)* and a second lesion in the right ischium. **B,** A posterior planar scintiphotograph reveals increased activity at the right iliac crest *(arrow)* and a generalized increase within the right ischium.

Continued.

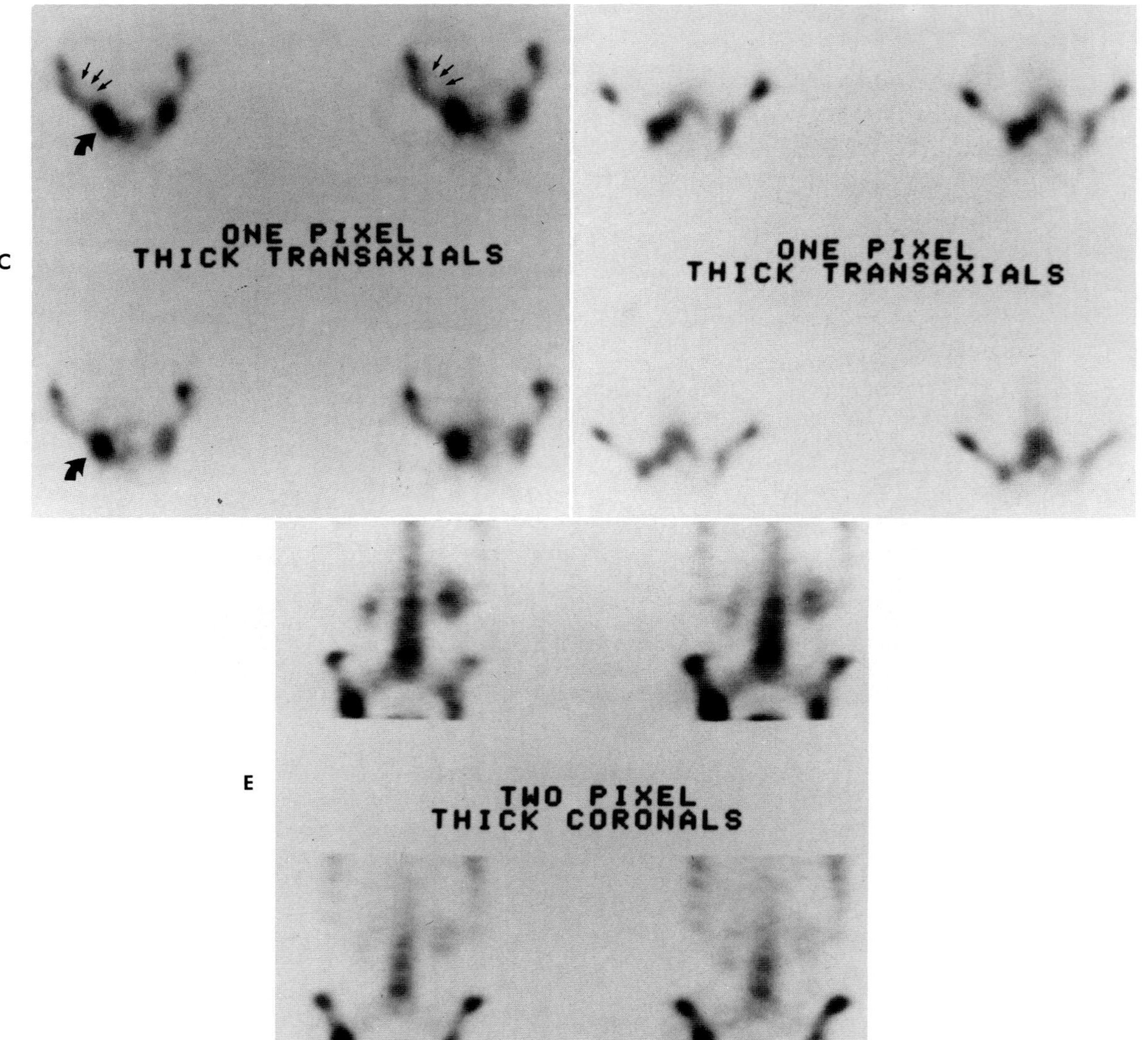

FIGURE 3-2, cont'd. **C,** Transaxial single photon emission computed tomographic (SPECT) images at the level of the iliac fossa show expansion of the right ilium with relatively normal intensity of tracer activity *(small arrows).* Also demonstrated is an abnormal increase in labeling of the right ilium at the sacroiliac joint compared to the left *(curved arrows).* **D,** Transaxial SPECT images at a more cephalic level reveal contiguous involvement of the right sacral ala and a distorted and photopenic (decreased activity) appearance of the left ilium. **E,** Coronal SPECT images confirm the right iliac destructive process as well as the abnormal appearance to the right ischium and lumbar vertebral bodies.

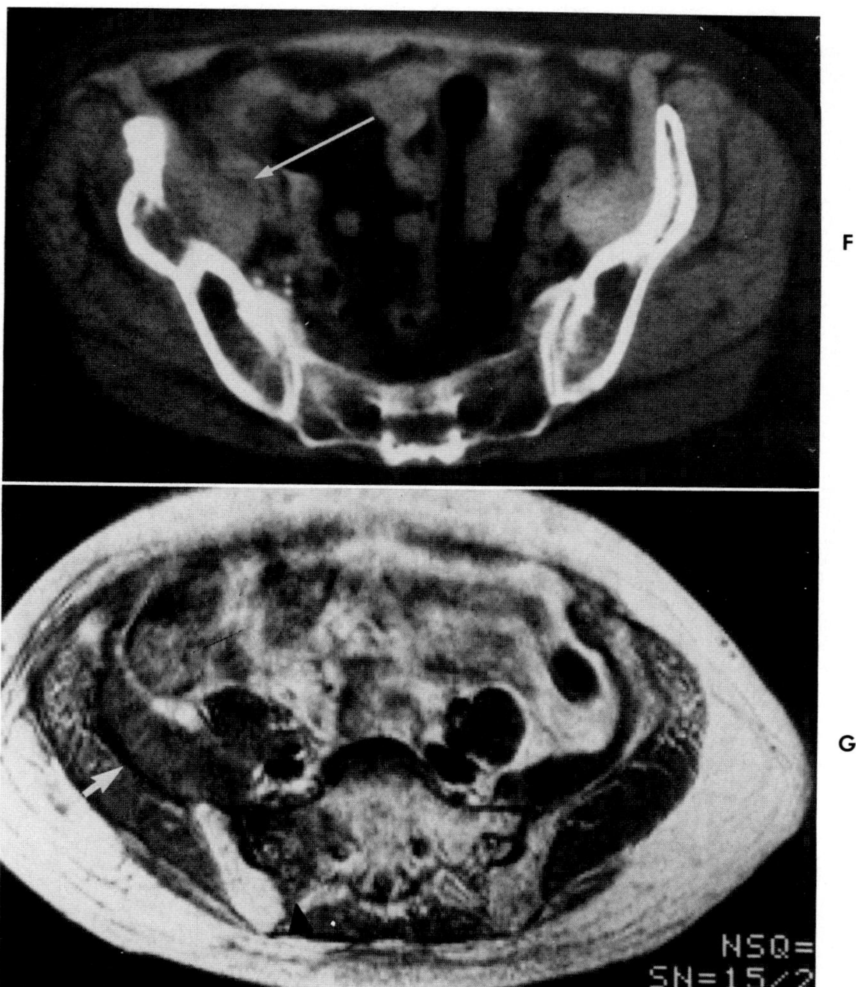

FIGURE 3-2, cont'd. **F,** A transaxial CT bone window image of the pelvis shows destruction in the medial aspect of the right ilium. An associated soft tissue mass extends posterior to the iliopsoas muscle *(arrow)*. **G,** A transaxial short–repetition time (short-TR) magnetic resonance image at the same level reveals focal areas of low signal intensity involving the right iliac wing *(white arrow)* and the right sacral ala *(black arrowhead)*, as well as a diffuse poorly defined low signal intensity in the left ilium compatible with marrow involvement. Note the soft tissue mass posterior to the iliopsoas tendon.

Continued.

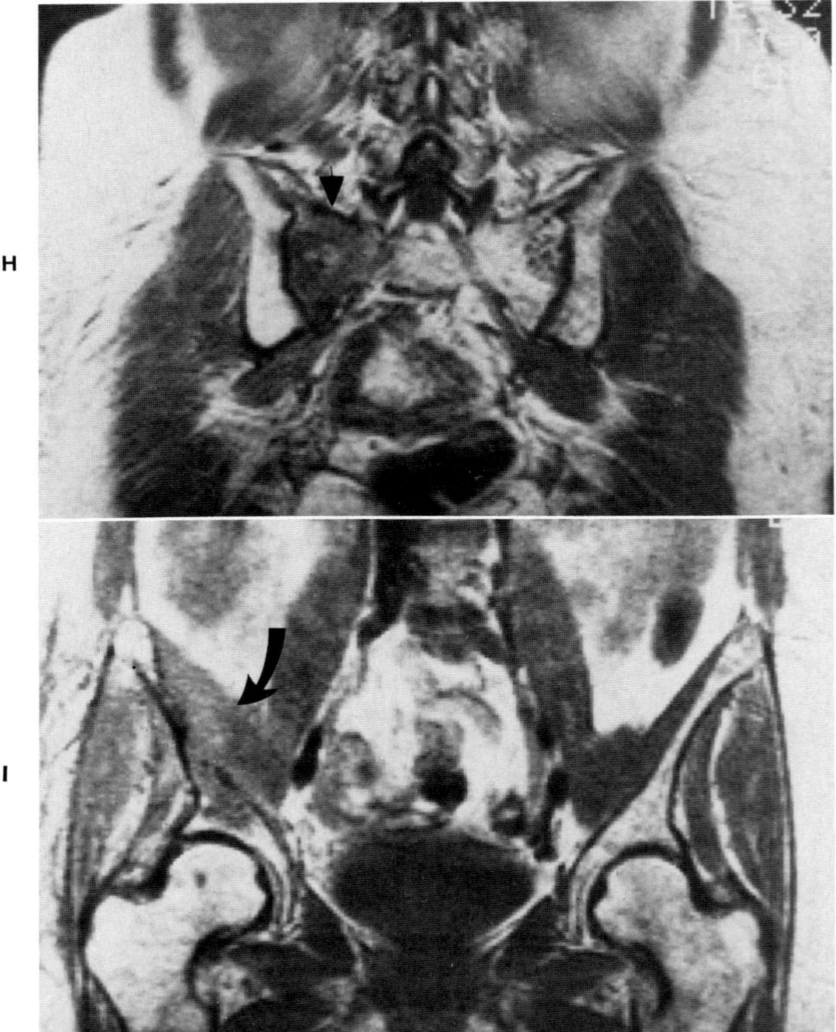

FIGURE 3-2, cont'd. **H,** A coronal short-TR magnetic resonance image through the sacral abnormality *(arrow)*. **I,** A more anterior coronal short-TR magnetic resonance image demonstrates the supraacetabular extent of the myelomatous marrow involvement and the associated soft tissue mass *(arrow)*.

primary care physician is the pivotal means by which the most effective diagnostic approach is utilized in each case.

The value of single photon emission computed tomography (SPECT), which dramatically improves contrast resolution over that of standard planar scintigraphy (Figs. 3-1 and 3-2), as well as the relative roles of x-ray computed tomography (CT) and magnetic resonance imaging (MRI) as correlative modalities are currently under extensive evaluation.

MALIGNANT METASTATIC DISEASE OF BONE

Overall, whole body bone scintigraphy is the most sensitive method for detecting skeletal metastases. Bone pain alone is an unreliable diagnostic index of both the presence and the extent of metastatic disease and is similarly of limited value in predicting response to therapy. Although nearly 75% of all cancer patients with symptoms of bone pain will also have abnormal scans, nearly 45% may be pain free at the time of strongly positive scintigraphic evidence of metastases.[5]

Laboratory values may remain normal, unless extensive bone destruction produces significant elevations in serum calcium and/or marked osteoblastic repair causes a diagnostic rise in alkaline phosphatase. Differences in measurement of serum calcium, phosphorus, and alkaline phosphatase in patients with and without scintigraphic evidence of metastases have not been shown to be statistically significant.[25] In patients with carcinoma of the prostate, for example, skeletal scintigraphy is both more sensitive and more specific in detecting metastases than are either alkaline or acid phosphatase measurements.[26]

SKELETAL SCINTIGRAPHY IN ADULTS WITH NONOSSEOUS PRIMARY NEOPLASMS

At a time when health care dollars are limited and growing numbers of patients are relying on fixed-cost third party coverage plans, the use of any low-yield diagnostic test requires accurate cost justification analysis. The use of skeletal screening at the time of initial detection of a nonosseous primary malignancy must be carefully evaluated in terms of patient symptoms, the specific primary tumor, its propensity for skeletal metastases, and the potential therapeutic implications of early detection of such metastases. The routine use of preoperative skeletal scintigraphy in patients with malignancies of the colon, uterus, and cervix should be discouraged. Scintigraphy in patients with these malignancies, which metastasize infrequently to bone, is best reserved for evaluation of specific symptoms or some change in clinical course of the disease.

Most controversial is the application of screening skeletal scintigraphy in patients with newly diagnosed primary malignancies known to metastasize frequently to bone. In particular, the diagnostic yield and value of preoperative skeletal imaging have been questioned in patients with carcinoma of the breast, lung, and prostate.[22] Although there is a wide range of reported true-positive findings in skeletal scintigraphy for patients with Stage I and Stage II carcinoma of the breast, it is generally held to be quite low (averaging 3% for Stage I and 7% for Stage II). This contrasts with the significantly higher yield in Stage III disease (about 25%).[13] However, Stage I and Stage II disease carries a reported incidence of 20% to 26% for conversion from a normal baseline radionuclide survey to an abnormal scan. Since such conversion correlates with an adverse prognosis, its accurate documentation is felt to be essential. Thus, despite the relatively low yield of preoperative skeletal scintigraphy in patients with Stage I and Stage II carcinoma of the breast, it may reorient the therapeutic approach away from mastectomy and more toward radiotherapy, chemotherapy, or hormonal therapy when positive. Such an approach is still cost effective if the average reported incidence of bone metastases in these stages is utilized. Similarly, preoperative studies are particularly desirable in patients with bronchogenic carcinoma, since documentation of skeletal metastases in this disease could preclude a relatively high-mortality surgical procedure.

Baseline skeletal scintigraphy is felt to be essential for patients with prostatic carcinoma, because of the high propensity of this condition to spread silently to the skeleton. Prostatic carcinoma has one of the highest reported incidences of positive skeletal scintigraphy (35%) at the time of initial staging.[13]

Baseline scintigraphy is invaluable in patients presenting with a primary malignancy known to metastasize frequently to bone (Table 3-1). It provides a cost-effective noninvasive assessment of the entire skeleton that

TABLE 3-1 Frequency of Skeletal Metastases from Soft Tissue Primary Neoplasms

Primary Malignancy	Skeletal Metastases	Type of Metastases
Breast	Very common	Lytic-mixed
Lung	Very common	Lytic
Prostate	Very common	Blastic
Kidney	Very common	Lytic-expanding
Hodgkin's	Very common	Lytic-mixed-blastic
Thyroid	Common	Lytic-expanding
Bladder	Infrequent	Lytic
Melanoma	Infrequent	Lytic-expanding

can detect clinically occult metastases as well as benign disease that might otherwise cause confusion on follow-up evaluation of a then symptom-ridden patient, and it serves as a baseline to which subtle or evolving abnormalities can be readily compared. Follow-up scintigraphy for the evaluation of therapeutic response should be performed at 3-to-6-month intervals. Successful responses to ionizing radiation and/or antimetabolite or hormonal therapy are characterized by a serial decrease in radiotracer intensity, with eventual disappearance of abnormal foci of activity. Even persistent but nonprogressive scintigraphic abnormalities are consistent with clinical remission and improved patient survival.

SKELETAL SCINTIGRAPHY FOR THE DETECTION OF METASTASES IN CHILDREN

The same factors of superior sensitivity and the ability to evaluate the entire skeleton, together with the relatively lower exposure to ionizing radiation than occurs with conventional radiographic evaluation, render radionuclide scanning the method of choice for detecting skeletal metastases in pediatric patients. Gilday et al.[12] compared the relative efficacy of radionuclide and radiographic skeletal surveys in detecting skeletal metastases prospectively in 159 children. Diagnoses included primary bone tumors, neuroblastoma, histiocytosis X, lymphoma, leukemia, fibrosarcoma, rhabdomyosarcoma, and retinoblastoma. Metastases were detected in 44 of the patients. Of these, 30 (or 68%) were demonstrated only by radionuclide imaging and 14 by a combination of radionuclide and roentgenographic techniques. There were no metastatic lesions detected by roentgenography alone. In this same series there were no false-negative scans in 30 patients with neuroblastoma (8 with metastases) or in 19 patients with histiocytosis X (3 with metastases).

Other series,[16,18] however, report that up to 77% of extremity lesions in neuroblastoma may be missed by scintigraphy, presumably because of the normal intense increase in tracer avidity for growing epiphyses and because of the often symmetrical distribution of metastatic deposits in the metaphyses of long bones. In one report on histiocytosis X,[24] scintigraphy was able to detect only 35% of radiographically demonstrable metastases.

CORRELATIVE DIAGNOSTIC IMAGING PROCEDURES

The low incidence of both false-negative and false-positive findings with skeletal scintigraphy in the detection of osseous metastases has been discussed. Although relatively infrequent, false-negative scans can often be attributed to an absence of or reduction in reactive bone formation induced by primarily lytic and more aggressive tumor deposits. For these reasons the extent of metastases from anaplastic tumors, carcinoma of the breast, neuroblastoma, multiple myeloma, solitary plasmacytoma, histiocytosis X, leukemia, lymphoma, and thyroid carcinoma may be underestimated by standard planar skeletal scintigraphy. Early experience with SPECT imaging of the skeleton suggests improved delineation of focal lesions with the usual pattern of increased tracer activity (Fig. 3-1) as well as detection of alterations in normal morphology by less reactive processes, such as multiple myeloma and plasmacytoma[14] (Fig. 3-2). Thus, when conventional scintigraphic skeletal surveys are negative or equivocal in the face of strong clinical suspicion or symptoms, further regional SPECT evaluation may provide improved positive and negative predictive values to this initial screening examination of the skeleton.

SPECT imaging requires a specialized gantry, allowing the otherwise conventional gamma camera detector to rotate circumferentially around the patient (Fig. 3-3, *A*). This angular information is processed by computer back-projection techniques similar to those employed by CT and MRI systems to generate tomograms or "slices" through the area of interest in the patient. SPECT images are typically constructed into transaxial, coronal, and parasagittal anatomical planes (Fig. 3-3, *B*), with slice thickness and image magnification varied as necessary to optimize resolution in the bone or region of interest. The improved detection of lesions is related primarily to increased contrast resolution (Fig. 3-3, *C*). Subsequent correlation with MR and CT images in similar planes of section provides the optimal evaluation of the extent and nature of a disease process.

Metastatic prostate carcinoma, as well as other primary malignancies, occasionally result in a "superscan" appearance of diffusely increased tracer activity without delineation of focal lesions (Fig. 3-4). Careful analysis of scintigraphic findings is required in such cases to avoid rendering a false-negative interpretation. Typically the diffusely increased skeletal activity produces a *steal* phenomenon, reducing the normal renal activity to a level that is barely perceptible or absent. Absence of renal activity can also occur without diffuse skeletal metastases in patients with poor renal function. In these cases, however, the inability to clear excess tracer from soft tissues generally produces a lower-quality image of the skeleton rather than the increased skeletal contrast apparent with the superscan of diffuse metastases.

The nonspecificity of scintigraphic abnormalities, particularly when they present as a solitary focus of increased tracer accumulation, requires careful evaluation and correlation with clinical (e.g., a history of prior trauma, surgery, other disease conditions) as well as roentgenographic findings to help differentiate the wide variety of benign conditions that may produce an identical appearance to that of a metastatic focus. Indeed, approximately one third of such solitary abnormalities detected by skeletal scintigraphy in patients with a primary malignancy have been shown to be secondary to benign processes.[2,18] If plain film roentgenographic findings in these cases are negative or equivocal, CT or MRI evaluation may determine whether the process is benign or malignant, thereby either obviating the need for or guiding subsequent percutaneous biopsy.

The advent of CT in the mid-1970s virtually revolutionized the practice of roentgenology. The technique utilizes a special gantry and finely collimated x-ray beams, which "slice" the patient, usually in the transaxial plane, allowing for tomographic reconstruction of each discrete slice so the cross-sectional anatomy at that level can be evaluated. Although computer reformations of several contiguous transaxial tomograms can be used to create coronal, sagittal, or oblique plane images, the results are usually disappointing in that considerable image degradation occurs. Direct sagittal and coronal plane imaging can be performed without this loss of resolution but requires often cumbersome patient positioning.

CT patterns of metastases are similar to those demonstrated by plain film roentgenography since both techniques depend on the interaction of x-rays with body tissues to produce an image. However, in addition to documenting the presence of suspected metastases and confirming the osteolytic or osteoblastic nature of the lesions, both CT and MRI may be useful in evaluating the medullary and extraosseous extent of the neoplasm.[10,11,15,28] A suspected early metastatic focus that is not visualized by conventional roentgenography may be confirmed by CT with special contrast adjustments on the computer image display to favor higher-density structures (such as bone and calcification) at the expense of the lower-density soft tissues. These "bone window" settings are used to demonstrate subtle osseous destruction, sclerosis, or focal increased medullary density (Figs. 3-2, *F*, and 3-5, *C*). Most metastatic deposits in the skeleton are intramedullary. Normal intramedullary CT density in the diaphyseal and metaphyseal regions of the appendicular skeleton is generally less than that in adjacent muscle because of the presence of marrow fat. Most cases of intramedullary tumor produce increased density on CT scans (Fig. 3-5, *C*).

In the evaluation of long bones for metastatic involvement, comparison with the density of the contralateral marrow space is useful. Careful positioning of the patient for comparison of CT density is important. CT density can be quantified in Hounsfield units (H).

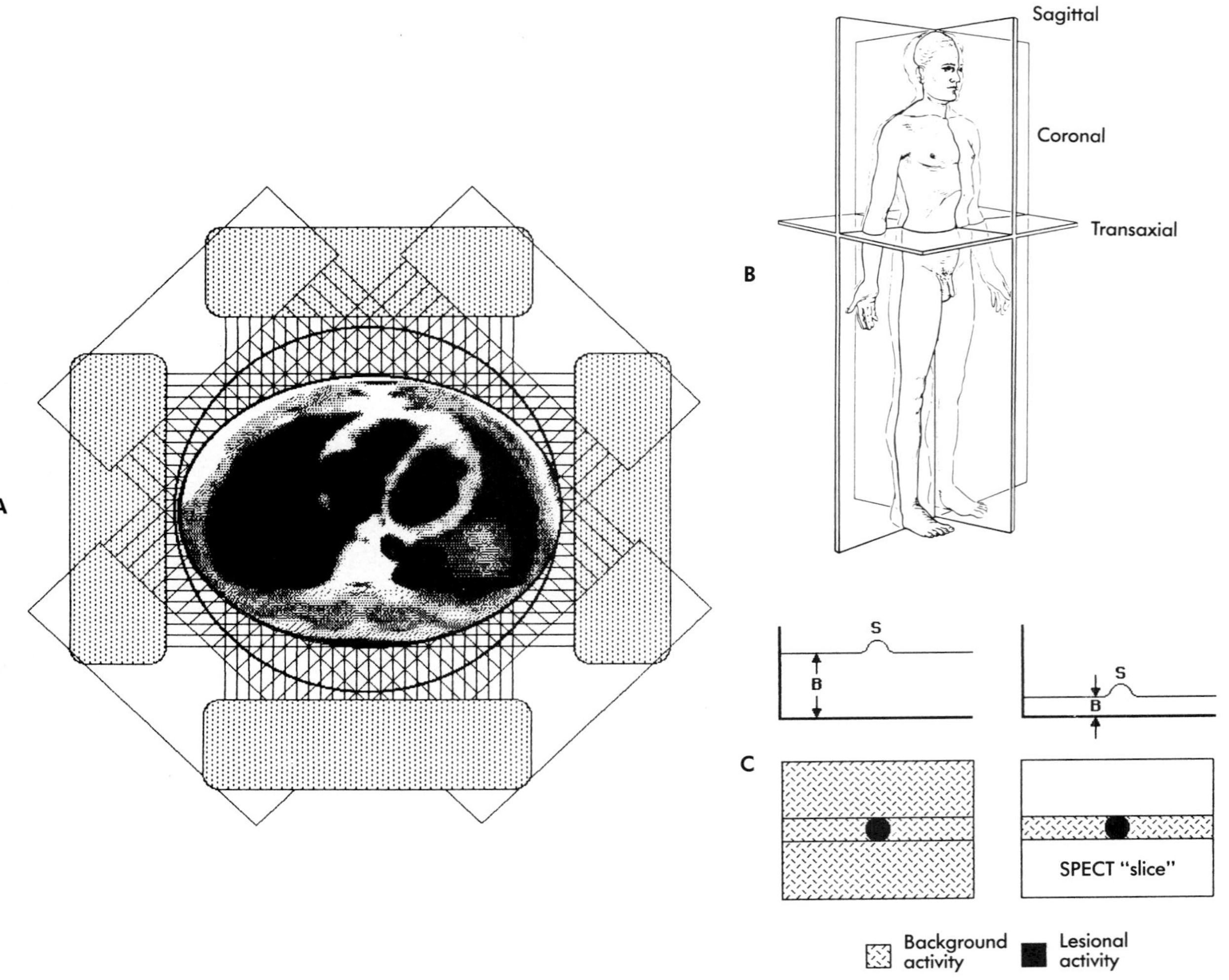

FIGURE 3-3 Single photon emission computed tomography (SPECT). **A,** The gamma camera detector rotates around the patient, acquiring multiple images at fixed angular intervals. **B,** Computer processing of the raw data allows for construction of tomographic slices into multiple planes through the body region of interest. **C,** Contrast resolution, depicted as signal-to-background (S/B), is clearly improved with computed tomographic imaging *(right)* as compared to standard planar imaging *(left)*.

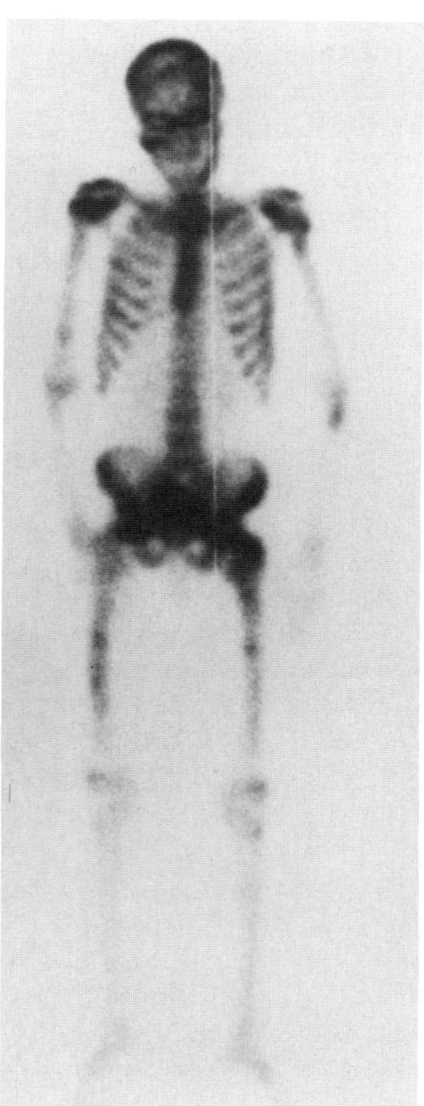

FIGURE 3-4 Prostatic carcinoma. An anterior whole body radionuclide image demonstrates the evolving "superscan" pattern of diffusely increased tracer labeling. In this case ribs, spine, and pelvis have become diffusely infiltrated by metastatic deposits. Only the appendicular skeleton contains multiple focal abnormalities; the more distal long bones are spared. In an older patient, as more disseminated disease involves the entire skeleton, the scan may be falsely interpreted as normal if subtle findings (e.g., decreased or absent renal activity and unusually well defined osseous structures) are not appreciated.

Although a difference of 20 H or greater in intramedullary density between limbs is abnormal, it is not specific for metastatic disease and can be caused by infection, hemorrhage, or radiation.[15]

Skeletal metastases are sometimes detected incidentally during the performance of a CT examination for another clinical problem. Bone metastases and other skeletal lesions may be overlooked if bone window images are not routinely reviewed.

CT is also well-suited to providing guidance for biopsy, the optimal surgical approach, or the design of radiation therapy ports. It is useful postoperatively as a baseline for later comparison if recurrence is suspected, or to monitor the response of tumor mass to therapy if local recurrence is a possibility. CT imaging may be hampered in this regard by the artifacts of metallic surgical clips, fixation apparatus, or prosthetic devices in the area of interest (Fig. 3-6).

MRI has become a commercially available imaging modality in the 1980s. Based on the well-known physicochemical principles of nuclear magnetic resonance (NMR), it requires high strength and high uniformity of magnetic fields to "align" the magnetic moments of the nuclei making up the tissue exposed to this external magnetic field. A radiofrequency (RF) signal is subsequently applied at 90 degrees to the external magnetic field and at the proper frequency to reorient the nuclear magnetic moments perpendicular to the magnetic field. After the RF signal is terminated, the nuclear magnetic moments gradually realign themselves with the external magnetic field. The rate of decay of perpendicular alignment (secondary to the perpendicular RF pulse) and the rate of growth of realignment to the external magnetic field (after termination of the RF signal) are tissue-specific parameters known as T2 and T1 respectively. The appearance of the computer-generated images can be varied by varying the repetition time (TR) of (i.e., the rate), or the interval between (TE), successive RF pulses.[29] Generally signal intensity increases with increasing concentration of "free" or mobile hydrogen nuclei (protons). Thus fluid and fatty tissue would produce high signal intensity whereas cortical bone would produce virtually no signal or MR images.

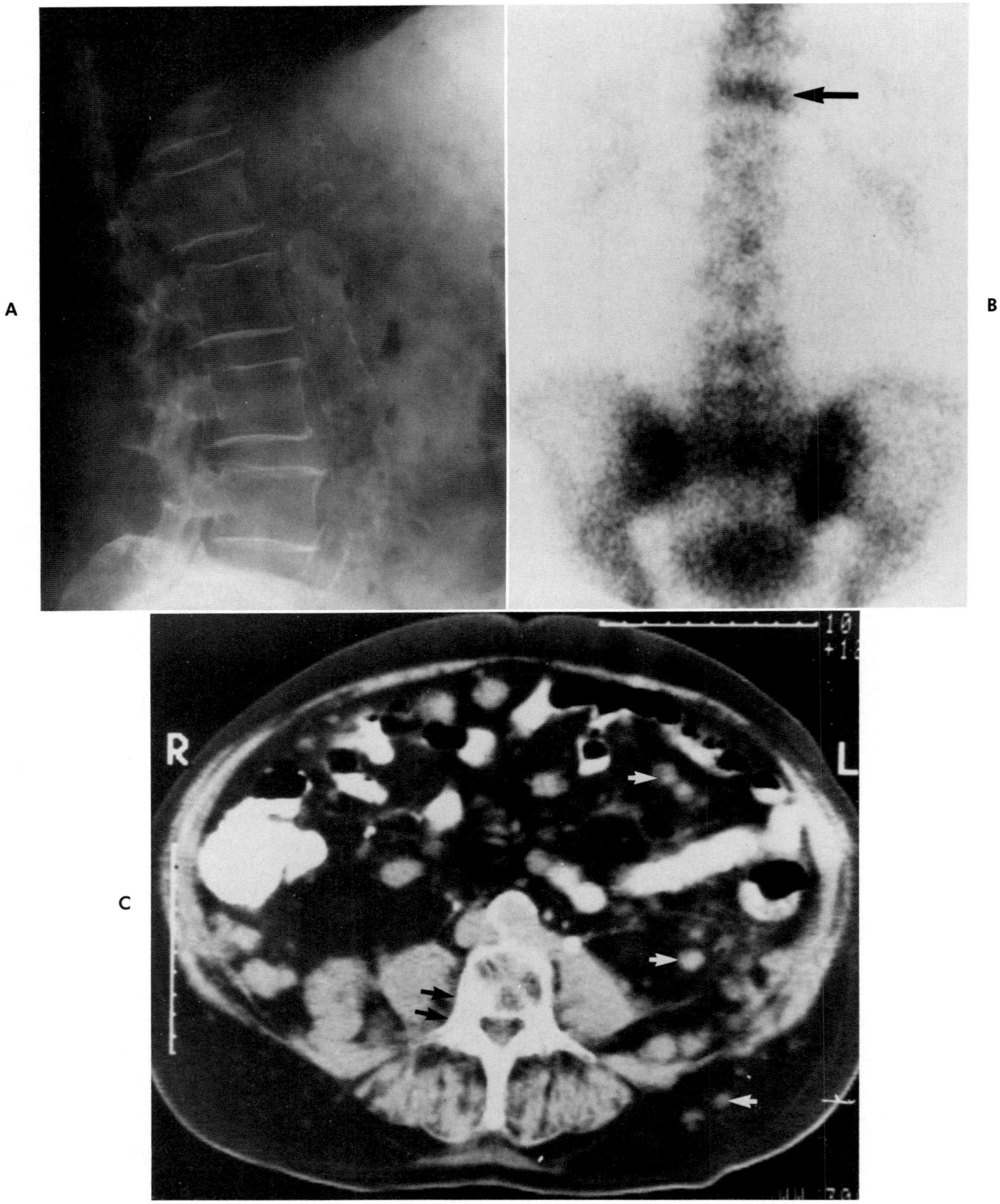

FIGURE 3-5 Lymphoma. **A,** A lateral roentgenogram of the thoracolumbar spine reveals generalized osteopenia with a compression fracture of T12. There is no evidence of any focal bone marrow abnormality. **B,** A posterior planar scintiphotograph shows abnormal tracer labeling *(arrow)* at the T12 level, consistent with a compression fracture. **C,** An axial CT scan through the L4 vertebral body demonstrates sclerosis of the right L4 pedicle and nonhomogeneity of the marrow space of L4 *(black arrows),* consistent with marrow involvement by lymphoma. Multiple mesenteric and subcutaneous lymph nodes can be seen *(white arrows).*

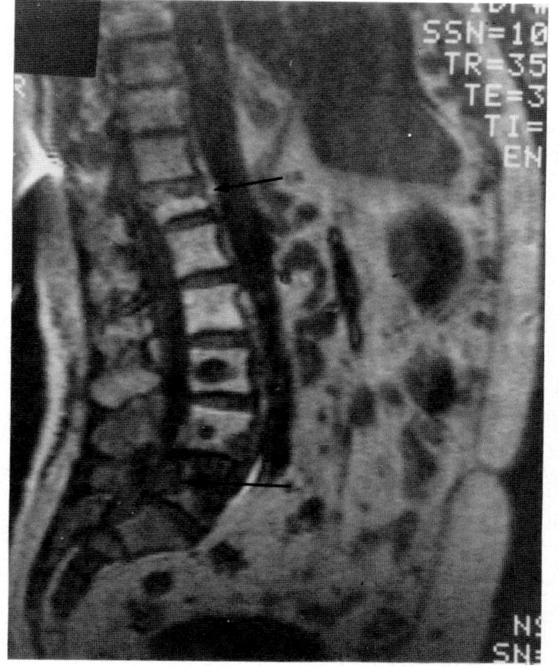

D

FIGURE 3-5 cont'd. **D,** A sagittal body coil short-TR magnetic resonance image from T9 through the sacrum shows focal areas of low signal intensity involving the marrow spaces of T12, L3 to L5, and the sacrum due to lymphoma. There is a pathological fracture of T12 *(short arrow)* with a posteriorly displaced fragment impinging on the conus of the spinal cord. High signal intensity occurs posterior to L4 through S1 *(long arrow)*, representing epidural tumor. On short-TR images the theca is normally of homogeneous low signal intensity. CT would have required intrathecal injection of metrizamide contrast medium to disclose this abnormality.

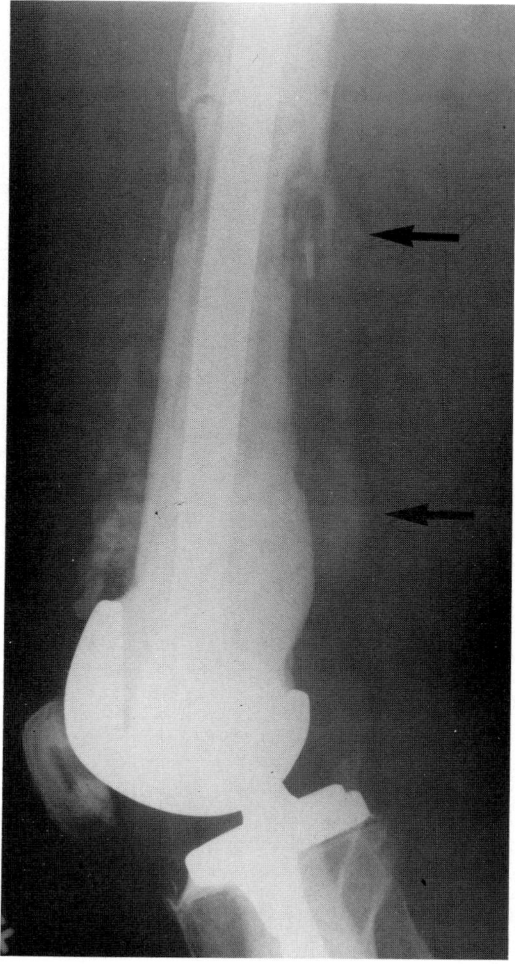

A

FIGURE 3-6 Recurrent osteogenic sarcoma. **A,** A lateral roentgenogram of the distal femur with a total knee prosthesis shows heterotopic calcification and two calcified soft tissue masses *(arrows)* originating from the posterior femoral metaphysis and distal diaphysis and indicating a possible recurrent tumor.

Continued.

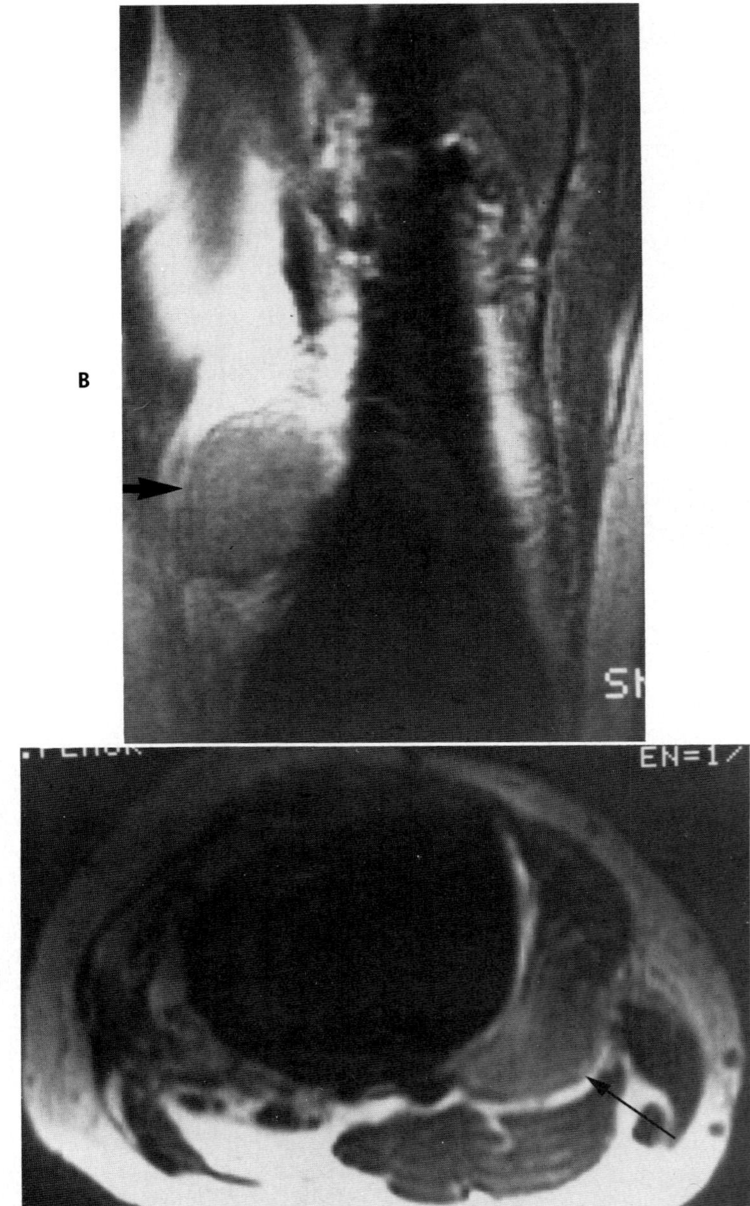

FIGURE 3-6, cont'd. **B,** MRI was performed next, since the metallic prosthesis would have produced significant artifacts on CT. A coronal short-TR (short repetition time) image demonstrates a mass of intermediate signal intensity *(arrow)* contiguous with the medial femoral metaphysis, which would be compatible with a recurrent osteogenic sarcoma. Because of the prosthesis, the femoral diaphysis and metaphysis have a decreased signal intensity with minimum peripheral field distortion artifact. **C,** A transaxial short-TR magnetic resonance image through the proximal femur reveals an area of higher signal intensity *(arrow)* than is seen through muscle, representing recurrent osteogenic sarcoma. This abnormal tissue has invaded the vastus medialis and extended into the sartorius.

The clinical applications of MRI are similar to those of CT and include confirmation of suspected metastatic bone lesions, setting of guidelines for surgery, and radiation therapy port planning. MR-directed biopsy is also possible, but currently this procedure is more readily performed with CT guidance. MRI is quite well suited for examination of the skeletal system. Image contrast varies with the strength of the magnetic field and the pulse sequence employed. Images are usually viewed in at least two planes, with instrument parameters of TR (repetition time) and TE (echo time) varied to provide maximum information about tissue characteristics in the area of abnormality.

The marrow space is the most frequent site of skeletal metastases. The detection of bone marrow abnormalities by MRI is a function of the change in appearance of infiltrated marrow. Normal marrow has high signal intensity in short-TR images (because of its short T1) and lower relative signal intensity in long-TR images. These signal characteristics are felt to be related to the presence of fat in the marrow space (Fig. 3-7).

Most tumors and pathological processes involving the marrow space have low signal intensity in short-TR images. This is the most sensitive sequence for the detection of marrow space disease, because of the marked contrast between the high signal intensity of normal marrow and the lower signal intensity of the infiltrative process (Figs. 3-2, *G* and *H*, and 3-5, *D*). The few exceptions to this pattern include subacute hemorrhage and metastatic melanoma, which produce high signal intensity in short-TR images (Fig. 3-8).

Tumors and other pathological processes have variable intensity in long-TR images. Their signal characteristics with these sequences vary depending on the type of tissue replacing normal marrow. Hemorrhage, necrosis, and inflammatory tissue will have high signal intensity in long-TR images. Fibrous tissue or sclerotic areas will have low signal

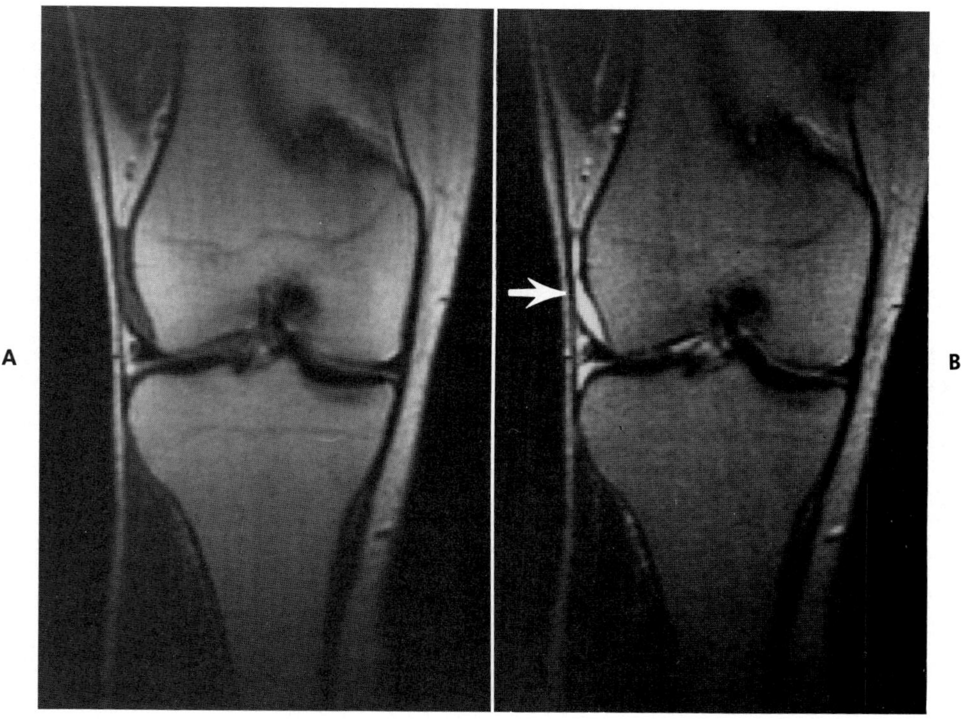

FIGURE 3-7 MRI examination of the knee. **A,** A coronal short–repetition time (short-TR) image through the knee shows homogeneous high signal intensity of normal bone marrow. **B,** A coronal long-TR image shows relatively lower signal intensity of bone marrow. Note the incidental knee effusion *(arrow)*.

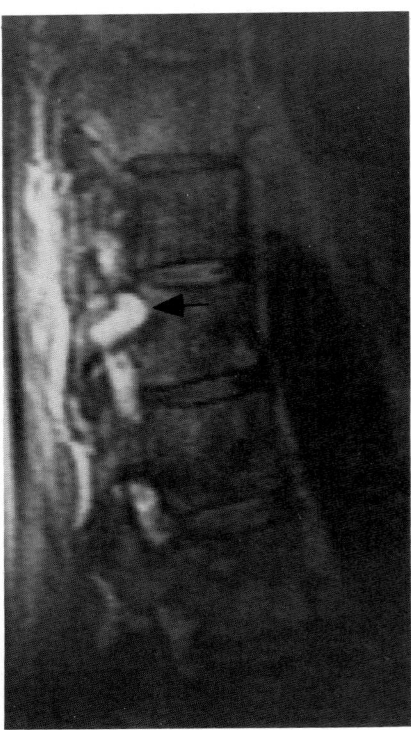

FIGURE 3-8 Prostatic carcinoma. A sagittal surface coil MR image of the thoracolumbar junction demonstrates a generalized low signal intensity of all visualized marrow spaces secondary to metastases. An area of high signal intensity in the left T10 pedicle *(arrow)* represents a hemorrhagic metastatic focus.

intensity in both long- and short-TR images.

MRI is superior to CT and other imaging modalities in demonstrating the presence and extent of tumor in bone marrow and its extraosseous soft tissue extension (Figs. 3-2 and 3-5). Marrow lesions are often not visible on plain roentgenograms and may be subtle on CT. The superiority of MRI is related to the superb contrast between tumor or inflammation and normal bone marrow, muscle, and extraosseous soft tissues.

MRI may be useful in distinguishing the demineralization of osteoporosis from the bone destruction of metastatic disease. Osteoporosis, especially if long-standing, produces multifocal areas of increased signal intensity in short-TR images because of fatty replacement of the affected marrow, rather than the decreased signal characteristics of most pathological tissue in image sequences with short-TR intervals. In a recent study[8] MRI was able to distinguish osteoporosis from multiple myeloma. Thus it may prove to be the preferred modality for evaluating multiple myeloma, which cannot always be differentiated from osteoporosis by CT.

MRI may also be useful in excluding as well as confirming the presence of skeletal metastases when scintigraphy or other diagnostic imaging findings are inconclusive. It has the added advantage of no demonstrable biohazard to patients, in contrast to known small but finite effects of ionizing radiation inherent in both x-ray (including CT) and scintigraphic evaluations.

Because of the lack of mobile protons in compact bone, the cortex has low signal intensity in both short- and long-TR images. Although cortical destruction can be demonstrated in MR images by disruption or attenuation of the cortical line of low signal intensity, CT and plain-film roentgenography are more sensitive in delineating cortical destruction because of their superior spatial resolution in compact bone.[4,30]

MRI is superior to CT in the evaluation of skeletal structures and soft tissues for recurrent tumor in the presence of metal clips, fixation devices, and prostheses. Although some artifacts such as field distortion and signal dropout (signal intensity falls to zero) are caused by these metal appliances, the magnitude of image degradation is much less than that manifested with CT. The only contraindication to MRI is the presence of ferromagnetic material (e.g., aneurysm clips) or a cardiac pacemaker, both of which might be caused to "torque" or move or be functionally altered by the required external magnetic field.

IMAGING ALGORITHM FOR EVALUATION OF SKELETAL METASTASES

The recommended approach to evaluation of the skeleton for possible metastatic disease is summarized in Fig. 3-9. Whole body scintigraphy is the most sensitive and cost-effective screening modality, with SPECT techniques recommended for additional yield in patients whose primary malignancy is known to produce mainly lytic or nonreactive metastases. Correlation of scintigraphic abnormalities or persistent clinical findings with plain roent-

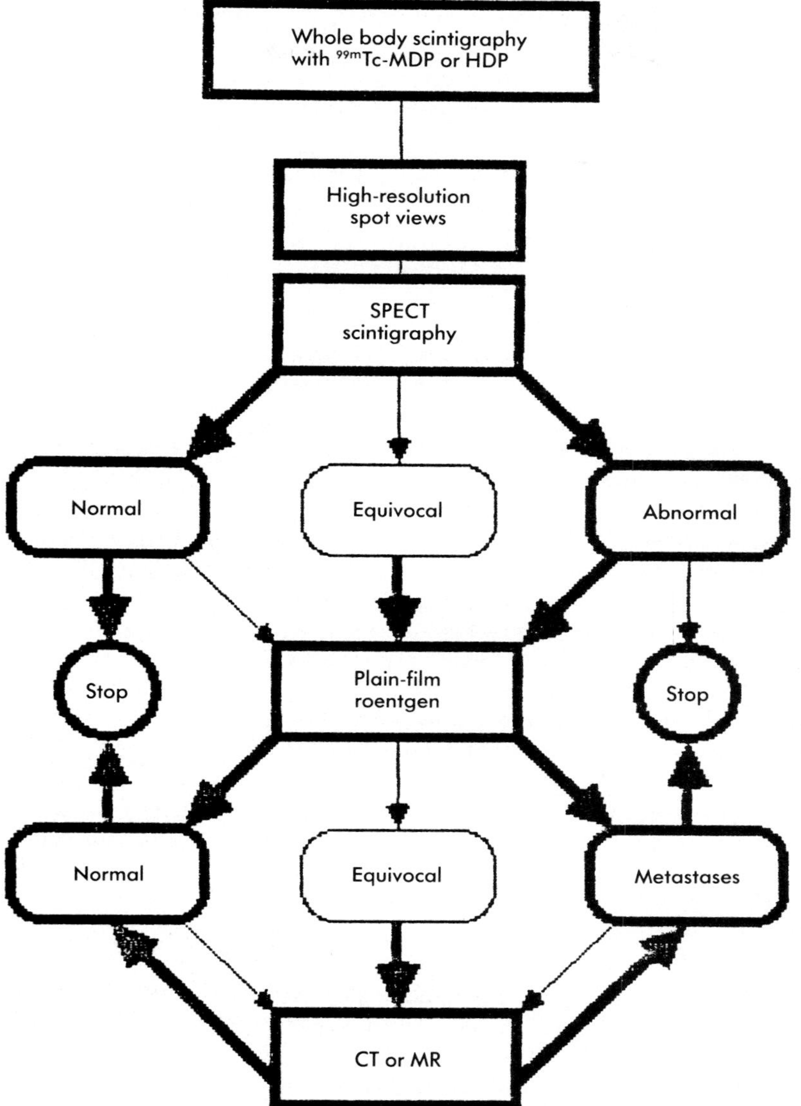

FIGURE 3-9 Diagnostic imaging algorithm. The more common or preferred pathways are in bold. The highly sensitive radionuclide survey is performed initially, allowing the entire skeleton to be evaluated. When state-of-the-art techniques, including SPECT, become widely available, the negative predictive value of scintigraphy will usually be sufficient to allow for termination of the work-up. When clinical signs or symptoms dictate, or when the primary malignancy is known to produce predominantly lytic metastases, negative scintigraphy is followed by a radiographic evaluation. Because of nonspecificity, abnormal or equivocal scintigraphic findings should always be correlated with a roentgenographic evaluation. MRI and CT are reserved for precise regional or directed evaluation, biopsy or surgical guidance, or radiation therapy. MRI and CT are superior for defining extraosseous and soft tissue extension and may provide diagnostic information when scintigraphy and plain roentgenograms are inconclusive. *^{99m}Tc-MDP* and *HDP* are medium-density and high-density technetium-99m planigraphic studies.

genograms is frequently sufficient to confirm or exclude metastatic disease. In patients with multiple myeloma, roentgenographic whole body surveys are usually preferred for initial evaluation because of the generally absent osteoblastic response to myelomatous deposits and the resulting failure of scintigraphy to detect many of these lesions accurately. If evaluation of a single anatomical region is desired and plain film roentgenography is not diagnostic, CT or MRI of the suspicious area may conclusively demonstrate or exclude skeletal metastatic involvement. MRI is more sensitive than CT for determining the extent of marrow and soft tissue involvement whereas CT is better for demonstrating a cortical lesion. MR and CT imaging is usually reserved for more precise regional or directed evaluation, guidance for biopsy or surgery, and/or assistance in planning appropriate radiation therapy when indicated. Occasionally MRI or CT will provide diagnostic information when scintigraphy and plain roentgenography are negative or equivocal in the face of persistent clinical findings. Both modalities are also superior in defining the extraosseous and soft tissue extension of tumor, often essential information for optimal treatment planning.

— REFERENCES

1. Bachman, A.L., and Sproul, E.E.: Correlation of radiographic and autopsy findings and suspected metastases in the spine, Bull. N.Y. Acad. Med. **31:** 146, 1955.
2. Bassett, L.W., et al.: Radionuclide bone imaging, Radiol. Clin. North Am. **19:**675, 1981.
3. Belliveau, R.E., and Spencer, R.P.: Incidence and sites of bone lesions detected by ^{99m}Tc polyphosphate scans in patients with tumors, Cancer **36:**359, 1975.
4. Bloem, J.L., et al.: Magnetic resonance imaging of primary malignant bone tumors, Radiographics **5:** 853, 1985.
5. Brady, L.W., and Croll, H.N.: The role of bone scanning in the cancer patient, Skeletal Radiol. **3:**217, 1979.
6. Citrin, D.L.: The role of the bone scan in the investigation and treatment of breast cancer, C.R.C. Crit. Rev. Diagn. Imaging **13:**39, 1980.
7. Citrin, D.L., et al.: The application of the ^{99m}Tc polyphosphate bone scan to the study of breast cancer, Br. J. Surg. **62:**201, 1975.
8. Daffner, R.H., et al.: MRI in the detection of malignant infiltration of bone marrow, A.J.R. **146:**353, 1986.
9. Donato, A.T., et al.: Bone scanning in the evaluation of patients with lung cancer, Ann. Thorac. Surg. **27:**300, 1979.
10. Genant, H.K., et al.: Computed tomography of the musculoskeletal system, J. Bone Joint Surg. **62A:** 1088, 1980.
11. Genant, H.K., et al.: Advances in computed tomography of the skeletal system, Radiol. Clin. North Am. **19:**645, 1981.
12. Gilday, D.L., et al.: Radionuclide skeletal survey for pediatric neoplasms, Radiology **123:**399, 1977.
13. Harbert, J.C.: Efficacy of bone and liver scanning in malignant disease: facts and opinions. In Freeman, L.M., and Weissmann, H.S., editors: Nuclear medicine annual, New York, 1982, Raven Press.
14. Hartshorne, M.F., et al.: Plasmacytoma of the lumbar spine by SPECT, Clin. Nucl. Med. **11:**65, 1986.
15. Helms, C.A., et al.: Detection of bone marrow metastases using computed tomography, Radiology **140:** 745, 1981.
16. Howman-Giles, R.B., et al.: Radionuclide skeletal survey in neuroblastoma, Radiology **131:**497, 1979.
17. Joo, K.G., et al.: Bone scintigrams: their clinical usefulness in patients with breast carcinoma, Oncology **36:**94, 1979.
18. Kaufman, R.A., et al.: False-negative bone scans in neuroblastoma metastatic to the ends of long bones, A.J.R. **130:**131, 1978.
19. Kirkman, S., and Henk, J.M.: The value of bone scanning in the staging of breast cancer, Clin. Radiol. **30:**11, 1979.
20. Krishnamurthy, G.T., et al.: Distribution pattern of metastatic bone disease. A need for total body skeletal image, J.A.M.A. **237:**2504, 1977.
21. McKillop, J.H., et al.: The prognostic and therapeutic implications of the positive radionuclide bone scan in clinically early breast cancer, Br. J. Surg. **65:**649, 1978.
22. McNeil, B.J.: Rationale for the use of bone scans in selected metastatic primary bone tumors, Semin. Nucl. Med. **8:**336, 1978.
23. O'Mara, R.E.: Bone scanning in osseous metastatic disease, J.A.M.A. **229:**1915, 1974.
24. Parker, B., et al.: Relative efficacy of radiographic and radionuclide bone surveys in detection of skeletal lesions of histiocytosis X, Radiology **134:**377, 1980.
25. Pistenma, D.A., et al.: Screening for bone metastases. Are only scans necessary? J.A.M.A. **231:**46, 1975.
26. Shafer, R.B., and Reinke, D.B.: Contribution of bone scan, serum acid and alkaline phosphatase, and radiographic bone survey to management of newly diagnosed carcinoma of the prostate, Clin. Nucl. Med. **2:**200, 1977.
27. Silberstein, E.B., et al.: Imaging of bone metastases ^{99m}Tc-Sn-EHDP (diphosphonate), F-18, and skeletal radiography, Radiology **107:**551, 1973.
28. Wilson, J.S., et al.: Computed tomography of musculoskeletal disorders, A.J.R. **131:**155, 1978.
29. Young, S.W.: Nuclear magnetic resonance imaging; basic principles, New York, 1984, Raven Press.
30. Zimmer, W.D., et al.: Bone tumors: Magnetic resonance imaging versus computed tomography, Radiology **155:**709, 1985.

CHAPTER 4

CLOSED BIOPSY

Tillman M. Moore

A biopsy is a surgical procedure to obtain tissue for histological diagnosis and can be performed by a variety of open or closed techniques. The term *closed* in this discussion will refer to percutaneous biopsy methods, which are particularly useful in the evaluation of patients with known or suspected metastatic cancer to the musculoskeletal system.

Almost all secondary malignant deposits of orthopaedic significance originate from carcinomas and have a strong predilection for skeletal rather than soft tissues. In view of the large mass of muscle in the body, the rarity of metastatic carcinomatous deposits in the soft tissues has never been adequately explained. Among the primary sarcomas of the musculoskeletal system, Ewing's sarcoma metastasizes frequently from its primary site to other bones or else is multicentric in origin. The same multicentric origin is undoubtedly true of many multiple myelomas, and serum immunoelectrophoresis or hematological bone marrow studies usually make biopsy of an associated bone lesion unnecessary. Carcinoma comprises well over 95% of all cancer, and when metastases are present the skeleton is often involved. It is in this group of patients that by closed biopsy one can obtain crucial information for confirmation of diagnosis, clinical staging, and management. Physicians and other workers responsible for any aspect of care of patients with primary and secondary musculoskeletal cancer should be aware of the advantages of closed biopsy and familiar with the instruments in common use.

HISTORY

The development of closed biopsy began at the turn of this century and has led to numerous techniques with an amazing diversity of equipment. According to Ackermann[1] the first set of bone biopsy instruments was patented by Barret in Great Britain in 1901. The first account of a closed biopsy of bone is probably the marrow aspiration done in 1908 by an Italian, Ghedini.[30] However, Seyfarth[71] in Germany is credited with the first sternal trephine biopsy, in 1923. Although "skinny" needle aspiration biopsy of bone tumors was initially used in the United States in 1936,[79] other authors had reported their experiences with aspiration biopsy techniques from 1930 to 1935.[12,45,48,75] Robertson and Ball[67] were among the first to report on aspiration biopsy of destructive spinal lesions, and Frankel[28] described his technique and experience almost 20 years later. Blady,[5] a radiologist, reported on an x-ray–guided aspiration biopsy in 1939, but it was not until 1970 that Lalli,[46] also a radiologist, introduced the use of an image intensifier for closed biopsy. Early in the decade of the 1940s a vacuum trepan instrument was introduced from Scandinavia by Christiansen,[11] and a trephine was developed in the United States by Turkel and Bethell.[77] Michele[54,55] designed a trephine instrument for biopsy of the vertebral body from a transpedicular approach in 1947, and the same year Frank Ellis[23] related his experiences with needle biopsy in Britain. Ray[66] modified the Valls angled guide for direct lumbar spine biopsies by aspiration in 1953, and Ackermann[1] designed a new trephine instrument and described his technique for vertebral biopsy 3 years later. He then summarized his experiences[2] in 635 cases in 1963. Two years after that Craig[14] reported on the use of a trephine set and in 1970 summarized his experience.[15] Ellis et al.[24] related their technique involving 1445 modified Silverman needle biopsies of bone and marrow in 1964. Deeley,[18] writing in Britain in 1972, reported on his drill biopsy technique for bone and 2 years later[19] authored a book reviewing biopsy instruments and techniques. De Santos and two groups of co-workers[20,21] related their experience at M.D. Anderson Hospital with closed biopsy in bone tumor patients, and in the same year (1979) I reported[56] on 500 closed biopsies of various musculoskeletal bone and soft tissue lesions from the Los Angeles County–University of Southern California Medical Center. By this time image intensifiers were in common use, representing a major advance over conventional roentgenographic and standard fluoroscopic techniques. The two decades from the mid-1960s to the mid-1980s have witnessed increasing interest and participation in bone biopsies by radiologists.*

TERMINOLOGY

The nomenclature of closed biopsy is confusing for several reasons. Authors have invented new terms or used imprecise or double names for their techniques or equipment. In fact, only two categories of closed biopsy exist: aspiration and core. Aspiration biopsy provides material that is most appropriately examined by cytological techniques; core biopsy provides material most appropriate for routine paraffin block processing. That aspiration biopsy will often obtain a small core of intact tissue and core biopsy will occasionally provide material for supplemental cytological examination should not interfere with precise nomenclature. Terms such as punch,[41] puncture,[48,68,69] drill,[7,19] trephine† and needle‡ serve only to complicate both the concept and the nomenclature of closed biopsy. In the interest of clarity, *needle* should be used for techniques utilizing needles (16 to 22 gauge) as the primary implement. All other techniques should then be designated *core,* regardless of the specific large-bore equipment utilized.

INDICATIONS FOR CLOSED BIOPSY

There are five general situations in which the question of possible musculoskeletal metastases is best resolved by closed biopsy. The *first* involves patients with a known primary malignancy who are also found to have a musculoskeletal lesion during initial diagnosis and staging. Exact identification of any suspected metastasis is crucial for correct staging and may influence management of the primary tumor, particularly if radical surgery is being considered. The *second* involves patients with known carcinoma who have been or are being treated and in whom a new bone or soft tissue lesion is found. This suggests treatment failure of the primary tumor if the patient was accurately staged at diagnosis. The implications are serious and may require change or reinstitution of chemotherapy or hormonal programs in addition to local treatment of the suspected metastasis. However, if some time has elapsed since diagnosis and treatment, it must be remembered that patients with one malignancy are at increased risk of a second primary tumor. The possibility of a radiation-induced sarcoma must be considered also. Moreover, the existence of a malignancy is no assurance that infectious, metabolic, traumatic, or degenerative musculoskeletal lesions will not occur, and these possibilities must be considered in differential diagnosis. The *third* involves patients who present with multiple skeletal lesions from an undiagnosed primary tumor (Fig. 4-1). If the primary tumor is not easily diagnosed by simple and inexpensive screening tests, biopsy must be considered to be the next, and often the most cost-effective, diagnostic procedure. The *fourth* category involves a small group of patients with known skeletal metastases already treated systemically and locally but in whom the response of the lesions is unclear. Biopsy is the only way to resolve the question immediately. A *fifth* category includes patients with localizable bone pain and in whom an isotopic bone scan shows one or more bony lesions.

Bone scan often shows an abnormality earlier

---

*References 3, 4, 13, 16, 17, 20, 21, 22, 32, 34, 35, 37, 38, 40, 46, 57, 65, 76.

†References 1, 2, 16, 17, 64, 72.

‡References 16, 17, 41, 44, 51, 66.

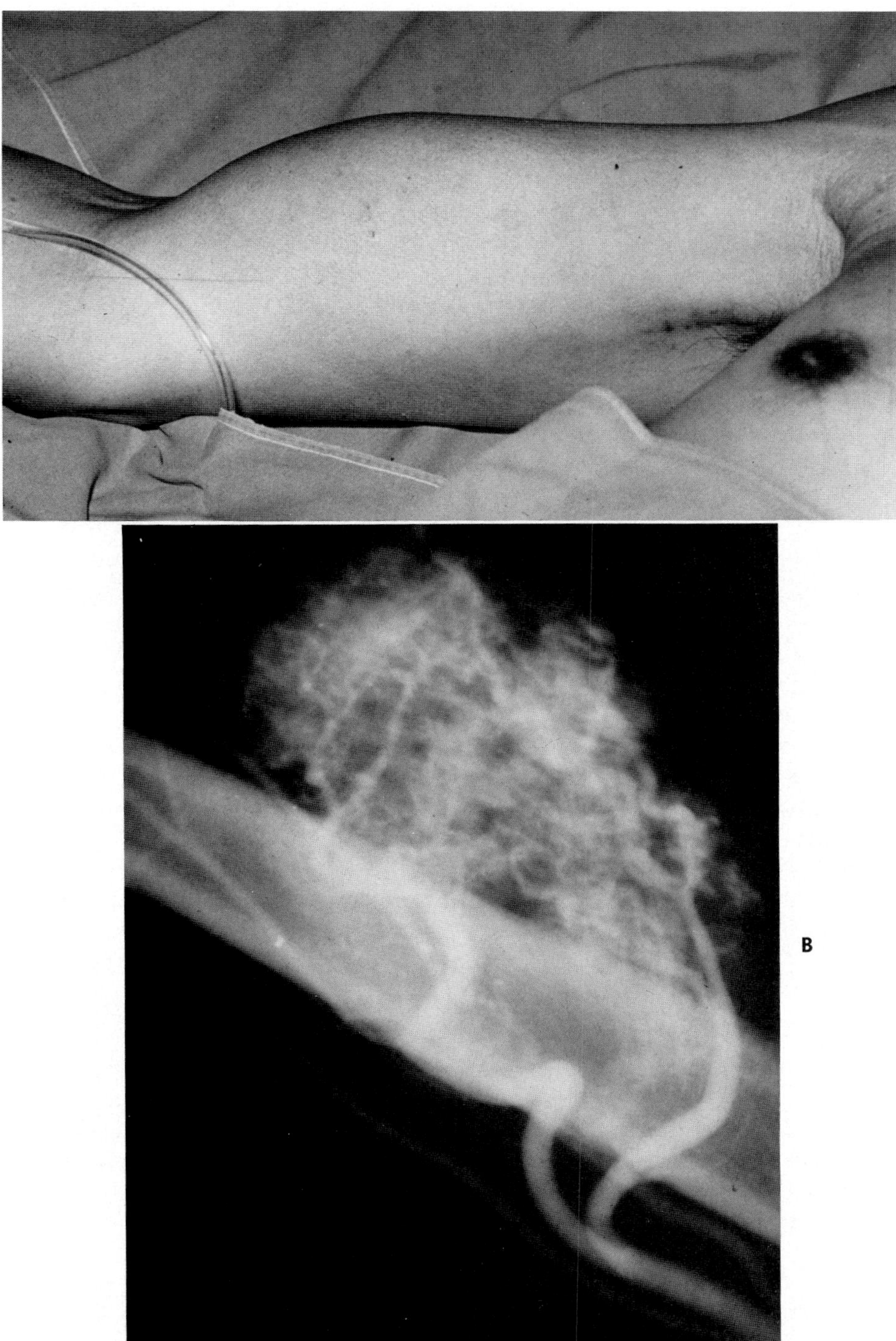

FIGURE 4-1 **A,** Right forearm of a patient with a slowly growing pulsatile mass in the right biceps present for 17 months. **B,** A brachial arteriogram demonstrated the mass to be quite vascular with abundant feeding vessels. A Travenol Tru-Cut biopsy through the long axis of the mass revealed a clear cell lesion histologically suggestive of renal carcinoma. Bleeding was controlled by elevation and local pressure.

Continued.

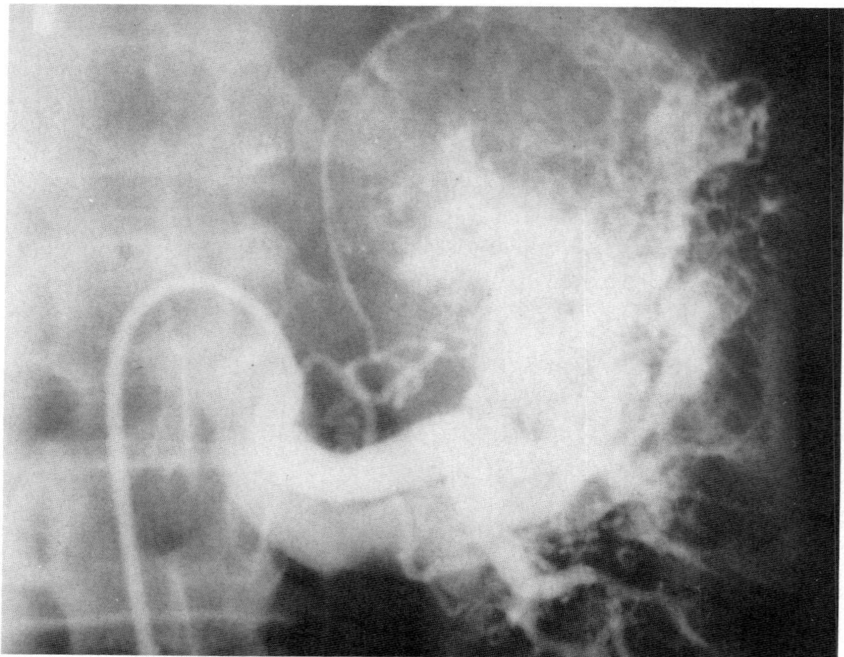

FIGURE 4-1, cont'd. **C,** A renal arteriogram subsequently revealed the primary tumor.

than plain roentgenograms do. Closed biopsy of a suspicious lesion noted by bone scan may be quite difficult if the lesion is not roentgenographically apparent (Fig. 4-2). In one comparative study,[13] however, successful biopsy was accomplished almost as often with radioisotopically located as with roentgenographically apparent lesions.

ADVANTAGES AND DISADVANTAGES OF CLOSED BIOPSY

For lesions of the musculoskeletal system there are many advantages of closed over open biopsy. With closed biopsy, local anesthesia generally is adequate unless the patient is uncooperative.* However, when infection is present, it may be difficult to obtain adequate anesthesia by local infiltration.[15] In most instances only closed biopsies of the thoracic spine or an occasional cervical biopsy from a transoral approach will require general endotracheal anesthesia.† In addition to this lowered anesthesia risk, closed biopsy techniques are preferable to open biopsy because there is less blood loss along with lessened time expenditure by the patient and doctor and a lessening of the risks of infection and wound healing problems. Chemotherapy and radiotherapy can be initiated much sooner after closed than after open biopsy. Reduced tumor contamination of surrounding tissues occurs with closed as compared to open biopsy, although that is not as important in metastatic disease as in primary tumors. From an economic viewpoint, then, improved medical resource utilization and lowered medical costs should result from closed biopsy in almost all circumstances.

The main disadvantage of closed biopsy is the small size of the tissue specimen obtained for study. The pathologist must be both competent and confident that an accurate histological diagnosis can be made from minute tissue samples. Slides of the primary tumor or of previous biopsies should be available for review. The pathologist must be aware of the clinical condition of the patient and have access to all roentgenograms, particularly those taken at the time of biopsy.

*References 1, 3, 14, 15, 20, 21, 31, 34, 56, 70.
†References 8, 26, 62, 63, 79.

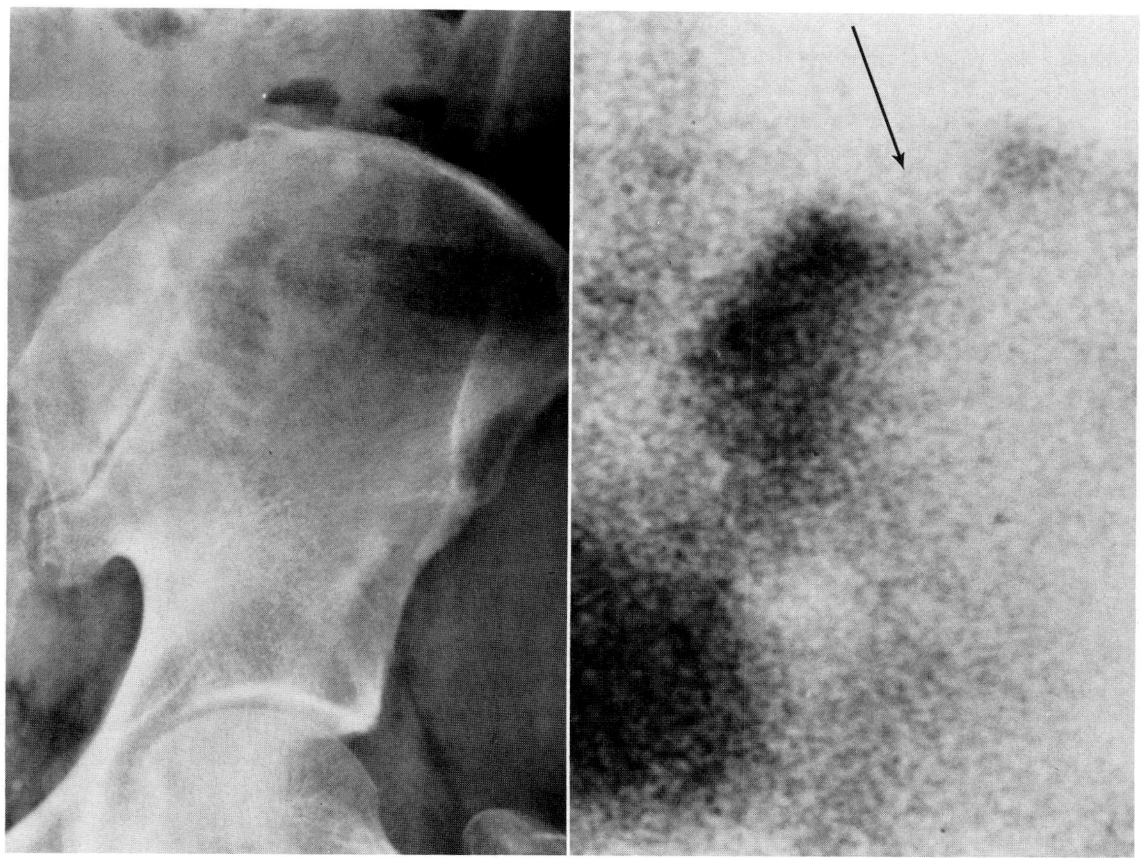

FIGURE 4-2 **A,** AP roentgenogram of a patient with known carcinoma of the pancreas and recurrent cholangitis who complained of pain and tenderness in the left iliac crest. Blastic changes were noted adjacent to the sacroiliac joint but no abnormalities in the region of tenderness. **B,** A technetium-99 scan revealed an area of decreased isotope concentration in the iliac crest *(arrow)*. This tissue was biopsied, and three Jamashidi cores revealed bone necrosis and adenocarcinoma. No organisms were cultured from the biopsy specimen.

Closed biopsy, like open biopsy, is not always successful. Sampling errors are still reported in recent series.[5,16,17,34] Closed biopsy is inexact even when roentgenographically controlled, and exact placement of the biopsy instrument does not always occur. Some lesions will be missed, and only reactive or normal tissue biopsied. This problem can be largely avoided by taking multiple tissue samples at each procedure and by obtaining a frozen section examination of the first or subsequent samples if necessary. The pathologist may make "touch" preparation slides if the tissue cannot be sectioned at the time of biopsy, smearing the surface of even a calcified specimen on a glass slide and examining that smear microscopically. If this produces cytological evidence of malignant cells, further diagnostic studies can proceed while more definitive histological evaluation awaits decalcification of the solid specimen. The pathologist may also wish to fix a portion of the biopsy material in glutaraldehyde should electron microscopic diagnosis be necessary in an unusual and complicated diagnostic problem.

When representative tissue is not obtained at biopsy or representative tissue is obtained but cannot be diagnosed by the pathologist, the closed biopsy must be considered a failure. In this event, further biopsy is mandatory and the patient must be so advised. If indications were originally present for biopsy, then failure of closed biopsy does not alter those indications and rebiopsy or open biopsy is appropriate. Weakening of bone by the biopsy, with the risk of consequent pathological fracture, has been considered a potential disadvantage of closed biopsy techniques by some clinicians. However, for a lesion to have been appreciable roentgenographically and thus accessible to biopsy, between 30% and 50% of the cortical matrix must have been destroyed and the risk of a latent pathological fracture must already exist. From a biomechanical viewpoint, even a small defect in the cortex of a long bone diminishes its resistance to torque by about 50%.[10,29,64] Moreover, one would anticipate that open bone biopsy would increase the risk of fracture because of the necessity of soft tissue stripping in addition to violation of the cortex. In fact, it is unlikely that any small biopsy, whether open or closed, significantly increases the risk of fracture in a bone already affected by lytic metastases. Open biopsy has been favored sometimes because the surgeon can select an unmineralized portion of the tumor for frozen section diagnosis and routine tissue processing without decalcification. If mineralized bone cores are obtained at closed biopsy, standard decalcification techniques result in delayed tissue processing. However, with a rapid decalcification process[3,4,43,56] bone tissue can be fully decalcified in a few hours instead of days or weeks and the material made available for pathological interpretation the following day, just as with soft tissue biopsy. This technique requires a knowledgeable and cooperative pathologist, because the biopsy material must be evaluated frequently during the rapid decalcification process. Excessive decalcification will produce cellular distortion, or "burning" of tissue, and the process must be terminated as soon as decalcification is complete.

CONTRAINDICATIONS TO CLOSED BIOPSY

There are only three contraindications to closed musculoskeletal biopsy, all of which are relative: the condition of the skin, a bleeding diathesis, and the requirement for open surgery.

The *condition of the skin* in the area of the contemplated biopsy is the first concern. Chronic draining sinuses and skin ulceration or cellulitis obviously are associated with the risk of implanting potentially infectious material into a bone lesion. This has not occurred in my experience and to my knowledge has not been reported, but it could theoretically cause a serious osteomyelitis. More subtly, the relative immune incompetence existing in many cancer patients, particularly if associated with bone marrow replacement by tumor or bone marrow depression from chemotherapy, predisposes to infection following biopsy. Such factors should be corrected, or at least improved as much as possible, prior to biopsy or a more appropriate biopsy site should be sought.

Any *bleeding diathesis* is of concern when closed biopsy is being considered, for hemorrhage can occasionally be a problem.[70] Many metastatic lesions are sufficiently hypervascular to be of concern even when hemostatic function is normal. Liver disease or infiltration by metastases may lower prothrombin levels, and bone marrow replacement or chemotherapeutic depression may impair platelet production or function. A rare paraneoplastic syndrome seen with lung and prostatic cancers[33] can also cause fibrinolysis. Closed biopsy must be approached cautiously unless these clotting deficiencies can be improved, and hematological evaluation should be obtained prior to biopsy if the procedure is imperative.

The third potential contraindication to closed biopsy exists when an *open surgical operation* will be required for treatment. For example, a frank or latent subtrochanteric pathological fracture of the femur in a patient with known carcinoma of the breast does not require closed biopsy under ordinary circumstances. Instead, the patient should be evaluated and prepared for surgery and a frozen section diagnosis accomplished by open biopsy. In the rare situation when a patient's medical condition will not allow surgery, a patient refuses operation, or a complicated procedure requires extensive planning or preoperative treatment such as embolization,[39] a preliminary closed biopsy still may be appropriate. Occasionally, when it can be anticipated that neither aspiration nor core biopsy will obtain sufficient tissue for special studies (e.g., estrogen receptors, lymphoma typing, immunoperoxidase determinations), open biopsy still is preferable.

PATIENT EVALUATION

From the previous discussion of clinical findings and indications it is apparent that both the patient's clinical condition and the information already available from laboratory, roentgenographic, and isotope studies must be carefully evaluated so one can be certain that closed biopsy is, in fact, necessary and the technique probably will be successful and uncomplicated. A specific history, physical examination, and review of laboratory studies will help to avoid or at least identify infection or bleeding problems. In the history the chronic use of aspirin or nonsteroidal anti-inflammatory medications should be noted because of their interference with hemostasis. A history of bruises, melena, menorrhagia, epistaxis, or hematuria suggests a latent or actual clotting problem. Allergies or an idiosyncratic reaction to local anesthetic agents must also be noted and provision made to manage any untoward event associated with their use. Physical examination should include evaluation for icterus, ecchymoses, or an enlarged liver. The biopsy site should be inspected for assurance that no local infectious process exists. If a significant soft tissue mass is noted, closed biopsy will likely be easier and as successful as biopsy of a skeletal lesion. Regional lympadenopathy may also suggest lymph node biopsy along with, or instead of, bone biopsy.

If the history and physical examination do not suggest a clotting deficit, biopsy is probably safe; but if the lesion is lytic, near major structures, or in the spinal column, screening clotting studies are essential. These include a smear for platelet estimation and a prothrombin or partial thromboplastin time. Depending on the clinical evaluation, a unit or two of whole blood can be ordered on a type-and-hold basis. If several skeletal lesions are shown on plain films or isotopic whole body bone scans, the most accessible lesion will generally be the safest. For example, a greater trochanteric or proximal humeral lesion would be preferred to a thoracic spinal or cranial location. Computed tomographic (CT) studies rarely are necessary for routine closed skeletal biopsies but have been reported to be helpful on occasion,[38] particularly if the regional anatomy is in question.

ARRANGEMENTS FOR BIOPSY

Specific tissue processing and preparation for frozen section diagnosis are the responsibility of the pathologist, who must be involved in biopsy planning and aware of clinical and roentgenographic findings. The pathologist should also be aware of radiotherapy and chemotherapy treatment, which may influence histological interpretation.

Almost all closed biopsies of skeletal lesions can be done with standard biplanar roentgenograms or with an image intensifier. Lesions that are difficult to visualize on plain films often are even more difficult to see on fluoroscopic image intensification. For any lesion in a dangerous anatomical location (e.g., the posterior aspect of a cervical vertebra, the anterior aspect of a lumbar vertebra, any part of the thoracic spine) or in a location invariably difficult to visualize on image intensifier (the ala of the sacrum), a CT-guided biopsy is preferable (Fig. 4-3). A discussion with the radiologist will be necessary to schedule the biopsy and decide who will actually perform it. As pointed out in the previous discussion, radiologists have become more interested in musculoskeletal biopsy and many recently trained radiologists are experienced and comfortable with closed biopsy techniques for several organ systems, including the musculoskeletal system. It has been stated that the radiologist can help decide which portion of a lesion should be submitted for biopsy to avoid necrotic tissue[32,35]; however, ordinarily it is easy to ensure that viable tissue has been obtained if multiple cores are taken and frozen section microscopy is used immediately. A surgical suite setting is not necessary for routine closed biopsy,[50,56,76] and standard resuscitative equipment available in any radiology department is adequate for untoward reactions to premedication or local anesthesia.

ANESTHESIA OPTIONS AND INDICATIONS

Aspiration biopsies do not always require premedication or local anesthesia,[4,22,40] but local infiltration anesthesia is helpful for aspiration

Text continued on p. 65.

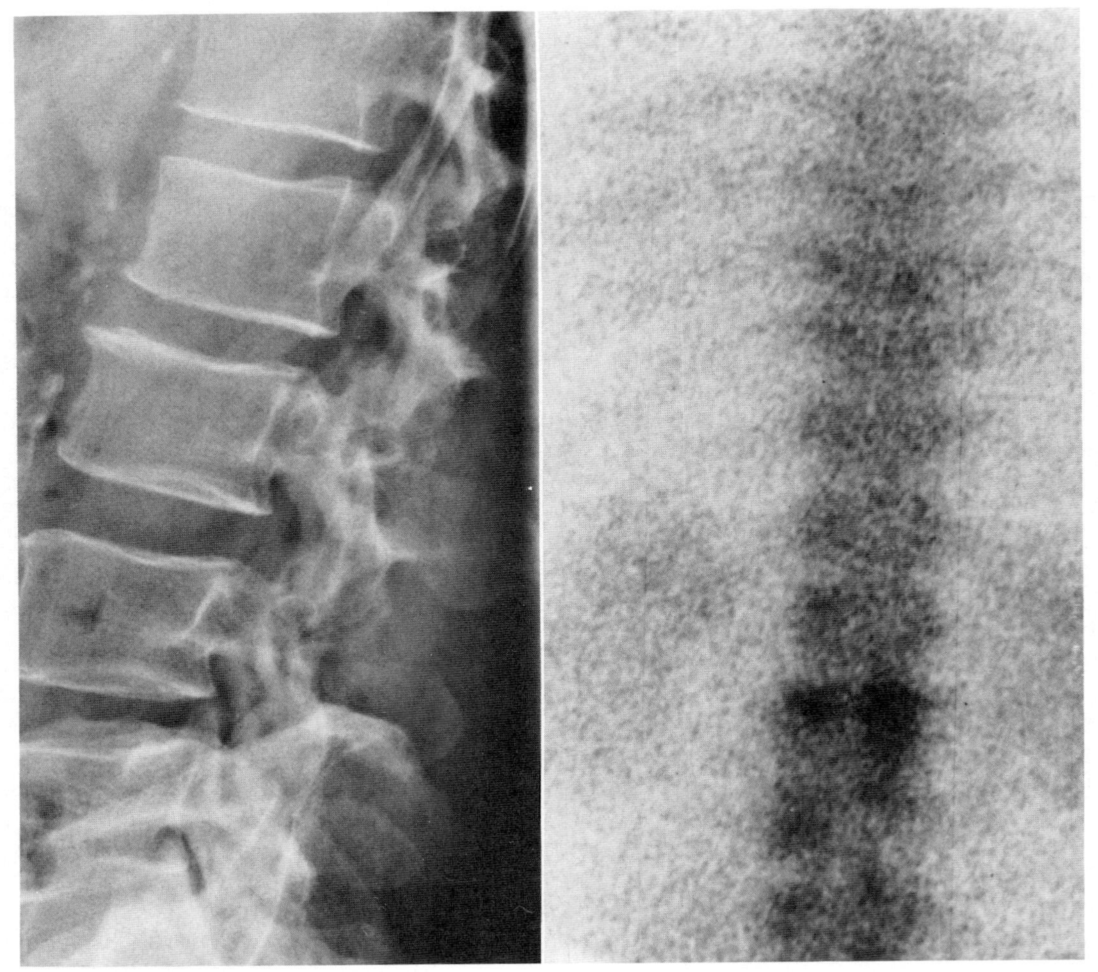

FIGURE 4-3 A patient with known breast carcinoma experienced mild lumbar pain, but the roentgenogram of her spine, **A,** showed no abnormalities. A technetium-99 scan, **B,** however, revealed markedly increased uptake in the L2 vertebral body. Then, 6 weeks after the isotope scan, her pain increased.

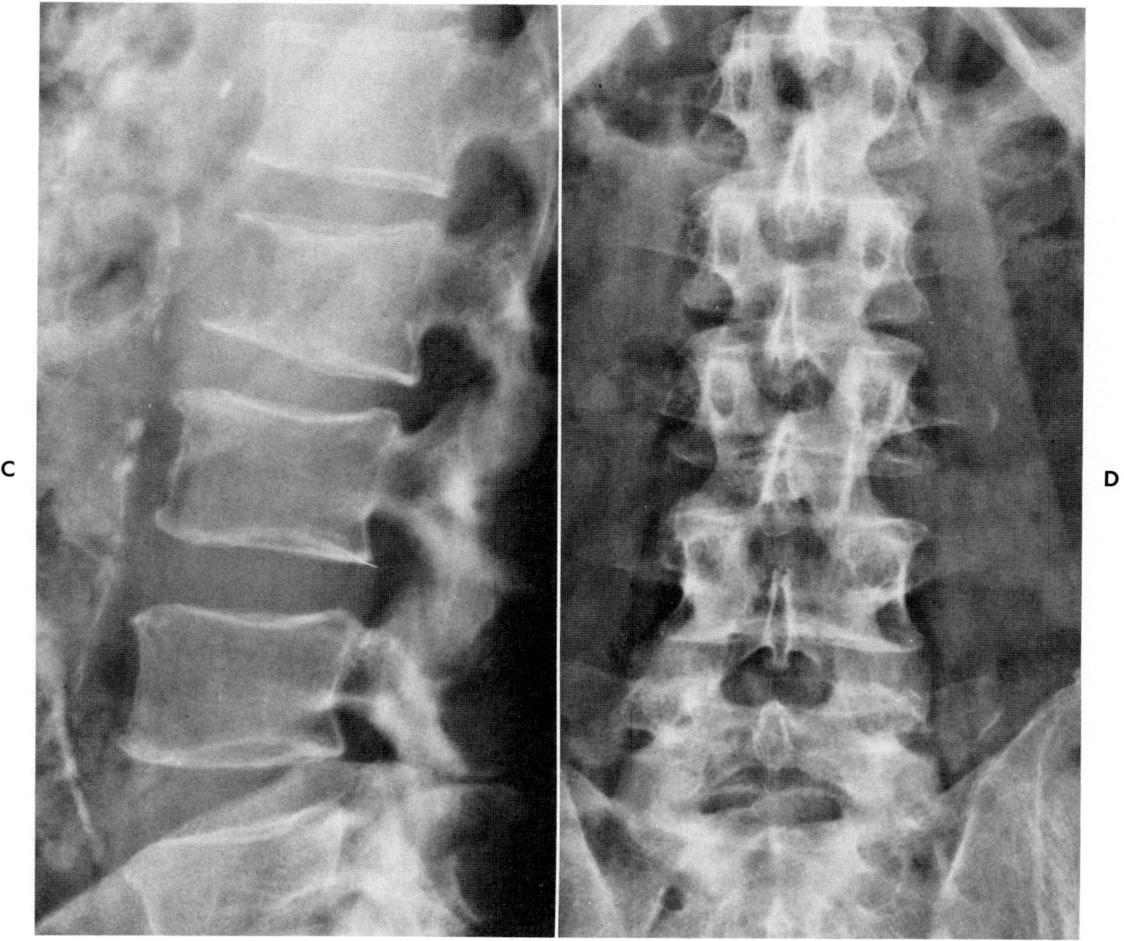

FIGURE 4-3, cont'd. Spinal roentgenograms, **C** and **D,** now revealed evidence of wedging of the L2 vertebral body and an obvious lytic lesion in the anterior vertebrae.

Continued.

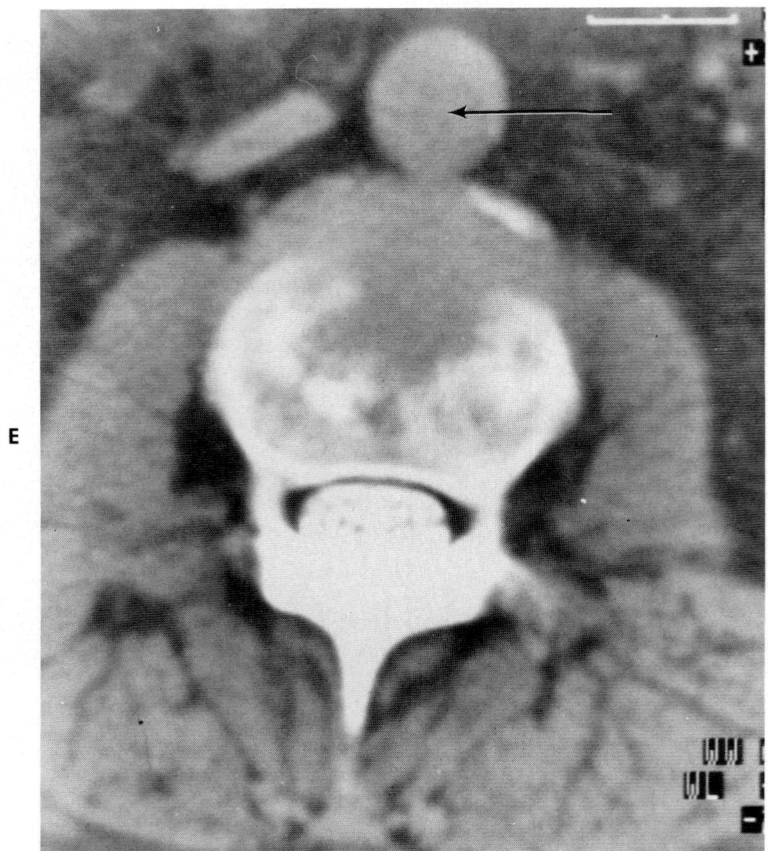

E

FIGURE 4-3, cont'd. A CT scan enhanced by metrizamide, **E,** confirmed the location of the lesion and defined the extent of a paravertebral soft tissue mass near the aorta *(arrow)*. Because of the proximity of the tumor mass to the aorta, it was felt that a CT-guided biopsy with a Craig trocar (Figs. 4-5 and 4-6) would be safer than to attempt the biopsy under image intensifier control.

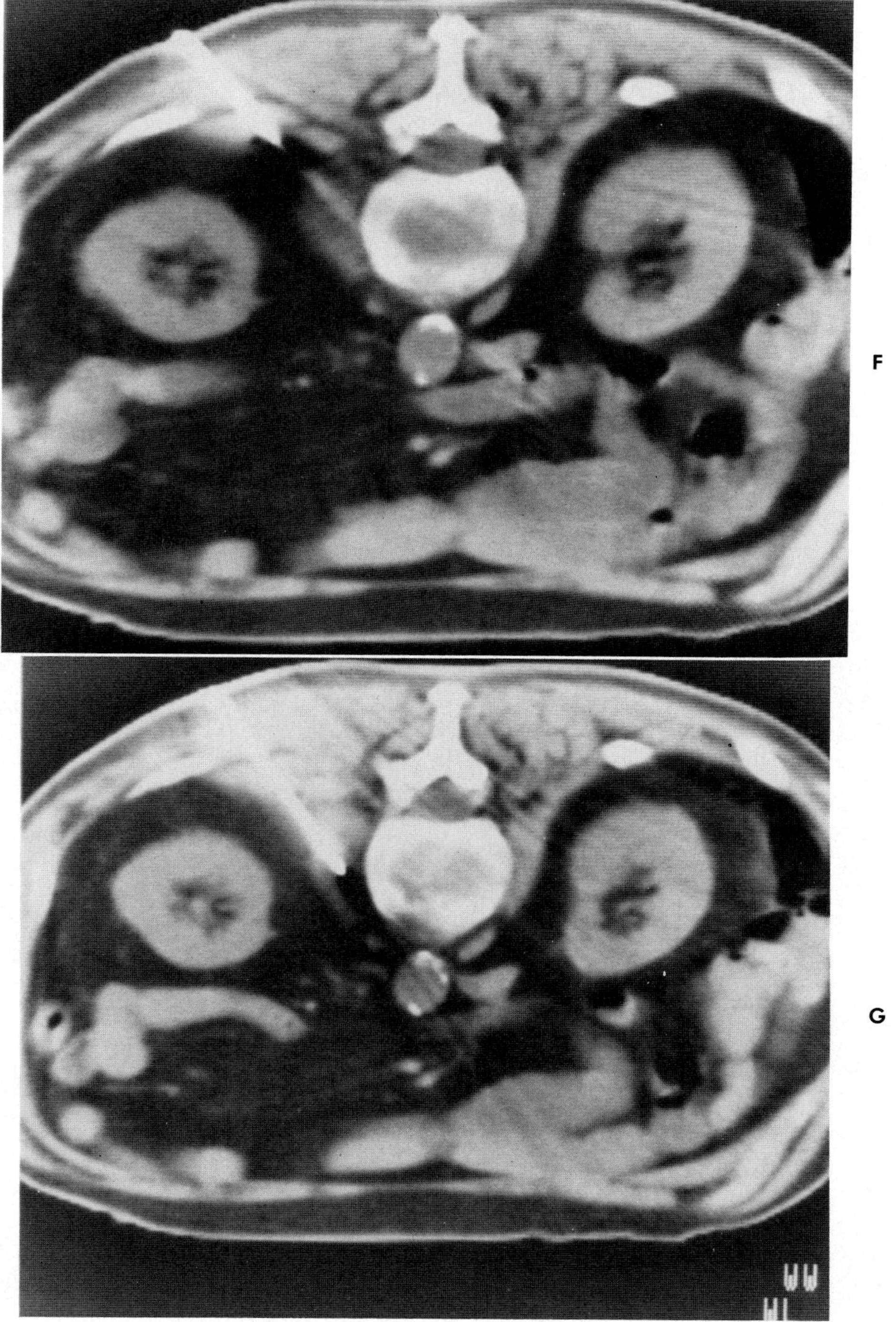

FIGURE 4-3, cont'd. On the first biopsy attempt, **F** and **G,** the needle tip was angled too far ventrally, directly toward the aorta. *Continued.*

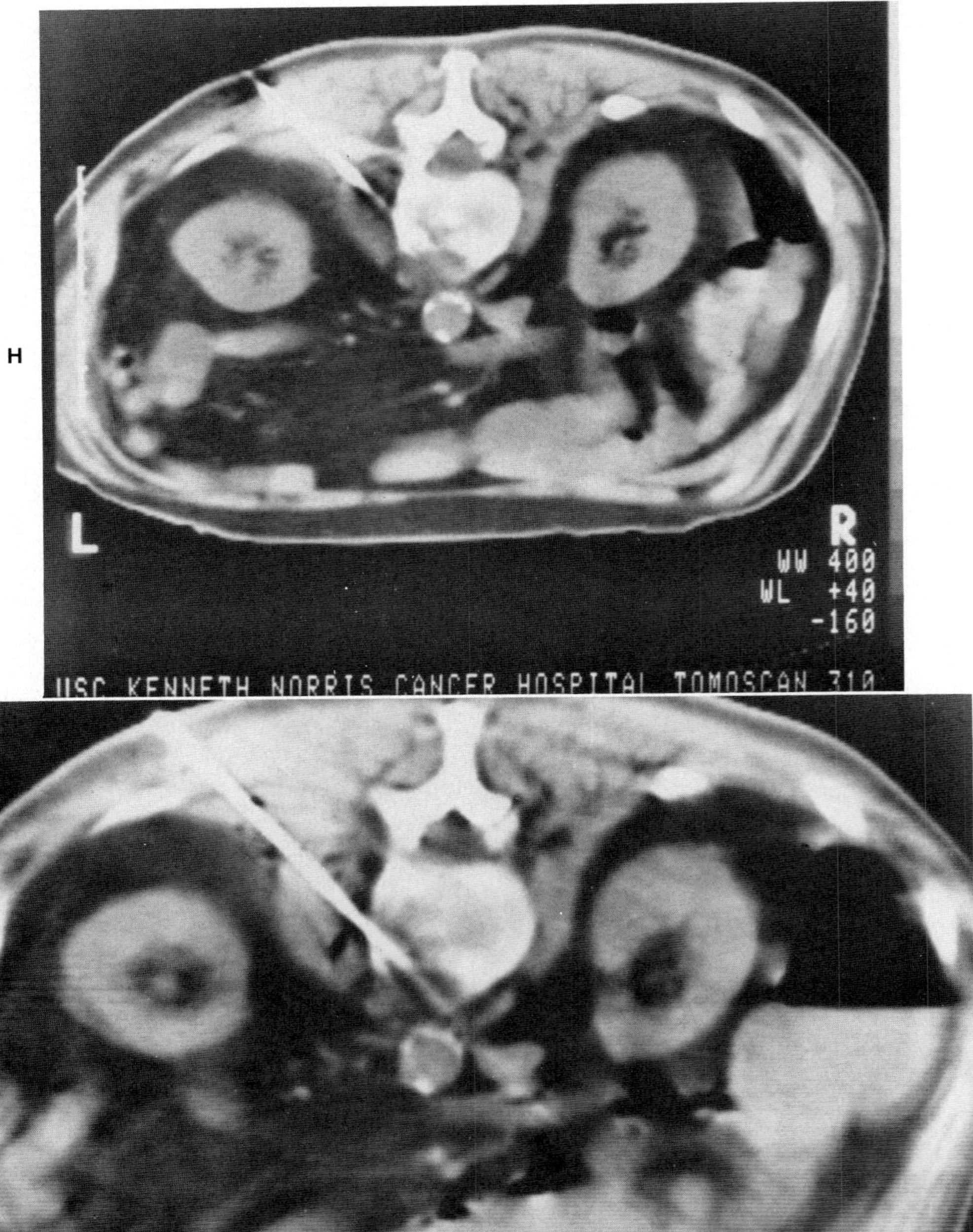

FIGURE 4-3, cont'd. The trocar was therefore redirected, **H** and **I,** and a safe and successful biopsy was accomplished.

or core biopsy in most cases. In general, premedication* with a narcotic and hypnotic[14,15] is helpful but it often prolongs the procedure and requires close monitoring of vital signs. A barbiturate will protect against local anesthetic overdose but not against idiosyncratic reactions. Skin, fascia, and periosteum are the major pain-sensitive structures; the periosteum, in particular, should be widely infiltrated with local anesthesia before biopsy. Procaine (Novocaine) has the greatest margin of safety per milligram, but lidocaine (Xylocaine) or other agents can be used if the volume is kept below 0.5 ml/kg of 1% solution. Epinephrine in combination with local anesthetic may have a theoretical advantage in an occasional case but has not been considered necessary. Brachial plexus, axillary, median, or ulnar conduction nerve blocks occasionally are useful in the upper extremity, as are sciatic, femoral, or peroneal blocks in the lower extremity. A Bier block, using double tourniquet and intravenous route, will occasionally be helpful but requires an emotionally mature patient who can understand and cooperate. General anesthesia is best for the child or young adolescent or an emotionally unstable adult.

EQUIPMENT AND TECHNIQUES

There are many original instruments available for closed biopsy, and most have been modified at least once. A partial listing includes Ackermann, Chiba, Corb, Craig, Deeley, Franseen, Hayes Martin, Gidlund, Jamshidi, Michele, Silverman, Turkel, Tru-Cut (Cook, Inc.), Valls, Vim Silverman, Vim Tru-Cut (Travenol), and Westerman-Jensen. I have found that four types of equipment will suffice for any routine skeletal or soft tissue biopsy. These include a spinal needle, a Tru-Cut instrument (Fig. 4-4), a Craig set (Figs. 4-5 and 4-6), and a hollow drill of some type for blastic metastases or medullary lesions beneath an intact cortex.

Aspiration or "skinny" needle biopsy for metastatic skeletal lesions (Fig. 4-7) is not used frequently now, being reserved instead for primary lesions in patients who are limb-salvage candidates. However, in some cases of primarily lytic metastases, histological examination of the minute tissue core can produce a definitive diagnosis. Adler and Rosenberger[4] use 22-gauge needles and report good results in lytic bone lesions. The reader is referred to the literature* for detailed discussions of this technique and its limitations in blastic and fibrous tumors. Equipment required includes the following:

1. An 18-gauge spinal needle with obturator
2. The 1% local anesthetic of choice
3. Plastic disposable syringe (10 ml)
4. Glass slides
5. A small vial of formaldehyde tissue fixative
6. A sheet of Telfa dressing
7. Saline
8. Aerobic and anaerobic culture tubes
9. Steri-Strips or Band-Aids
10. Occasionally a skin suture of choice

Remove the obturator and firmly attach the syringe to the spinal needle. Draw local anesthetic into the syringe, and with CT, biplanar roentgenographic, or image intensifier guidance if necessary direct the needle toward the lesion, infiltrating the agent as it advances. When a bone lesion is reached, the periosteum is liberally infiltrated and any remaining local anesthetic is discarded. Strong suction is then provided by withdrawing the plunger, and the needle tip is moved back and forth several times through the lesion. Suction is released before the needle is extracted. It is not necessary that blood or tissue fragments be drawn into the syringe for a successful biopsy. If the syringe is empty when withdrawn, remove it, fill it with air, reattach it, and eject the contents of the needle onto one or more slides. Use another slide to smear the material as for a blood smear. If blood has been withdrawn into the syringe, eject it onto a Telfa pad and empty the needle with a syringe of air. Before discarding the syringe and needle, flush it by aspirating a few drops of saline and eject the retained material into formalin or onto a glass slide to be smeared. Clotted blood expelled onto Telfa should be submitted,[12,42] because microscopic fragments of tumor are often present in the clot. A Gram stain and anaerobic and aerobic cultures should be an integral part of any biopsy. Acid-fast and fungus cultures should also be obtained.

*References 4, 5, 16, 17, 34, 42, 56, 76.

*References 6, 20, 22, 27, 40-42, 49, 61, 62.

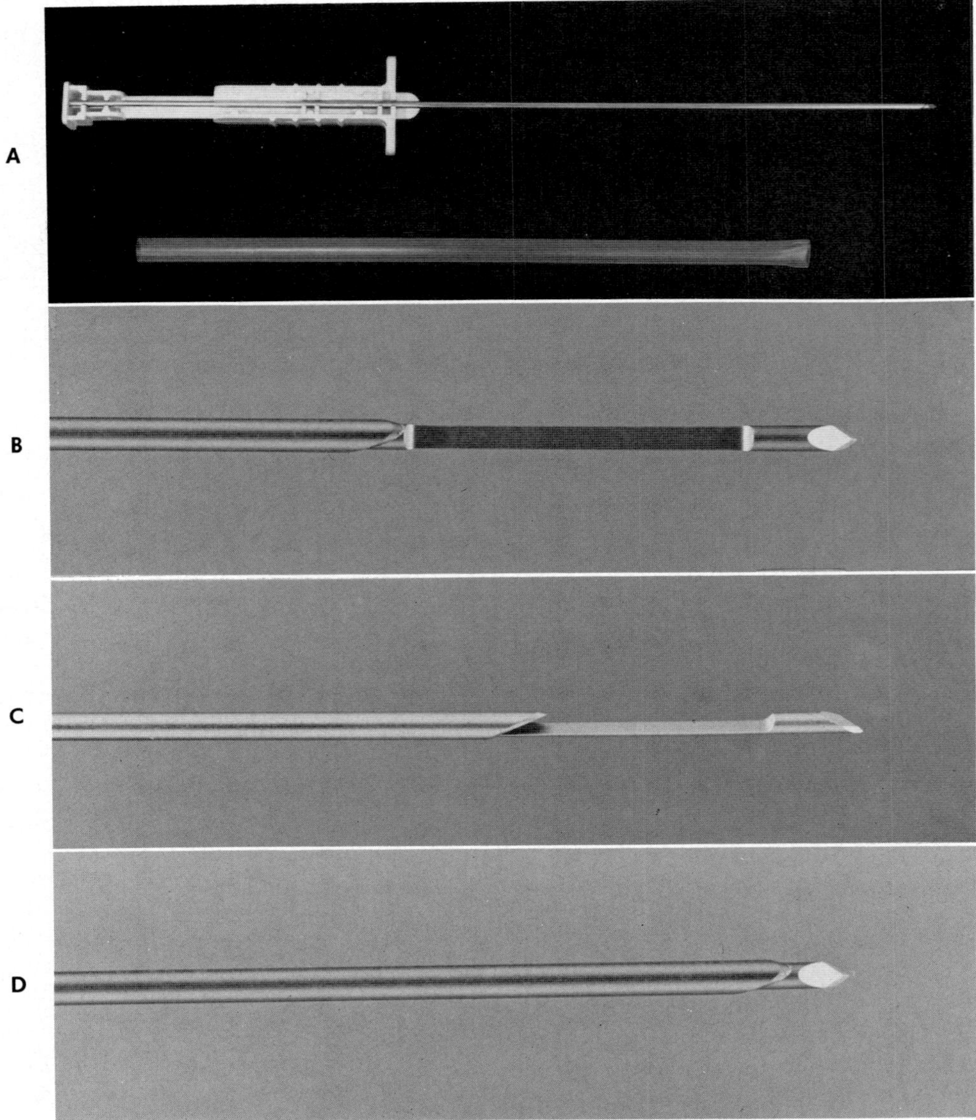

FIGURE 4-4 **A,** The Tru-Cut (Travenol) sterilely packaged disposable instrument is excellent for soft tissue and lytic bone biopsies. A plastic sheath protects the thin pointed obturator and the cutting edge cannula. **B,** A detailed view shows the cannula fully retracted to expose the specimen notch. **C,** Cannula partially closed. **D,** Cannula completely closed. The obturator and cannula handles can be separated if desired, allowing retrieval of multiple cores while the cannula remains within the lesion.

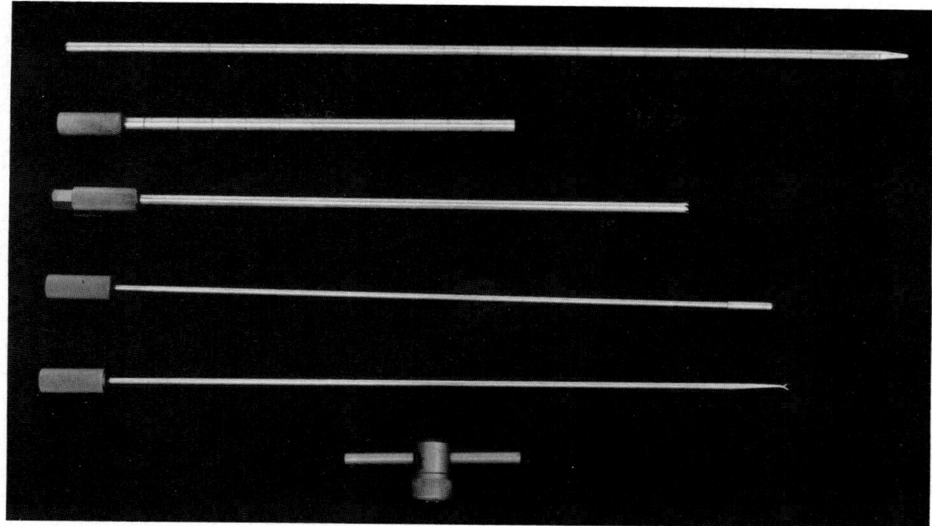

FIGURE 4-5 Essential components of the Craig biopsy set. *Top* to *bottom,* Calibrated trocar, calibrated cannula, cutter, obturator, worm, and wrench.

A sterile disposable Travenol Tru-Cut instrument is useful for some metastatic bone lesions, particularly those that are largely lytic (see Fig. 4-8). For biopsy with the Tru-Cut device the only equipment required in addition to that just listed is a no. 11 stab blade. The instrument is relatively large (13 gauge), but skin penetration is facilitated by a preliminary 3 to 4 mm stab incision. This rarely requires a suture and can be closed with a Steri-Strip or Band-Aid. The apparatus has been successfully used for percutaneous biopsy of prostatic, maxillary and mandibular,[58] lung, and more recently primary musculoskeletal soft tissue[56] tumors and with relatively solid tumors should deliver a core of tissue approximately 20 mm in length and 1 mm in diameter. The Tru-Cut instrument consists of only two parts: a sharp pointed obturator with a 20 mm bar connecting it to a rod and a plastic handle. The pointed end, narrow bar, and rod all slide within a hollow cannula that has a sharpened cutting edge. The sleeve is also attached to a separate plastic handle. The set is available in various lengths. An instruction sheet packaged with each instrument describes two techniques for its use depending on whether the cannula or the obturator is kept stationary during biopsy (Fig. 4-4).

The best cores are obtained by the following method:

The closed instrument is advanced to the lesion by palpation or under roentgenographic control.

The obturator is fully advanced into the lesion and held stationary as the cutting cannula is advanced.

Any tissue falling into the slot behind the pointed tip of the obturator will be sheared off and trapped by the cutting edge of the hollow cannula.

If the tumor is soft, mucoid, or bloody, the biopsy material can be placed in formalin and smeared on slides.

For biopsy of bone lesions the instrument should be used *only* for very lytic lesions. The obturator end can bend and become caught, making its removal from bone difficult or impossible (Fig. 4-4).

The first Tru-Cut core is submitted for frozen section evaluation to ensure that viable lesional tissue is being retrieved. If so, a few more cores of tissue are removed and placed in formalin for routine processing.

The instrument can be extracted with each biopsy core, or the cannula and obturator can be separated and the cannula left in place while the obturator extracts multiple cores.

If multiple cores are to be obtained through the cannula, tissue yield is higher if the cannula is rotated 90 degrees after each biopsy.

For core biopsy of soft tissue masses the Vim Tru-Cut instrument is ideal.

The Craig biopsy instrument can be used for lytic, mixed lytic-blastic, and minimally blastic lesions in cancellous bone. Nothing is required in addition to the materials listed previously except the Craig set. Frederick Craig[14,15] developed this set for freehand vertebral biopsy under biplanar roentgenographic control (Figs. 4-5, 4-6, 4-9, and 4-10). It has been helpful in biopsy of metastatic, primary, and other lesions in many locations, in addition to those of the spine.[25,41,56] It is best used for cancellous bone biopsy adjacent to vital structures. For example, material from the scapula, pelvis, proximal humerus, tibia and femur, distal radius, and distal femur and tibia can be safely retrieved with the Craig set. Subcutaneous locations (e.g., clavicle, calcaneus, rib, metacarpals, metatarsals, distal fibula, even phalanges) are also easily biopsied using only the cutter. There are six working components (Figs. 4-5 and 4-6) and a tray for sterilization.

The advantage of the Craig biopsy set over the Tru-Cut instrument is that the trocar is blunt and thus unlikely to injure vital structures during insertion. All trephination is done within a protective cannula. In addition, the Craig cutters are hollow and any bleeding is readily apparent. Blood and tissue can also be aspirated with a syringe fitted to the cutter. Much larger specimens are obtained than with the Tru-Cut biopsy instrument. When the Craig cutter is filled with specimen, a core 25 × 3.5 mm is obtained (roughly 15 times larger in volume than that obtained with the Tru-Cut instrument). A worm-tipped trocar can be used to grasp soft tissue, which can be either retrieved through the cutter or maintained within the cutter as it is removed (Fig. 4-6, *B*). A blunt obturator can also be used to show how much tissue is within the cutter as well as dislodge a bone core from the cutter after biopsy.

In the original sets there were two cutters, a smooth knife-edge type for lytic lesions and a toothed type for mixed lytic-blastic or blastic cancellous lesions. Current instruments have cutters that are thin and inadequate for cortical or sclerotic bone biopsy (Fig. 4-6, *B*); therefore, when blastic cancellous lesions must be biopsied, a hexagonal wrench has been added that fits the cutters (Fig. 4-5) and enhances the surgeon's

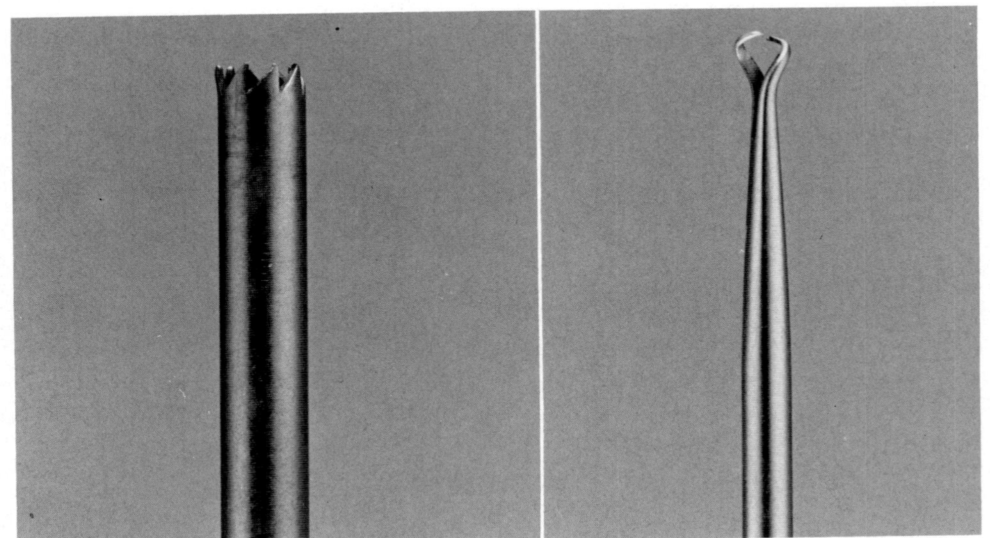

FIGURE 4-6 **A,** Detailed view of the Craig trocar, which cuts when turned clockwise but dulls quickly in cortical bone. **B,** The worm is used to grasp soft tissue in the cutter when turned between 90 and 180 degrees. If it is turned beyond 180 degrees, its teeth tend to cut through the specimen.

ability to twist the device and obtain core samples. There is no provision for power (although several adaptations have been made).

In subcutaneous locations the technique for obtaining biopsy cores is simple:

Infiltrate the skin and periosteum with local anesthetic or establish some type of conduction anesthesia.

Make a 4 to 5 mm incision in the skin and continue it to include periosteum.

Apply the cannula directly to the lesion and hold it firmly in place.

Insert a cutter (Fig. 4-6, *A*) and spin it clockwise with your fingers or turn it with the wrench. Use the obturator to check on the length of the tissue core.

If a core of bone is to be taken, rock the cutter and cannula back and forth to break the core at its base and remove the cutter keeping the cannula in place for subsequent biopsies.

When the first core has been obtained, roll it along one glass slide (to make a "touch prep" for cytological examination) and along a second slide (for Gram stain evaluation).

Cut two 1 mm slices of the core with the stab blade and drop them into aerobic and anaerobic culture tubes.

Place a second 1 mm slice in a tube for fungus and acid-fast culture.

A 1 mm cube of tissue can be placed in glutaraldehyde fixation for electron microscopic study if desired.

The obturator can be used to extrude the bone core from the cutter. If a lesion is purely lytic, a smooth cutter can be used similarly but the core of tissue will probably not be trapped within it. The worm can then be dropped into the cutter and turned 90 to 180 degrees to catch the soft tissue (Fig. 4-6, *B*). A syringe can also be attached and suction continued during removal of the cutter. The newer Craig sets do not include a smooth cutter.

For deeper locations under CT, biplanar roentgenographic, or image intensification guidance, infiltrate the skin, fascia, and periosteum with local anesthetic or use conduction anesthesia.

Make a skin incision and twist the blunt trocar in to contact the lesion.

Slip the cannula over the trocar and advance it to bone by spinning it through the tissue.

Hold the cannula firmly in place, remove the trocar, and insert a cutter.

The biopsy can then proceed as previously described.

It is important that during this last maneuver the cannula not be allowed to slip from contact with the bone. One wants to avoid injury to the surrounding soft tissue, maintain the original roentgenographically controlled position of the device, and ensure that the original biopsy site can be reentered to obtain further cores through the same hole. Moreover, if bleeding occurs, one can then be assured that it is from the biopsy defect alone. To assure fixation of the cannula after the first core, immediately reinsert the trocar through the cannula and into the bone defect. This will also serve as an effective tamponade to control bleeding. If bleeding persists, use the square end of the trocar to insert Gelfoam plugs cut with the trephine or rolled between your fingers into the site and pack them into the lesion. Surgicel can also be used to plug the lesion in the same manner.

Recently I have used an Intracath plastic sheath and needle to perform closed needle biopsies, particularly in primary tumors. If bleeding occurs after recovery of the specimen, the needle is reinserted into the plastic sheath and touched lightly with a Bovie tip. This has the theoretical advantage of destroying local tumor cells and the practical advantage of minimizing bleeding and spread of tumor cells along tissue planes because of continued bleeding.

Because skeletal metastases tend to occur in cancellous bone of the spine, pelvis, and ribs and the proximal long bones, it is rarely necessary to biopsy through intact cortical bone. When metastases lodge in diaphyseal bone, the cortex is usually softened by thinning and tumor invasion and the Craig set ordinarily serves well. In the unusual situation of a medullary tumor within relatively intact cortex, a long-shank 7/64-inch drill bit will fit the Craig cannula,[22] allowing the cortex to be penetrated. A regular Craig cutter then can be inserted into the lesion. On occasion, however, heavier biopsy instruments are necessary and may also be required if metastases are purely blastic. I have used three types of instruments, with varying degrees of success: one hand powered, one optionally powered by hand or air, and a third air powered.

1. The first, a Michele trephine,[54] is a heavy-duty hollow instrument that can be used successfully for biopsy of cortical or dense sclerotic bone. Unfortunately, however, it is difficult now to acquire and probably is not available in most hospitals. It also is difficult to insert safely through overlying soft tissue because the large cutting teeth are exposed; however, twisting it counterclockwise through muscle and fascia minimizes damage. When the rounded bone surface is contacted, the twisting direction is reversed to a clockwise cutting direction. Unless this trephine is rigidly stabilized, the eccentric contact of the teeth tend to spin it off the bone. Success requires a firm grip and an obstinant attitude.
2. The second tool, a simple hollow drill, generally is more widely available and can be used with hand or air power. It has the same disadvantage as the Michele trephine. However, the preliminary insertion of a large Steinmann pin will both serve as a roentgenographic locator and help stabilize the trephine.
3. Recently a counterrotating drill[69] has been devised with diameters of 4.8, 6.4, and 9.5 mm that its designers claim has significant advantages over previous similar instruments. The Corb biopsy instrument (air powered) retrieves a core diameter almost three times the size of that retrieved by the Craig instrument. It has a blunt probe and a cannula that helps stabilize the instrument on the bone surface during rotation of the hollow drills. The gearbox and counterrotating hollow drills require cautious use and fastidious cleansing.

None of these three instruments ensures that the biopsy will be simple or safe, but each does facilitate penetration of cortical or sclerotic bone, following which further sampling of the lesion can be accomplished by using conventional Craig instruments. Occasionally a pituitary rongeur or angled curet will prove useful for retrieving tissue from the medullary canal.

BIOPSY IN SPECIFIC ANATOMICAL LOCATIONS

Certain generalizations apply to any invasive procedure and should be considered in planning closed biopsy. If more than one lesion is present, as expected in 75% to 90% of patients, the safest and most accessible lesion should be selected for biopsy. Cutting biopsy instruments should be directed away from vital structures when possible (Fig. 4-7) and, if adjacent to them, should be inserted parallel to neurovascular structures or tangential to pleura, dura, and pharynx. Biopsy of pulsatile lesions or those demonstrating a bruit should be approached with a skinny needle (Fig. 4-8), provision made for transfusion, and the patient considered for general anesthesia with tourniquet hemostasis if the lesion is appropriately situated.

Cranium. Cranial metastatic lesions only rarely require biopsy; other sites are usually more available and are preferable. Neuroblastoma in the child and any of the most common adult carcinomas may metastasize to the skull. Skinny needle aspiration or Tru-Cut core biopsy is adequate if a palpable mass is present, but the biopsy should be done *tangentially* to the skull. The galea aponeurotica is dense and well innervated, requiring careful field block surrounding any tumor located there. Depending on the tumor location, an occipital nerve block may be helpful. Mild postbiopsy finger pressure for 3 to 5 minutes will minimize bleeding. Metastases to the facial bones are rare, but in such cases alternative sites for biopsy should be sought.

Upper Three Cervical Bodies. C1 to C3 are approached by a transoral open[8,26,74] or closed[78] technique. Patient cooperation is difficult and general anesthesia with intubation or even tracheostomy is necessary. Biopsy location is best appreciated by palpation of the ring of the first cervical vertebra, but needle position must be roentgenographically confirmed. Infection can be a problem following biopsy,[26] and it is advisable to give preoperative and intraoperative systemic antibiotics.[8] Bonney and Williams[8] also used topical antibiotics prior to closure.

Lower Cervical Bodies. C4 through C7 can be approached laterally along a straight line beginning at the mastoid process and paralleling the spine. The head and neck must be in a neutral position. Roentgenography with image-intensifier control may be used. From the mastoid line a guide needle is directed slightly anteriorly. More posterior penetration along this line will encounter the lateral masses and the partially exposed vertebral artery. A paresthesia may be produced in the brachial plexus, usually indicating that the needle is directed too posteriorly. At the other

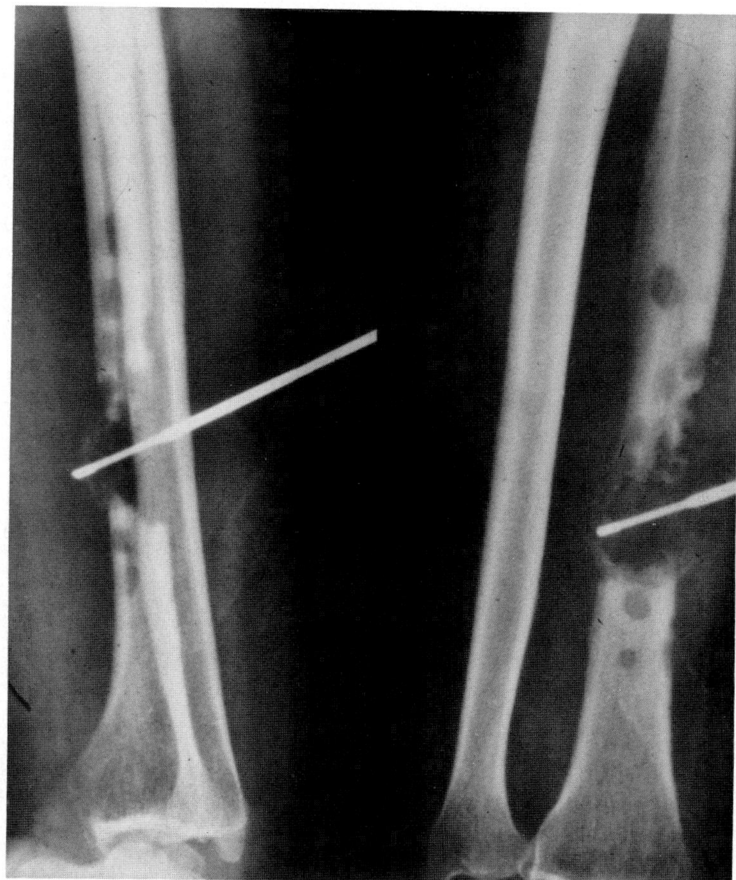

FIGURE 4-7 Multiple lytic abnormalities in the radius of a patient many years after breast carcinoma had been diagnosed. A Travenol Tru-Cut biopsy was obtained and the histological diagnosis was adenocarcinoma consistent with a breast primary. The biopsy was uncomplicated. Ideally, however, the instrument should have been introduced in a plane more parallel to the bone and to the radial artery.

extreme the pharynx may be penetrated if the needle is angled too far anteriorly.

An anterolateral approach can also be used. The anterior border of the sternocleidomastoid muscle is identified by inspection and palpation. The surgeon's fingers retract this muscle and the underlying carotid sheath posteriorly. At the same time the larynx and pharynx are displaced medially by the extended fingers. Through this essentially avascular interval the skin and subcutaneous tissues can be depressed against the anterior cervical vertebral bodies. No vital structures lie between the skin and these vertebrae provided the surgeon's fingers sense the pulsation of the carotid artery laterally. When the biopsy instrument has contacted bone and is stabilized, its position and level can be confirmed with biplanar or image-intensifier roentgenography prior to biopsy (Fig. 4-9). The patient should be carefully observed for a few hours to ensure that there is no bleeding into the neck tissues or injury to the pharynx. Dysphagia occasionally develops but should diminish over the following 24 hours.

Clavicle and Scapula. Clavicular and most scapular biopsies ordinarily do not require roentgenographic control because they are superficial and have easily palpable landmarks. They also are difficult to visualize by roentgenography, even with image intensification. Biopsy of the lateral third of the clavicle is safely performed by directing the instrument laterally or posterolaterally.

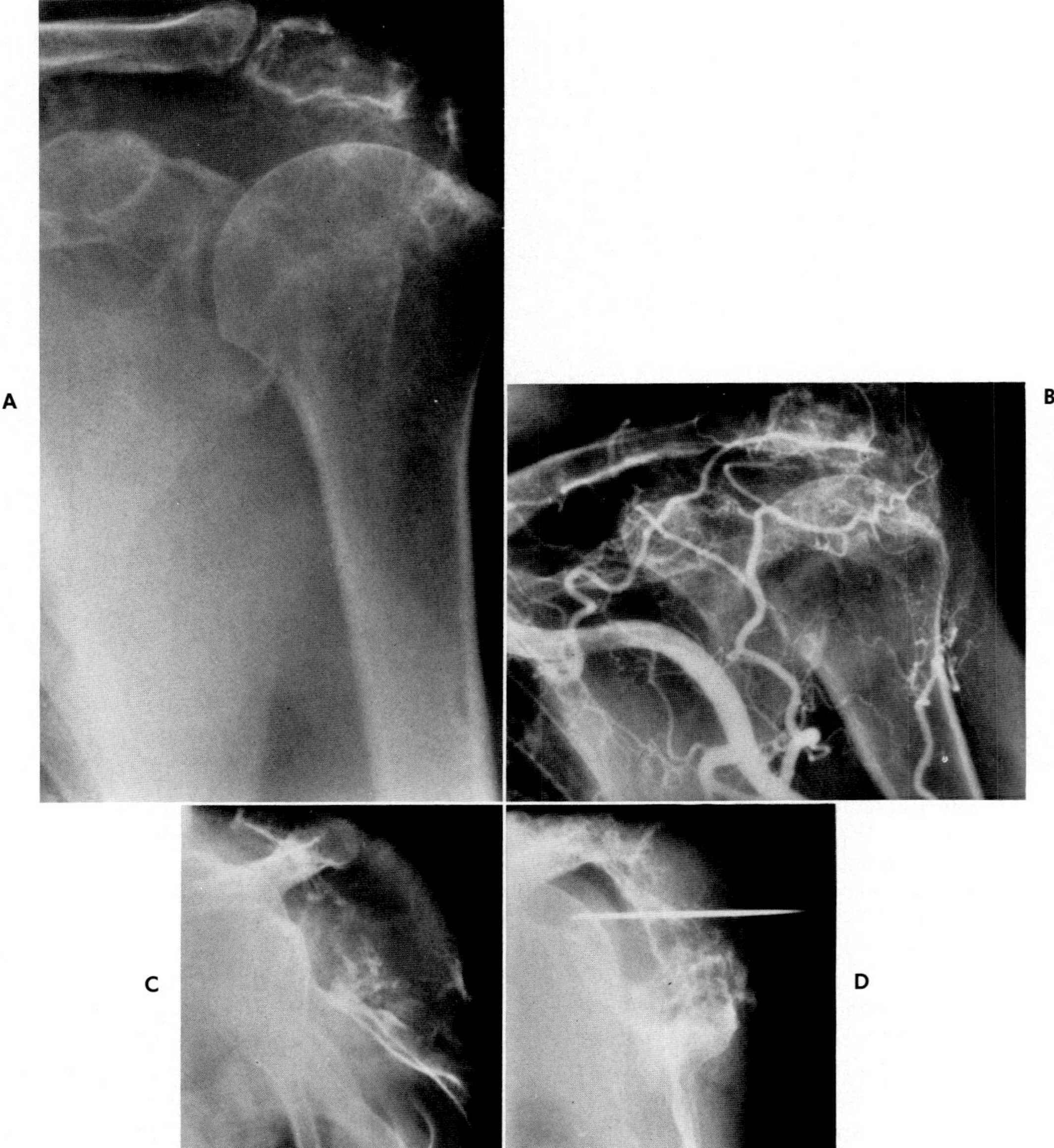

FIGURE 4-8 An AP roentgenogram, **A,** of the left shoulder of a 42-year-old man with a 3-month history of local pain showed evidence of an aneurysmal destructive acromial lesion. An arteriogram, **B,** revealed moderate vascularity and a pattern suggestive of neoplasm. In an effort to minimize bleeding, an aspiration biopsy, **C** and **D,** was selected and the cytological diagnosis was poorly differentiated squamous cell carcinoma. Although no primary malignancy was noted despite a thorough evaluation, ultimately an occult bronchogenic carcinoma was discovered.

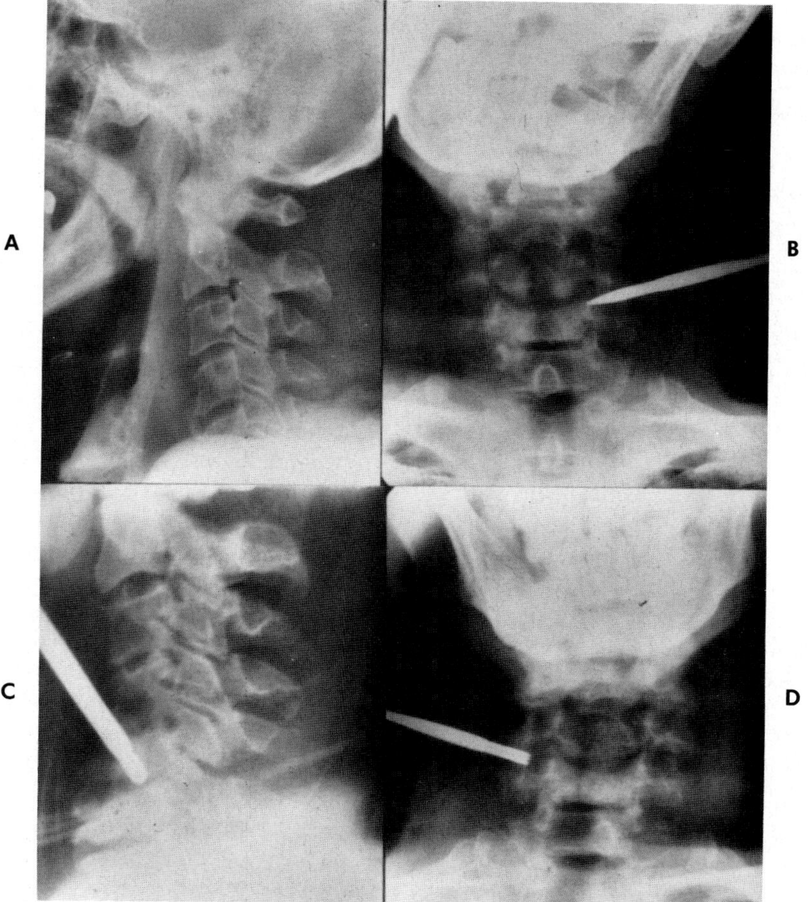

FIGURE 4-9 **A,** Lateral roentgenogram of the cervical spine in a young male drug abuser also suffering from Stage IIIA follicular lymphoma. Neck pain and fever developed while the patient was receiving chemotherapy. Note the loss of the normal lordotic curve as well as the anterior soft tissue mass. **B,** A Craig trocar and cannula were inserted through an anterolateral approach to the C6 vertebral body. **C** and **D,** The instrument has been positioned for the biopsy. Despite premedication and local anesthesia, the procedure was painful and the patient uncooperative. The position of the cannula on bone was lost twice because of motion, but eventually a core of soft tissue and bone was obtained without undue complications. The core showed granulation tissue and osteomyelitis. Culture disclosed *Pseudomonas.* This patient would have been better managed by aspiration under general anesthesia.

The medial clavicle should be biopsied as nearly parallel to its axis as possible because of the proximity of the great vessels. The body of the scapula should be approached tangentially when possible. Immobilization can be achieved by placing the patient in the prone position with arms crossed overhead. The spine of the scapula and the acromion are easily palpable and should not be difficult to identify or biopsy (Fig. 4-8). The neck of the scapula can be approached safely medial to the junction of the body and neck of the acromion or via an axillary route with the arm abducted, again under roentgenographic control.

Biopsy of the humeral head and neck is uncomplicated unless the axillary or radial nerve is inadvertently blocked by local anesthesia. In this event it is safer to reposition the biopsy after return of nerve function. The axillary nerve lies approximately 3 cm below the acromion in an adult, and this area should be avoided by moving the skin entry distally and angling the biopsy instrument superiorly.

Thoracic Vertebrae. The bodies of the thoracic vertebrae are approached through a rather narrow corridor between the pleura and the dura.

Although there are several reports of successful and relatively uncomplciated biopsy of T1 through T9 or T10,* I know of several cases of paraplegia or paraparesis following attempted biopsy of the thoracic spine. Transpedicular biopsy is preferred (as described in Chapter 12). This method is essentially an open biopsy, because the dorsal elements are exposed as for a conventional laminectomy.

The increasing availability of CT-guided biopsy[73] and the participation of radiologists in the procedure† probably will make thoracic spinal biopsy safer, simpler, and faster than in the past. However, several detailed descriptions of thoracic spinal biopsy using standard biplanar roentgenographic or image-intensifier control are available.[1,14,15,63] Under general anesthesia the patient is positioned prone on an image table or a regular operating table with a cassette tunnel beneath the chest and provision for a lateral cassette holder. A C-arm image intensifier will expedite the procedure. After determining the level and position of biopsy, the surgeon makes a skin wheal about 4 cm from the midline,[63] always medial to the angle of the rib,[14] and advances a probing spinal needle under roentgenographic control at about 35 degrees from the sagittal (vertical) plane toward the midline of the body (Fig. 4-10). It must be emphasized that this angle should not be with the plane of the back but rather *with the vertical plane of the dorsal spinous processes.* Thirty-five degrees from the plane of the back will direct the biopsy instrument *too superficially,* placing the spinal cord in jeopardy. The great vessels and the azygos and hemiazygos vessels are within 7 cm of the skin, particularly in a small thin patient. In children or infants extreme caution must be exercised to prevent unnecessary penetration. As the needle is advanced, the neck of the rib may be encountered and the needle should then be directed cephalad to contact the vertebral body. Advance of the biopsy instrument should be carefully checked every 1 to 2 cm by an image intensifier. Chest auscultation and percussion should be assessed as soon as the patient is extubated, and a sitting PA chest film obtained in the recovery room to ensure that a pneumothorax has not occurred.

Thoracolumbar Vertebrae. Biopsy from T10 through L4 is of less concern if established instruments and technique are used. The patient is prone or lateral with provision for biplanar roentgenographic or image-intensifier control. Generally local anesthesia is adequate and preferred.

For biopsy of the lower three thoracic bodies the skin entry is made approximately 5 cm lateral to the spinous process. For biopsy of the L1 through L4 vertebral bodies the biopsy instrument is inserted between 6 and 7 cm lateral to the tip of the spinous process and at an angle of 35 degrees. As the needle is advanced, the transverse spinous process is often encountered and it may be necessary to angle the needle somewhat cephalad to reach the side of the vertebral body (Fig. 4-10). Biplanar roentgenography or image intensification is used at each step to guide the exploring needle or probe. If the lesion is anterior in the vertebral body, a CT-guided biopsy will be safer because of the proximity of the large vessels (Fig. 4-3).

At the level of the L5 vertebral body the posterior spine of the ilium protrudes varia-

*References 14, 15, 31, 56, 63.

†References 3, 4, 16, 17, 20, 21, 38, 40, 42, 47.

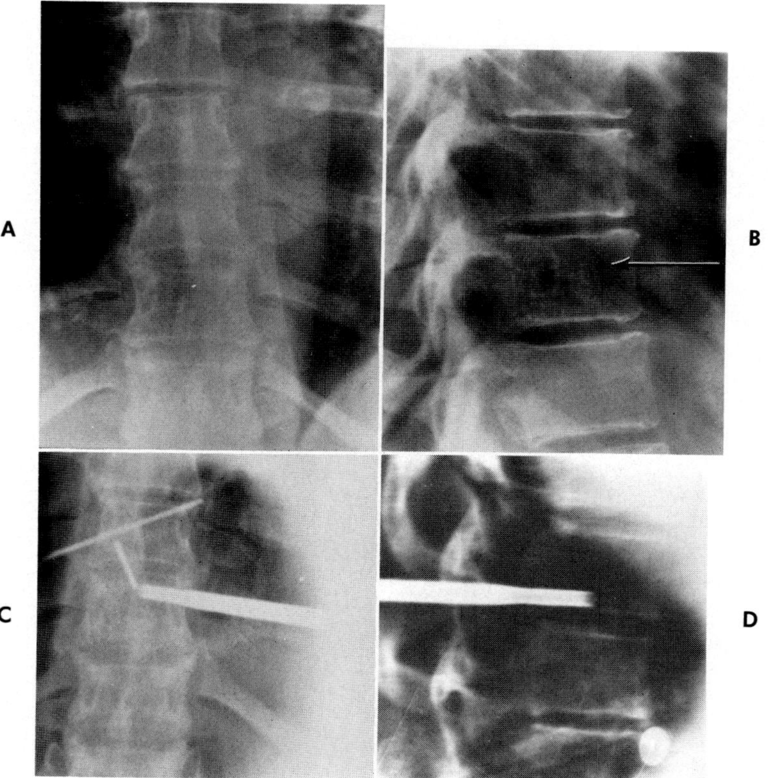

FIGURE 4-10 **A** and **B,** AP and lateral roentgenograms of the thoracic spine in a patient with known carcinoma-in-situ of the cervix and progressive spinal pain. Lytic changes within the body of T10 are apparent *(arrow)*. **C** and **D,** On the AP view the T9 vertebral level has been marked with needles and the Craig instrument inserted into the body of T10. Good tissue was obtained and a diagnosis of benign hemangioma confirmed.

bly, depending on the sex and habitus, and may block a standard 6 to 7 cm lateral entry site. The needle then must be inserted more medially and directed caudad to reach the L5 body. However, at this caudad and more acute angle the biopsy instrument is more likely to impinge on the nerve root. Not surprisingly, injury to nerve roots in the lumbar region are more common and more serious than in the thoracic spine. Local anesthesia for lumbar spine biopsy is preferable to general anesthesia because it allows the patient to sense proximity of the biopsy instrument to the nerve root. When the patient complains of root pain during placement of the biopsy instrument, the instrument tip usually needs to be directed more laterally. If the root cannot be bypassed, it may be necessary to discontinue the biopsy attempt from that side. Biopsy in the face of persistent root pain produced by an exploring needle or Craig trocar can lead to permanent disability if the lumbar nerve root is damaged.[56,75]

There is another caveat with regard to biopsy technique in the lumbar spine. If the exploring spinal needle or Craig cutter produces root pain, observation and aspiration should be done to determine whether spinal fluid can be obtained. If so, the site and angle should be changed or the biopsy attempted from the opposite side or rescheduled depending on the amount of root pain, the amount of spinal fluid, and the urgency of the biopsy. If spinal fluid is obtained, post–spinal surgical precautions should be observed for at least 24 hours and the patient then tested by sitting and standing so the possibility of a continuing spinal fluid leak can be ruled out. Experience with chemonucleolysis techniques will make the biopsy surgeon more confident,

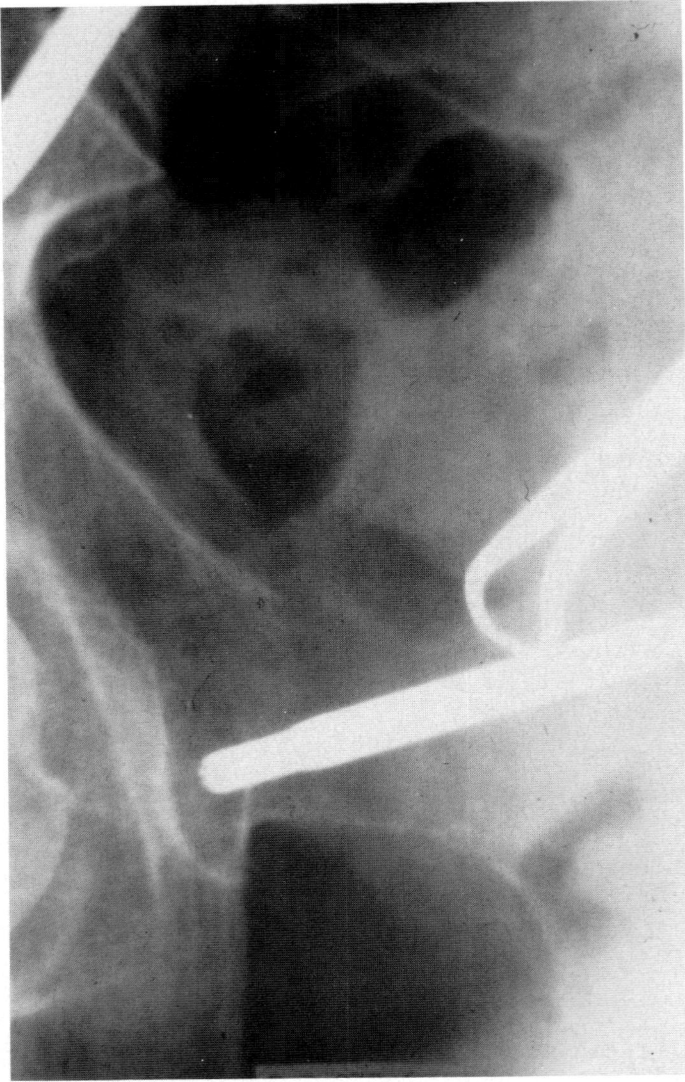

FIGURE 4-11 The Craig set is particularly useful and safe when biopsy material must be obtained near a major vital structure. In this case a lytic lesion of the superior pubic ramus is to be examined. The blunt trocar is guided under image intensifier control down to the bone. The cannula is then inserted over the trocar and twisted to become impacted on bone. As long as the cannula is held firmly against bone, the cutter can cut only bone and the adjacent vessels and nerves will not be injured.

and a minor change in directing the instrument from the disc space to the adjacent vertebral body should be easy.

Sacrum and Pelvis. Biopsy of the sacrum and pelvis is usually straightforward. A lateral view of the distal sacrum is not difficult with roentgenographic or image intensifier control, but the proximal sacrum and alae are harder to visualize on a lateral projection. For the remainder of the pelvis, AP and oblique projections will help locate the lesion and the subsequent biopsy better than will standard lateral views. However, this requires more careful evaluation of spatial relationships than for standard 90-degree biplanar evaluation. The patient is placed prone for sacral and posterior iliac wing biopsies, supine or lateral for supraacetabular biopsies, and supine for superior pubic ramus (Fig. 4-11) and pubic body biopsies. Biopsy of the inferior pubic

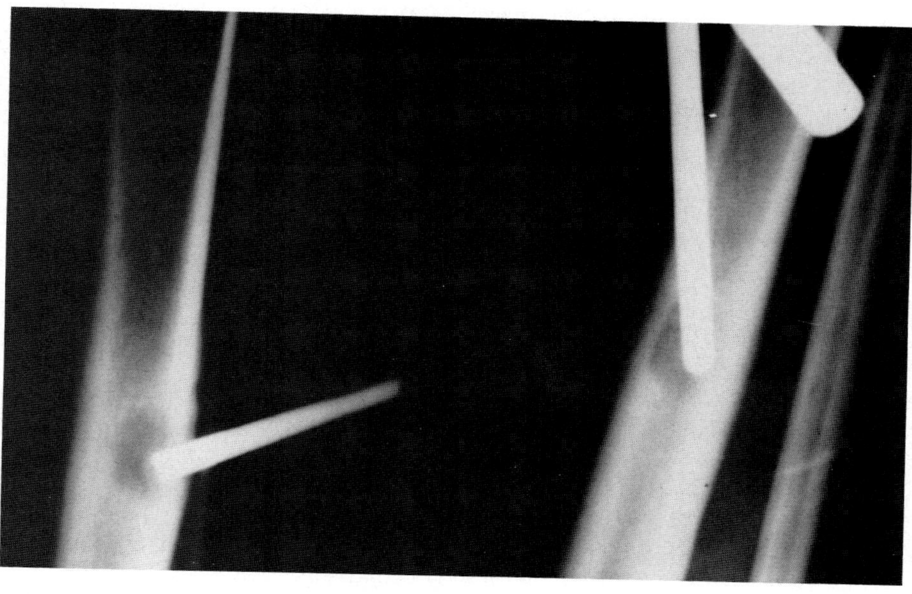

FIGURE 4-12 AP and lateral roentgenograms of the midtibial diaphysis in an 80-year-old man with a known hard prostatic nodule but normal acid phosphatase levels. He had been feeling night pain in the tibia. The intact tibial cortex was broached with a Michele trephine, a diagnosis of lymphangioma of bone was made, and the pain disappeared promptly after the biopsy.

ramus and ischial tuberosity can be done in stirrups, or with an assistant holding the leg flexed and abducted, but I prefer the prone jackknife position. AP and oblique roentgenograms are useful for documenting the location of the biopsy. Biopsy of the femur and tibia (Fig. 4-12) should pose no problem if anatomical and biomechanical factors are considered in planning and implementing the biopsy.

COMPLICATIONS AND THEIR MANAGEMENT

Any surgical treatment exposes the patient to a risk of complications, but a low complication rate is clearly one of the many advantages of closed biopsy over standard open biopsy. For example, no serious complications were encountered by Adapon[3] or Hardy et al.[38] in a total of 41 CT-guided spinal biopsies. Murphy et al.[57] and nine other authors reported no significant complications in 913 trocar biopsies. Ottolenghi[62] reported no complications after 1078 spinal aspiration biopsies. In less experienced hands, however, and depending on the site biopsied, major or minor complications can be anticipated in up to 1% of cases. A complication rate of 0.2% was calculated by Murphy et al.[57] from a review of literature at the time of their study. Complications include pneumothorax after rib biopsy[13,34,70] and after thoracic spine biopsy[17,22,31,60] and direct or indirect spinal cord injury.[48] Cauda equina and nerve root and peripheral nerve injuries also may occur.[56] Infection is very rare, two instances having occurred in 600 biopsies reviewed by Griffiths.[34] Biopsy of tubercular abscesses has been reported to produce draining sinus tracts,[17] but I have not observed infection as a complication in well over 500 core biopsies, including tuberculous abscesses.[56] Postbiopsy fracture is also rare, but one case[51] is reported. Hemorrhage[70] is possible, and some bleeding is not uncommon,[17,34] particularly in biopsy of metastases from renal cell carcinoma, known to be highly vascular (Fig. 4-1). Seeding of the biopsy track with tumor cells[17] is one theoretical complication, especially in primary tumors, but this has not occurred despite attempts in animal models[20] or been observed in clinical practice.* In the ordinary biopsy of metastatic disease to bone, local

---

*References 12, 20, 25, 36, 61, 62.

seeding is of no practical concern. If necessary to excise the biopsy site, it can be simply identified with a nonabsorbable skin suture and later widely excised en bloc at definitive surgery.

In the past the success rates for closed biopsies have ranged from 67%[44,56] to 80% or better,[3,4,13,16-19] and in recent series by radiologists using computed tomography[20,22] have approached 90%. Schajowicz and Hokama[69] reported a 74% success rate in 7165 aspiration biopsies. As further experience accumulates, instrumentation improves and becomes standardized, and imaging techniques are more sensitive, it can be anticipated that the success rate of closed biopsy should approach or equal that of open biopsy. Roentgenographic imagers with increasing interest in biopsy will be particularly helpful in evaluating the difficult lesion (Fig. 4-3) and should improve the overall success rate and safety of closed biopsy, especially in the thoracic spine. Although early concern was apparent in the literature regarding the use of ferromagnetic devices within the strong magnetic field necessary for magnetic resonance imaging,[53,59] there seems to be no practical contraindication to the use of current biopsy instruments in combination with MRI. The major obstacle is the increased imaging time necessary for MRI when compared to computed tomography. However, the ability of MRI to image multiple planes, provide improved resolution, and distinguish tissue characteristics may well offer additional closed biopsy advantages in the future.

— REFERENCES

1. Ackermann, W.: Vertebral trephine biopsy, Ann. Surg. **143:**373, 1956.
2. Ackermann, W.: Application of the trephine for bone biopsy. Results in 635 cases, J.A.M.A. **184:**11, 1963.
3. Adapon, B.D., et al.: CT-guided closed biopsy of the spine, J. Comput. Assist. Tomog. **5**(1):73, 1981.
4. Adler, O., and Rosenberger, A.: Fine needle aspiration biopsy of osteolytic metastatic lesions, A.J.R. **133:** 15, 1979.
5. Blady, J.V.: Aspiration biopsy of tumors in obscure or difficult locations under roentgenoscopic guidance, A.J.R. **42:**515, 1939.
6. Boland, P.J., et al.: Metastatic disease of the spine, Clin. Orthop. **169:**95, 1982.
7. Bond, W.: A simple drill biopsy apparatus, Br. J. Radiol. **24:**214, 1951.
8. Bonney, G., and Williams, J.P.R.: Trans-oral approach to the upper cervical spine, J. Bone Joint Surg. **67B:**691, 1985.
9. Burn, J.I., et al.: Drill biopsy and dissemination of cancer, Br. J. Surg. **55:**628, 1968.
10. Burstein, A.H., et al.: Bone strength: the effect of screw holes, J. Bone Joint Surg. **54A:**1143, 1972.
11. Christiansen, H.: An aspiration trepan for tissue biopsy, Acta Radiol. **21:**349, 1940.
12. Coley, B.L., et al.: Diagnosis of bone tumors by aspiration, Am. J. Surg. **13:**215, 1931.
13. Collins, J.D., et al.: Percutaneous biopsy following positive bone scans, Radiology **132:**439, 1979.
14. Craig, F.S.: Vertebral body biopsy, J. Bone Joint Surg. **38A:**93, 1956.
15. Craig, F.S.: Metastatic and primary lesions of bone, Clin. Orthop. **73:**33, 1970.
16. Debnam, J.W., and Staple, T.W.: Trephine bone biopsy by radiologists, Radiology **116:**607, 1975.
17. Debnam, J.W., and Staple, T.W.: Needle biopsy of bone, Radiol. Clin. North Am. **13:**157, 1975.
18. Deeley, T.J.: The drill biopsy of bone lesions, Clin. Radiol. **23:**536, 1972.
19. Deeley, T.J.: Needle biopsy, London, 1974, Butterworth.
20. De Santos, L.A., et al.: The value of percutaneous needle biopsy in the management of primary bone tumors, Cancer **43:**735, 1979.
21. De Santos, L.A., et al.: Percutaneous biopsy of bone in the cancer patient, A.J.R. **130:**641, 1978.
22. El-Khoury, G.Y., et al.: Fine needle aspiration biopsy of bone, J. Bone Joint Surg. **65A:**522, 1983.
23. Ellis, F.: Needle biopsy in the clinical diagnosis of tumours, Br. J. Surg. **34:**240, 1947.
24. Ellis, L.D., et al.: Needle biopsy of bone and marrow, Arch. Intern. Med. **114:**213, 1964.
25. Evarts, C.M.: Diagnostic techniques. Closed biopsy of bone, Clin. Orthp. **107:**100, 1975.
26. Fang, H.S.Y., and Ong, G.B.: Direct anterior approach to the upper cervical spine, J. Bone Joint Surg. **44A:**1588, 1962.
27. Frable, W.J.: Technique of thin needle aspiration biopsy. In Bennington, J.L., editor: Major problems in pathology, Vol. 14, Bone and soft tissue tumors, Philadelphia, 1983, W.B. Saunders Co.
28. Frankel, C.J.: Aspiration biopsy of the spine, J. Bone Joint Surg. **36A:**69, 1954.
29. Frankel, V.H., and Nordin, M.: Basic biomechanics of the skeletal system, Philadelphia, 1980, Lea & Febiger.
30. Ghedini, G.: Studi sulla patologia del midullo osseo umano vivente. 1, Puntura esplorativa tecnica, Gazz. Osp. Milano **29:**140, 1908.
31. Gladstein, M.D., and Grantham, S.A.: Closed skeletal biopsy, Clin. Orthop. **103:**75, 1974.
32. Golimbu, C., et al.: Use of CT guided percutaneous bone biopsy in staging of genitourinary tumors, Urology **22:**322, 1983.
33. Greenberg, E., et al.: A review of unusual systemic manifestations associated with carcinoma, Am. J. Med. **36:**106, 1964.
34. Griffiths, H.J.: Interventional radiography: the musculoskeletal system, Radiol. Clin. North Am. **17:**475, 1979.

35. Haaga, J.R., and Alfidi, R.J.: Precise biopsy localization by computered tomography, Radiology **118:**603, 1976.
36. Hajdu, S.I., and Melamed, M.R.: Needle biopsy of primary malignant bone tumors, Surg. Gynecol. Obstet. **133:**829, 1971.
37. Hanafee, W.N., and Tobin, P.L.: Closed biopsy by a radiologist, Radiology **92:**605, 1969.
38. Hardy, D.C., et al.: Computed tomography in planning percutaneous bone biopsy, Radiology **134:**447, 1980.
39. Harrington, K.D.: The management of acetabular insufficiency secondary to metastatic malignant disease, J. Bone Joint Surg. **63A:**653, 1981.
40. Harter, L.P., et al.: CT guided fine needle aspirations for diagnosis of benign and malignant disease, A.J.R. **140:**363, 1983.
41. Hartman, J.T., and Phalen, G.S.: Needle biopsy of bone, J.A.M.A. **200:**201, 1967.
42. Hewes, R.C., et al.: Percutaneous bone biopsy: the importance of aspirated osseous blood, Radiology **148:**69, 1983.
43. Johnston, A.D.: Pathology of metastatic tumors in bone, Clin. Orthop. **73:**8, 1970.
44. Kendall, P.H.: Needle biopsy of the vertebral bodies, Ann. Phys. Med. **5:**236, 1960.
45. Kirschner, M.: Die Probebohrung, Schweiz. Med. Wochenshr. **65:**28, 1935.
46. Lalli, A.F.: Roentgen-guided aspiration biopsy of skeletal lesions, J. Can. Assoc. Radiol. **21:**71, 1970.
47. Lodwick, G.S.: The radiologic diagnosis of metastatic cancer in bone in tumors of bone and soft tissue. University of Texas, M.D. Anderson Hospital and Tumor Institute, Chicago, 1965, Year Book Medical Publishers, Inc.
48. Martin, H.E., and Ellis, E.B.: Biopsy by needle puncture and aspiration, Ann. Surg. **92:**169, 1930.
49. Martin, H.E., and Ellis, E.B.: Aspiration biopsy, Surg. Gynecol. Obstet. **59:**578, 1934.
50. Matthews, L.S., and Braunstein, E.M.: A counter rotating power drill for needle biopsy, Clin. Orthop. **184:**217, 1984.
51. Mazet R., and Cozen, L.: The diagnostic value of vertebral body needle biopsy, Ann. Surg. **135:**245, 1952.
52. McLaughlin, R.E., et al.: Quadriparesis after needle aspiration of the cervical spine. Report of a case, J. Bone Joint Surg. **58A:**1167, 1976.
53. Mechlin, M., et al.: Magnetic resonance imaging of post-operative patients with metallic implants, A.J.R. **143:**1281, 1984.
54. Michele, A.A., and Krueger, F.J.: Vertebral body trephine biopsy, Public Health Rep. **62:**1166, 1947.
55. Michele, A.A., and Krueger, F.J.: Surgical approach to the vertebral body, J. Bone Joint Surg. **31A:**873, 1949.
56. Moore, T.M., et al.: Closed biopsy of musculoskeletal lesions, J. Bone Joint Surg. **61:**375, 1979.
57. Murphy, W.A., et al.: Percutaneous skeletal biopsy 1981—a procedure for radiologists—results, review, and recommendations, Radiology **139:**545, 1981.
58. Najjur, T.A., and Gaston, G.W.: Biopsy technique for fibro-osseous and osteolytic lesions of the jaws, Oral Surg. **44:**177, 1977.
59. New, P.F.J., et al.: Potential hazards and artifacts of ferromagnetic and non-ferromagnetic surgical and dental materials and devices in nuclear magnetic resonance imaging, Radiology **147:**139, 1983.
60. Nordenström, B.: Percutaneous biopsy of vertebrae and ribs, Acta Radiol. [Diagn.] **11:**113, 1971.
61. Ottolenghi, C.E.: Diagnosis of orthopaedic lesions by aspiration biopsy, J. Bone Joint Surg. **37A:**443, 1955.
62. Ottolenghi, C.E.: Aspiration biopsy of the spine: technique for the thoracic spine and results of twenty-eight biopsies in the region and overall results of 1050 biopsies of other spinal segments, J. Bone Joint Surg. **51A:**1531, 1969.
63. Ottolenghi, C.E., et al.: Aspiration biopsy of the cervical spine: technique and results in thirty-four cases, J. Bone Joint Surg. **46A:**715, 1964.
64. Paterson, C.R.: Trephine biopsy of bone: technique and indications, Br. J. Hosp. Med. **9:**342, 1973.
65. Rabinov, K., et al.: The role of aspiration biopsy of focal lesions in lung and bone by simple needle and fluoroscopy, A.J.R. **101:**932, 1967.
66. Ray, R.D.: Needle biopsy of the lumbar vertebral bodies. A modification of the Valls technique, J. Bone Joint Surg. **35A:**760, 1953.
67. Robertson, R.C., and Ball, R.P.: Destructive spine lesions. Diagnosis by needle biopsy, J. Bone Joint Surg. **17:**749, 1935.
68. Schajowicz, F., and Derqui, J.C.: Puncture biopsy in lesions of the locomotor system. Review of results in 4050 cases, including 941 vertebral punctures, Cancer **21:**531, 1968.
69. Schajowicz, F., and Hokama, J.: Aspiration (puncture or needle) biopsy in bone lesions, Recent Results Cancer Res. **54:**139, 1976.
70. Schneider, R.: Percutaneous needle bone biopsy, Orthop. Rev. **12:**119, 1983.
71. Seyfarth, C.: Die Sturnum Trepanation, eine enfache Methode zur diagnostischen Entnahme von Knochenmark bei Lebenden, Dtsch. Med. Wochenschr. **49:**180, 1923.
72. Siffert, R.S., and Arkin, A.M.: Trephine biopsy of bone with special reference to the lumbar vertebral bodies, J. Bone Joint Surg. **31A:**146, 1949.
73. Sim, F.H.: Metastatic bone disease and myeloma. In Evarts, C.M., editor: Surgery of the musculoskeletal system, vol. 4, sect. 11, New York, 1983, Churchill Livingstone, Inc.
74. Southwick, W.O., and Robinson, R.A.: Surgical approaches to the vertebral bodies in the cervical and lumbar regions, J. Bone Joint Surg. **39A:**631, 1957.
75. Stewart, F.W.: The diagnosis of tumors by aspiration, Am. J. Pathol. **9:**801, 1933.
76. Tehranzadeh, J., et al.: Closed skeletal needle biopsy: review of 120 cases, A.J.R. **140:**113, 1983.
77. Turkel, H., and Bethell, F.H.: Biopsy of bone marrow performed by a new and simple instrument, J. Lab. Clin. Med. **28:**1246, 1943.
78. Valls, J., et al.: Aspiration biopsy in diagnosis of lesions of vertebral bodies, J.A.M.A. **136:**376, 1948.
79. Warren, S., and Meissner, W.A.: Neoplasms. In Anderson, W.A.D., editor: Pathology, ed. 5, St. Louis, 1966, The C.V. Mosby Co.

PART II

MEDICAL THERAPY

CHAPTER 5

IRRADIATION FOR BONE METASTASES

As noted in Chapter 1, there were 910,000 new cases of cancer reported in the United States in 1985, of which 120,000 were breast cancers. Approximately 7,000,000 patients are living with cancer metastases, and more than half of these have had metastases to bone. Although their disease may be controllable for variable lengths of time, only in the rare situation of a solitary metastasis is the condition curable. Consequently, the primary objective of treatment for the great majority of patients with bone metastases is the relief of pain, and irradiation is the most effective means of achieving this. Johnson et al.[15] reviewed a 12-year experience in the management of osseous metastases from breast cancer. They noted that the frequency of bone pain relief as a function of treatment was 73% for irradiation, 46% for adrenocorticosteroid therapy, 37% for chemotherapy, and 30% for hormonal manipulation.

The largest segment of the radiation oncologist's practice is directed toward palliative control of bone pain. Because such treatment rarely is curative, and generally has little if any influence on the overall duration or ultimate course of the disease, it should be designed to give the maximum benefit with the least morbidity and the easiest logistics.

The common practice of treating painful bone lesions with increments of several hundred centigrays* daily over a number of weeks recently has been reassessed. As we shall see in this chapter, many radiation oncologists have been active in evaluating shorter overall protraction with higher incremental doses. The reduction in time expenditure by the physician and the technologist (plus the machine time) is an obvious economic advantage. The reduction in hospitalization and patient transportation is both an economic and a humanitarian gain.

Unfortunately, however, the problem is not so simple as merely to say the shorter and easier the therapy the better. Some patients have tumor metastases that are relatively radioresistant (Table 5-1). Patients with lung metastases, for example, enjoy good to excellent pain relief only about one quarter of the time whereas those with pain from myeloma, lymphoma, or breast, colon, or prostate metastases can look forward to pain relief approximately 75% of the time. Often patients with widespread bone metastases cannot tol-

*A centigray (cGy) is the currently accepted term for radiation absorbed dose (rad).

TABLE 5-1 **Percentage Response to Treatment by Primary Tumor**

Site	Good or Excellent	Fair	None
Breast	73	17	10
Lung	28	28	44
Colon	75	—	25
Prostate	67	11	22
Other	88	6	6

erate intense wide-field irradiation because their hematopoietic system may already be depleted by their disease or by ancillary chemotherapy. Patients in whom bone metastases develop within an already irradiated field usually cannot be reirradiated unless their life expectancy is quite brief because of the risks to skin or soft tissues less resilient than bone to the devascularizing effects of irradiation. As this chapter will demonstrate, there is some evidence that short-term intense irradiation, although as effective as long-term treatment in achieving pain relief, is associated with a higher incidence of late recurrence of tumor foci, pain, and the need for re-treatment.

PRINCIPLES OF RADIOBIOLOGY

Prior to 1950 most radiation therapy was administered using orthovoltage equipment with beam energies in the range of 100 to 400 kV. A theoretical advantage of this was that within the energy range there was an increased radiation absorption in bone as compared to surrounding soft tissue structures. However, tumor dosages and the consequent efficacy of treatment were severely limited by the poor tolerance of skin at these low energy levels. With the advent of cobalt-60 teletherapy units and later of high-peak (up to 35 MeV) linear accelerator units, higher doses of radiation could be delivered safely to deep-lying structures such as bone without major limitations from skin and soft tissues. For more superficial bone structures, such as ribs, orthovoltage radiation may still be appropriate.

There has been a revival of interest in the use of radiation sources introduced into tissues (interstitial) or body cavities (intracavitary). This interest has been generated, in part, by the development of radioactive isotopes (i.e., iridium-192 and iodine-125) that can be used in highly adaptable, flexible, custom-made applicators. Such clinical use, which usually requires an operative procedure, can deliver very focal radiation doses that are relatively high compared to the doses inadvertently received by the surrounding normal tissues.

Radiosensitivity is a measure of susceptibility to injury by ionizing radiations. This injury may be lethal to the cell by interrupting its capacity to replicate indefinitely (reproductive death) or through metabolic incapacitation. Radioresistance is the reciprocal of radiosensitivity and therefore is relative rather than absolute. These terms are frequently misused in clinical oncology because of the misconception that the rate of gross reduction in size of the tumor is a measure of the effectiveness of irradiation. Such gross response depends not only on cellular susceptibility to damage but also on other factors, such as the rate of clearance of dead cells and the proportion of intercellular components.

It has been demonstrated[17] that interference with the blood supply of a radiosensitive tissue diminishes its radiosensitivity. Whether the radiosensitivity of the tumor cells is actually altered or not, inadequate blood supply (resulting from edema, atrophy, previous surgical interventions, or previous irradiation) definitely lessens the radiocurability of an otherwise amenable tumor. Laboratory studies have shown that normal and malignant cells are similar in most regards. Their greatest sensitivity is during mitosis and their least is during the period of DNA synthesis. Between sequential applications or fractions of ionizing radiations, separated by several hours or more, there is repair of sublethal damage, with duplication of undamaged tumor cells and consequent partial repopulation of the cancer. Whereas normal tissues are considered to be uniformly well oxygenated, tumors have a certain proportion of cells (perhaps as large as 20%) that are hypoxic. Reduction in the proportion of oxygenated cells improves the proximity of the hypoxic cells to their vascular supply, allowing an improvement in their oxygenation and a consequent increase in their radiosensitivity.[17] This phenomenon of increased radiosensitivity with cell recovery became the basis of the protracted fractionation method of treatment adopted in the 1930s.

PRETREATMENT EVALUATION

Before the initiation of radiotherapy, it is essential that the accuracy of the diagnosis and the scope of the malignancy be carefully assessed. On occasion, there is pressure from a patient, his or her family, and/or the physician to irradiate an inoperable, unbiopsied, presumed (but often undiagnosed) lesion for the sake of the psychological benefits such efforts may afford all involved. Obviously such a course is ill-considered, and the short- or long-term ill effects almost always overbalance any possible emotional boost. In addition, the possibility that the alleged metastasis may actually be a benign anomaly, such as an area of pagetoid bone, fibrous dysplasia, or even infection, cannot be excluded in the absence of a biopsy, except in patients with a well-documented and previously histologically confirmed metastasis. As demonstrated in Fig. 9-1, *C*, sclerotic or lytic defects and even a pathological fracture may occur in previously irradiated bones with areas radiographically suggestive of recurrent metastases. Not infrequently, such areas may in reality represent regions of progressive radiation osteitis or osteonecrosis, with the fracture being the result of irradiation rather than an indication for further treatment. Once such a bone lesion has been misdiagnosed as a metastasis and subjected to a course of irradiation, that diagnosis becomes effectively established and legitimized and the patient's future course of medical treatment, perhaps including hormonal manipulations, chemotherapies, etc., may depend on that error. Consequently, in almost every questionable case, a biopsy of a suspicious bone lesion should be performed, often by percutaneous trocar (Chapter 4). Histological identification of tumor type and assessment of tumor cell activity within a particular tumor type (grading) are useful pretherapeutic predictors of biological behavior. However, such evidence is a poor predictor of radioresponsiveness or radiocurability.

If metastasis to bone is confirmed, it is important to determine whether it is as a solitary tumor or whether multiple lesions are present. Patients with a single bone metastasis often are candidates for an aggressive treatment course, perhaps including surgical excision as well as irradiation, in an effort to effect a cure. When palliation becomes the obvious goal, the aim of irradiation changes to local control of pain rather than permanent tumor ablation. The most sensitive diagnostic modality for separating patients with a solitary metastasis from those with multiple lesions is the bone scan, using technetium-99m phosphate. Comparison with previous bone scans often is valuable in helping to differentiate between benign lesions, sequelae of prior irradiation or surgery, and new metastatic foci. On occasion, CT scanning or MR imaging may be necessary to define the extent of paraosseous soft tissue masses and the relationship of bony metastatic foci to major vessels, the spinal cord, or the bowel or bladder. CT scanning may also be helpful in tumor localization and biopsy trocar placement during the establishment of a histological diagnosis.

Hortobagyi et al.[13] attempted to clarify which diagnostic studies are most accurate in determining objective responses to radiation over and above a patient's clinical response. They discovered that although the bone scan was more sensitive in reflecting the presence of bone metastases it was less specific than plain or CT-directed roentgenography in demonstrating improvement after irradiation. There was concordance between clinical and radiographic findings, indicative of either improvement or progression of metastatic disease, in 80% to 90%, but between scan and clinical findings this dropped to only 55% to 72%. Alkaline phosphatase (AP) levels were obtained serially before and after radiotherapy and in general showed a gradual decline in patients who responded clinically to treatment. However, the pattern was inconsistent from one patient to another and had little prognostic value. Serial lactic dehydrogenase concentrations could not be correlated with either clinical or radiographic findings. Serial carcinoembryonic antigen (CEA) levels consistently reflected the clinical course and were much the most accurate laboratory prognosticator of patient response.

On the basis of this study, Hortobagyi et al.[13] recommended the following approach for optimum detection of osseous metastases and monitoring response to therapy in patients with metastatic breast cancer:

1. Baseline evaluation of all patients should include roentgenographic and scintigraphic bone surveys and a determination of alkaline phosphatase and CEA levels.
2. If all baseline tests are normal, then periodic surveillance (every 3 mo) of AP and CEA levels and a bone scan are adequate. If skeletal pain develops without bone scan abnormalities, roentgenographic evaluation of apparently involved areas will be needed.
3. If the initial bone scan is positive and

roentgenograms are negative, then repeat bone scans and roentgenograms of areas found to be abnormal by bone scan, along with the biochemical tests, should be performed every 2 to 3 months.

4. If the initial bone scan is negative and roentgenograms are positive, then serial roentgenography should be utilized.
5. If both the initial scan and the roentgenograms are positive, roentgenography is the method of choice for evaluating response to therapy.
6. When progressive disease or new osseous lesions are believed to have developed, a roentgenogrpahic skeletal survey including all symptomatic areas should be obtained. If this is inadequate to explain the symptoms, a bone scan should be performed.

Although roentgenographic, scintigraphic, and laboratory evaluations are helpful in following a patient's response to treatment, the relief of bone pain remains both the main indication and the primary yardstick for measuring the efficacy of palliative irradiation. Consequently, several investigators[10,13,15,19] have attempted to analyze and quantify the components of that symptom (pain) to be able to assess their treatment protocols better. The Radiation Therapy Oncology Group (RTOG) pain rating system (box) reflects the importance not only of pain severity but also of pain frequency and the analgesic requirements for its control. In a randomized prospective study of 1016 patients treated for a primary indication of pain,[19] they demonstrated that both the pain score and the narcotic score before treatment were excellent prognosticators of the likelihood of relief after irradiation. Thus patients with an initial pain score or narcotic score of 9 were less likely to achieve partial or complete relief than were those with a score of 4 or 6. The site of the primary tumor also had a considerable effect on the frequency of pain relief. The site of the treated metastasis, however, had no significant effect on the rate of relief, nor did the duration of pain prior to treatment, the presence of prior internal fixation at the study site, or the use of steroid or chemotherapy treatment during the study period.

PAIN RATING SYSTEM (Radiation Therapy Oncology Group)

Measures
- Severity of pain at treatment site
  - 0, None
  - 1, Mild
  - 2, Moderate
  - 3, Severe
- Frequency of pain at treatment site
  - 0, None
  - 1, Occasional (less than daily)
  - 2, Intermittent (at least once a day)
  - 3, Constant (most of the time)
- Type of pain medication administered
  - 0, None
  - 1, Analgesic (aspirin, Bufferin, Anacin, Darvon)
  - 2, Mild narcotic (0.5 gr codeine, Percodan, etc.)
  - 3, Strong narcotic (1 gr or more codeine, morphine, Demerol, etc.)
- Frequency of pain medication administration
  - 0, None
  - 1, Less than daily
  - 2, Once per day
  - 3, More frequently than once per day

Score (Pain severity × Pain frequency)
Narcotic (Medication type × Medication frequency)

Modified from Tong, D., et al.: Cancer **50:**893, 1982.

TIMING AND DURATION OF IRRADIATION

An ongoing controversy rages within the radiotherapy community concerning whether short-term, high-increment, but low–total dose irradiation should be used for most patients with bone metastases or whether a long-term, higher-dose, multiple-fraction course is preferable. In general, those who advocate short-term therapy contend that it maximizes the promptness and frequency of pain relief while minimizing inconvenience and expense to the patient. Those who advocate long-course treatment protocols do not debate the promptness of benefit from short-term therapy, nor do they disagree that it is psychologically and financially preferable to a longer treatment course; however, they do contend that the incidence of late recurrence of pain and the need for re-treatment are much higher after short-term than after long-term therapy.

Short-Term Therapy. As already noted, the RTOG carried out a prospective randomized study[12,19] using pain relief as the parameter of success to determine whether a short- or a long-term protocol for radiation was more efficacious. They subdivided the patients into those with a solitary bone metastasis and those with multiple bone metastases, and they reported significant differences in the proportion of each group who experienced relief depending on the primary site of the original tumor (Table 5-2). The study population consisted of patients with a painful bone metastasis of the femur, humerus, pelvis, or dorsal or lumbar spine documented by roentgenograms and/or bone scan. In addition, all patients satisfied the following requirements: a pain or narcotic score of at least 4; an expected survival of at least 3 months; no prior irradiation to the study site; and no new cheomotherapy within 2 weeks of the start of treatment.

The results of the study with regard to relief of pain are summarized in Table 5-3. Approximately 90% of the patients eventually

TABLE 5-2 **Pain Relief with Treatment of Different Types of Cancer**

	Disease Characteristics		
Primary Site	**Solitary Metastasis (no./percent)**	**Multiple Metastases (no./percent)**	**Total (no./percent)**
Lung	49/34	139/22	188/24
Prostate	6/4	103/16	109/14
Breast	45/31	246/39	291/38
Other	40/28	127/20	167/22
Unknown	4/3	13/2	17/2
	144/100	628/100	772/100

From Hendrickson, F.R., et al.: In Weiss, L., and Gilbert, H.A., editors: Bone metastases, Boston, 1981, G.K. Hall & Co.

TABLE 5-3 **Patients Who Experienced Relief from Irradiation (Centigrays)**

	Level		
	Minimal (%)	**Partial* (%)**	**Complete (%)**
Solitary metastasis			
4050/3 wk	68/74 (92)	61/72 (85)	45/74 (61)
2000/1 wk	65/72 (90)	59/72 (82)	38/72 (53)
TOTAL	133/146 (91)	120/144 (83)	83/146 (57)
Multiple metastases			
3000/2 wk	153/167 (92)	143/165 (87)	96/167 (57)
1500/1 wk	127/143 (89)	121/142 (85)	70/143 (49)
2000/1 wk	138/155 (89)	126/152 (83)	87/155 (56)
2500/1 wk	129/148 (87)	114/147 (78)	72/148 (49)
TOTAL	547/613 (89)	504/606 (83)	325/613 (53)

Modified from Tong, D., et al.: Cancer **50:**893, 1982.

Note: In this table a patient is counted as experiencing relief if he ever reports improvement during the intrastudy or follow-up periods.

*Patients who did not have an initial pain score of at least 4 were not evaluated for partial relief.

TABLE 5-4 Irradiation of Multiple Bone Metastases

Patients	Treatment (cGy)	Percent Requiring Re-treatment*
132	3000/2 wk	8
108	1500/1 wk	18
119	2000/1 wk	13
113	2500/1 wk	14

*Most failures occurred within the first 12 months after therapy.

TABLE 5-5 Irradiation of Solitary Bone Metastases

Patients	Treatment (cGy)	Percent Requiring Re-treatment*
67	4050/3 wk	9
60	2000/1 wk	22

*Most failures occurred within the first 12 months after therapy.

TABLE 5-6 Equivalent Doses Necessary to Produce Skin Desquamation

Treatments	Dose (cGy)	Total (cGy)
1	1400	1400
2	850	1700
4	500	2000
9	250	2250
16	150	2400

TABLE 5-7 Outcome Versus Time Dose Factor (TDF)

Dosage (cGy)	TDF	Complete Combined, Pain + Narcotic (%)
Solitary Metastasis		
270 × 15	78	38/69 (55)
400 × 5	48	25/68 (37)
Multiple Metastases		
300 × 10	62	72/158 (46)
300 × 5	31	48/135 (36)
400 × 5	48	59/147 (40)
500 × 5	67	39/137 (28)

Modified from Blitzer, P.H.: Cancer **55:**1468, 1985.

experienced at least minimal relief of pain, and 54% obtained complete relief. There was no difference between the two groups with regard to the degree of relief, but those receiving 1500 to 2500 cGy over 1 week enjoyed a significantly more rapid relief of pain than did those having a 2- or 3-week course of radiation. There also were no significant differences in the relapse rates among the various treatment groups, although follow-ups averaged only 2 months. The incidence of pathological fracture through the area irradiated was significantly higher in patients receiving 4050 cGy (18%) than in those who received only 2000 cGy (4%).

Many other authors* have reported generally similar pain relief results, but several[3,18] have also reported disturbingly high tumor recurrence rates (requiring re-treatment) in patients treated with short-term protocols and followed for many months. Schocker et al.,[18] for example, reported a linear increase in the percentage of patients requiring re-treatment as the dose of irradiation given and the time span for treatment decreased (Table 5-4). The majority of patients requiring re-treatment were those with osseous metastases from breast carcinoma (24%), reflecting the fact that the average life-span of these patients is considerably longer than of patients with other tumors. The difference between the percentage of patients with solitary metastases who required re-treatment after short therapy courses and those requiring re-treatment after long therapy courses was even more striking (as summarized in Table 5-5).

Long-Term Therapy. These relatively high recurrence and re-treatment rates for bone metastases managed by short-term therapy have prompted several investigators[3,7,18] to advocate the more conventional, higher-dose, longer-fractionation protocol (e.g., 2500 to 3000 cGy in 15 to 20 sessions) for patients with a prolonged life expectancy. Skin, lung, and gastrointestinal tolerance also is better after irradiation over such long periods with small fractionations (Table 5-6). Thus, not only is the likelihood of the need for re-treatment reduced but the tolerance of radiosensitive nor-

*References 1, 2, 6, 14, 18, 20.

mal structures is improved if re-treatment does become necessary. Certainly, if re-treatment is required for a lesion originally given a short concentrated course of irradiation, the re-treatment should be in small increments over a prolonged period.

Blitzer[3] also has raised the issue of whether the long-term pain relief afforded by concentrated irradiation is indeed equivalent to that afforded by conventional multifraction irradiation. By reanalyzing the RTOG data just discussed and by projecting survival courses after the completion of treatment, he demonstrated that *complete* and lasting pain relief improved in direct proportion to the duration of therapy and to the number of fractions administered (see box and Table 5-7).

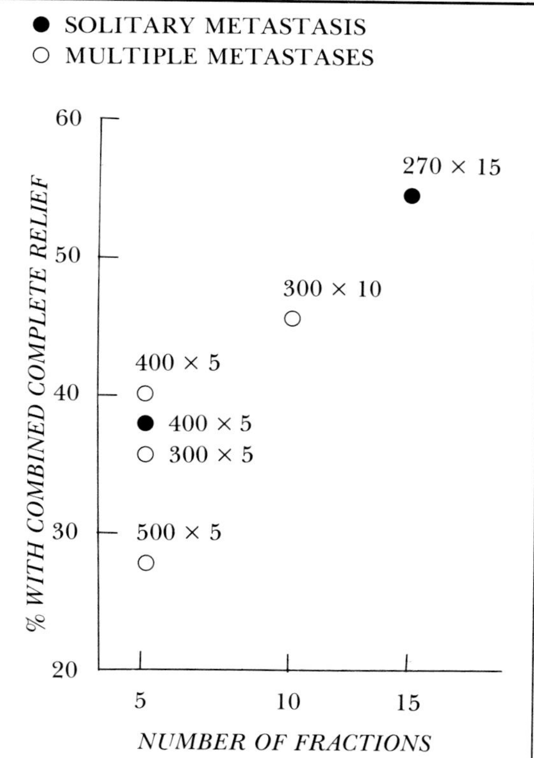

Number of fractions versus complete combined relief. Percent of patients achieving complete combined relief (both narcotic score and pain score falling to zero) plotted versus the number of fractions of irradiation for the solitary and multiple metastases groups. Next to each point is the dose per fraction (in cGy) times the total number of fractions. (From Blitzer, P.H.: Cancer **55:**1468, 1985.)

Hemibody Irradiation (HBI). Only 11 years after the discovery of x-rays by Roentgen, Dessauer (in 1907) made the first attempt at total body irradiation (TBI) using the so-called "x-ray bath" in an attempt to control pain in a patient with widespread osseous metastases.[8] The radiobiological rationale for this type of treatment was later established[5] by the observation that a single dose of 300 cGy has a cell lethality of perhaps 90% but 700 to 800 cGy has a lethality of 99.5% or better. Thus, if a tumor has a doubling time of 3 months, a remission of approximately 30 months might be anticipated following 700 to 800 cGy. For doubling times of 6 months or longer the equivalent remission might be even more significant, on the order of 5 years. Unfortunately, total body irradiation with 800 cGy is in the lethal range for bone marrow and cannot be tolerated. Subsequent investigators established that 500 cGy TBI in one treatment had a probable lethal effect of 90% but that a high-energy cobalt-60 source with 300 cGy was well tolerated, at least initially, with minimal morbidity. Even at this lower dosage, however, bone marrow suppression often was severe.

Then it was discovered that when 10% of the marrow was protected from the radiation hematopoietic recovery was possible. This observation led to an initial trial of hemibody irradiation.[9] The protocol for the technique presumed that with an appropriate interval between two half-body doses the unirradiated marrow could circulate and repopulate the areas that had been lethally irradiated. At the same time it is also rationalized that the more fixed metastatic cancer deposits would be less likely to migrate than would the labile bone marrow cells and that during the interval between the two fractions no appreciable reseeding of the cancer would occur. Obviously the patient with a slowly growing cancer would do better with this approach than would one whose tumor was more virulent.

The current protocol for HBI[8] involves arbitrary division of the body at the umbilicus into two half-body fields. A single dose of 600 to 1000 cGy is given, usually first to the upper half; then the lower half is irradiated after a recovery time of 4 to 6 weeks. The course is invariably associated with bone marrow depression after each half-body dose, with recovery generally occurring in 2 to 3 weeks. In addition, a wide variety of other sequelae may occur (summarized in Table 5-8). Potentially the most serious of these involves the lung parenchyma. Radiation damage results from microvascular endarteritis and alveolar cell damage. Acute radiation pneumonitis, characterized by increasing cough and dyspnea and with typical roentgenographic changes, develops in approximately 20% of patients, occurring at a mean of 100 days and proving fatal within 2 weeks in 84% of patients affected. Acute radiation sickness occurs in 90% of patients with HBI, beginning approximately 1 hour after therapy and usually lasting about 4 to 6 hours. This is manifested by nausea, diarrhea, anorexia, dry mouth, and change in taste.

In view of the multiplicity of sequelae and the potential complications of this technique, its use should be reserved for patients with very widespread bone metastases, severe and poorly controlled pain, and a limited life expectancy. Within that select and obviously debilitated group the results have been surprisingly good. In 100 consecutive patients with widespread breast cancer osseous metastases, 91% enjoyed complete or partial pain relief and two thirds of these had continuing benefits for at least half of their remaining life (Table 5-9). In terms of actual time, however, that period averaged only 3 months.[18]

Other Radiation Techniques. The availability of radioisotopes and hyperthermic perfusion has broadened the applicability of cancer radiotherapy.

TABLE 5-8 **Side Effects and Complications Following Hemibody Irradiation**

Area Affected	Sequela	Onset	Duration
Head and Neck			
Hair	Epilation	2 wk	12 wk (regrowth)
Parotid gland	Parotitis	8 hr	24-48 hr
	Dryness	24 hr	4 wk
Mucosa	Mucositis	3 wk	2 wk
	Herpes labialis	2-3 da	1-2 wk
Taste	Alteration	24-48 hr	4 wk
Upper Torso			
Digestive tract	Nausea, vomiting	50 ± 20 min	5-6 hr
	Diarrhea	2 hr	5-12 hr
	Esophagitis	1-2 wk	1-3 wk
	Anorexia	1-2 da	4 wk
Bone marrow	Depression	12-21 da	2-3 wk (recovery)
Lung	Pneumonitis	8-36 wk	1-2 wk (fatal)
	Erythema	24 hr	24-48 hr
Skin	Dry desquamation	3 wk	2 wk
Lower Torso			
Digestive tract	Nausea, vomiting	70 ± 14 min	5-6 hr
	Diarrhea		
	Acute	2 hr	5-12 wk
	Delayed	3 da	1-2 wk
Bone marrow	Depression	12-21 da	2-3 wk (recovery)
Bladder*	Dysuria	3 da	1-2 wk
Vagina*	Vaginitis	1-2 wk	2-4 wk

Modified from Fitzpatrick, P.J.: In Weiss, L., and Gilbert, H.A., editors: Bone metastases, Boston, 1981, G.K. Hall & Co.
*Rare

Intercavitary irradiation with radioactive isotopes has been mentioned earlier in this chapter. We prefer to use iridium-192 beads in flexible plastic catheters that are then placed within the bed of a resected tumor (Fig. 12-11, *E*). The local intensity of irradiation is approximately 30 times higher than what can be achieved by external beam methods although the depth of penetration of the source is only about 8 to 9 mm into the adjacent soft tissues.

Hyperthermic limb perfusion may occasionally be an effective adjunct to external beam irradiation. Heat both kills cells directly at temperatures above 104° F and alters cellular radiosensitivity. The hyperthermia is an attractive modality with ionizing radiation because it blocks radiation-induced sublethal damage and is not adversely affected by cellular hypoxia.[17]

The ability of ^{32}P to concentrate in growing tumors and bone metastases has been exploited in a number of patients, principally those with breast and prostatic cancer. Parathormone is used to produce a rebound deposition of radioactive phosphorus in bone. In the case of prostatic tumors, testosterone also has the capability of potentiating uptake.[21] The ^{32}P is given in a range of 10 to 20 millicuries in divided doses. The overwhelming majority of patients so treated enjoy an excellent response in terms of pain relief, such relief being more predictable with blastic than with lytic lesions. Unfortunately, most patients also experience fairly severe discomfort during the initial phase of treatment and usually demonstrate a transient hematological depression after the treatment.

TABLE 5-9 Overall Pain Relief Following Hemibody Irradiation in 100 Breast Carcinoma Patients

	Upper or Lower Half		Upper and Lower Halves	
Complete	11	(53%)	29	(91%)
Partial	13		21	
No benefit	11	(47%)	4	(9%)
Worse	5		0	
Unknown	5		1	
	45		55	

Modified from Fitzpatrick, P.J.: In Weiss, L., and Gilbert, H.A., editors: Bone metastases, Boston, 1981, G.K. Hall & Co.

COMPLICATIONS OF IRRADIATION

As reviewed in Table 5-8, a wide variety of minor and transient complications can occur after hemibody irradiation for osseous metastases. The incidence and severity of these are directly related to the size of the radiation field and the dose administered at any sitting.

The serious complications of severe and even fatal pneumonitis and irreversible hematopoietic depression can be avoided. The sequelae of radiation myelopathy, bowel stenosis, and laryngeal stenosis are quite rare following bone irradiation and generally are avoidable if areas are not reirradiated or radiation fields allowed to overlap. The complications of osteonecrosis, radiation osteitis, and pathological fracture are not common, but their incidence is difficult to predict and they are therefore less easily avoided.

Osteonecrosis after prophylactic or postoperative irradiation of femoral head and neck lesions occurs in approximately 5% of cases. Its incidence is not directly related to radiation dosage or to the schedule of administration. Presumably the complication occurs because of radiation vasculitis and secondary vascular obstruction in the end-arterioles of the femoral head. Proximal femoral replacement is the only reasonable way of managing osteonecrosis if collapse of bone occurs.

Radiation osteitis also occurs as a result of devascularization of bone; but, in addition, it can result directly from radiation-induced osteoblast and osteocyte necrosis. When severe, the bone becomes brittle because of osteoclastic resorption of dead lamellae. As already noted, the changes perceived roentgenographically may be confused with those of recurrent metastatic disease. Differentiation obviously is essential; osteitis precludes, recurrence may call for, further irradiation. Whereas ordinary bone is relatively radioresistant, necrosis, fracture, and infection begin to occur at dose levels between 7000 and 8000 cGy. Osteocytes and blood vessel endothelial cells apparently cannot proliferate on demand at as high a rate as the stem cells in the bone marrow and intestine. Even if the osteocytes were capable of division after intense irradiation, changes in vasculature and stroma in the haversian canals would impede the transport of oxygen and other vital nutrients.

It is more important to recognize in the treatment of large tumors that, when the recommended tumoricidal dose approximates 7000 cGy, the risk of bone injury is high. The probability of bone injury can be especially high if the tumor is surrounded by bony structures (e.g., a T_4 carcinoma of the oral cavity). In this situation bone usually receives the same dose as the tumor. Occasionally, however, a small segment of bone may receive an even higher dose than the tumor; and, it has been shown,[4] radiation injury may frequently develop from a small localized area receiving such a dose. For this reason other types of treatment (e.g., surgery or chemotherapy) should be considered in conjunction with radiation of such bone-enclosed tumors to permit the use of lower radiation doses. In doing this, one must be careful that the chemotherapy or surgery does not also lower the threshold of normal tissues to radiation injury.

At lower doses, and particularly in the 3000 to 4000 cGy range, bone has an excellent potential for recovery. The reparative process following radiation therapy has been summarized by Matsubayashi.[16] In his study bone specimens obtained at autopsy were used to evaluate the histopathological effect of irradiation, and the results were correlated clinically with roentgenograms of living patients. The reparative process involves several steps—first degeneration and necrosis of the cancer cells occurs, followed by replacement with fibrous tissue; collagen fibers then aggregate within the loose fibrous stroma, which contains a rich blood supply; these fluffy strands of aggregated collagen fibers become calcified and mineralized, and through this process woven bone trabeculae are formed and there is osteoblastic recovery; finally, the woven bone structure matures and is replaced by lamellar bone.

The incidence of radiation-induced sarcomas is very rare in the modern age of cobalt-60 teletherapy and other megavolt devices. When this complication does occur, it appears many years after the irradiation and, consequently, is of little concern in the palliative treatment of patients with bone metastases.

As described in Chapters 8 through 12, pathological fracture can occur through irradiated bone despite, or even because of, the irradiation. In most instances there has been sufficient destruction of bone before irradiation commenced that a pathological fracture develops in spite of the irradiation and before bone repair can begin (Fig. 11-9, *C* to *E*). However, it must be recognized that during the initial phase of radiation therapy (usually in the first 10 da of a conventional 4-to-5-week 4500 cGy course), a hyperemic softening of bone occurs that actually increases the risk of pathological fracture temporarily. Occasionally this effect may be quite pronounced, particularly in the periacetabular bone, producing a marked softening and then a protrusio deformity of the affected bone (Fig. 9-3, *A* and *B*). This hyperemic effect should be anticipated in every patient with an impending fracture and often is an indication for prophylactic internal fixation of the affected bone before a course of radiation therapy is begun.

Once a pathological fracture does occur, the proper sequencing of irradiation and internal fixation is somewhat controversial. On the one hand, many radiotherapists feel that preoperative irradiation is appropriate to reduce the risk of tumor dissemination by the operation or of local recurrence in the incision postoperatively. In my opinion, these risks are remote. In our series of 399 patients undergoing internal fixation for pathological long bone fractures,[11] only one patient suffered a local recurrence and she had been irradiated immediately postoperatively. Much more important is the fact that if an operative site has been irradiated within 2 weeks of internal fixation bleeding from bone and soft tissues often (but unpredictably) tends to be accentuated. Moreover, the likelihood of wound healing problems and infection clearly is higher if the tissues have recently been irradiated. For these reasons, I advocate internal fixation of actual or impending pathological fractures *before* irradiating the area. Ideally, a period of 2 to 3 weeks should elapse postoperatively to give the greatest assurance of uncomplicated wound healing.

CONCLUSION

The pathophysiology of osseous metastases involves the hematogenous deposition of tumor emboli in the bone or marrow capillaries. If the "soil" is acceptable, the deposit proliferates and destroys bone by both direct tumor invasion and the stimulation of bone osteoclast activity. In general, the rate of growth of metastatic foci is faster than that of the primary neoplasm. This may be related to the more aggressive behavior of a subclone of the original neoplasm or to a general reduction in the body's defense mechanism as the disease progresses. The local destruction of bone leads to a stimulation of the bone repair process, with the ultimate roentgenographic and isotope image being the net interaction of the two processes. The symptom of pain comes primarily from increased internal pressure on the periosteum and a structural weakness of the bone, particularly where weight-bearing is concerned.

Patient management will relate to the extent of disease and particularly the involvement of life-critical organs, the availability of effective systemic agents, and the severity of the local symptoms. With widespread disease or involvement of the visceral organs critical to life, systemic management is appropriate, particularly if effective agents are available. In many situations, local irradiation to the life-threatening site is also appropriate. With less extensive disease and particularly with significant localized pain or impending fracture, aggressive local treatment is appropriate.

How best to administer that treatment depends on the anticipated sensitivity of the tumor type, the extent of osseous metastases, and the projected life-span of the patient. At one end of the spectrum is the individual with a solitary metastasis from a lesion long ago controlled by surgical extirpation. Such a patient is best treated by local irradiation for cure (on average a 4-to-5-week course of 5000 cGy) followed by wide operative resection. Much more common is the individual with an extended prognosis and with several recognized but widely disseminated metastases but with only one of these lesions painful or at risk of pathological fracture. For example, many patients with disseminated breast cancer fit this description. To minimize the risk of recurrence and the need for re-treatment, this individual probably is best served by irradiation of the entire affected bone to a total dose of 2500 to 3000 cGy over a 3-week period. Next in order is the individual with widespread disease, with a limited life expectancy, and with a painful metastatic focus poorly controlled by chemotherapy or analgesics. For this patient local irradiation at the minimum dose necessary to relieve pain should give the optimum in symptomatic relief with minimal depression of the bone-healing capacity. A single dose of 400 to 600 cGy or briefly fractionated treatment to 1000 cGy may well be appropriate. Treatment with limited doses and limited volumes will permit re-treatment if ever necessary and if the patient survives long enough for this to be of concern. It also will preserve the maximum bone marrow tolerance for systemic chemotherapy. Finally, the unusual patient with a brief life expectancy and with widely disseminated painful osseous metastases should be considered for HBI. Although this technique is associated with a large number of transient complications, it may be the only effective means of affording reasonable pain relief during the person's remaining life-span.

REFERENCES

1. Allen, K.L., et al.: Effective bone palliation as related to various treatment regimens, Cancer **37:**984, 1976.
2. Ambral, A.: Single dose and short high dose fractionation radiation therapy for osseous metastases. In Weiss, L., and Gilbert, H.A., editors: Bone metastases, Boston, 1981, G.K. Hall & Co.
3. Blitzer, P.H.: Reanalysis of the RTOG study of the palliation of symptomatic osseus metastasis, Cancer **55:**1468, 1985.
4. Cheng, V.S.T., et al.: Osteoradionecrosis of the mandible resulting from external megavoltage radiation therapy, Radiology **112:**685, 1974.
5. Cunningham, J.R, et al.: A simple facility for whole-body irradiation, Radiology **78:**941, 1962.
6. Delclos, L., et al.: Palliative irradiation in breast cancer, Radiology **83:**272, 1964.
7. Dutreix, J.: Clinical and radiobiologic bases of concentrated irradiation for rapid palliation of bone metastases. In Weiss, L., and Gilbert, H.A., editors: Bone metastases, Boston, 1981, G.K. Hall & Co.
8. Fitzpatrick, P.J.: Wide-field irradiation of bone metastases. In Weiss, L., and Gilbert, H.A., editors: Bone metastases, Boston, 1981, G.K. Hall & Co.
9. Fitzpatrick, P.J., et al.: Half-body radiotherapy of advanced cancer, J. Can. Assoc. Radiol. **27:**75, 1976.
10. Gillick, L.S., et al.: Technical report no. 185R, final analysis RTOG protocol no. 74-02, Boston, May, 1981, Department of Biostatistics, Sidney Farber Cancer Institute.
11. Harrington, K.D., et al.: Methylmethacrylate as an adjunct in internal fixation of pathological fractures. Experience with 399 patients, J. Bone Joint Surg. **58A:**1047, 1976.

12. Hendrickson, F.R., et al.: Palliation of osseous metastases: preliminary report. In Weiss, L., and Gilbert, H.A., editors: Bone metastasis, Boston, 1981, G.K. Hall & Co.
13. Hortobagyi, G.N., et al.: Osseous metastases of breast cancer, Cancer **53:**577, 1984.
14. Jensen, N., et al.: Single dose radiaton of bone metastases, Acta Radiol. [Ther.] **15:**337, 1976.
15. Johnson, M.: Osseous metastases and mammary cancer, Arch. Surg. **101:**578, 1970.
16. Matsubayashi, T.: The reparative process of metastatic bone lesions after radiotherapy, Jap. J. Clin. Oncol. **11**(suppl.):253, 1981.
17. Parker, R.G.: Principles of radiation oncology. In Haskell, C.M., editor: Cancer treatment, ed. 2, Philadelphia, 1985, W.B. Saunders Co.
18. Schocker, J.D., et al.: Radiation therapy for bone metastasis, Clin. Orthop. **169:**38, 1982.
19. Tong, D., et al.: The palliation of symptomatic osseous metastases: final results of the study by the Radiation Therapy Oncology Group, Cancer **50:**893, 1982.
20. Vargha, Z., et al.: Single dose radiation therapy in the palliation of metastatic bone disease, A.J.R. **93:**1181, 1969.
21. Wizenberg, M.J.: The philosophy and economics of palliative radiotherapy for bone metastases. In Weiss, L., and Gilbert, H.A., editors: Bone metastases, Boston, 1981, G.K. Hall & Co.

CHAPTER 6

CHEMOTHERAPY AND HORMONAL MANAGEMENT

Steven B. Newman

Metastases to bone occur commonly with primary tumors of the breast, lung, prostate, kidney, and thyroid gland, and less commonly with tumors arising in the urinary bladder, uterus, stomach, colon and rectum, head, and neck[15] (Table 6-1).

The pattern of spread to bone is determined by the venous drainage of the primary tumor site. Prostatic carcinoma, for example, drains through the pelvic veins to Batson's paravertebral plexus and predictably metastasizes to the pelvis, femur, vertebral bodies, and bones of the skull. Primary lung tumors drain through the pulmonary arterial and venous circulation and tend to metastasize in a more generalized fashion.

The most common resulting symptom is pain, which can be incapacitating in and of itself. Bone destruction by a malignant neoplasm can also cause significant structural instability and adjacent tissue compression depending on the site. Such complications are almost always managed surgically or with radiation therapy as opposed to chemotherapeutic or hormonal agents.

In the past 20 years there has been a substantial increase in the use of chemotherapeutic and hormonal agents in the treatment of solid tumors. In some tumor types a significant benefit in symptom control, disease-free interval, and overall survival can be expected through the proper use of these agents. It is, therefore, critical to understand the available agents and their mechanism of action, indications for use, and expected side effects.

TABLE 6-1 **Incidence of Skeletal Metastases at Autopsy**

Primary Site	Percent
Breast	50-70
Prostate	40-80
Lung	30-60
Thyroid	30-50
Kidney	30-40
GI tract	5-15
Unknown	10-20

PRINCIPLES OF CHEMOTHERAPY

In 1898 Paul Erhlich described the first alkylating agents, thereby initiating the modern era of chemotherapy. Erhlich actually used the word "chemotherapy" in referring to drugs used to treat parasitic infection. In 1910 he completed synthesis of an arsenical salversan (the savior of mankind) used to treat trypanosomiasis.[30]

Alkylating agents were further developed for chemical warfare during World War II, and this led to the observation that exposure caused bone marrow and lymphoid hypoplasia. The alkylating agents were first used in humans with malignant lymphoma in 1943 at Yale University and the results (reporting transient remission) were published in 1946.[17] Table 6-2 illustrates the drugs developed since that time currently in clinical use.

Fifteen thousand new potentially useful agents are screened annually in rodents with transplantable tumors. Further testing is then done on 500 to 1000 of these compounds using human tumor xenografts in immune-incompetent mice and mouse tumor panels. Following approval by the Food and Drug Administration, toxocology testing is done to determine a lethal dose (LD) in 10%, 50%, and 90% of subjects tested. Human testing generally starts at 10% of the LD in rodents.

Four phases of human testing occur. Phase I trials are performed on patients with advanced cancer no longer responsive to conventional therapy and are designed to test toxicity and dose tolerance. Phase II studies assess dose response and the specific types of tumors that respond. Phase II is also performed on patients no longer responsive to conventional therapy. Phases III and IV are generally performed on previously untreated patients in a randomized controlled fashion to assess the agent in question as compared to standard available therapy. Drug testing from conception to marketing takes approximately 10 years in the United States.

Basic Biological Principles. The ideal chemotherapeutic agent would selectively kill tumor cells while sparing normal host cells. Cancer implies uncontrolled cell growth. In the early stages cancer cell growth is exponential. As the tumor becomes clinically palpable, single-cell growth remains exponential but the mass-doubling time progressively diminishes as the growth constant decreases. This is referred to as Gompertzian function.

For most chemotherapeutic agents there is a direct relationship between dose and cell kill, and for any given dose a fixed percentage of cells are killed. Assuming this in Gompertzian growth kinetics, it is possible to see that the smaller the tumor the greater will be the chance of response to chemotherapy. As the tumor mass gets smaller, the doubling time shortens and more cells become metabolically active (and therefore more sensitive to the effects of chemotherapy). Conversely, the larger the tumor the greater the likelihood of drug resistance. Since metastases are often smaller than the primary tumor site, they theoretically will be more sensitive to chemotherapy.[43]

Fig. 6-1 illustrates the cycle through which all dividing mammalian cells go during replication. This cycle and the biological principles just described can be applied to understanding the mechanism of action of the different classes of chemotherapeutic and hormonal agents.

Alkylating Agents. Historically the alkylating agents were the first group of nonsteroid

TABLE 6-2 **Chronology of Anticancer Drug Development***

Year	
1949	Nitrogen mustard
1953	Methotrexate, mercaptopurine
1954	Busulfan
1955	Chlorambucil
1959	Cyclophosphamide, thiotepa
1961	Vinblastine
1962	5-Fluorouracil
1963	Vincristine
1964	Melphalan, actinomycin-D
1969	Cytosine arabinoside
1973	Bleomycin
1974	Doxorubicin, mitomycin-C
1977	BCNU, CCNU (carmustine, lomustine)
1978	Cisplatin
1983	VP-16-213 (etoposide)

*Total number of anticancer chemotherapeutic agents FDA approved for use as of 1/1/86 = 36.

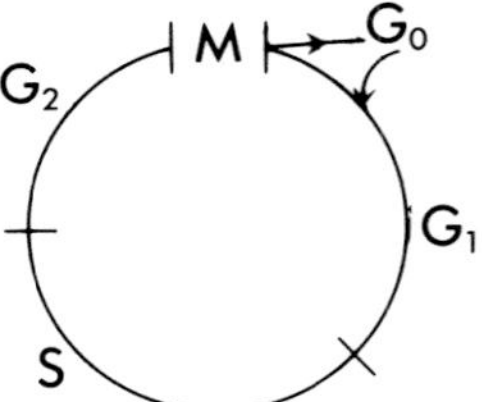

FIGURE 6-1 The cell cycle. *M,* Mitosis, cell division; G_0, No growth or cell differentiation, cell death: G_1 first growth phase, diploid DNA; *S,* DNA synthesis; G_2 second growth phase, tetraploid DNA.

compounds to show significant antitumor activity. As previously discussed, they were found to produce lymphoid aplasia and to cause regression of lymphoid malignancy in rodent models.

The antitumor effect is produced by the covalent bonding of an alkyl group to part of the DNA molecule, thus interfering with DNA function.[29] The no. 7 nitrogen of guanine is the most common site of alkylation (approximately 90%). Other sites include the no. 1 N of guanine, the no. 1, 3, and 7 Ns of adenine, and the 3 N of cytosine (Fig. 6-2). Alkylation of nucleic acids causes DNA breakage, misreading of the genetic code, and cross-linking.

Fig. 6-3 illustrates the conventional alkylating agents by structure. Side group substitutions can both change the bioavailability of the drug and influence the expected side effects. Of the classical alkylating agents, cyclophosphamide and melphalan are the two most likely to be encountered in regimens used to treat patients with bone metastases.

Also included among alkylating agents are the nitrosoureas (Fig. 6-4) and cisplatin.

The nitrosoureas are lipid soluble and are used mainly in the treatment of lymphomas, primary central nervous system malignancies, gastrointestinal cancers, and melanoma. For the surgeon, the most important point to remember in caring for patients treated with a nitrosourea is that delayed myelosuppression (4 to 6 weeks after therapy) occurs consistently. In addition, the effects and side effects are cumulative and more profound in patients treated concomitantly with other chemotherapeutic agents.

Cisplatin is a heavy metal compound that has gained wide clinical use in the past 10 years. In aqueous solution an activated and charged complex is formed that can attack nucleophilic sites on DNA or RNA and form covalent links in a manner similar to that of conventional alkylating agents (Fig. 6-5). Cisplatin can be curative in the treatment of testicular germ cell neoplasms and highly effec-

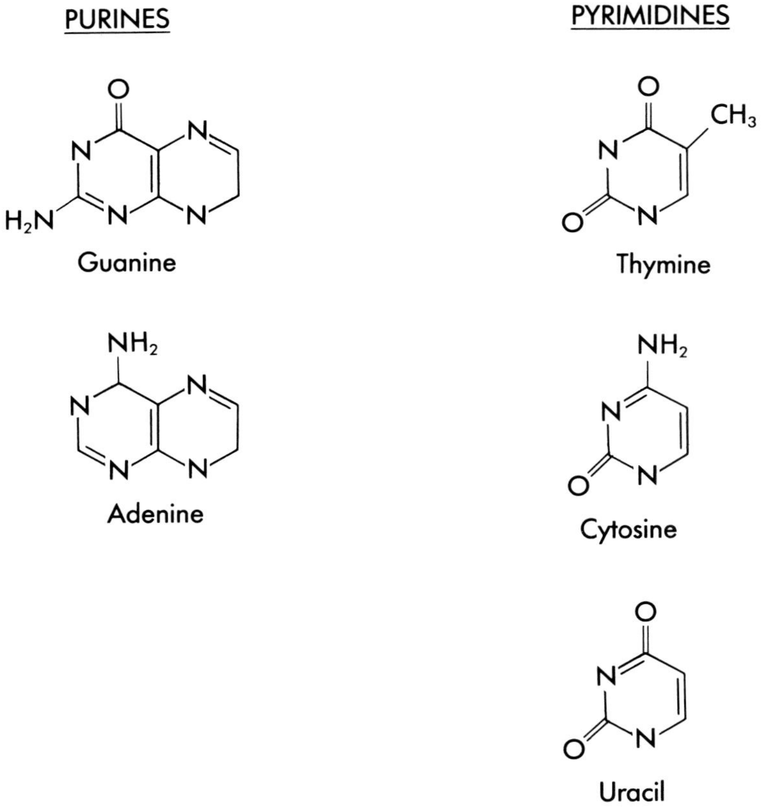

PURINES

PYRIMIDINES

Guanine

Thymine

Adenine

Cytosine

Uracil

FIGURE 6-2 Conventional alkylating agents.

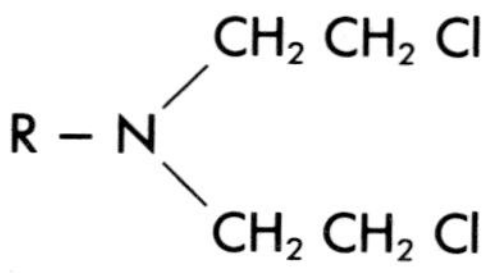

$$R-N\begin{matrix}CH_2CH_2Cl\\CH_2CH_2Cl\end{matrix}$$

R	
CH_3 —	Nitrogen Mustard
NH_2 / CH_2CH_2—(phenyl)— with C bearing NH_2 and COOH	Melphalan
HOOC $(CH_2)_3$—(phenyl)—	Chlorambucil
H_2C ring with CH_2—O—P(=O)— and CH_2—NH—P	Cyclophosphamide

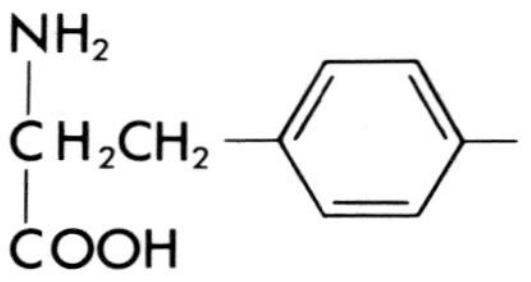

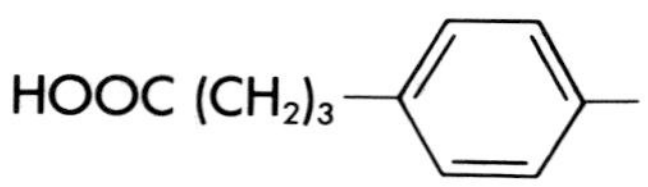

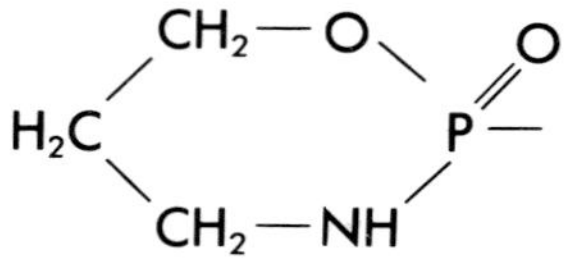

$CH_3OSO_2(CH_2)_4OSO_2CH_3$
Busulfan

FIGURE 6-3 Building blocks of DNA and RNA.

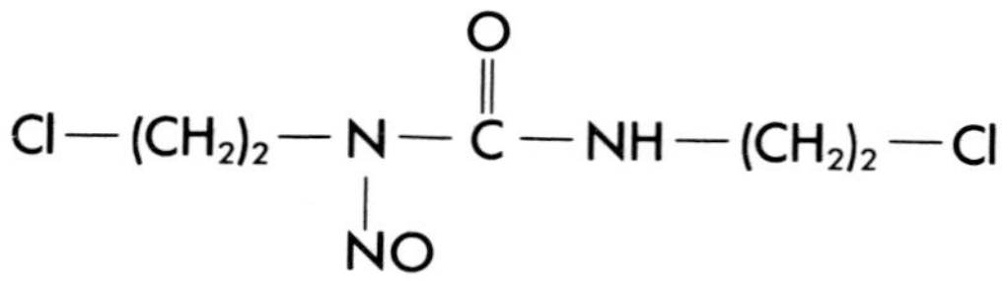

$Cl-(CH_2)_2-N(NO)-C(=O)-NH-(CH_2)_2-Cl$ Carmustine (BCNU)

$Cl-(CH_2)_2-N(NO)-C(=O)-NH-$(cyclohexyl) Lomustine (CCNU)

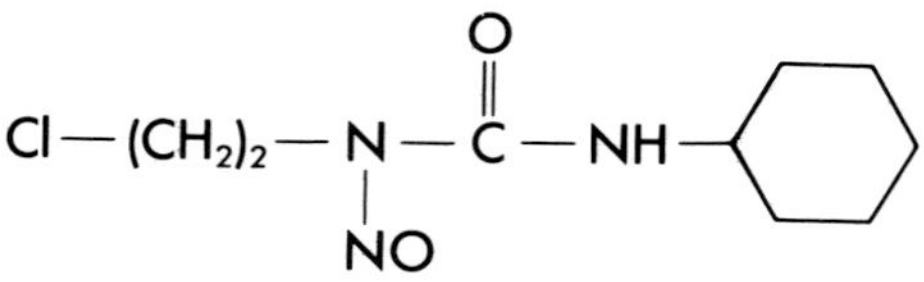

FIGURE 6-4 Chlorethyl nitrosoureas.

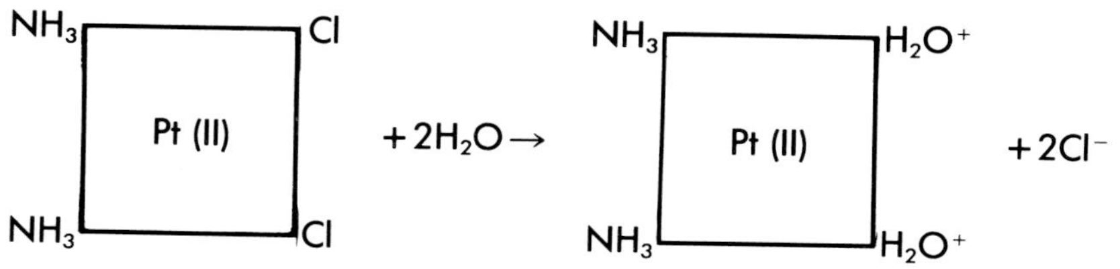

FIGURE 6-5 Cisplatin activation in aqueous solution.

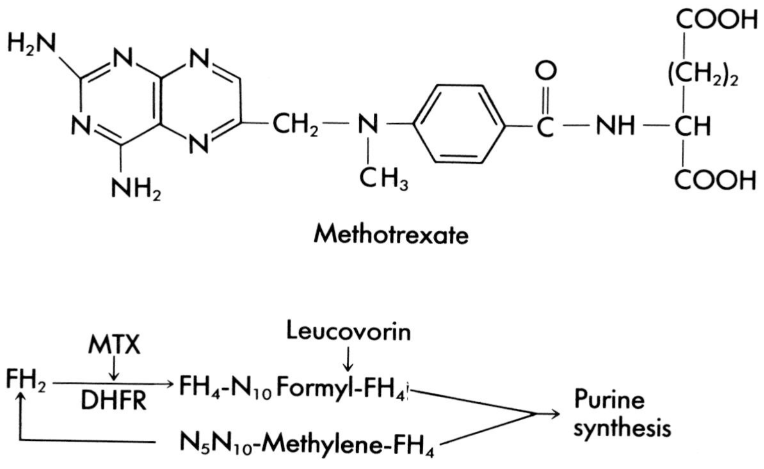

FIGURE 6-6 Methotrexate structure and site of action. *MTX,* Methotrexate; *FH_2,* dihydrofolate; *FH_4,* tetrahydrofolate; *DHFR,* dihydrofolate reductase.

tive in the treatment of disseminated transitional cell carcinoma of the urinary bladder and collecting system, ovarian cancer, head and neck cancer, and bronchogenic carcinoma.

Antimetabolites. Antimetabolites are agents with antitumor activity. They act as false substrates in the synthesis of DNA, RNA, and protein.

Methotrexate exerts antitumor activity by interfering with folic acid metabolism. Folic acid is responsible for 1-carbon transfers in purine biosynthesis. Methotrexate blocks the enzyme dihydrofolate reductase (DHFR), required to keep folate in the reduced state. DHFR is also necessary in maintaining thymidylate synthesis (Fig. 6-6).

In addition, high doses of methotrexate have been used with citrovorum factor rescue. This is based on the concept that methotrexate entry into cells is carrier mediated and the tumor cells do not transport the drug intracellularly as effectively as normal host cells do. When exceptionally high doses are used, methotrexate can be forced into the tumor cell by a concentration gradient. Leucovorin (N_5-formyl FH_4) (citrovorum) is then given in low doses and "rescues" the normal cells, which effectively transport the rescue factor as they would methotrexate, thereby leaving tumor cells with a lethal concentration of methotrexate intracellularly. This sequential treatment eliminates significant bone marrow toxicity and allows the drug to be given during times of myelosuppression. The technique has been used primarily in the treatment of lym-

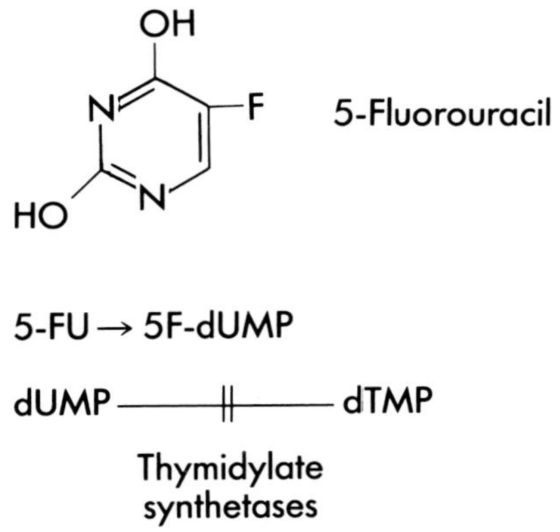

5-Fluorouracil

5-FU → 5F-dUMP

dUMP ——‖—— dTMP

Thymidylate synthetases

FIGURE 6-7 Structure and site of action of 5-fluorouracil.

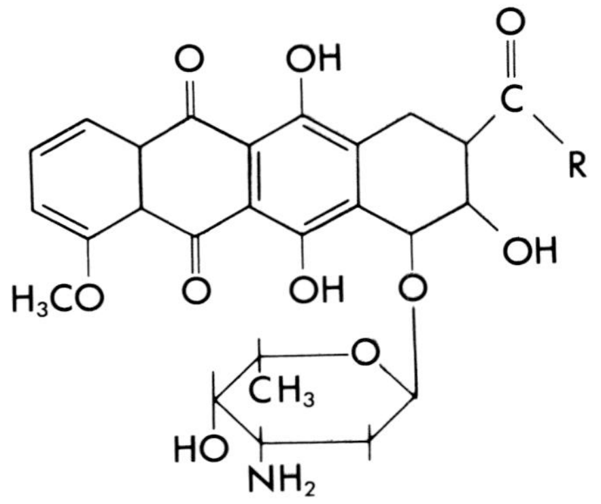

FIGURE 6-8 Structure of anthracyclines.

phoma, primary central nervous system tumors, and primary bone and soft tissue tumors.

5-Fluorouracil (Fig. 6-7) is a pyrimidine analog synthesized as a chemotherapeutic agent by Dr. Charles Heidelberg in the late 1950s. It is activated and incorporated into deoxyuridine monophosphate (dUMP) to make 5-fluoro-deoxyuridine monophosphate (5F-dUMP), which inhibits the enzyme thymidylate synthetase. Thymidylate synthetase is necessary for the conversion of dUMP to deoxythymidine monophosphate (dTMP) in pyrimidine and, ultimately, for the synthesis of DNA. 5-FU is active against primary gastrointestinal malignancies as well as breast, ovarian, and prostatic carcinomas. In recent years efforts have been made to increase the antitumor activity of 5-fluorouracil without increasing its toxicity. Continuous infusion (IV or IA) over 5 days, although technically feasible, has not been shown to be essentially more effective than weekly bolus injections. Whereas the described myelosuppression is somewhat less than with conventional use, the toxic effects on the mucous membrane (stomatitis, diarrhea) are comparable.

The other antimetabolites commonly used in clinical practice are cytosine arabinoside (pyrimidine analog) and 6-mercaptopurine and 6-thioguanine (purine analogs). These are effective in the treatment of hematological malignancies and are listed in Table 6-3.

Antitumor Antibiotics

Anthracyclines. The anthracyclines are produced by *Streptomyces peucetius.* Their basic structure is an anthraquinone nucleus with an amino sugar (Fig. 6-8). The most important mechanism of action of anthrocyclines is intercalation, whereby the drug inserts itself between base pairs in the DNA strands and lies perpendicular to the long axis of the double helix. The intercalation causes partial unwinding of the DNA helix, strand breakage, impaired DNA template formation, and therefore disruption of DNA, RNA, and protein synthesis.[35] These changes also account for the mutagenic and carcinogenic potential of the drug.

Another mechanism by which anthracyclines act is free radical formation.[33] The drug is reduced by the microsomal enzyme P-450 reductase to a semiquinone radical, which reacts with oxygen to form a superoxide. The reaction can take place on cell membranes, mitochondria, and submitochondrial particles, and the generated superoxide radicals cause oxidative damage to cell membranes and DNA. It is unclear how much this mechanism contributes to the antitumor effect of the anthracyclines. What is clear, however, is that the mitochondria-rich heart muscle can be easily damaged by superoxide radicals. There are studies[49] to suggest that free radical scavengers such as α-tocopherol (vitamin E) decrease pathological evidence of damage on exposure to anthracyclines.

Free radical formation has been identified as a cause of the cardiac toxicity associated with anthracycline use. Generally, cardiac toxicity falls into two categories: The first is acute, unrelated to cumulative drug dose, and manifests itself as atrial arrhythmias or supraventricular tachycardias, less commonly as ventricular arrhythmias or acute cardiac failure.[10] Acute congestive heart failure is thought to be due to a pericarditis-myocarditis with significant drop in the ejection fraction. The pathological changes are similar to those seen in chronic anthracycline cardiac toxicity; and, although the acute damage may leave a permanent defect in myocardial function, it does not necessarily predict the development of the chronic form of anthracycline cardiac toxicity. The second chronic anthracycline-related cardiac toxicity occurs in 1% to 10% of patients who receive greater than 550 mg/M^2 of the drug (450 mg/M^2 if there has been prior chest or mediastinal radiation therapy in excess of 2000 cGy* recent or remote). Patients at high risk of cardiac toxicity are generally over the age of 70 and have preexisting heart disease or essential hypertension or are receiving concurrent chemotherapy with cyclophosphamide or mitomycin-C. The incidence of toxicity increases linearly after these cumulative doses are exceeded.

The pathological changes seen in anthracycline cardiac toxicity are necrosis and vacuolization of the sarcoplasmic reticulum (SR).[6] The SR is a major site of calcium binding, which is critical in the control of myocardial contraction. In addition, there are direct effects on the uptake and release of calcium by the mitochondrial membrane.

Clinically the symptoms encountered are those of congestive heart failure. They can be assessed noninvasively by means of both echocardiography and radionuclide cardiography. The echocardiogram is used to measure ventricular volumes and fractional shortening in approximately 60% of adults. If the estimated fractional shortening is less than 30%, significant cardiomyopathy is likely to be present. Far more accurate is the radionuclide cardiogram, whereby ventricular volumes and ejection fraction during rest and exercise can be measured. A 15% drop in the ejection fraction from pretreatment levels, an ejection fraction of less than 40%, or a failure to increase the ejection fraction by 5% with exercise suggests cardiomyopathy. The most reliable studies for assessing a doxorubicin effect on the myocardium are cardiac catheterization and endomyocardial biopsy. Catheterization gives the full range of chamber pressures and the cardiac index. A resting cardiac index of less than 2.5 or an exercise index of less than 5 indicates pathological changes. An endomyocardial biopsy with a histological grading of vacuolization and necrosis correlates extremely well with the risk of congestive heart failure.[1,9]

Prevention of cardiac toxicity by prophylactic use of digitalis, histamine blockers, ubiquinones, and free radical scavengers such as N-acetylcysteine and α-tocopherol has been effective in animal models but not in human beings at the present time.[33] Weekly administration of low-dose (10 to 15 mg/M^2) doxorubicin as opposed to monthly standard dose injection (40 to 60 mg/M^2) has also been reported to lessen the incidence of cardiac toxicity.[47]

The treatment of cardiac toxicity is twofold. First is immediate discontinuation of the drug at the earliest signs of congestive heart failure (tachycardia, shortness of breath, unexplained cough, S_3 gallop). Second is administration of inotropic agents (digitalis) and diuretics. These measures will cause stabilization or improvement in some patients. Unfortunately, many cases are refractory to all measures and symptomatic congestive heart failure persists.

Bleomycin. Bleomycin is a complex polypeptide derived from *Streptomyces verticellus.* Its mechanism of action is by production of single- and double-strand breaks in DNA. This is mediated by free radicals produced by bleomycin-Fe(II) complexes. Cells appear to be most susceptible to bleomycin in the G_2 phase of the growth cycle. Prolonged exposure causes increased cell kill and DNA breakage; hence the rationale for long-term intravenous infusion (6 to 96 hr) or intramuscular injection. The most important side effects of bleomycin are fever, chills and rare anaphylaxis. These are not dose related and, for this reason, a one-unit test dose is often given before standard infusion or injection. The fevers and chills generally respond to acetaminophen and an antihistamine but may require meperidine or morphine sulfate. Anaphylaxis is treated in the usual fashion with epinephrine, airway protection, etc.

The most common side effect of bleomycin

*The centigray (cGy) is the currently used designation for radiation absorbed dose.

is a dose-related interstitial pneumonitis that ultimately results in pulmonary fibrosis, occurring in 3% to 5% of patients who receive less than 450 mg of bleomycin and at least 10% of those in whom this dose is exceeded. Significant risk factors include advanced age, chronic obstructive pulmonary disease, prior radiation therapy, and high-dose bolus injections (greater than 25 mg/M^2). The pathology is inflammation of the pulmonary arterioles with proliferation of alveolar macrophages. This results in pulmonary fibrosis and clinical changes of restrictive lung disease.

Roentgenographically the picture is one of interstitial infiltrates usually starting in the lower lobes. The roentgenographic changes may be subtle and may occur late in the clinical course. A gallium scan often reveals increased pulmonary activity. Pulmonary function studies show decreased diffusion of carbon monoxide (Dl_{co}), a reduction in lung volumes, and arterial oxygen desaturation. Although both corticosteroids and nonsteroidal antiinflammatory agents have been used to treat bleomycin pulmonary toxicity, there has been little success in reversing the fibrotic changes.[51]

Of special concern to the surgeon is the fact that patients who have been treated with bleomycin are at an unusually high risk of postanesthesia respiratory failure. Such patients are very sensitive to high concentrations of inspired oxygen, and are best managed with lower oxygen concentrations and with special care to avoid pulmonary fluid overload.[16]

Mitomycin-C. Mitomycin-C is produced by the fungus *Streptomyces caespitosus.* Its structure is depicted in Fig. 6-9. The mechanism of its action is uncertain; but it is thought to alkylate, cross-link, and cause single-strand breakage of DNA.[11]

Mitomycin-C causes delayed myelosuppression similar to that seen with nitrosoureas.

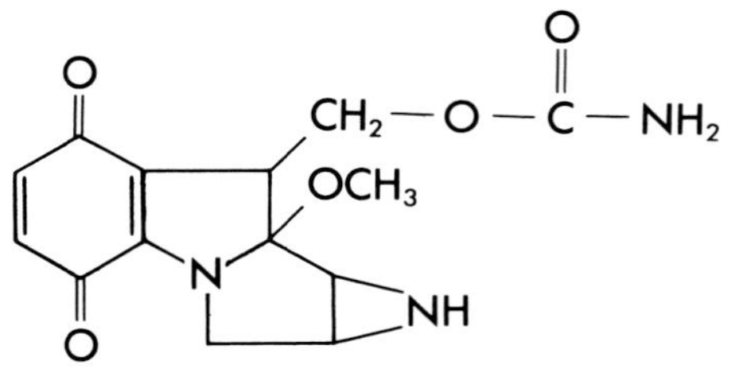

FIGURE 6-9 Structure of mitomycin-C.

The nadir occurs 4 to 6 weeks after administration. Reversible renal failure has been reported in patients receiving over 100 mg total dose of mitomycin. The drug is also thought to increase the risk of cardiac toxicity when given with an anthracycline. Recently a rare thrombotic thrombocytopenic purpura–like syndrome has been reported[19] with mitomycin-C administration. The outcome of this complication is usually fatal.

Mithramycin. Mithramycin is derived from *Streptomyces plicatus.* Although it has virtually no use as an antineoplastic agent, it is extremely effective in treating hypercalcemia associated with malignancy. This use is particularly relevant to patients with extensive bone metastases.

Mithramycin binds the guanine-cytosine base pairs in DNA. At high concentrations it can inhibit DNA-directed synthesis of RNA and protein. The hypocalcemia occurring with mithramycin is from inhibition of bone resorption through toxic effects on osteoclasts. There is a fall in serum and urinary calcium and a decrease in alkaline phosphatase activity. The hypocalcemic effect occurs within 24 to 48 hours and can be profound with associated tetany. Twenty-five micrograms per kilogram given once or twice weekly is usually adequate for control of hypercalcemia.

Side effects associated with mithramycin include thrombocytopenia, hepatotoxicity, renal toxicity, a severe hemorrhagic diathesis with abnormal platelet function, depletion of liver-dependent coagulation factors, and increased fibrinolytic activity similar to that occurring in disseminated intravascular coagulation.

Plant Alkaloids. Two classes of plant alkaloids are available for use as antineoplastic agents: the vinca alkaloids (vincristine, vinblastine, vindesine) and the epipodophyllotoxins (VP-16-213, VM-26). Both classes are used in the treatment of lymphoma, lymphoid leukemia, testicular neoplasms, and small cell carcinomas of the lung.

The vinca alkaloids exert their activity through binding to tubulin and disrupting mitotic spindle formation. The epipodophyllotoxins are thought to inhibit DNA-dependent RNA polymerase and nucleoside incorporation into DNA and RNA.

Vincristine causes very little myelosuppres-

TABLE 6-3 **Selected Major Antineoplastic Agents**

	Routes	Excretion	Acute Toxicity WBC	Plt	GI	Nadir (da)	Other Toxic Effects	Indications
Alkylating Agents								
Melphalan	p.o.	R	++	++	+	10-15	Secondary leukemia	Multiple myeloma, breast and ovarian cancers
Chlorambucil	p.o.	R	++	++	+	10-15	Secondary leukemia	Chronic lymphocytic leukemia, lymphoma, ovarian cancer
Busulfan	p.o.	R	+++	+++	+	15-20	Pulmonary fibrosis, secondary leukemia	Chronic myelogenous leukemia, myeloproliferative disorders
Nitrogen mustard	IV	R	+++	+++	+++	7-10	Vesicant dermatitis, secondary leukemia, neurological alopecia	Hodgkin's lymphoma, sclerosing agent for malignant effusions
Cyclophosphamide	p.o., IV	R*	+++	+	++	7-10	Hemorrhagic cystitis, alopecia, inappropriate ADH (unclear whether increased synthesis or heightened end-organ sensitivity), pneumonitis, secondary leukemia	Hematological malignancy; breast, lung, ovarian, and prostatic carcinomas; sarcomas
BCNU (carmustine)	IV	R	+++	+++	++	20-30	Pulmonary fibrosis, renal failure, prolonged myelosuppression	Multiple myeloma, brain cancer, lymphoma, melanoma, colorectal cancer
CCNU (lomustine)	p.o.	R	+++	+++	++	20-30	Pulmonary fibrosis, renal failure, prolonged myelosuppression	Small-cell lung cancer, lymphoma, brain cancer, colorectal cancer
Cisplatin	IV	R*	++	++	+++	10-15	Renal failure, neuropathy, hearing loss	Germ cell cancer, lung, head and neck, urinary bladder, prostatic, ovarian, and uterine cancers

*Requires dose modification with abnormal renal function.
†Requires dose modification with hepatic dysfunction.
Code:

p.o., Oral	WBC, White blood cell
IV, Intravenous	Plt, Platelet
IM, Intramuscular	GI, Gastrointestinal (nausea and/or vomiting)
SQ, Subcutaneously	0, Rare to none
IA, Intraarterial	+, Mild
R, Renal	++, Moderate
H, Hepatic	+++, Marked

Continued.

TABLE 6-3 **Selected Major Antineoplastic Agents—cont'd**

	Routes	Excretion	Acute Toxicity WBC	Plt	GI	Nadir (da)	Other Toxic Effects	Indications
Antimetabolites								
Methotrexate	p.o., IV, IM	R*	++	+	+	7-10	Stomatitis, diarrhea, hepatic fibrosis, renal failure, dermatitis, conjunctivitis, pneumonitis	Breast, lung, germ cell, uroepithelial, cervical, and head and neck cancers; hematological malignancy
5-Fluorouracil	IV, p.o. IA	R†	++	+	+	7-10	GI mucositis, diarrhea, dermatitis, photosensitivity, conjunctivitis, cerebellar ataxia	Breast, GI, uroepithelial, prostatic, ovarian, head and neck, and uterine cancers; sclerosis of malignant effusions
Cytosine arabinoside	IV	R†	+++	+++	++	7-10	Mucositis, cholestasis, neurotoxicity	Hematological malignancy, lymphoma
Antibiotics								
Doxorubicin (Adriamycin)	IV, IA	H,R†	+++	+++	+++	7-10	Stomatitis, alopecia, cardiomyopathy	Breast, lung, GI, and uroepithelial cancers, hematological malignancy, lymphoma, sarcoma
Actinomycin-D	IV	H, R*†	+++	+++	+++	7-10	Mucositis, alopecia	Germ cell tumors, choriocarcinoma, sarcoma
Bleomycin	IV, IM, SQ	R	0	0	0/+	—	Fever, dermatitis, pulmonary fibrosis	Squamous cell cancer, lymphoma, testicular cancer
Mitomycin-C	IV	R	+++	+++	++	20-30	Pulmonary fibrosis, pneumonitis, renal cumulative myelosuppression	GI and breast cancers
Mithramycin	IV	R*	++	++	+	7-10	Hypocalcemia	Hypercalcemia
Plant Alkaloids								
Vincristine	IV	H†	+	+	+	7	Alopecia, neurotoxicity	Lymphoma, lung and breast cancers, sarcoma
Vinblastine	IV	H, R†	+++	++	+	7	Alopecia, neurotoxicity	Breast cancer, germ cell neoplasm, lymphoma, choriocarcinoma
VP-16-213	IV	H, R†	+++	++	++	7-10	Alopecia, neurotoxicity	Lung cancer, lymphoma

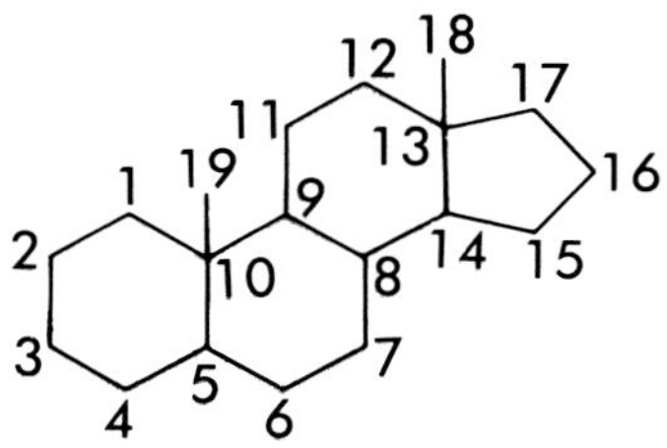

FIGURE 6-10 Basic steroid nucleus (cyclopentane-perhydrophenanthrene).

sion. However, because it binds the tubulin-rich neuronal axon fibers, it is associated with significant neurotoxicity. This can cause peripheral neuropathy (motor or sensory), autonomic neuropathy (ileus, urinary retention, orthostatic hypotension), or cranial neuropathy (diplopia, facial paralysis). In contrast, vinblastine, VP-16-213, and VM-26 cause severe leukopenia and mucositis and little neurotoxicity in standard doses (Table 6-3).

Steroids. There are five major classes of steroid hormones: cortisol, estradiol, progesterone, testosterone, and aldosterone. Four of these play an important role in cancer treatment.* All endogenous steroids are derived from cholesterol. The basic steroid nucleus is shown in Fig. 6-10. The adrenal glands synthesize and secrete all five classes of steroids. The testes and ovaries secrete androgens and estrogens respectively.

For the most part, steroids circulate bound to plasma-binding proteins. They are transported to a target tissue, which contains intracellular receptors. A hormone receptor complex is formed in the cytoplasm, undergoes activation, and then is transported to the nucleus. The precise effect of the steroid receptor complex on the cell genome is unclear. The complex binds DNA, causing mRNA synthesis. The translation of mRNA to different proteins mediates the ultimate steroid effect.

Glucocorticoids. Glucocorticoids are synthesized in the zona fasciculata of the adrenal cortex. Synthesis is controlled by pituitary adrenocorticotrophic hormone (ACTH).

*Aldosterone does not.

TABLE 6-4 **Major Effects of Glucocorticoids**

Physiological	Pharmacological
Increased glycogenolysis	Hyperglycemia
Increased glyconeogenesis	Decreased collagen formation
Increased protein catabolism	Impaired wound healing
Decreased protein synthesis	Volume overload
Sodium retention	Congestive heart failure
	Hypokalemia
	Antiinflammatory effect
	Immune suppression
	Proximal muscle weakness
	Decreased calcium absorption

TABLE 6-5 **Common Glucocorticoid Preparations**

USP Name	Trade Name	Dose (mg)
Hydrocortisone	Solu-Cortef	20
Prednisone	Meticorten	5
Methylprednisolone	Medrol	4
Triamcinolone	Aristocort	4
Dexamethasone	Decadron	0.75

Glucocorticoids travel in the peripheral circulation bound to albumin and cortisol-binding globulin (CBG). The bound corticoid is inactive but becomes active on dissociation to a free cortisol. The physiological and pharmacological effects and side effects of glucocorticoids are listed in Table 6-4. The commonly available steroid preparations are listed in Table 6-5. Glucocorticoids are most commonly used in the treatment of lymphoma, lymphoid leukemia, and myeloma and are occasionally used in the treatment of bone metastases from breast and prostatic carcinoma.

Androgens. Androgens are anabolic steroids synthesized primarily in the testes, and less in the ovaries and adrenal glands. Testicular secretion is under the control of the pituitary tropin luteinizing hormone (LH). Although 95% of circulating testosterone is protein bound, its effect is mediated by the free hormone. The effects of androgens are as follows: male sexual differentiation, initiation of spermatogenesis, male libido, male secondary sex characteristics (beard, voice, muscle mass), and an increase in red blood cell mass. In females these can cause ambiguous genitalia, clitoromegaly, hirsutism, precocious puberty, acne, and increased muscle mass when androgens are given in pharmacological doses. Androgens are used in the treatment of metastatic breast cancer.

Recently two antiandrogens have become clinically available for the treatment of metastatic prostate carcinoma, leuprolide and flutamide. They are analogs of luteinizing hormone–releasing hormone (LHRH), a hypothalamic peptide that controls pituitary LH secretion, and they significantly lower circulating testosterone levels by blocking LH-directed testosterone secretion. They compare favorably with both orchiectomy and diethylstilbestrol (DES) in the treatment of prostatic carcinoma but they lack the significant side effects of those modalities. (See later discussion of prostatic carcinoma.)

Estrogens. Estrogens are female sex hormones secreted by the ovaries and adrenal cortices. Ovarian estrogen synthesis is regulated by LH and follicle-stimulating hormone FSH. The physiological effects of estrogens are initiation and maintenance of the female genitalia and secondary sexual characteristics. Pharmacological doses can cause breast enlargement, darkening of the nipples, an increase in body fat, and the retention of sodium in female and male patients. Estrogens are used in the treatment of prostatic carcinoma and breast cancer.

Antiestrogens. Antiestrogens are nonsteroidal weakly estrogenic compounds that competitively bind the cytoplasmic estrogen receptor sites. Two drugs in this class are available: clomiphene, for stimulation of ovulation, and tamoxifen, for cancer treatment. Tamoxifen is used in the treatment of advanced estrogen receptor–positive breast cancer. Its side effects are those of estrogen deficiency and include nausea, hot flashes, atrophic vaginitis, dry skin, and visual blurring.

Progestins. Progesterone is synthesized in the ovaries and secreted by the corpora lutea. It is also synthesized in the adrenal glands, testes, and placenta. Its primary role is the maintenance of pregnancy. It also promotes the secretory phase of the endometrium and the proliferation of mammary acini. It is both antiestrogenic and weakly antiandrogenic. Naturally occurring progestins are not clinically useful in cancer treatment. Megestrol acetate (Megace), medroxyprogesterone (Provera), and hydroxyprogesterone (Delalutin) are active synthetic products; Megace is commonly used in the treatment of breast cancer and endometrial cancer, and less enthusiastically in renal cell carcinoma.

Aminoglutethimide. Aminoglutethimide is a potent inhibitor of steroid biosynthesis. It suppresses the converison of cholesterol to pregnenolone, which is the first step in the synthesis of adrenal steroids. The synthesis of cortisol, progesterone, testosterone, and estrogen is also affected. Because adrenal suppression is near complete, glucocorticoid and mineralocorticoid replacement is imperative. Expected side effects include lethargy, visual blurring, and skin rash, all of which resolve with adequate cortisol replacement and time. Aminoglutethimide has been approved for use in the treatment of breast cancer.

TREATMENT OF SPECIFIC TUMORS

The primary objectives of chemotherapy or hormonal manipulation in the treatment of patients with bone metastases are the palliation of pain and the maintenance of a high quality of life for as long as possible. Candidates for chemotherapy or hormonal treatment include patients with diffuse bone metastases with or without other organ system involvement. Patients with destructive lesions in weight-bearing bones or critical support structures often should be stabilized with local surgical and/or radiotherapeutic measures prior to consideration for systemic therapy.

Breast Cancer

Cancer of the breast occurs in approximately one out of every 10 adult women in the United States. There are over 100,000 new cases and 30,000 deaths annually from it. Important risk factors are prolonged unopposed estrogen stimulation (early menarche, late first parity), family history of breast cancer, and low-dose ionizing radiation exposure (10 to 1000 cGy). The relationship of benign breast disease and exogenous estrogen supplementation to breast cancer remains controversial.

The prognosis for women with breast cancer is related to the size of the primary tumor, the nodal involvement, the woman's menstrual status, the tumor estrogen and progesterone receptor activity, and the presence or absence of metastases. The most common sites of metastases,[20] documented in large autopsy series, are shown in Table 6-6.

The options for treatment of breast cancer with bone metastases include surgical stabilization of the bone, radiation therapy, hormonal therapy, and chemotherapy or some combination thereof. Indications for surgery and radiation are discussed elsewhere in this book.

Oophorectomy. Castration was previously the initial treatment of choice for premenopausal women with metastatic breast cancer. Using hormone receptors as a predictor, one can expect a 60% response rate in patients with hormone receptor–positive tumors treated by castration. Response rates are highest in patients with bone and soft tissue metastases and lowest in those with visceral metastasis. If successful, castration causes a response lasting 12 to 14 months. Response to oophorectomy predicts a 40% to 50% chance of responding to a second hormonal manipulation at the time of progression.[36]

Adrenalectomy. The rationale behind adrenalectomy in patients with breast cancer is to lower estrogen levels even further following castration; and, in fact, previous responders to oophorectomy show a 40% to 50% response to adrenalectomy. Bone and soft tissue metastases react better to adrenalectomy than do visceral metastases; thus this procedure should not be undertaken in a patient with liver, pulmonary, or central nervous system metastases.[13,42] Recently, medical adrenalectomy using aminoglutethimide has largely replaced surgical removal of the adrenal glands in the treatment of metastatic breast cancer. The mechanism of action of aminoglutethimide and its expected side effects have been described previously. Medical therapy has the same expected response rate and duration of response as does surgical ablation.[50]

Hypophysectomy. Hypophysectomy produces the same effect as adrenalectomy in hormone receptor–positive and postmenopausal women with metastatic breast cancer. A 40% to 50% response rate can be predicted from hypophysectomy as the primary treatment and a 40% response rate in previous responders to hormonal manipulation. One problem with hypophysectomy is incomplete ablation, probably explaining the slight superiority of surgical or medical adrenalectomy. In addition to corticosteroid and mineralocorticoid replacement, exogenous thyroid hormone is required after hypophysectomy.[24]

Hormonal Therapy. Observations of breast cancer growth patterns and potential hormonal dependency date back to the 1800s. In 1836 Cooper noted an increased growth rate of primary breast cancer in premenopausal women and decreased growth rate postmenopausally. Based on observations of Schinzinger in 1889, Bateson performed the first oophorectomy in 1896; and in 1900 Boyd reported a 35% improvement in patients undergoing oophorectomy for metastatic breast carcinoma.[8] Based on these early observations, modern approaches to the hormonal manipulation of patients with breast cancer have developed.

Hormone Receptors. As discussed earlier in this chapter, hormone receptors are specific proteins that bind a specific steroid and transfer it to the cell nucleus where it acts. In breast cancer tissue, the two specific measurable receptors are the estrogen receptor protein and the progesterone receptor protein.

TABLE 6-6 **Frequency of Breast Cancer Metastases by Site at Autopsy**

	Percent
Lymph node	60-75
Lung	60-70
Liver	55-65
Bone	45-75
Pleura	25-50
Adrenal gland	30-50
Skin-subcutaneous	25-35
Brain	20-25
Ovary	10-20

Each has an independent prognostic significance. The receptors are quantitated in femtomoles per milligram of tissue. For the estrogen receptor protein, less than 3 femtomoles is considered negative, 3 to 10 is borderline, and over 10 is positive. For the progesterone receptor protein, less than 5 femtomoles is considered negative whereas greater than 5 is positive. Approximately 65% of postmenopausal women are hormone receptor positive while only 20% to 30% of pre- and perimenopausal women have hormone receptors. Response to hormonal therapy based on estrogen and progesterone receptor proteins is shown in Table 6-7. Approximately 85% of patients with hormone receptor positivity in the primary tumor will have hormone receptor positivity at biopsied metastatic sites. Visceral metastases in general have the lowest estrogen and progesterone receptor protein values whereas bone and soft tissue metastases tend to have the highest values.

Estrogens. Until recently, congugated estrogens were the most commonly used hormonal agents in the treatment of metastatic breast cancer. In unselected postmenopausal women a 30% response rate is expected. In estrogen receptor–positive (ER+) females one can expect a response rate of 50%. The mechanism of action of additive estrogens in ER+ women is unclear because one would assume, at least theoretically, that they would enhance tumor growth. Nonetheless, receptor positivity predicts a favorable response to estrogen therapy.

Two interesting phenomena associated with estrogen treatment are the "flair" reaction and rebound regression. The former is an acute exacerbation of bone pain with or without hypercalcemia starting shortly after the initiation of treatment. The reaction generally predicts a favorable response. Treatment of symptoms should be undertaken while the estrogens are continued. Rebound regression refers to tumor response after the stopping of estrogen in a patient who shows signs of progression on treatment. As is the case with other hormonal maneuvers, a response to estrogen therapy generally predicts a 30% to 40% chance for a response to secondary hormonal manipulation after failure.[4,24,28]

Antiestrogens. Tamoxifen is the most widely used antiestrogen in the treatment of metastatic breast cancer. Expected response rates in unselected patients are 40%. Based on ERP and PRP values, significant responses to tamoxifen in patients with metastatic breast cancer can be predicted (Table 6-7). These rates are similar to the ones expected with ablative or additive treatment, but the minimal side effects of tamoxifen make it an attractive first-line agent. It can take 8 to 10 weeks to achieve a response; and, as with other hormonal maneuvers, bone and soft tissue metastases respond more favorably than do visceral metastases, lasting generally 12 to 14 months.[26]

A newer approach to antiestrogen therapy is the use of leuprolide. It has shown response in 40% to 45% of patients with metastatic breast cancer and may prove to be more effective than tamoxifen in premenopausal women. Its mechanism of GnRH antagonism produces medical castration rather than blocking of peripheral estrogen receptors. Results with this agent are strictly preliminary, and it has not been released for use in the treatment of breast cancer at the present time.

Progestational Agents. Medroxyprogesterone acetate and megestrol acetate are active agents in the treatment of metastatic breast cancer and show response rates, remission durations, and palliative effects similar to those achieved with estrogen or antiestrogen treatment. Progesterones can induce a response in up to 30% of previously treated patients.[38]

Androgens. Androgens are comparable to estrogens and progestins in the treatment of breast cancer with bone metastases. They are thought to be less effective in postmenopausal

TABLE 6-7 Predicted Response to Hormonal Therapy Based on Estrogen and Progesterone Receptor Status

Receptor	Percent
ER+ PR+	75
ER+ PR−	60
ER− PR+	40
ER− PR−	10

ER, Estrogen receptor protein.
PR, Progesterone receptor protein.
+, Greater than 10 femtomoles per milligram.
−, Greater than 5 femtomoles per milligram.

women or in women with soft tissue metastases and should not be given to anyone who has enjoyed a previous response to oophorectomy (presumably because of the secondary conversion of androgenic to estrogenic compounds peripherally).

Chemotherapy. Breast cancer is one of the most responsive of the nonhematological solid tumors to systemic chemotherapy. The prognostic factors predicting a response to chemotherapy are shown in Table 6-8. Single agents with reported response rates are listed in Table 6-9. The agents most commonly used alone or in combination are doxorubicin (Adriamycin, A), cyclophosphamide (C), 5-fluorouracil (F), and methotrexate (M). These agents appear to be non–cross resistant and can be used sequentially. The expected response rate is higher in previously untreated patients and lower in patients who have received therapy. The reported duration of response to single agents is 4 to 8 months. In contrast to hormonal therapy, single-agent chemotherapy is less effective against bone and soft tissue metastases than against visceral metastases.

In 1966 Greenspan[18] reported a 60% response rate in women with disseminated breast cancer treated by 5-FU, methotrexate, thiotepa, prednisone, and testosterone. In 1969 Cooper[12] reported a 90% response rate in hormone-resistant patients treated with cyclophosphamide, methotrexate, 5-fluorouracil, vincristine, and prednisone. Since that time numerous combination regimens have been used (Table 6-10). The critical points are that (1) combination therapy produces higher response rates and longer remissions than do single agents; (2) Adriamycin-containing regimens produce a higher objective response rate than do non–Adriamycin-containing regimens, but overall survival is comparable regardless of the program used; (3) alternating non–cross-resistant combination regimens does not appear to be superior to using standard CMF or FAC programs in either the

TABLE 6-8 **Prognostic Factors in Predicting Response to Chemotherapy of Breast Cancer**

Poor Response
Extensive disease
Poor performance status
Pancytopenia
Abnormal liver function tests
Low sodium albumin
Prior chemotherapy or radiation therapy

Favorable Response
Long disease-free interval
Good performance status
Dominant local disease

No Influence
Age
Menstrual status
Primary tumor size
Axillary node status
Family history

TABLE 6-9 **Response Rates to Single-Agent Chemotherapy of Metastatic Breast Cancer**

	Dose Range and Route (mg/M²)	Percent
Doxorubicin (Adriamycin)	60-75 IV q. 3 wk.	35-50
Methotrexate	30-40 IV weekly	30-40
Cyclophosphamide	300 IV weekly 100 p.o. daily	30-50
5-Fluorouracil (5-FU)	600 IV weekly	25
L-Phenylalanine mustard (L-PAM)	6 p.o. daily × 5 da q. 4 wk.	20-25
Vinblastine	1-2 mg/da × 5 da by continuous IV infusion q. 2-3 wk.	20-30
Vincristine	1.4 IV weekly	15-20

TABLE 6-10 **Combination-Chemotherapy Regimens in Metastatic Breast Cancer**

	Dose (mg/M²)	Response (complete and partial) (%)
Cyclophosphamide	100 p.o. da 1-14	50
Methotrexate	40 IV da 1, 8	
5-Fluorouracil	600 IV da 1, 8 (q. 4 wk)	
Cyclophosphamide	80 p.o. daily	50
Methotrexate	20 IV weekly	
5-Fluorouracil	500 IV weekly	
Vincristine	1 IV weekly	
Prednisone	30 p.o. daily × 5 da	
Adriamycin (doxorubicin)	40 IV da 1	80
Cyclophosphamide	200 p.o. da 3-6 (q. 3 wk)	
5-Fluorouracil	500 IV da 1, 8	65
Adriamycin (doxorubicin)	50 IV da 1	
Cyclophosphamide	500 IV da 1 (q. 4 wk)	
Vinblastine	2 mg by continuous IV infusion daily × 4 da	30
Mitomycin-C	10 IV da 1	

remission rate or the overall survival; (4) third-line therapy with vinblastine and mitomycin-C produces a 25% to 35% response rate in patients previously treated with a CMF or FAC program.[21]

Combined Hormonal Therapy and Chemotherapy. Combined-modality therapy in patients with metastatic breast cancer remains controversial. Theoretically a patient with ER+ and PR+ tumors treated with two effective modalities should enjoy an improved response rate and survival. The superiority of endocrine and chemotherapy together over endocrine therapy alone has been shown in selected studies.[25] However, others believe that tamoxifen decreases the number of cells going into the active cell cycle and, therefore, decreases the efficacy of chemotherapeutic agents. The latter effect is theoretical and has not been substantiated at the present time.

SELECTION OF THERAPY

A reasonable approach to patients with metastatic breast cancer who are candidates for systemic therapy is outlined in Table 6-11.

Breast Cancer in Men

Breast cancer in men is uncommon in the United States, and occurs at a rate of 1% of that seen in women. Factors predisposing to breast cancer in men are hyperestrogenemia, Klinefelter syndrome, and chronic gynecomastia. Prognostic factors are similar to those in women, as is the pattern of metastases. Initial treatment of metastatic disease is orchiectomy with an expected response rate of 50% to 60% reflecting the high percent of hormone receptor–positive tumors. Response duration is variable. In responders adrenalectomy (medical or surgical) is a reasonable second-line therapy. The systemic chemotherapeutic agents available to treat metastatic breast cancer in men are the same as in women, and the expected response rate, duration of response, and survival are similar.

Prostatic Carcinoma

Cancer of the prostate is the third most common cause of cancer death (after lung and colorectal cancer) in men in the United States; 75,000 new cases and 27,000 deaths are reported annually. The incidence in black males is approximately 1.6:1 over that in white males, and there has been little change in incidence over the past four decades. Bone is by far the most common site of metastases in prostatic cancer. Bone metastases are present in 20% to 30% of patients at the time of diag-

TABLE 6-11 Selection of Therapy in Metastatic Breast Cancer

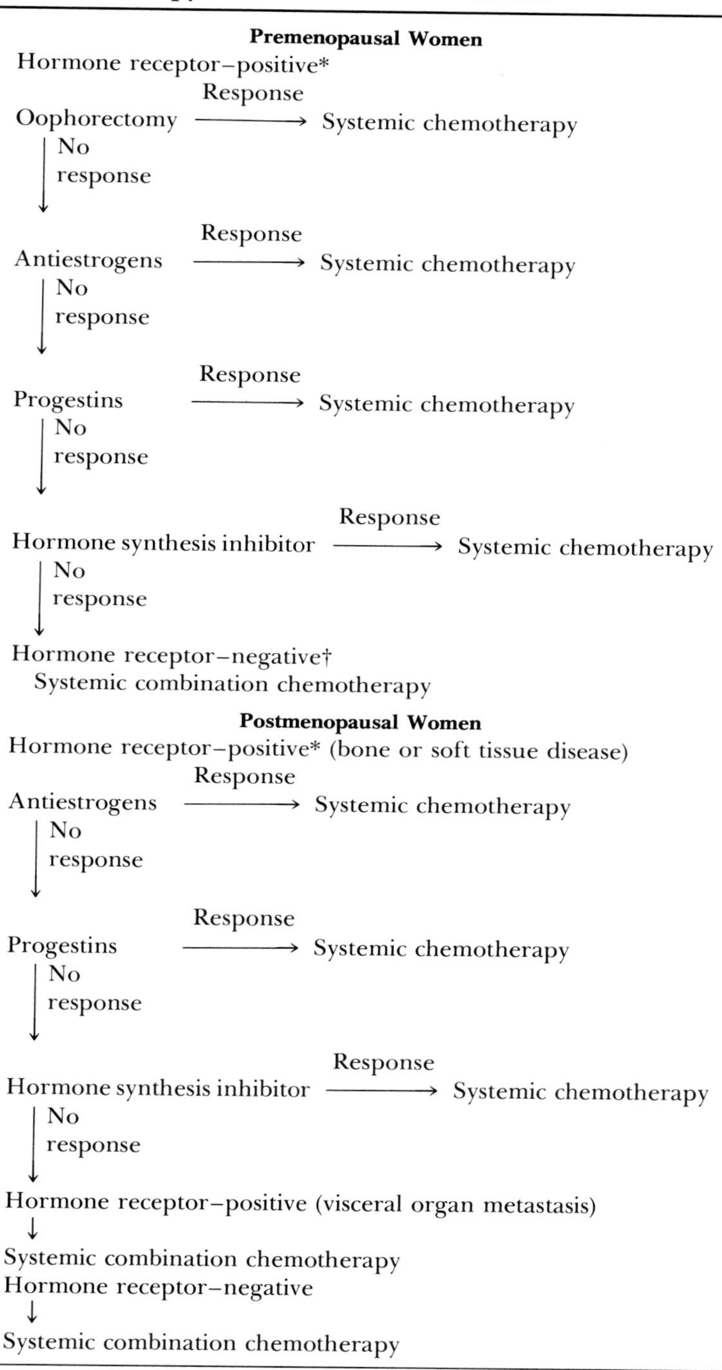

Premenopausal Women

Hormone receptor–positive*

Oophorectomy —Response→ Systemic chemotherapy
↓ No response
Antiestrogens —Response→ Systemic chemotherapy
↓ No response
Progestins —Response→ Systemic chemotherapy
↓ No response
Hormone synthesis inhibitor —Response→ Systemic chemotherapy
↓ No response

Hormone receptor–negative†
Systemic combination chemotherapy

Postmenopausal Women

Hormone receptor–positive* (bone or soft tissue disease)

Antiestrogens —Response→ Systemic chemotherapy
↓ No response
Progestins —Response→ Systemic chemotherapy
↓ No response
Hormone synthesis inhibitor —Response→ Systemic chemotherapy
↓ No response

Hormone receptor–positive (visceral organ metastasis)
↓
Systemic combination chemotherapy

Hormone receptor–negative
↓
Systemic combination chemotherapy

*To either estrogen receptor protein or progesterone receptor protein (or both).
†To neither estrogen receptor protein nor progesterone receptor protein.

nosis and up to 70% of patients in autopsy series. The incidence of bone metastases at presentation has decreased over the past 20 years, perhaps owing to public and physician awareness.

Hormonal Therapy. Hormonal therapy remains the cornerstone of treatment for metastatic prostate cancer. In 1941 Huggins and Hodges[22] at the University of Chicago performed orchiectomy on patients with prostatic carcinoma demonstrating tumor regression and decrease in serum acid phosphatase activity. They also showed that the administration of exogenous estrogens caused a similar clinical and chemical response. The guiding principle for all hormonal manipulations used in treating prostatic cancer is the lowering of circulating testosterone levels.

Orchiectomy removes 95% of circulating testosterone. Exogenous estrogen suppresses pituitary gonadotropin, which is responsible for stimulating testicular androgen synthesis. Estrogens can also block testosterone uptake by prostatic tissue and also will increase testosterone binding to plasma proteins, rendering less free testosterone available for peripheral effects. Although equivalent clinical effects are seen with 1 mg of DES daily, 3 mg/day is recognized to consistently lower testosterone to castration levels.

Androgen synthesis and peripheral testosterone action can be altered by several additional compounds. Progestational agents (such as megestrol or cyproterone) block peripheral binding of testosterone to target tissues. Aminoglutethimide blocks all adrenal steroid synthesis and can be used to obliterate adrenal androgens in previously castrated patients. Leuprolide, a GnRH agonist, causes an initial increase in gonadotropins followed by a decrease that lasts as long as the drug is administered. Flutamide is a nonsteroidal pure antiandrogen with estrogenic side effects. Orchiectomy, DES, and leuprolide can all be expected to produce a 70% to 85% response rate (complete and partial) with an expected 5-year survival from the time of metastases in 30% of cases. Aminoglutethimide produces a 20% to 30% response in previously castrated patients (medical or surgical) at the time of progressive disease.

Recently results comparing complete androgen blockade (orchiectomy or leuprolide with flutamide) and standard DES orchiectomy therapy have shown a significantly higher response rate in the complete androgen blockade group. It is difficult to draw conclusions from these data[27] because the number of patients is small and follow-up is short (less

TABLE 6-12 **Response Rates in Single-Agent Chemotherapy of Metastatic Prostate Cancer**

	Percent*
Cyclophosphamide	30-40
Adriamycin (doxorubicin)	20-25
5-Fluorouracil	10-40
Lomustine (CCNU)	20-30
Estramustine	20-30
Cisplatin	15-30

*Includes complete response, partial response, and disease stabilization.

TABLE 6-13 **Combination-Chemotherapy Regimens in Metastatic Prostate Cancer**

	Response Rate* (%)	Median Duration (mo)
5-Fluorouracil Adriamycin (doxorubicin) Cyclophosphamide	20-50	6
Adriamycin (doxorubicin) Cyclophosphamide BCNU (carmustine)	30	5
Cyclophosphamide Methotrexate 5-Fluorouracil	40-50	5

*Includes complete responses, partial responses, and disease stabilization.

than 24 mo). The natural history of the disease is extremely variable. Furthermore, subjective improvement does not always correlate with improvement in either serum alkaline phosphate elevations or bone scan results. Although rapid objective response is desirable, clinical palliation and subjective patient improvement should remain the critical objectives until clear-cut benefit and improvement in survival can be shown.

Chemotherapy. The role of chemotherapy in metastatic prostate cancer remains controversial. Chemotherapy is almost always reserved for second-line treatment after hormonal therapy fails. Single-agent and combination regimens for hormone-resistant prostatic cancer[48] are shown in Table 6-12. Combination-chemotherapy regimens are shown in Table 6-13.[48] There are no data to support the concept that any of these agents prolong survival after the failure of hormonal manipulation. Since the majority of patients show increasing metastases to bone, pain is the predominant problem and radiation therapy often is effective for palliation. When chemotherapy is given, it is usually in end-stage patients who are less likely to respond to any therapeutic maneuvers because of poor previous responses. Based on the foregoing, chemotherapy should be considered for palliation of bone metastases if hormonal maneuvers fail and metastatic progression is not in a site amenable to radiation control. Single-agent therapy using Adriamycin, cisplatin, or 5-fluorouracil is a reasonable first step before attempting a combination regimen.

Modality Selection. At the time that bone metastases are documented, the initial therapeutic maneuver should be hormonal manipulation. Orchiectomy is highly effective, with the fewest side effects. If orchiectomy is undesirable or refused, DES 3 mg/day is begun. Leuprolide (with 2 to 3 wk of concomitant antiandrogen therapy) is comparable in its efficacy to DES, but DES is far less expensive at the present time. As metastases progress, secondary hormonal treatment with flutamide or aminoglutethimide may further lower androgen levels and yield a clinical improvement. High-dose pulsed estrogen therapy with DES diphosphate (Stilphostrol) often is extremely effective in patients with bone pain in whom initial hormonal therapy fails. When all hormonal maneuvers are exhausted, single-agent or combination chemotherapy can be used if desired.

TABLE 6-14 **Selected Characteristics of Bronchogenic Carcinoma by Cell Type**

	Incidence (%)	Resectability (%)	Nodal Involvement (%)	Patient Never Smoked (%)	Extrathoracic Metastasis at Autopsy (%)	Bone Metastasis at Autopsy (%)	Overall 5 yr Survival (%)
Epidermoid	33	60	42	9	25-50	20	25
Adenocarcinoma	25	38	41	64	50-75	36	12
Large cell	16	38	42	14	50-75	30	13
Small cell undifferentiated	25	11	72	3	75-95	37	1

Lung Cancer

There are 130,000 new cases and 110,000 deaths from bronchogenic carcinoma annually in the United States. Most cases (60% to 70%) are inoperable at the time of presentation, and the majority of patients die from metastatic disease. There are four major histological subtypes of bronchogenic carcinoma: epidermoid (squamous), adenocarcinoma, large cell, and small cell. Their characteristics are outlined in Table 6-14. The approach to treatment of epidermoid carcinoma, adenocarcinoma and, large-cell carcinoma are similar and all are distinctly different from the treatment for small cell carcinoma.

Non–Small Cell Bronchogenic Carcinoma (NSBC). Bone metastases occur in 30% to 35% of patients with NSBC. The most frequent associated complaint is pain. The goal of treatment when bone metastases are present is palliation, because cure generally is not achievable. Radiation therapy is the most effective local modality and should be used when possible. If multiple bone metastases are present, systemic chemotherapy should be considered. The single agents with known activity against NSBC are listed in Table 6-15. It is unfortunate that response rates are low, with an expected duration of only 2 to 4 months, and no significant increase in survival has been reported. Popular combination regimens are shown in Table 6-16. In contrast to single-agent protocols, the combination-chemotherapy regimens have a slightly higher response rate and show some (though modest) prolongation of survival.

In lung cancer patients with bone metastases the major objective often is maintaining stability and relief of pain in weight-bearing bones. Surgery and radiation therapy, respectively, are the modalities of choice in this setting. The single most important determinant in predicting a response to any treatment modality is the performance status at the time that treatment is initiated.

Small-Cell Lung Carcinoma (SCLC). SCLC presents with metastases outside the hemithorax of origin in 50% of patients. Based on clinical and autopsy studies, the frequency of bone metastases is approximately 35%. Unlike many metastatic solid tumors, the majority of bone metastases are not painful and pathological fractures are rare. For this reason a bone scan is a reasonable screening test at the time of diagnosis even in the absence of symptoms or elevation of the alkaline phosphatase. Interestingly, carcinoembryonic antigen (CEA) is elevated in 88% of patients with extensive disease and may be a useful marker to monitor response if it is elevated at presentation.

Unlike NSBC, small-cell lung carcinoma is best treated with chemotherapy. The most active single agents are shown in Table 6-17. As with other chemotherapy-responsive solid tumors, combination regimens with SCLC have been shown to be far superior to single-agent therapy. Frequently used combination regimens are shown in Table 6-18. Response rates and expected survival correlated directly with the extent of disease noted at presentation and with the performance status. The use of alternating non–cross-resistant regimens as initial therapy remains controversial and to date has shown no significant advantage over single-agent therapy in terms of remission or overall survival. Once initial therapy has failed, survival is limited. Second-line chemotherapy withVP-16-213, cisplatin, and other agents, if not used in the primary treatment, has shown variable response rates. However, impact on palliation and survival remains questionable. Radiation therapy is extremely effective in treating painful bone metastases and can be used concomitantly with chemotherapy initially or at the time of progression.

Colorectal Carcinoma

There are 140,000 new cases and 60,000 deaths from colorectal cancer reported annually in the United States. Disseminated disease develops in approximately half the patients. By far, the most common metastatic site is the liver. Bone metastases are present in 20% of patients at autopsy. The use of chemotherapy in colorectal cancer has been disappointing, at best. 5-Fluorouracil is the standard drug used and has been administered weekly, consecutively for 5 days, by bolus injection, or by continuous infusion regionally (IV or IA). Regardless of the route of administration, the expected response rate with it has been 15% to 40% and the impact on survival insignificant.[5] Combination-chemotherapy regimens using nitrosourea, 5-fluorouracil, and vincristine have produced response rates of up to 40%.[14] However, in comparing combination regimens with 5-

TABLE 6-15 Response Rates to Single-Agent Chemotherapy in Metastatic Non–Small Cell Bronchogenic Carcinoma

	Percent
Cisplatin	25-35
Adriamycin (doxorubicin)	18
VP-16-213	18
Mitomycin-C	25
Cyclophosphamide	10
Methotrexate	10

TABLE 6-17 Response Rates to Single-Agent Chemotherapy in Small-Cell Lung Carcinoma

	Percent
VP-16-213	45
Cyclophosphamide	35
Adriamycin (doxorubicin)	35
Vincristine	30
Methotrexate	30
CCNU (lomustine)	15

TABLE 6-16 Combination-Regimen Chemotherapy in Metastatic Non–Small Cell Bronchogenic Carcinoma

	Response (%)*	Median Survival (mo)
Cisplatin Vindesine	43	14 (+)
Cisplatin VP-16-213	37	16
5-Fluorouracil Adriamycin (doxorubicin) Mitomycin-C	36	9 (+)
Adriamycin (doxorubicin) CCNU (lomustine)	35	10
Cyclophosphamide Adriamycin (doxorubicin) Methotrexate Procarbazine	31	13

*Complete and partial responses.

TABLE 6-18 Combination-Regimen Chemotherapy in Small-Cell Lung Carcinoma

	Dose (mg/M²)	Response* (%)	Median Survival with Extensive Disease (wk)
Cyclophosphamide Adriamycin (doxorubicin) VP-16-213	1000 IV da 1 45 IV da 1 50 IV da 1-5 (repeat q. 28 da.)	75	40
Methotrexate Vincristine Cyclophosphamide Adriamycin (doxorubicin)	50 IV da 1 1.4 IV da 1 500 IV da 1 30 IV da 1 (repeat q. 21 da.)	70	42
Cyclophosphamide Vincristine Adriamycin (doxorubicin)	1000 IV da 1 1 IV da 1 40 IV da 1 (repeat q. 21 da.)	56	24
Cyclophosphamide CCNU (lomustine) Methotrexate	700 IV da 1, 22 70 IV da 1 50 IV da 1, 22 (repeat q. 42 da.)	50	36

*Complete and partial responses.

fluorouracil alone, there has been no evidence of improved overall response or survival with the more aggressive regimens.[32] For patients with painful bone metastases, radiation therapy remains the treatment of choice. Chemotherapy also can be used, but with the expected limitations described.

Urinary Tract Cancer

Urinary tract cancers include malignancies of the kidney, ureter, bladder, and urethra. There are approximately 60,000 new cases annually (bladder 40,000) and 20,000 reported deaths (bladder 11,000, kidney and others 9000).

Adenocarcinoma accounts for nearly all renal carcinomas in adults. There is a 30% incidence of bone metastases during the course of the disease. Although it was originally thought that patients with only osseous metastases had an improved prognosis compared to those with parenchymal disease, it is now clear that the number of metastatic sites and the biological grade of the tumor appear to determine the prognosis. The most frequent symptoms of bone metastasis are pain, and radiation therapy is the most reliable palliative maneuver. There are no chemotherapeutic agents with known significant activity in renal adenocarcinoma. Vinblastine, CCNU (lomustine), and hydroxyurea have been shown to produce response rates of 15% to 25% in small groups of patients. Initial reports of progestational agents showing significant activity in advanced disease have not been substantiated. More encouraging are reports using leukocyte and recombinant interferon. Since 1983, over six centers[37] have shown that approximately 35% of patients with measurable metastatic disease can benefit from the use of interferon. Further studies are underway to confirm these initial reports.

Transitional cell carcinoma (TCC) of the urinary bladder, ureter, and renal pelvis has been found to respond to several chemotherapeutic agents, and cisplatin has emerged as the single most important agent in its treatment. The dose of 70 mg/M^2 is standard, and response is expected in 3 to 6 weeks. Most remissions last 3 to 6 months, although some lasting over 1 year have been reported. Methotrexate in standard or high-dose regimens produces responses in 25% to 30% of patients, with a similar expected duration of remission. Single-agent and combination chemotherapy regimens[40,44,50] for treating TCC are shown in Table 6-19. These results are encouraging; and combination therapy should be considered as the treatment of choice in disseminated TCC with bone involvement, if surgical stabilization or radiotherapy for prompt pain control is not indicated.

TABLE 6-19 **Response Rates to Single-Agent and Combination-Regimen Chemotherapy in Transitional Cell Carcinoma**

	Percent*
Single-Agent	
Cisplatin	35
Cyclophosphamide	30
Methotrexate	30
Adriamycin (doxorubicin)	25
Mitomycin-C	20
5-Fluorouracil	20
Vinblastine	15
Combination-Regimen	
Cisplatin Adriamycin (doxorubicin) Cyclophosphamide	40-50
Cisplatin Methotrexate Vinblastine	40-80
Methotrexate Vinblastine Adriamycin (doxorubicin) Cisplatin	40-90

*Complete and partial responses.

Plasma Cell Myeloma

Plasma cell neoplasms represent an uncontrolled proliferation of B-lymphocytes. They are usually associated with a monoclonal spike of immunoglobulin on serum protein electrophoresis or on immunoelectrophoresis of serum or urine (M-protein). Disease entities associated with an M-protein include benign monoclonal gammopathy, cold agglutinin syndrome, amyloidosis, and other lymphoproliferative disorders.

Plasma cell neoplasms may produce whole immunoglobulin or a fragment thereof (heavy-chain or light-chain fragments). There are 10,000 new cases and 7500 deaths of plasma cell myeloma reported annually. The disease incidence increases with age, the mean at diagnosis being 65 years. The incidence in American blacks is twice that in the white population.

Plasma cell myeloma cannot truly be considered as a metastatic tumor to bone; rather it is a primary hematological malignancy arising most commonly in the bone marrow. The disease can be unifocal (solitary plasmacytoma) but more frequently is multifocal in distribution. Plasmacytoma can also occur in extramedullary sites, usually the upper air passages, lymph nodes, spleen, bronchi, and lungs.

Approximately 70% of patients with plasma cell myeloma present with bone pain. Roentgenograms may show generalized osteoporosis or, more commonly, a purely lytic lesion of bone. This presentation associated with a serum or urine M-spike and plasmacytosis in the bone marrow is diagnostic for plasma cell myeloma. If the skeletal lesions are osteoblastic, metastatic carcinoma must be ruled out, because myeloma lesions are almost always purely lytic.

Treatment should be tailored to the extent of disease. If a solitary plasmacytoma of bone is confirmed, primary radiation is the treatment of choice. An M-spike present at diagnosis should disappear with such therapy. If this does not occur, multifocal disease should be suspected and treated as indicated.

Plasma cell myeloma is a systemic disease and ideally requires chemotherapy for adequate control. The general principles of treatment are similar to those for other chemotherapy-responsive tumors. Critical lesions in weight-bearing bones should be treated with surgery or radiation. Otherwise, chemotherapy is the modality of choice. In the early stages of plasma cell myeloma the disease is often responsive to oral alkylating agents or prednisone. Table 6-20 outlines the common chemotherapy regimens used in treating myeloma.[2,3,39] It is unclear whether more aggressive multidrug regimens are significantly better than alkylating agents and corticosteroid alone. Although the response rate (measuring the M-protein quantitatively) with multidrug chemotherapy may be higher, overall survival is not significantly prolonged when compared to alkylating agent and corticosteroid therapy. The course of plasma cell myeloma is extremely variable, and there is often a lengthy indolent phase, especially in patients presenting at an advanced age. In these patients minimal or no therapy may be needed, often for several years. Once the disease becomes more aggressive or after initial chemotherapeutic maneuvers fail, the disease usually is fatal within 6 months.

Plasma cell myeloma is exquisitely radiosensitive, and painful or destructive lesions in weight-bearing bones should be treated with radiation alone or concomitantly with chemotherapy.

Malignant Lymphoma

Malignant lymphoma is a neoplastic process involving lymphocytes, most commonly in the lymph nodes, spleen, or bone marrow. The clinical spectrum is vast. Presentation of primary lymphoma in an extranodal site accounts for approximately 20% of cases. The gastrointestinal tract, lung, genitourinary tract, and central nervous system are the most common extranodal sites. Only 5% of extranodal lymphomas occur in bone (1% of all such lesions). The most common site is the femur, but lymphoma can present in any bone.

Once the diagnosis of lymphoma in bone is confirmed, a complete staging work-up to determine extent of disease is critical. Staging procedures include a detailed history and physical examination, complete blood count, sedimentation rate, chemistry evaluation of liver and renal function, chest roentgenogram, chest and abdominal CT scans, bone marrow aspirate, and bone core biopsy. Depending on the site of disease, a nuclear scan (^{99m}Tc) of the bone, a lymphangiogram, or a gallium scan may be useful. The necessity of a staging laparotomy is controversial and beyond the scope of this text.

If after complete staging the disease is apparently confined to one site (Stage IE), radiation is the treatment of choice. If two or more lesions are demonstrated, the patient must be considered to have Stage IV disease and should be treated with local radiation and systemic chemotherapy. Similarly, if progression of a primary nodal lymphoma causes destructive lesions in bone, the treatment should include a combined-modality ap-

TABLE 6-20 **Single-Agent and Combination-Regimen Chemotherapy in Myeloma**

	Dose (mg/M²)	Response (%)*	Median Survival (mo)
	Single-Agent		
Cyclophosphamide	1000 IV q. 3 wk 250 per da × 4 (q. 3 wk)	24-40	NR
Melphalan	9 per da × 4 (q. 4 wk)	25-40	18
BCNU (carmustine)	150 IV q. 4-6 wk	30	NR
Prednisone	60 p.o. daily	30	NR
	Combination-Regimen		
Melphalan Prednisone	8 per da × 4 da p.o. 60 per da × 4 da p.o. (q. 4 wk)	53	37
Vincristine Melphalan Cyclophosphamide Prednisone	1 mg IV da 1 5 per da × 4 da p.o. 100 per da × 4 da p.o. 60 per da × 4 da p.o.	53	40
Vincristine Cyclophosphamide Adriamycin (doxorubicin) Prednisone	1 mg IV da 1 100 per da × 4 da p.o. 30 per da × 4 da p.o. 60 per da × 4 da p.o.	53	40
Vincristine BCNU (carmustine) Adriamycin (doxorubicin) Prednisone	1 mg IV da 1 30 IV da 1 30 IV da 1 60 per da × 4 da p.o.	53	40
Vincristine Adriamycin (doxorubicin) Dexamethasone	0.4 mg/da IV × 4 da (continuous infusion) 9 per da IV × 4 da (continuous infusion) 40 mg/da × 4 da; d 1, 9, 17 (repeat q. 28 da)†	70	NR

*50% or greater reduction in M-protein.
†Used as second line treatment in alkylating agent failures.
NR, Not reported.

proach with radiation and chemotherapy.[45]

There are numerous chemotherapeutic regimens that can be utilized in the treatment of lymphoma. The drugs vary depending on the histological type of lymphoma and the extent of disease. The agents most commonly used include cyclophosphamide, doxorubicin, vincristine, methotrexate, bleomycin, and corticosteroids. Aggressive combination regimens may be expected to produce remission in 70% to 90% of patients and should be administered by a qualified hematologist-oncologist. Five-year "cures" are reported in 50% to 95% of patients depending on the extent of disease at presentation and the treatment modality.[7] However, it is important to emphasize that most patients with malignant lymphoma of bone will have more extensive disease and unless they are treated aggressively and all occult disease eradicated the desired cure rates will not be forthcoming.

Metastatic Carcinoma of Unknown Primary Origin

Five percent of carcinoma patients present with metastases of unknown origin; and of these, 5% to 25% will have bone metastases. Bone pain or pathological fracture is the most common presenting symptom, and the most likely primary tumor sites are the lung (squamous cell carcinoma, adenocarcinoma, small cell carcinoma), breast, prostate, ovary, GI tract (adenocarcinoma), and epidermis (melanoma). Diffuse bone marrow involvement may be seen in 10% to 15% of patients with metastases of unknown origin (with or without discrete cortical bone metastases).

The prognosis for survival of patients presenting with bone metastases of unknown primary origin is only 3 to 6 months, and 85% of patients die within 1 year. Identification of the primary site does not affect the prognosis; the primary site is identified in only 15% to 20% of patients prior to death, even after an extensive antemortem search. The most important information in determining the prognosis is the correct histology of the metastasis. Treatment is based on the histological diagnosis rather than on the presumed primary site. Anaplastic small-cell carcinoma, breast carcinoma, prostatic carcinoma, and ovarian carcinoma can all present as metastases with no apparent primary site, and each tumor may exhibit significant responses to chemotherapy or hormonal manipulation in some instances. Based on the location of the bone metastasis and the roentgenographic characteristics and histological features of the biopsy, a rational decision about chemotherapy or radiation therapy can be made.

SPECIAL CONSIDERATIONS

Surgical Debulking. Debulking of most tumors metastatic to bone generally is not indicated. Although radiation, chemotherapy, and hormonal therapy are presumably more effective against a small tumor burden, more often the potential benefits are outweighed by the morbidity of surgery and in the delay in the initiation of radiation or chemotherapy imposed by surgery. This is especially true of chemotherapy-sensitive tumors (small cell carcinoma of lung, breast cancer, lymphoma).

When a pathological fracture has already occurred or there is significant cortical erosion in a weight-bearing bone, internal fixation is required. At the time of surgery, debulking of the surrounding tumor is desirable if technically feasible.

Intraarterial Infusions. The concept of intraarterial delivery of high concentrations of chemotherapy to a tumor has great theoretical advantages. It has been explored most extensively with intrahepatic infusions of chemotherapeutic agents in the treatment of primary or metastatic tumors of the liver. Improved response rates in these patients have been reported, although significant prolongation of survival has not been demonstrated.[34] In children with osteogenic sarcoma, intraarterial infusion of chemotherapy has been used successfully.[23] In metastatic tumors to bone, however, there is no role for intraarterial chemotherapy at the present time.

REFERENCES

1. Alexander, J., et al.: Serial assessment of doxorubicin cardiotoxicity with quantitative radionuclide angiocardiography, N. Engl. J. Med. **300:**278, 1979.
2. Alexanian, R., and Preicer, R.: Chemotherapy for multiple myeloma, Cancer **53:**583, 1984.
3. Alexanian, R., et al.: Prednisone pulse therapy for refractory melanoma, Blood **62:**572, 1983.
4. Alexleuz-Figusch, J., and Van Gilse, H.A.: Flare and rebound regressions in the hormonal therapy of breast cancer, Rev. Endocr. Rel. Cancer **21:**5, 1985.
5. Ansfield, R., et al.: A phase III study comparing the clinical utility of four regimens of 5-fluorouracil, Cancer **39:**34, 1977.
6. Billingham, M.E., et al.: Anthracycline cardiomyopathy monitored by morphologic changes, Cancer Treat. Rep. **62:**865, 1978.
7. Bonadona, G.: Chemotherapy of malignant lymphomas, Semin. Oncol. **12**(suppl. 6):1, 1985.
8. Boyd, S.: On oophorectomy in cancer of the breast, Br. Med. J. **2:**1161, 1900.
9. Bristow, M.R., et al.: Adriamycin cardiomyopathy: evaluation by phonography, endomyocardial biopsy, and cardiac catheterization, Ann. Intern. Med. **88:**168, 1978.
10. Bristow, M.R., et al.: Early anthracycline cardiotoxicity, Am. J. Med. **65:**823, 1978.
11. Cooke, S.T., and Bradner, W.T.: Mitomycin-C—a review, Cancer Treat. Rev. **3:**121, 1976.
12. Cooper, R.: Combination chemotherapy in hormone resistant breast carcinoma, Proc. Am. Assoc. Cancer Res. Am. Soc. Clin. Oncol. **10:**15, 1969. (Abstract.)
13. Dao, T.L., and Huggins, C.: Metastatic cancer of the breast treated by adrenalectomy, J.A.M.A., p. 1793, 1957.
14. Falkson, G., and Falkson, H.C.: 5-Fluorouracil, methyl-CCNU, and vincristine in the treatment of advanced colorectal cancer, Cancer **38:**1468, 1976.
15. Galasko, C.B.: Anatomy and pathway of skeletal metastasis. In Weiss, L., and Gilbert, H.A., editors: Bone metastasis, Boston, 1981, G.K. Hall & Co.
16. Gocdiner, P.L., et al.: Factors influencing post-operative morbidity and mortality in patients treated with bleomycin, Br. Med. J. **1:**1664, 1978.
17. Goodman, L.S., et al.: Nitrogen mustard therapy. Use of methyl bis (B-chloroethyl) amine hydrochloride and tris (B-chloroethyl) amine hydrochloride for Hodgkin's disease lymphosarcoma, leukemia, certain allied muscle tumor disorders, J.A.M.A. **132:**126, 1946.

18. Greenspan, E.M.: Combination cytotoxic chemotherapy in advanced disseminated breast carcinoma, J. Mt. Sinai Hosp. **33:**1, 1966.
19. Gulati, S.C., et al.: Microangiopathic hemolytic anemia observed after treatment of epidermoid carcinoma with mitomycin-C and 5-fluorouracil, Cancer **45:**2252, 1980.
20. Haagenson, C.D.: Disease of the breast, ed. 2, Philadelphia, 1971, W.B. Saunders Co.
21. Harris, J.R., et al.: Cancer of the breast. In DeVito, V.T., editor: Cancer: principles and practice of oncology, ed. 2, Philadelphia, 1985, J.B. Lippincott Co.
22. Huggins, C., and Hodges, C.V.: Studies on prostatic cancer. The effects of castration, of estrogen, and of androgen injection on serum phosphatases in metastatic carcinoma of the prostate, Cancer Res. **1:**293, 1941.
23. Jaffe, N., et al.: Chemotherapy for primary osteosarcoma by intra-arterial infusion, Cancer Bull. **36:** 37, 1984.
24. Kennedy, B.J.: Hormonal therapies in breast cancer, Semin. Oncol. **1:**119, 1974.
25. Kiang, D.T., et al.: A randomized trial of chemotherapy and hormonal therapy in advanced breast cancer, N. Engl. J. Med. **313:**1241, 1985.
26. Kiang, D.T., and Kennedy, B.J.: Tamoxifen (antiestrogen) therapy in advanced breast cancer, Ann. Intern. Med. **87:**687, 1977.
27. Labrie, F., et al.: New approach in the treatment of prostate cancer: complete instead of only partial withdrawal of androgens, Prostate **4:**579, 1983.
28. Legha, S.S., et al.: Hormonal therapy of breast cancer: new approaches and concepts, Ann. Intern. Med. **88:**69, 1978.
29. Ludlum, D.B.: Aklylating agents and nitrosureas. In Baker, F.F., editor: Cancer: a comprehensive treatise, vol. 5, New York, 1973, Plenum Press, Inc.
30. Marshall, E.: Historical perspectives in chemotherapy. In Gordin, A., and Hawking, I.F., editors: Advances in chemotherapy, vol. 1, New York, 1964, Academic Press, Inc.
31. Minna, J.D., et al.: Cancer of the lung. In DeVito, V., editor: Cancer: principles and practice of oncology, ed. 2, Philadelphia, 1985, J.B. Lippincott Co.
32. Moertel, C.G.: Chemotherapy of gastrointestinal cancer, N. Engl. J. Med. **299:**1049, 1978.
33. Myers, C.E.: Antracyclines. In Chabner, B., editor: Pharmacologic principles of cancer treatment, Philadelphia, 1982, W.B. Saunders Co.
34. Oberfield, R.A.: Intra-arterial hepatic infusion chemotherapy in metastatic liver cancer, Semin. Oncol. **10:**206, 1983.
35. Patel, D.J., and Canuel, L.L.: Anthracycline antitumor antibiotic nucleic acid interactions, Eur. J. Biochem. **90:**247, 1978.
36. Puga, F.J., et al.: Therapeutic oophorectomy in disseminated carcinoma of the breast, Arch. Surg. **111:** 877, 1976.
37. Quesada, J.F., et al.: Phase II study of interferon alpha in metastatic renal-cell carcinoma: a progress report, J. Clin. Oncol. **3:**1086, 1985.
38. Ross, M.B., et al.: Treatment of advanced breast cancer with megastrol acetate after therapy with Tamoxifen, Cancer **49:**413, 1982.
39. Salmon, S.E., et al.: Alternating combination chemotherapy and levamisole improves survival in multiple myeloma, J. Clin. Oncol. **1:**453, 1983.
40. Samuels, M.L., et al.: Cytoxan, adriamycin and cisplatinum (cisSCA) in metastatic bladder cancer, Proc. Am. Assoc. Cancer Res. **21:**137, 1980.
41. Santen, R.J., et al.: Randomized trial comparing surgical adrenalectomy with aminoglutethimide plus hydrocortisone in women with advanced breast cancer, N. Engl. J. Med. **305:**545, 1981.
42. Silverstein, M.J., et al.: Bilateral adrenalectomy for advanced breast cancer: a 21 year experience, Surgery **77:**825, 1979.
43. Skipper, H.E., et al.: Experimental evaluation of potential anticancer agents. XIII. On the criteria and kinetics associated with "curability" of experimental leukemia, Cancer Chemother. Rep. **35:**1, 1964.
44. Sternberg, C., et al.: Methotrexate, vinblastine, adriamycin, and cis-platin (M-VAC) for transitional cell carcinoma (TCC) of the urothelium, Proc. Am. Soc. Clin. Oncol. **3:**156, 1984.
45. Sweet, D.L., et al.: Histiocytic lymphoma (reticulum-cell sarcoma) of bone, J. Bone Joint Surg. **63A:**79, 1981.
46. Tannock, I.F.: Is there evidence that chemotherapy is of benefit to patients with carcinoma of the prostate? J. Clin. Oncol. **3:**1013, 1985.
47. Torti, F.M., et al.: Reduced cardiotoxicity of doxorubicin delivered on a weekly schedule. Assessment by endomyocardial biopsy, Ann. Intern. Med. **99:** 745, 1983.
48. Torti, F.M., et al.: Treatment of prostate cancer, Clin. Cancer Briefs **3:**3, 1982.
49. Wang Y.M., et al.: Effect of vitamin E against adriamycin-induced toxicity in rabbits, Cancer Res. **40:** 1022, 1980.
50. Yagoda, A.: Chemotherapy of metastatic bladder cancer, Cancer **45:**1879, 1980.
51. Yagoda, A., et al.: Bleomycin: an antitumor antibiotic. Clinical experience in 274 patients, Ann. Intern. Med. **77:**861, 1972.

GENERAL REFERENCES

Bone metastasis, Stoll, B.A., and Parbhoo, S., editors, New York, 1983, Raven Press.
Cancer: principles and practice of oncology, DeVito, V.T., et al., editors, Philadelphia, 1985, J.B. Lippincott Co.
Cancer treatment, Haskell, C.M., editor, Philadelphia, 1984, W.B. Saunders Co.
Manual of bedside oncology, Casciato, D.A., and Lowitz, B.B., editors, Boston, 1983, Little, Brown & Co.
Pharmacologic principles of cancer treatment, Chabner, B.A., editor, Philadelphia, 1982, W.B. Saunders Co.
Principles of cancer treatment, Carter, S.K., et al., editors, New York, 1982, McGraw-Hill, Inc.

CHAPTER 7

CONTROL OF PAIN

Alexander Mauskop   Kathleen M. Foley

In both adults and children with cancer, bone metastases are the most common cause of pain. In fact, pain is the most frequent and characteristic of the presenting symptoms. Although bone metastases occur with all tumor types, 70% of patients will have breast, lung, or prostatic cancer. The pain is of several types: acute, associated with a pathological fracture; chronic, associated with far-advanced widely disseminated bone metastases; or incidental, occurring with acute pain on movement.

Tumor involvement of bone produces pain in one of two ways[3]: either by direct involvement of bone, with activation of nociceptors locally, or by compression of adjacent nerves, soft tissues, and/or vascular structures. The pain is characteristically dull and aching, progressive in intensity, lasting for several weeks to months, and of a focal, radicular, or referred type. For example, in the presence of vertebral body metastases[14] the pain is focal with tenderness to percussion over the vertebral body, radicular with radiation anteriorly along the intercostal neves (most commonly in the thoracic area), or referred with manifestations in a distant site (as occurs with L1 metastases, in which it is referred to the sacroiliac joint). Similarly, metastases in the proximal femur may be associated with local pain in the hip, radicular pain if there is compression of the sciatic nerve, or referred pain to the knee. Recognition of the radicular and referred types of pain patterns is important in evaluating the exact site of the bone metastases.[14,38]

A series of common pain syndromes occurs in patients with cancer and bone metastases, and it is critical that a clear diagnosis of the nature and site be established before treatment is undertaken.[17] It is well recognized that the best way to manage bone pain is to treat its cause, and an accurate diagnosis is critical to this approach. It is particularly essential in evaluating patients with vertebral metastases, in whom pain may be only the earliest symptom preceding neurological compromise, which, if not properly diagnosed, may progress to irreversible neurological deficits including paraplegia and quadriplegia from local epidural extension or spinal cord compression.[26] Eighty-five percent of patients with epidural spinal cord compression originally had vertebral metastases.

MECHANISMS OF BONE PAIN

The underlying physiological and neuropharmacological mechanisms of bone pain are not fully understood. Anatomical studies[3] have demonstrated that there are both myelinated and unmyelinated nerve fibers present in bone, most dense in the region of compact bone. The periosteum and all the structures of the joints except the articular cartilage are pain sensitive, whereas the cortex and

Supported in part by a grant from the U.S. Public Health Service (CA 32897) and from the Patricia Drake Hemingway Fund.

Dr. Mauskop is supported in part by a National Research Service Award (CA 09461).

bone marrow are considered to be pain insensitive.[8,38] The vascular supply to bone has its own nerve fiber network, but to what extent these nerves play a role in the generation of pain remains undefined.

The current hypothesis is that bone pain is somatic. It originates from the activation of free nerve endings within bone, which in turn activate unmyelinated C and myelinated A-delta fibers. These two types of peripheral nerve fibers mediate information into the central nervous system via the dorsal root ganglia entering the spinal cord in the dorsal horn, where specific laminae (I and V) receive the nociceptive input. Nociceptors in bone, like those in other comparable tissue, can be activated by both mechanical and chemical stimulation. Pressure and distortion of receptors occur with an enlarging tumor and are the explanation for pain in certain types of bone tumors. To what extent chemical factors cause activation of nociceptors in bone is not fully understood, but there is a series of metabolic changes that occurs in bone that might account for nociceptive stimulation.

One hypothesis for the origin of bone pain relates to the role of prostaglandins in the metastatic process and comes from several lines of evidence. It is well recognized that metastatic tumor in bone is associated with at least two processes, active bone destruction and new bone formation. Several investigators[22,59,60] have demonstrated that prostaglandins are important in the osteolytic and osteoblastic effects of bone metastases. The specific prostaglandins E_1 and E_2 appear to be most involved in the pathology of metastatic bone disease, and they are known to be potent agents in producing hyperalgesia.[12] In both clinical and experimental studies, drugs that inhibit prostaglandin synthesis have also been demonstrated to inhibit pain and in some instances to inhibit tumor growth in bone as well.* Prostaglandins also mediate the hormonal responses of certain tumors (e.g., the effects of prolactin on breast cancer cells[63]), further suggesting the pivotal role that prostaglandins play in the mechanism of bone pain. It is not clear, however, whether it is new bone formation, with associated prostaglandin release, or bone destruction that causes bone pain.

*References 5, 23, 59, 60, 69.

Although the prostaglandin hypothesis has received a great deal of attention, there are other factors that may influence or control the appearance of pain in patients with metastatic bone disease. For example, in patients with a variety of metastatic tumors and multiple myeloma, osteoclast activating factor (OAF), a nonprostaglandin substance, is thought to be the pain-producing agent.[30] Other chemical factors (including acetylcholine, histamine, serotonin, bradykinin, and substance P) can produce excitation in nociceptors. Substance P is comparable to prostaglandin in that it both sensitizes nociceptors and causes plasma extravasation through an increase in the permeability of capillary walls. The action of substance P presumably increases the access of blood-borne substances to the terminals of nociceptors and, in turn, promotes the activation of nociceptors. The presence of bone macrophages and circulating factors such as calcitonin, changes in the host cells, variations in calcium metabolism, and alterations in the hormone receptor status of metastatic tumor cells are all components that play a role in the production of pain in metastatic bone disease.[2]

Endocrine manipulation, including the use of diethylstilbestrol, steroids, and hypophysectomy[46,51] and the administration of levodopa,[47,48,73] has been reported to relieve pain in patients with both endocrine- and non–endocrine-responsive bone disease, a fact that supports the concept that hormonal interactions also are important in producing bone pain. There is an important clinical dilemma, however: some patients with metastatic tumor complain of significant pain while others rarely do. Further understanding of how analgesics and other antitumor agents are associated with pain relief in patients with bone metastases will enhance our ability to manage these situations more effectively.

MANAGEMENT OF METASTATIC BONE PAIN

Prior to the introduction of successful antitumor therapy, or when treatment of the cause of pain has failed, appropriate management is imperative and requires a multidimensional approach. Treatment of the primary tumor with radiation therapy, chemotherapy, or hormonal manipulation and orthopaedic stabilization represent first-line approaches to the management of tumor-induced bone pain.

Analgesic Drug Therapy

Drug therapy with nonnarcotic, narcotic, and adjuvant analgesics represents the mainstay of pain management,[15,70] and the aim is to provide sufficient relief to allow the patient to tolerate any necessary diagnostic and therapeutic procedures and to remain functioning with minimal discomfort and side effects. In the patient with far-advanced disease, pain control should provide sufficient comfort to allow him to function at the level he chooses and to die relatively pain free.

Because bone pain is often multifocal and therefore less amenable to specific anatomical anesthetic and neurosurgical approaches, drug therapy often becomes the primary treatment of choice. The rational use of analgesics falls within the purview of any physician caring for such patients, and the choice of drug or type of drug must be individualized and the dose titrated for each patient.

Nonnarcotics. The nonnarcotic nonsteroidal antiinflammatory drugs (NSAIDs) include aspirin, acetaminophen, and ibuprofen (Table 7-1). In the management of mild to moderate pain, nonnarcotic analgesics should be tried initially.

Aspirin, the prototypical NSAID, is the standard against which all antiinflammatory agents are measured. Some authors[36,37] have suggested that the enteric coated form of aspirin should be the nonnarcotic analgesic of choice. However, because cancer patients are at increased risk of bleeding from disease and treatment-related thrombocytopenia, acetaminophen is preferable, despite its relatively weaker antiinflammatory activity.

In contrast to the other nonnarcotics, acetaminophen produces less gastric irritation, erosion, and bleeding, although in rare instances it has caused thrombocytopenia. Ibuprofen, fenoprofen, diflunisal, naproxen, and naproxen sodium have been approved by the Food and Drug Administration for use as analgesics in mild to moderate pain. These drugs have a higher analgesic potential than does aspirin and, with the exception of mefenamic acid (which can be given only for a week at a time), are better tolerated than aspirin.[37] They differ primarily in their chemical formulas, pharmacokinetics, and duration of action. Ibuprofen and fenoprofen have a short duration of action whereas diflunisal and naproxen have a longer half-life and are longer acting.

Indomethacin has both analgesic and antiinflammatory effects that are greater than those of aspirin, and it has also been shown[5] to reduce elevated serum calcium levels in patients with metastatic cancer. However, almost 50% of patients taking it experience untoward effects (prompting discontinuance of the drug in 20%). Furthermore, gastric ulceration, frontal headache, and hematopoietic reactions may complicate its use.

Despite the fact that all these drugs have a comparable mechanism of action, the patient receiving inadequate analgesia from one NSAID may often obtain much better relief from another.[36] It is impossible to predict which drug will be more effective for or better tolerated by a particular individual.

An effect directly on the inflammatory process is thought also to be the mechanism of analgesia of the NSAIDs. In clinical use it is

TABLE 7-1 **Nonnarcotic and NSAIDs for Mild to Moderate Cancer Pain**

	Dose (mg)	Approximate Plasma Half-Life (hr)
*Aspirin	650-1300 q. 4-6 h.	3-5
*Acetaminophen	325-650 q. 4 h.	1-4
*Ibuprofen	200-600 q. 4-6 h.	2
*Fenoprofen	200-600 q. 6 h.	2
*Diflunisal	500-1000 q. 12 h.	8-12
*Naproxen	250 q. 12 h.	13-14
*Naproxen sodium	275 q. 4 h.	13-14
Indomethacin	50-200 q. d.	4.5

*Approved by the FDA for analgesic use.

suggested that they be administered on a regular basis so their efficacy can be assessed. Unlike the narcotic analgesics, NSAIDs do not induce tolerance and physical or psychological dependence. However, they do have ceiling effects. (For example, with aspirin once the dose has been titrated above 1300 mg there is no additional analgesic effect.) Thus in the clinical setting, each patient should have an adequate trial of one or several NSAIDs for 2 or 3 days and if inadequate analgesia results or the side effects become intolerable a narcotic analgesic combination be started.

Combinations of Nonnarcotics and Narcotics. The several fixed nonnarcotic-narcotic combinations available include codeine, oxycodone, or propoxyphene with either aspirin or acetaminophen (Table 7-2).

Numerous studies[13,32] have demonstrated that nonnarcotic analgesics combined with narcotics produce an additive analgesic effect. However, combinations of more than one NSAID do not provide heightened analgesia and may, in fact, counteract each other by competing for protein binding. Analgesic mixtures containing codeine and propoxyphene (see box) are thought to have a lower abuse potential than preparations containing oxycodone. The advantages of these preparations are that the number of tablets a patient must take at one time is reduced and analgesics that work by different mechanisms can be combined in a single tablet. For example, the nonnarcotic analgesic works on peripheral mechanisms of pain while the narcotic works by activation of opiate receptor sites in the central nervous system. The major disadvantage of this combination is that when one needs to escalate the dose of the narcotic the added dose of the NSAID may become excessive. If this problem develops and the pain remains poorly controlled, more potent narcotic analgesics should be used.

Narcotic Analgesics. The commonly used narcotic analgesics are listed in Table 7-3. In discussing the use of these drugs (see box), it is important to recognize that there is no therapy more dependent on the prejudice of the prescribing physician than the use of narcotic analgesics in acute and chronic pain management. Traditionally the narcotic analgesics have been used to manage only acute pain.

TABLE 7-2 **Oral Nonnarcotic and Narcotic Analgesics for Mild to Moderate Pain**

	Route	Equianalgesic Dose*	Duration (hr)	Plasma Half-Life (hr)	Comments
Aspirin	p.o.	650	4-6	3-5	Standard for nonnarcotic comparison; GI and hematological effects limits its use in cancer patients
Acetaminophen	p.o.	650	4-6	1-4	Weak antiinflammatory effects; safer than aspirin
Codeine	p.o.	32	4-6	3	Biotransformed to morphine; available in combinations with nonnarcotic analgesics
Propoxyphene	p.o.	65	4-6	12	Biotransformed to potentially toxic metabolite norpropoxyphene; used in combination with nonnarcotic analgesics
Pentazocine	p.o.	30	4-6	2-3	Psychotomimetic effects with escalation of dose; available only in combinations with naloxone or aspirin
Meperidine	p.o.	50	4-6	3-4	Biotransformed to active toxic metabolite, normeperidine; produces myoclonic seizures

Adapted from Foley, K.M.: N. Engl. J. Med. **313:**84, 1985.
*Relative potency of drugs compared to aspirin for mild to moderate pain.

COMBINATIONS OF NONNARCOTIC WITH NARCOTIC ANALGESICS FOR CANCER PAIN

Codeine combinations
- Empirin with codeine
  - Aspirin—325 mg
  - Codeine phosphate
    - No. 2—15 mg
    - No. 3—30 mg
    - No. 4—60 mg
- Tylenol with codeine
  - Acetaminophen—300 mg
  - Codeine phosphate
    - No. 1—7.5 mg
    - No. 2—15 mg
    - No. 3—30 mg
    - No. 4—60 mg

Oxycodone combinations
- Percodan
  - Oxycodone hydrochloride—4.5 mg
  - Oxycodone terephthalate—0.38 mg
  - Aspirin—325 mg
- Tylox
  - Oxycodone hydrochloride—4.5 mg
  - Oxycodone terephthalate—0.38 mg
  - Acetaminophen—500 mg
- Percocet
  - Oxycodone hydrochloride—5 mg
  - Acetaminophen—325 mg

Propoxyphene combinations
- Darvon with A.S.A.
  - Propoxyphene hydrochloride—65 mg
  - Aspirin—325 mg
- Darvon-N with A.S.A.
  - Propoxyphene napsylate—100 mg
  - Aspirin—325 mg
- Darvocet-N 100
  - Propoxyphene napsylate—100 mg
  - Acetaminophen—650 mg

PRACTICAL USE OF NARCOTIC ANALGESICS

Start with a specific drug for a specific type of pain.

Know the pharmacology of the drug prescribed.
- Difference between potency and efficacy
- Duration of the analgesic effect
- Pharmacokinetics of the drug
- Equianalgesic dose and route of administration

Adjust the route of administration to the patient's needs.

Administer the analgesic on a regular basis after initial titration of the dose.

Use drug combinations to provide additive analgesia and reduce side effects (e.g., nonsteroidal antiinflammatory drugs, an antihistamine [hydroxyzine], an amphetamine [Dexedrine]).

Avoid drug combinations that increase sedation without enhancing analgesia (e.g., a benzodiazepine [Diazepam], a phenothiazine [chlorpromazine]).

Anticipate and treat the side effects.
- Sedation
- Respiratory depression
- Nausea and vomiting
- Constipation

Watch for the development of tolerance.
- Switch to an alternative analgesic.
- Start with half the equianalgesic dose and titrate for pain relief.

Prevent acute withdrawal.
- Taper the dose of a narcotic slowly.
- Use diluted naloxone (0.4 mg/10 ml saline) to reverse respiratory depression in the physically dependent patient.
- Administer cautiously.

Adapted from Foley, K.M.: N. Engl. J. Med. **313:**84, 1985.

TABLE 7-3 Oral and Parenteral Narcotic Analgesics for Severe Pain

	Route	Equianalgesic (mg) Dose*	Duration (hr)	Plasma Half-Life (hr)	Comments
Narcotic Agonists					
Morphine	IM	10	4-6	2-3.5	Standard for comparison; available in slow-release tablets
	p.o.	60	4-7		
Codeine	IM	130	4-6	3	Biotransformed to morphine; useful as initial narcotic analgesic
	p.o.	200†	4-6		
Oxycodone	IM	15			Short acting; available as 5 mg dose in combination with aspirin and acetaminophen
	p.o.	30	3-5	—	
Heroin	IM	5	4-5	0.5	Illegal in U.S.; high solubility for parenteral administration
	p.o.	60	4-5		
Levorphanol (Levodromoran)	IM	2	4-6	12-16	Good oral potency; requires careful titration in initial dosing because of drug accumulation; more soluble than morphine
	p.o.	4	4-7		
Hydromorphone (Dilaudid)	IM	1.5	4-5	2-3	Available in high-potency injectable form (10 mg/ml) for cachectic patients and as rectal suppositories
	p.o.	7.5	4-6		
Oxymorphone (Numorphan)	IM	1	4-6	2-3	Available in parenteral and rectal suppository form only
	p.o.	10	4-6		
Meperidine (Demerol)	IM	75	4-5	3-4 (normeperidine 12-16)	Contraindicated in patients with renal disease; accumulation of active toxic metabolite, normeperidine, produces CNS excitation
	p.o.	300†	4-6		
Methadone (Dolophine)	IM	10		15-30	Good oral potency; requires careful titration in initial dosing to avoid drug accumulation
	p.o.	20			

Adapted from Foley, K.M.: N. Engl. J. Med. **313**:84, 1985.

*Based on single-dose studies in which an IM dose of each drug listed was compared to morphine for the establishment of its relative potency. Oral doses are those recommended when changing from parenteral to oral routes. For patients without prior narcotic exposure, the recommended oral starting dose is 30 mg for morphine, 5 mg for methadone, 2 mg for levorphanol, and 4 mg for hydromorphone.

†Initial oral doses of these drugs are listed in Table 7-2.

Because of the misconception by both clinicians and patients that *physical dependence* and *addiction* (psychological dependence) are interchangeable terms, the use of narcotic analgesics in patients with acute as well as chronic pain remains inadequate. The long-term use of narcotic analgesics in cancer patients is associated with the development of tolerance and physical dependence, but psychological dependence (addiction) rarely appears.[35]

Tolerance is a state in which escalating doses of drug are needed to maintain an analgesic effect. In patients with cancer pain, tolerance is not a limiting factor in providing adequate pain relief. Its development is dependent on a series of factors, the most important of which appears to be progression of the disease.[35] Escalating pain is associated with a more rapid escalation of drug dose.

Physical dependence is characterized by the

TABLE 7-3 **Oral and Parenteral Narcotic Analgesics for Severe Pain—cont'd**

	Route	Equianalgesic (mg) Dose*	Duration (hr)	Plasma Half-Life (hr)	Comments
Mixed Agonist-Antagonists					
Pentazocine (Talwin)	IM p.o.	60 180†	4-6 4-7	2-3	Limited use in cancer pain; psychotomimetic effects with dose escalation; available only in combination with naloxone, aspirin, or acetaminophen; may precipitate withdrawal in tolerant patients
Nalbuphine (Nubain)	IM p.o.	10 —	4-6	5	Not available orally; less psychotomimetic effects than pentazocine; may precipitate withdrawal in tolerant patient
Butorphanol (Stadol)	IM p.o.	2 —	4-6	2.5-3.5	Not available orally; psychotomimetic effects; may precipitate withdrawal in tolerant patients
Partial Agonist					
Buprenorphine (Temgesic)	IM s.l.	0.4 0.8	4-6 5-6	?	Not available in U.S. in sublingual form; no psychotomimetic effects; may precipitate withdrawal in tolerant patients

onset of acute symptoms of withdrawal if the narcotic is suddenly stopped or a narcotic antagonist is administered. This occurs, for example, if a cancer patient receiving a narcotic stops taking it when the pain has been effectively managed by some other approach.

Psychological dependence or addiction is separate from physical dependence and tolerance and is a concomitant of drug abuse whose characteristics are craving for the drug and overwhelming involvement in obtaining and using it for reasons other than control of pain.

When pain is adequately treated, almost all cancer patients will rapidly decrease their use of drug. This has been demonstrated clinically in the care of patients with cancer and pain and suggests that psychological dependence is not a necessary consequence of chronic narcotic intake. The long-term use of narcotic analgesics administered orally to manage cancer pain is now advocated, and several reviews* have discussed this approach.

Depending on their ability to bind to opiate receptors, the narcotic analgesics basically are subdivided into two classes (Tables 7-2 and 7-3): the narcotic agonists and the narcotic antagonists. The narcotic agonist drugs (e.g., morphine) bind to specific opiate receptors. The narcotic antagonist drugs block the effect of morphine at its receptors. In addition, there are mixed agonist-antagonist drugs. These are of limited use in cancer patients because they produce psychotomimetic effects with increasing doses and are available only parenterally. (For example, pentazocine exists only in combination with naloxone, as-

*References 15, 32, 45, 50, 67, 76.

pirin, or acetaminophen.) Because of their narcotic antagonist properties, these drugs also tend to precipitate withdrawal in narcotic-dependent patients. Some of the important principles that must be followed in using narcotic analgesics effectively[17] are briefly considered here and in the box on p. 125.

There is no best choice of narcotic analgesic for cancer pain. Rather, several narcotic drugs are commonly used. The Brompton cocktail,[76] heralded by the English hospice movement, contained morphine or heroin, cocaine, phenothiazine, and alcohol in a liquid solution that was used to ease the pain of cancer patients with far-advanced disease. Recent studies[34,75] have demonstrated that an oral narcotic alone is just as effective and have suggested that the use of mixed liquid combinations be discouraged.

Certain narcotics should be avoided in the management of chronic cancer pain. Repetitive administration of meperidine (Demerol) is associated with accumulation of its active toxic metabolite, normeperidine. Normeperidine has a half-life of 12 to 16 hours, and its accumulation induces the neurological symptoms of hyperactivity (subtle mood effects, tremors, multifocal myoclonus, and seizures).[33] Therefore meperidine should not be used chronically in this group of patients.

For moderate to severe pain morphine, hydromorphone, levorphanol, and methadone are the most commonly used drugs. Table 7-3 lists their equianalgesic doses. The relative potencies of these agents are based on single-dose studies. Lack of attention to the equianalgesic doses when switching from one medication to another or from one route of administration to another often leads to unnecessary recurrence of the patient's pain. Likewise, a lack of attention to the pharmacokinetic parameters of the agent can lead to excessive side effects from drug accumulation. For example, methadone and levorphanol have a long plasma half-life, and repeated administration can cause excessive sedation and respiratory depression.[11,72] These side effects are easily avoided by adjusting the dose to the patient's individual needs and by administering the drug during its initial titration on a p.r.n. rather than a fixed schedule. It takes four to five half-lives to reach a steady-state analgesic effect. Therefore drugs that have a long plasma half-life may require several days to reach their steady-state level, in contrast to morphine and hydromorphone, which have a short plasma half-life and reach their steady-state level within 24 hours (and whose efficacy and side effects can thus be assessed quite rapidly).

When titrating doses for a patient who has been receiving one type of narcotic analgesic chronically and who is then switched to another narcotic in an attempt to provide better analgesia, the physician should start with *half the equianalgesic dose* of the new drug. This information has been gained empirically and also is based on the somewhat controversial idea that cross tolerance is not complete[15,32] and the relative potency of the narcotic analgesics may change with repetitive dosing.

Route of Administration. An important factor in the use of analgesic drug therapy is the recognition that the route of administration must be adjusted to an individual patient's needs. The oral route of administration is both the easiest and the most widely applicable. However, there is a wide variety of alternative routes that can be employed to meet the needs of any given patient. Drugs administered orally have a longer duration of effect but a slower onset of action than do parenterally administered drugs. Consequently, for the patient requiring immediate relief, parenteral administration, either intramuscularly or intravenously, is preferred. The rectal route is suitable for patients who are unable to take drugs orally or in whom parenteral administration is contraindicated. More recently, continuous subcutaneous infusions[6,10] have been used for patients who are unable to take drugs orally or in whom a bleeding diathesis or cachexia limits the use of repetitive parenteral injections. Continuous IV infusions[21,49,57] also allow rapid titration of analgesic in patients with severe pain. By maintaining a steady-state level, it is possible to impart satisfactory pain relief without significant side effects. Both the continuous subcutaneous and the continuous IV infusion methods obviate the typical bolus effect that occurs following intermittent intramuscular or intravenous injections. This effect is characterized by excessive sedation and/or the early return of pain before the next analgesic dose is given. Guidelines for these methods of drug administration have been published recently.[10,58]

The use of epidural, intrathecal, or intraventricular administration of narcotic analgesics* minimizes the distribution of drug to receptors in the brain stem and cerebral hemispheres, thereby avoiding the side effects of systemic administration. Localized selective analgesia is produced without motor blockade. The efficacy of these approaches appears to be based on the concept that narcotic drugs bind to opiate receptors in the spinal cord and this binding, in turn, suppresses the firing of spinothalamic tract neurons in response to noxious stimuli.[80] The clinical efficacy of continuous intrathecal infusions using the Infusaid Pump has been studied in patients with cancer pain.[7] The clinical and pharmacokinetic data obtained demonstrated that profound analgesia can be produced with small doses of morphine. The intrathecal route also has been advocated[9,44] because the dose and subsequent systemic uptake with epidural administration are much higher. Both epidural and intrathecal methods are associated with rostral redistribution of the drug and with central side effects, including rare respiratory depression and occasional nausea.[44] Tolerance also occurs and is most problematical in patients with progressive disease. Considerable cross tolerance is induced by systemic narcotics, making it difficult to determine the proper timing for these techniques.[25,44]

The exact place for epidural, intrathecal, and intraventricular administration in metastatic bone pain remains to be clarified and compared to standard therapy with oral narcotic analgesics.

Method of Administration. It is important to administer the analgesic on a regular basis after initial titration of the dose. This allows maintenance of the patient's pain at a tolerable level and also enables a smaller amount of drug to be taken in a 24-hour period.

The availability of an oral slow-release morphine preparation[78] with 8-to-12-hour effectiveness has given patients greater freedom from repetitive dosing, especially during the night. This drug appears to be both safe and efficacious, but studies assessing its efficacy for pain relief are currently in progress.

Use of Combination Drugs. As already noted, the use of a combination of drugs may enable the prescribing physician to increase the analgesic effects without requiring an escalation of the narcotic dose. There are several combinations that produce additive analgesic effects. These include a narcotic with a nonnarcotic (e.g., aspirin, acetaminophen, ibuprofen), a narcotic plus an antihistamine (specifically 100 mg of hydroxyzine), or a narcotic plus an amphetamine (10 mg of parenteral Dexedrine).[1,13,19]

In clinical practice hydroxyzine (25 mg) has been used on a regular basis and anecdotal observations show it to be effective. Similarly an amphetamine (Dexedrine) in 2.5 to 5 mg doses twice daily has been effective in reducing narcotic sedation in patients who were receiving adequate analgesia but were excessively sedated. Certain combinations that do not provide additive analgesia are (1) a narcotic plus a benzodiazepine and (2) a narcotic plus a phenothiazine. In controlled studies assessing the analgesic properties of these two drugs with narcotics,[24,31] additive sedative effects without improved analgesia were noted.

Narcotic Side Effects. There is a wide variety of side effects that occur with the use of narcotics in the management of bone pain. These include sedation, respiratory depression, nausea, vomiting, and constipation.

SEDATION. It is not uncommon for patients to become sedated within the first 24 to 48 hours when switched to a new drug. Tolerance to the sedative effects of most narcotics develops before the maximal analgesic effects are achieved, the initial sedative effect often clearing rapidly.

RESPIRATORY DEPRESSION. Tolerance to the respiratory depressant effects occurs rapidly and provides a protective mechanism to the patient receiving analgesics for pain.

When narcotic analgesics are used on a long-term basis in patients with cancer pain, respiratory depression does not represent a significant clinical problem because other toxic effects of the drug (e.g., sedation) appear first. However, in patients with compromised pulmonary function the use of drugs with a short rather than a long half-life probably is indicated because of drug accumulation. Obviously in the presence of a compromised respiratory status secondary to obstructive

*References 7, 9, 26, 42, 44, 54.

pulmonary disease, it is important to know the patient's pulmonary function values as the drug is titrated. In our experience no significant problems with adequately managing this group of patients have arisen although titration has been slower in some instances.

Nausea and Vomiting. The narcotic analgesics often produce nausea and emesis, but again tolerance to this effect soon develops, usually rapidly enough that it can be prevented by an antiemetic initially. If the combination of an antiemetic and a narcotic is ineffective, however, an alternative narcotic of a different congener must be tried (for instance, switching from morphine to methadone).

Constipation. All the narcotic analgesics produce constipation, and it is therefore imperative that the patient be started on an adequate bowel regimen before beginning long-term narcotic therapy and that larger doses of cathartics be prescribed than those recommended for conventional hospital care. Bulk and high-fiber diets, in combination with senna derivatives and cathartics, usually will provide adequate control of constipation.[43,76]

Tolerance. As already discussed, tolerance to the analgesic effects of a drug does develop and when this occurs the physician can switch to an alternative narcotic analgesic and usually gain a useful effect because of the lack of complete cross tolerance. When switching, the equianalgesic dose should be calculated and then halved to provide the appropriate starting dose.[32]

To prevent acute withdrawal, patients chronically receiving narcotic analgesics should be slowly tapered off the drug if their pain has been effectively treated. This can be done by maintaining 10% of the previous daily regimen. However, for patients in whom respiratory depression develops during chronic narcotic administration, the use of diluted doses of naloxone (0.4 mg in a 10 ml syringe of saline) is the recommended approach, titrating the amount to the individual patient. Using this approach, we have prevented patients from suffering acute withdrawal reactions, with recurrence of pain and the onset of psychotomimetic symptoms. We advise a slow titration in patients who are tolerant to narcotics until an adequate respiratory rate is achieved. In patients receiving drugs with a long plasma half-life (e.g., methadone or levorphanol) a naloxone infusion may be necessary to provide a sustained antagonist effect.

These guidelines notwithstanding, the management of pain with narcotic analgesics remains problematical. Much of the difficulty arises from differences in the responses of individual patients to equivalent drug doses. However, attention to the principles just outlined will allow the physician readily to care for any patient with chronic cancer pain requiring narcotic analgesics.

Adjuvant Drugs. Along with the nonnarcotic and narcotic analgesics there is a series of adjuvant analgesic drugs that have been effective in specific pain syndromes or have been used to treat some of the side effects and symptoms associated with narcotic analgesics. Any attempt to develop guidelines for the use of these adjuvant drugs in clinical cancer pain management, however, must be prefaced by certain caveats.[18] To begin with, the drugs have been developed for clinical indications other than analgesia. Also, except for methotrimeprazine (a phenothiazine analgesic), they are not as effective in relieving pain as are the narcotic analgesics. In many instances there are no efficacy studies for their coanalgesic properties, particularly in cancer patients.

The choice of an adjuvant drug must be individualized using the simplest and most potent combination of drugs.

Steroids. In the management of pain from metastatic bone disease, steroids have been the most commonly used adjuvant drug. Although the mechanism by which they induce pain relief is not understood, it is thought that they have an antiinflammatory and an antitumor effect. In epidural spinal cord compression,[25] for example, 85% of patients receiving 100 mg of dexamethasone as part of their regular therapy protocol reported significant pain relief with marked reduction in analgesic requirements.

Steroids have both specific and nonspecific benefits in managing acute and chronic cancer pain. Their ability to produce euphoria and increased appetite and weight gain contributes greatly to the cancer patient's sense of well-being. Several studies[65,66] have demonstrated prolonged survival time and reduced narcotic doses for control of pain in terminal cancer patients receiving steroids.

The dose of corticosteroids depends on

the clinical situation. In patients with epidural cord compression and pain[25] the initial treatment using 100 mg of IV dexamethasone followed by a tapering schedule, with maintenance at 16 mg of dexamethasone during radiation therapy, achieved significant pain reduction. Both prednisolone and dexamethasone have been used in this population, but there are no comparative studies to show that an equivalent dose of dexamethasone has a more specific effect than one of prednisolone in the treatment of bone pain. Dexamethasone does have approximately seven times the antiinflammatory activity of prednisolone, however, and no mineralocorticoid activity.

In a prospective survey on the use of corticosteroids for pain control in patients with advanced cancer,[76] dexamethasone seemed to be more effective than prednisolone against nerve compression pain; however, there was no statistical difference against bone pain, and the incidence of side effects was broadly similar, the most common one being oral candidiasis. In patients receiving steroids the use of nonsteroidal antiinflammatory drugs should be markedly limited, for this combination may place the patient at greater risk of gastrointestinal side effects, specifically gastric ulceration and GI bleeding. Consequently, we discontinue the NSAID in any patient taking steroids for analgesia or symptom relief.

Antidepressants. Another group of drugs that have been very effective in the management of bone pain is the tricyclic antidepressants (TCAs). These drugs work as coanalgesics and also have been demonstrated to possess analgesic properties of their own.[79] The analgesic effects of amitryptyline (the TCA of choice) are mediated by its heightening of serotonin activity within the central nervous system. Animal studies have demonstrated the direct analgesic effect of these drugs, with amitryptyline showing the greatest potency, and the drugs have also been reported to enhance morphine analgesia in cancer patients. Amitryptyline is an effective analgesic quite independent of its antidepressant capability and has been used in the treatment of patients with postherpetic neuralgia and in others with diabetic neuropathy. It is most valuable when used as a nighttime medication, because it is also a potent sedative.

The starting dose of amitryptyline is 25 mg p.o. for the average patient, although 10 mg is safer for an elderly one. Slow escalation to 50 or 75 mg p.o. is usually associated with lesser hypnotic effects. In patients with symptoms of depression, doses up to 150 or 200 mg p.o. per day may be required. Amitryptyline is the commonly recommended sleeping medication for cancer patients because of its ability to enhance analgesia and because of its sedative properties.

Antihistamines. The antihistamines, specifically hydroxyzine, also have analgesic properties. Beaver and Feise[1] reported that 100 mg of parenteral hydroxyzine had analgesic activity approaching that of 8 mg of parenteral morphine. When combined with morphine, hydroxyzine has additive analgesic effects[27]; the sedative effects of the combination, however, are only slightly greater than those of morphine alone. In the management of an anxious and nauseated patient with pain, hydroxyzine serves multiple purposes because of its antiemetic and antianxiety properties. We regularly use 25 to 50 mg as a coanalgesic with a narcotic and have found the combination to be effective, but controlled studies for these doses are lacking.

Phenothiazines. Methotrimeprazine (Levoprome) is the phenothiazine drug with the most prominent analgesic properties. In single-dose studies of patients with postoperative cancer pain and with chronic pain of various causes, 15 mg IM of Levoprome was equivalent to 15 mg of IM morphine. In our experience[15] methotrimeprazine is best used to manage cancer bone pain in special circumstances. For example, in the patient tolerant of narcotic analgesics it offers an alternative method of producing analgesia; in the patient with associated bowel obstruction and pain it obviates the constipatory effects of narcotics; in the patient with respiratory compromise it counters the respiratory depressant effects of the narcotics; in the patient with pain and narcotic-induced nausea, vomiting, or anxiety it acts as both an analgesic and as an antiemetic and sedative drug. The physician should begin with a test dose of 5 mg IM to see whether it produces significant sedation or hypotension. Doses of 10 to 20 mg IM are the standard, but individual variations in response may be marked. The side effects of methotrimeprazine include postural hypotension and excessive sedation. Tolerance develops to these effects with repeated administration. Extrapyramidal effects also occur, but their incidence has not been well studied.

Chorpromazine,[31] another phenothiazine derivative widely used in the treatment of patients with terminal illness and cancer pain, does not produce additive analgesia. Its primary usefulness is as a tranquilizer,[24] although it has also been used as an antiemetic. Because it possesses minimal analgesic properties, it should not be used in that capacity; rather, methotrimeprazine should be used in its stead for patients with pain.

Anticonvulsants. The anticonvulsant drugs, specifically phenytoin and carbamazepine, have been most useful in the treatment of patients with certain chronic pain states of nerve origin (e.g., postherpetic neuralgia, diabetic neuropathy, deafferentation pain).[71] They have not been effective in patients with bone pain, except when it is associated with a radiculopathy, and even then have been of only questionable efficacy. We have found carbamazepine to be specifically useful in managing acute shocklike neuralgia in patients with cranial or high cervical neck pain caused by either tumor infiltration or traumatic neuroma. It has also been useful in patients with phantom limb pain secondary to traumatic neuroma. Neither phenytoin nor carbamazepine, however, has been effective in controlling the burning dysesthetic pains associated with other nerve injury; they have been useful only in the paroxysmal pains.

Doses for carbamazepine begin at 100 mg p.o. per day and slowly increase to 800 mg day over a 7-to-10-day period. Blood counts should be taken before drug therapy is started, 2 weeks after initiation of therapy, and at regular intervals during therapy to assess the potential for neutropenia. This effect is idiosyncratic, but in our experience cancer patients are at greater risk of suppression of their WBC count because of compromised bone marrow from previous therapy as well as tumor infiltration.

There is a variety of other agents that have been suggested as effective in the management of bone pain and cancer. Haloperidol (Haldol),[28] a butyrophenone, may be useful both as a coanalgesic and to treat side effects in patients receiving methadone. In a study of 56 patients receiving methadone for the treatment of cancer pain,[4] 24 also received Haldol: 10 for the management of confusion and hallucination, 11 for "overwhelming" pain, and 3 for control of nausea and vomiting; the authors suggested various roles for haloperidol. Haldol is the most widely used agent in the management of major psychiatric disorders, and it is the drug of choice in the medical management of acutely psychotic cancer patients or patients with an agitated delirium.

Amphetamines. Dextroamphetamine (Dexedrine) in a dose of 10 mg IM[19] has been demonstrated to produce additive analgesic effects when combined with morphine in single-dose studies of postoperative pain. The drug appears to act by reducing the sedative effects of the narcotic. In our experience the amphetamines are best used to counteract sedation in the patient receiving adequate analgesia but who is incapacitated by the sedative side effects. In oral doses of 2.5 to 5 mg twice a day, patients report improvement in their sedation. Controlled studies of the chronic use of Dexedrine in cancer patients with pain are lacking, however.

Cocaine. Among other drugs considered to play a role in the treatment of patients with cancer and bone pain is cocaine, which was initially reported by Snow[68] to be effective in combination with opium for pain associated with malignancy. In experimental studies cocaine potentiates morphine analgesia by blocking the reuptake of serotonin. Twycross,[75] evaluating the role of cocaine in the Brompton cocktail, reported that introducing cocaine in 10 mg increments per dose resulted in a small but statistically significant increase in alertness whereas stopping cocaine had no detectable effect. However, in the only controlled study of morphine and cocaine,[34] Kaiko et al. showed that there were no additive analgesic effects with cocaine and cocaine alone had no analgesic properties at the 10 mg oral dose used in the study.

• • •

In summary, these are some of the adjuvant analgesic drugs that have been used or suggested as potentially useful in the management of bone pain and cancer. However, further studies are needed to define the role of many of these drugs in the management of this group of patients.

Multidisciplinary Approaches to Pain Management

There is a well-defined role for physical therapy and for anesthetic, neurosurgical, and behavioral techniques in the management of patients with bone pain (see box).

Physical Therapy. Physical therapy plays a major role in rehabilitating patients. The use of appropriate splinting, bracing, and progressive exercise programs with support devices as needed greatly improves patient ambulation. Transcutaneous electrical stimulation (TENS)[39,77] has been most useful in managing focal pain syndromes, which usually are of neuropathic origin, but it has not been studied in bone pain except indirectly through its use in patients with associated radiculopathy. TENS involves the application of low- and high-intensity stimulation to peripheral nerves to selectively activate the large-diameter fibers and thus "close the gate" to pain perception. TENS is reported to be effective in 75% to 80% of patients with acute pain and is a safe and noninvasive approach. The analgesia that results, however, is transient and its role is therefore limited.

MULTIDISCIPLINARY APPROACHES TO CANCER PAIN

- Analgesic drug therapy
  - Nonnarcotic analgesics
  - Narcotic analgesics
  - Adjuvant analgesics
- Physical therapy
  - Exercise
  - Bracing
  - Stabilization
  - TENS
- Anesthetic methods
  - Trigger point injections
  - Peripheral nerve blocks
  - Epidural-intrathecal blocks
  - Chemical hypophysectomy
  - Nitrous oxide
- Neurosurgical methods
  - Epidural, intrathecal, intraventricular catheters for narcotic administration
  - Cordotomy
  - Hypophysectomy
- Behavioral approaches
  - Relaxation therapy
  - Biofeedback
  - Cognitive behavioral training
  - Hypnosis
  - Music therapy

Anesthetic Methods. Anesthetic procedures are most useful for managing local pain before nerve injury develops into a deafferentation state. Although they have been widely heralded, controlled studies of their effectiveness compared to that of other methods of pain control are lacking. In patients with bone pain the most commonly employed procedures are local triggerpoint injection, peripheral nerve block, and epidural or intrathecal block.

Trigger point injections involve the use of either saline or a short-acting local anesthetic deposited in a focal area of muscle spasm and resulting in significant local pain relief. On occasion such relief will persist long after the local pharmacological effects of the agent have been exhausted.

Peripheral nerve blocks are used both diagnostically, to identify a nerve distribution, and therapeutically, to interrupt the transmission of pain within a predetermined distribution. They are most effective in managing acute radicular pain associated with a rib fracture or with nerve root compression or to assess whether a permanent block will offer a patient adequate pain relief. The limitation of these procedures is that each peripheral nerve subserves sensory function over multiple levels, requiring multiple nerves to be blocked for adequate pain control. These procedures do not provide pain relief for vertebral body lesions because the vertebral bodies have bilateral innervation, which would require bilateral and extensive blocking.

Epidural and intrathecal blocks are used to provide relief from vertebral or sacral metastases or from so-called "midline" pain. Intermittent or continuous epidural infusions of local anesthetics have been used for the temporary management of these difficult pain syndromes.[56] Their advantage is that they do not result in cross tolerance with narcotic analgesics and can thus provide effective temporary pain relief for the patient who is already tolerant of these agents. Attempts to use epidural or intrathecal neurolytic blocks for permanent relief of pain may produce motor weakness and autonomic dysfunction, and tachyphylaxis can develop after continuous administration. The techniques, indications, dilutions, and concentrations of neurolytic agents vary from investigator to investigator,[18] with satisfactory results having been reported in 22% to 80% of patients and permanent side effects (e.g., urinary or rectal incontinence, motor weakness, paresthesias) in 1% to 13%. The procedures are most effective in patients who have sacral destruction with bowel and bladder incontinence and leg weakness. However, these patients are also candidates for bilateral cordotomy, which is a more reliable and effective procedure.

Chemical hypophysectomy, a technique involving the injection of alcohol into the sella turcica under roentgenographic control, has received attention as a method of easing pain in patients with widespread bone metastases. Initial studies[51] reported dramatic relief in 60% of 600 patients, but a more recent investigation[46] has stated that relief varies between 35% and 74%. The mechanism of analgesia may be related in part to the tracking of alcohol up the pituitary stalk and the consequent disruption of the hypothalamic-thalamic endorphinergic pain pathway. The lack of detail in the clinical data and information on the endocrine status of such patients limits critical assessment of the technique, and in many patients pain relief occurs independently of tumor regression. Chemical hypophysectomy does not appear to be technically superior to transphenoidal hypophysectomy in relieving pain. The incidence of diabetes insipidus is between 10% and 20% for both procedures. Some authors have criticized the use of hypophysectomy solely as a pain-relieving procedure, making its use controversial at best. Additional clinical studies should help to clarify this controversy.

Nitrous oxide[20] is used to manage chronic pain from tumor progression in the dying patient. It is most helpful in cases of specific incident pain, and it can be administered with oxygen via a nonrebreathing face mask in concentrations ranging from 25% to 75% often in combination with systemic narcotics. The patient remains alert during its use.

Neurosurgical Methods. The neurosurgical approaches for managing cancer pain include two major categories of procedures: neuroablative and neurostimulatory. With neuroablative procedures, surgical or radiofrequency lesions are made along pain pathways. With neurostimulatory procedures, electrodes are stereotactically placed to activate pain inhibitory pathways. Unfortunately, the use of neurosurgical procedures in the cancer patient remains a dilemma for both patients and physicians. Historically, neurosurgical procedures for cancer pain have been performed late in the course of the patient's illness, often in a debilitated patient. The development of overriding medical problems has thwarted full evaluation of their effectiveness and duration of action. Patients with cancer, and their physicians, often are unwilling to consider neuroablative or neurostimulatory procedures and their associated risks before trying more traditional therapy and analgesic regimens. Thus neurosurgical procedures are often a last resort, and this fact has made evaluation of their effectiveness difficult.

Guidelines for using neurosurgical intervention include an adequate prior trial of conventional methods of pain relief and a full awareness by the patient of the potential risks and benefits of the planned procedure. At the present time the two most common neurosurgical procedures for pain relief are cordotomy and the placement of epidural, intrathecal, and intraventricular catheters for narcotic drug delivery. A cordotomy[40,53,62] interrupts the anterolateral spinothalamic tract in the cervical or thoracic region and may be performed by a percutaneous stereotactic or an open surgical technique. It is most useful in managing unilateral pain below the waist. Initial complications include paresis (5% of patients), ataxia (20%), and urinary dysfunction (10%). Late complications occur in only 5%. Although initial pain relief from cordotomy is experienced by 90% of the patients, this figure drops to 80% at 3 months. At the end of 1 year approximately 40% of patients report a return of pain. The pain develops on the side opposite the cordotomy in 7% to 10% of patients and is referred to as "mirror" pain.

Patients with midline or bilateral pain need bilateral cordotomies. These may be done at different levels to obviate respiratory difficulties, specifically phrenic nerve paralysis, that may occur with high cervical lesions. In patients requiring bilateral cordotomies a high cervical percutaneous cordotomy is done on one side and an open high thoracic cordotomy on the other. In patients with upper extremity pain a high cervical cordotomy is particularly effective. The advantage of a percutaneous cordotomy is that it avoids general anesthesia and a prolonged period of recuperation while allowing careful monitoring of the effects on the lesion with the patient awake. In the management of midline pain from vertebral body disease or of bilateral sacral pain, bilateral cordotomies can often provide dramatic relief, allowing the patient to sit pain free when he was previously unable to move without excruciating discomfort. In our experience patients are more willing to undergo neurosurgical procedures when other attempts at pain relief have failed or when all primary modalities of therapy have been tried. Significant pain relief can be obtained by cordotomy, and this procedure should be encouraged for patients even with far-advanced disease, emphasizing that the dramatic relief will be associated with a marked improvement in the quality of life.

Behavioral Approaches. Interventions designed to modify problems in the attitude and behavior of cancer patients regarding the global experience of pain and distress are made through the application of specific mental and behavioral techniques.[74] These can take place in individual therapy sessions or in group sessions, and they help patients cope with the pain as well as the functional adjustments to living with a chronic impediment due to the disease or its treatment. These interventions may be useful as an adjuvant therapeutic modality and can easily be combined with drug therapy and with anesthetic, neurosurgical, or physical therapy approaches.

Behavioral techniques include relaxation training, cognitive and behavioral training, biofeedback, hypnosis, and music therapy. They can give the patient an increased sense of control by reducing his feelings of hopelessness and helplessness. The effectiveness of any one of these techniques compared to another or to standard medical or surgical regimens is unknown, and few controlled studies have been performed. Patients are taught the techniques and then are urged to use them independently. Relaxation training can be given by all health care professionals. Other behavioral approaches require biophysical instrumentation or more specialized skills. Cognitive and behavioral training provides the patient with a variety of strategies to divert his attention from the pain, facilitate his tolerance of pain, and increase his perceived sense of self-control and adaptive functioning. Music therapy[52] has been used in hospitals and hospice settings, alone and combined with relaxation training and hypnosis, to augment the effectiveness of these techniques. Hypnosis[29] has been studied most extensively and is widely used in the treatment of acute and chronic cancer pain. Studies report that 50% of patients may obtain some pain relief but indicate that there is no single effective hypnotic procedure.

All behavioral techniques appear to reduce pain by mechanisms that are in part related to their ability to modulate the affective response to painful stimuli.

SUMMARY

Pain, one of the most feared concomitants of cancer and metastatic bone disease, may be the single most important factor limiting the patient's quality of life. Its management should be possible with the variety of approaches just described. Careful definition of the nature of the pain, aggressive attempts to treat its cause, and the use of a multidisciplinary approach toward the management of the pain will greatly improve the overall course of any patient with bone metastases.

REFERENCES

1. Beaver, W.T., and Feise, G.: Comparison of analgesic effects of morphine sulfate, hydroxyzine, and their combination in patients with postoperative pain. In Bonica, J.J., and Albe-Fessard, D., editors: Advances in pain research and therapy, New York, 1976, Raven Press.
2. Bockman, R.S., and Myers, W.P.L.: Osteotropism in human breast cancer. In Day, S.B., et al., editors: Cancer invasion and metastases: biologic mechanisms and therapy, New York, 1977, Raven Press.
3. Bonica, J.J.: The management of pain, Philadelphia, 1953, Lea & Febiger.
4. Breivik, H., and Rennemo, F.: Clinical evaluation of combined treatment with methadone and psychotropic drugs in cancer patients, Acta Anaesthesiol. Scand. **74**(suppl.):135, 1982.
5. Brodie, G.N.: Letter: Indomethacin and bone pain, Lancet **1:**1160, 1974.
6. Campbell, C.F., et al.: Continuous subcutaneous infusion of morphine for the pain of terminal malignancy, Ann. Intern. Med. **98:**51, 1983.
7. Coombs, D.W., et al.: Relief of continuous chronic pain by intraspinal narcotics infusion via an implanted reservoir. J.A.M.A. **250:**2336, 1983.
8. Cooper, P.R., et al.: Morphology of the osteum, J. Bone Joint Surg. **48B:**1239, 1966.

9. Cousins, M.J., and Mather, L.E.: Intrathecal and epidural administration of opioids, Anesthesiology, **61:**276, 1984.
10. Coyle, N., et al.: Continuous subcutaneous infusions of opiates in cancer patients with pain, Oncol. Nurs. Forum **13:**53, 1986.
11. Ettinger, D.S., et al.: Important clinical pharmacologic considerations in the use of methadone in cancer patients, Cancer Treat. Rep. **63:**457, 1979.
12. Ferreira, S.H., et al.: The hyperalgesic effects of prostacycline and prostaglandin E2, Prostaglandins **16:**31, 1978.
13. Ferrer-Brechner, T., and Ganz, P.: Combination therapy with ibuprofen and methadone for chronic cancer pain, Am. J. Med. **77:**78, 1984.
14. Foley, K.M.: Pain syndromes in patients with cancer. In Bonica, J.J., et al., editors: Advances in pain research and therapy, New York, 1979, Raven Press.
15. Foley, K.M.: The practical use of narcotic analgesics, Med. Clin. North Am. **66**(5):1091, 1982.
16. Foley, K.M.: Adjuvant analgesic drugs in the management of cancer pain. In Aronoff, G.M., editor: Relief of chronic pain, Boston, 1983, Addison Wesley.
17. Foley, K.M.: Assessment of pain. In Twycross, R.G., editor: Clinics in oncology. Pain relief in cancer, Philadelphia, 1983, W.B. Saunders Co.
18. Foley, K.M.: The treatment of cancer pain, N. Engl. J. Med. **313:**84, 1985.
19. Forrest, W.H., Jr., et al.: Dextroamphetamine with morphine for the treatment of postoperative pain, N. Engl. J. Med. **296:**712, 1977.
20. Fosburg, M.T., and Crone, R.K.: Nitrous oxide analgesia for refractory pain in the terminally ill, J.A.M.A. **250:**511, 1983.
21. Fraser, D.G.: Intravenous morphine infusion for chronic pain, Ann. Intern. Med. **93:**781, 1980.
22. Galasko, C.S.B.: Mechanisms of bone destruction in the development of skeletal metastases, Nature [Lond.] **263:**507, 1976.
23. Gasic, C., et al.: Anti-metastatic effect of aspirin, Lancet **2:**932, 1972.
24. Gordon, R.A., and Campbell, M.: The use of chlorpromazine in intractable pain associated with terminal carcinoma, Can. Med. Assoc. J. **75:**420, 1956.
25. Greenberg, H.S., et al.: Epidural spinal cord compression from metastatic tumor: results from a new treatment protocol, Ann. Neurol. **8:**361, 1980.
26. Greenberg, H.S., et al.: Benefit from and tolerance to continuous intrathecal infusion of morphine for intractable cancer pain, J. Neurosurg. **57:**360, 1982.
27. Halpern, L.W.: Psychotropics, ataractics, and related drugs. In Bonica, J.J., et al., editors: Advances in pain research and therapy, New York, 1979, Raven Press.
28. Hanks, G.W., et al.: The myth of haloperidol potentiation, Lancet **2:**523, 1983.
29. Hilgard, E.R., and Hilgard, J.R.: Hypnosis in the relief of pain, Los Altos, Calif., 1975, William Kaufmann, Inc.
30. Horton, J.E., et al.: Bone resorbing activity in supernatant fluid from cultured human peripheral blood leukocytes, Science **177:**793, 1972.
31. Houde, R.W., and Wallenstein, S.L.: Analagesic power of chlorpromazine alone in combination with morphine, Fed. Proc. **14:**353, 1955. (Abstract.)
32. Inturrisi, C.E.: Narcotic drugs, Med. Clin. North Am. **66**(5):1061, 1982.
33. Kaiko, R.F., et al.: Central nervous system excitatory effects of meperidine in cancer patients, Ann. Neurol. **13:**180, 1983.
34. Kaiko, R.F., et al.: Cocaine and morphine interaction in acute and chronic cancer pain, Pain. In press, 1986.
35. Kanner, R.M., and Foley, K.M.: Patterns of narcotic drug use in a cancer pain clinic, Ann. N.Y. Acad. Sci. **362:**162, 1981.
36. Kantor, T.G.: Control of pain by nonsteroidal antiinflammatory drugs, Med. Clin. North Am. **66**(5): 1053, 1982.
37. Kantor, T.G.: Nonsteroidal anti-inflammatory analgesic agents in management of cancer pain. In Hospital practice. The management of cancer pain, New York, 1984, HP Publishing.
38. Kellgren, J.G.: On the distribution of pain arising from deep somalic structures with charts of segmental pain areas, Clin. Sci. **435:**303, 1939.
39. Keravel, Y., et al.: Long term results of TENS in peripheral nerve lesions, Pain **2**(suppl.):S73, 1984.
40. Levin, A.B.: Techniques and results of cordotomy in patients with pain of benign and malignant origin. In Rizzi, R., and Visentin, M., editors: Pain therapy, Amsterdam, 1983, Elsevier Biomedical Press.
41. Lipton, S.: Percutaneous cordotomy. In Wall, P.D., and Melzack, R., editors: Textbook of pain, New York, 1984, Churchill Livingstone, Inc.
42. Lobato, R.D., et al.: Intraventricular morphine for control of pain in terminal cancer patients, J. Neurosurg. **59:**627, 1983.
43. Maguire, L.C., et al.: Prevention of narcotic induced constipation, N. Engl. J. Med. **305:**1654, 1981.
44. Max, M.B., et al.: Epidural and intrathecal opiates: cerebrospinal fluid and plasma profiles in patients with chronic cancer pain, Clin. Pharmacol. Ther. **38:** 631, 1985.
45. McGivney, W.T., and Crooks, G.M.: The care of patients with severe chronic pain in terminal illness, J.A.M.A. **251:**1182, 1984.
46. Miles, J., and Lipton, S.: Mode of action by which pituitary alcohol injection relieves pain. In Bonica, J.J., et al., editors: Advances in pain research and therapy, New York, 1976, Raven Press.
47. Minton, J.P.: The response of breast cancer patients with bone pain to L-dopa, Cancer **33:**358, 1974.
48. Minton, J.P., et al.: L-Dopa effect in painful bony metastases, N. Engl. J. Med. **294:**340, 1976.
49. Miser, A.W., et al.: Continuous intravenous infusion of morphine sulfate for control of severe pain in children with terminal malignancy, J. Pediatr. **96:** 930, 1980.
50. Moertel, G.G.: Treatment of cancer pain with orally administered medications, J.A.M.A. **244:**2448, 1980.
51. Moricca, G.: Chemical hypophysectomy for cancer pain. In Bonica, J.J., editor: Advances in neurology, New York, 1974, Raven Press.
52. Munro, S., and Mount, B.: Music therapy in palliative care, Can. Med. Assoc. J. **119:**1029, 1978.

53. Nathan, P.W.: Results of antero-lateral cordotomy for pain in cancer, J. Neurol. Neurosurg. Psychiatr. **26**:353, 1963.
54. Onofrio, B.M., et al.: Continuous low-dose intrathecal morphine administration in the treatment of chronic pain of malignant origin, Mayo Clin. Proc. **56**:516, 1981.
55. Payne, R., and Foley, K.M.: Advances in the management of cancer pain, Cancer Treat. Rep. **68**:173, 1984.
56. Pilon, R.N., and Baker, A.R.: Chronic pain control by means of an epidural catheter, Cancer **37**:903, 1976.
57. Portenoy, R.K., et al.: Continuous intravenous infusions of opiates in cancer pain: review of 46 cases and guidelines for use, Cancer Treat. Rep. **70**:575, 1986.
58. Portenoy, R.K., et al.: Back pain in the cancer patient: an algorithm for evaluation and management, Neurology **37**:134, 1986.
59. Powles, T.J., et al.: Inhibition by aspirin and indomethacin of osteolytic tumor deposits and hypercalcemia in rats with Walker tumor and its possible application to human breast cancer, Br. J. Cancer **28**: 316, 1973.
60. Powles, T.J., et al.: Factors influencing development of bone metastases. In Day, S.B., editor: Cancer invasion and metastasis: biologic mechanisms and therapy, New York, 1977, Raven Press.
61. Robbie, D.S.: A trial of sublingual buprenorphine in cancer pain, Br. J. Clin. Pharmacol. **7**(suppl. 3):315S, 1979.
62. Rosomoff, H.L.: Percutaneous radiofrequency cervical cordotomy for intractable pain. In Bonica, J.J., editor: Advances in neurology, New York, 1974, Raven Press.
63. Sacks, P.V.: Letter: Prolactin, prostaglandin, and bone pain of metastatic breast cancer, Lancet **2**: 1385, 1974.
64. Sawe, J., et al.: Patient controlled dose regimen of methadone for chronic cancer pain, Br. Med. J. **282**:771, 1981.
65. Schell, H.W.: The risk of adrenal corticosteroid therapy in far advanced cancer, Am. J. Med. Sci. **252**: 641, 1966.
66. Schell, H.W.: Adrenal corticosteroid therapy in far advanced cancer, Geriatrics **27**:131, 1972.
67. Shimm, D.S., et al.: Medical management of chronic cancer pain, J.A.M.A. **241**:2408, 1979.
68. Snow, H.: The opium-cocaine treatment of malignant disease, Br. Med. J. **1**:1019, 1897.
69. Stoll, B.A.: Indomethacin in breast cancer, Lancet **2**:384, 1973.
70. Swerdlow, M.: Anticonvulsant drugs and chronic pain, Clin. Neuropharmacol. **7**:51, 1984.
71. Swerdlow, M., and Stjernsward, J.: Cancer pain relief—an urgent problem, World Health Forum **3**: 325, 1982.
72. Symonds, P.: Methadone and the elderly, Br. Med. J. **1**:512, 1977.
73. Tolis, G.J.: L-Dopa for pain from bone metastases, N. Engl. J. Med. **292**:1353, 1975.
74. Turk, D.C., et al.: Pain and behavioral medicine, New York, 1983, The Guilford Press.
75. Twycross, R.G.: Value of cocaine in opiate containing elixers, Br. Med. J. **2**:1348, 1977.
76. Twycross, R.G., and Lack, S.A.: Symptom control in far-advanced cancer. Pain relief, London, 1983, Pitman Books.
77. Ventafridda, V., et al.: Transcutaneous nerve stimulation in cancer pain. In Bonica, J.J., editor: Advances in cancer pain, New York, 1979, Raven Press.
78. Walsh, T.D.: Controlled study of slow release morphine for chronic pain in advanced cancer, Pain **2**(suppl.):S202, 1984.
79. Walsh, T.D.: Antidepressants in chronic pain. In Walsh, T.D., editor: Clinical neuropharmacology, New York, 1983, Raven Press.
80. Yaksh, T.L.: Spinal opiate analgesia: characteristics and principles of action, Pain **11**:293, 1981.

PART III

ORTHOPAEDIC RECONSTRUCTION

CHAPTER 8

MANAGEMENT OF LOWER-EXTREMITY METASTASES

The femur accounts for 61% of all long-bone pathological fractures, with the peritrochanteric area accounting for almost 80% of those (Table 8-1). Only 39 of the 399 pathological long-bone fractures summarized in Table 8-1 occurred distal to the knee or elbow, and 36 of these were in the proximal tibial metaphysis. On the rare occasion when metastases in the foot bones progress sufficiently to cause a fracture, they will heal almost invariably following local irradiation and external splintage. In more than 15 years' experience treating long-bone metastases, we have had only one such fracture requiring operative intervention. This was an aneurysmal lytic metastasis from a renal carcinoma involving the distal half of the fifth metatarsal. Because of extensive bone destruction the fifth ray remained painful and unstable even after local irradiation and ultimately required a ray resection. The foot healed, and the patient was able to function well thereafter.

TABLE 8-1 **Distribution of 399 Pathological Lower-Extremity Fractures**

Location		Number
Femur		258
Femoral neck	69	
Peritrochanteric	50	
Subtrochanteric	84	
Femoral shaft	38	
Supracondylar	17	
Acetabulum		34
Tibia		31
Humerus		68
Forearm		8
	TOTAL	399

Most patients suffering a long-bone pathological fracture have widespread malignant disease, but it is wrong and unkind to regard this misfortune as a terminal event warranting only the simplest of symptomatic treatment. As already noted in Chapter 1, many patients suffering long-bone fractures from metastases can be expected to survive for more than a year following their fracture. Among the most commonly afflicted groups (those with breast carcinoma, lymphoma, or myeloma) more than 75% will be alive 1 year after their fracture, and the average survival will be 21 months.

Nonoperative Management. Because the majority of pathological fractures involve the proximal femur and because bracing of such fractures is cumbersome at best and rarely successful in debilitated patients, the decision to treat the fractures nonoperatively generally means treatment simply by bedrest. Effective prolonged fracture immobilization in bed is difficult to achieve, and adequate relief of pain impossible except with large doses of narcotic analgesics. Moreover, the existence of an unstable fracture, particularly of the femur, seriously interferes with attempts to achieve pain relief by local irradiation. A plaster hip spica cast is required to immobilize the limb sufficiently for transfer of the patient to and from the radiotherapy unit. Under such circumstances morbidity from supervoltage irradiation greatly increases. The usual skin-sparing effect is lost because electron buildup occurs as the beam traverses the cast.[44]

Few malignant pathological fractures treated conservatively can be expected to heal. Fractures of the femoral neck almost invariably fail to unite,[16] whereas those involving the trochanteric or subtrochanteric areas proceed to bony union in less than one out of four patients.[4,16]

However, the most compelling argument against attempting to treat such patients with bedrest is based on the multiplicity of medical complications that accompany such management. In addition to the deterioration in cardiorespiratory and gastrointestinal functions befalling any debilitated person who is immobilized, these patients suffer an extremely high incidence of skin breakdown, particularly over the buttocks and sacrum, because of their unwillingness to turn frequently and thus aggravate their fracture pain. Furthermore, these patients are subject to two complications peculiar to their systemic malignancy and particularly accelerated by enforced immobility: diffuse intravascular coagulopathy and malignant hypercalcemia.

Diffuse intravascular coagulopathy (DIC) occurs not infrequently in healthy young patients subjected to massive trauma with multiple long-bone fractures. However, it is unusual with single-bone fractures, except from certain malignant pathological conditions (particularly metastatic carcinoma of the prostate and lymphoma or myeloma when managed by prolonged recumbency).

A more common serious sequela of enforced immobilization in these patients is the development of extreme hypercalcemia.[35,52] The clinical manifestations of hypercalcemia are protean and may involve many organ systems. In severe disorders a syndrome characterized by abdominal pain, intractable vomiting, profound weakness, and severe dehydration with rapid deterioration of renal function may develop. Progression of the disorder may result in coma and death. Administration of phosphate infusions with or without steroids[42] is the treatment of choice for this condition.

To understand the significance of serum calcium measurements in these patients, it is important that one determine the relative contributions of potentially toxic ionized calcium and of metabolically inert protein-bound calcium to that measurement. For each increment or decrement in serum albumin or globulin of 1 g/100 ml, the serum calcium value decreases approximately 0.8 mg/100 ml. Thus, in a debilitated cancer patient with hypoproteinemia, even a moderate elevation in measurable serum calcium concentrations may represent a dangerously high level of free ionized calcium.

The most common cause of hypercalcemia in patients with a malignant pathological fracture is the mobilzation of ionized calcium from the fracture site and from other areas of bone metastases. With bedrest, the resorption of calcium from bone increases rapidly and within 24 hours the full-blown hypercalcemia syndrome may be apparent. Occasionally, serious hypercalcemic states develop because of a parathormone-like chemical secreted by the malignant tumor either at its primary origin or from its bone metastasis. Hypernephroma and bronchogenic carcinoma account for 60% of such cases, and again their effect tends to be accentuated in immobilized patients. Finally, induced hypercalcemia secondary to long-term hormonal therapy, particularly with androgenic hormones, accelerates dramatically in patients on enforced bedrest.

Operative Management. Because of all the problems inherent in nonoperative treatment of pathological lower-extremity fractures, their management today is surgical whenever possible—by prosthetic replacement in the case of femoral neck fractures, by internal fixation of other fractures when appropriate—all in the interest of early mobilization of the patient. If secure fixation of the fracture or of the prosthesis can be achieved, the patient may continue to be ambulatory or semiambulatory and usually will be free of pain.

The following criteria should be met, however, before any patient is considered for conventional open fracture fixation or prosthetic replacement:

1. A life expectancy of at least 2 months and a general condition good enough to tolerate major surgery
2. The expectation that the procedure will expedite mobilization of the patient and facilitate general care

3. The quality of bone both proximal and distal to the fracture site adequate to support metallic fixation or secure prosthetic seating

Unfortunately, in a significant number of patients, sufficiently extensive destruction of bone precludes secure immobilization of the fracture by conventional methods of internal fixation, and a long bone of the lower extremity with a pathological fracture must remain non–weight bearing until the fracture heals. In some cases, because bone destruction by the malignant process continues unabated, stability may never be achieved and the patient will become bedridden (Fig. 8-1). Any motion at the fracture site continues to cause pain, and the worsening complications of enforced bedrest lead to early death from cardiac or renal sequelae.

Prior to 1970, when methylmethacrylate was introduced as a means of augmenting conventional fixation, at least 25% of all patients

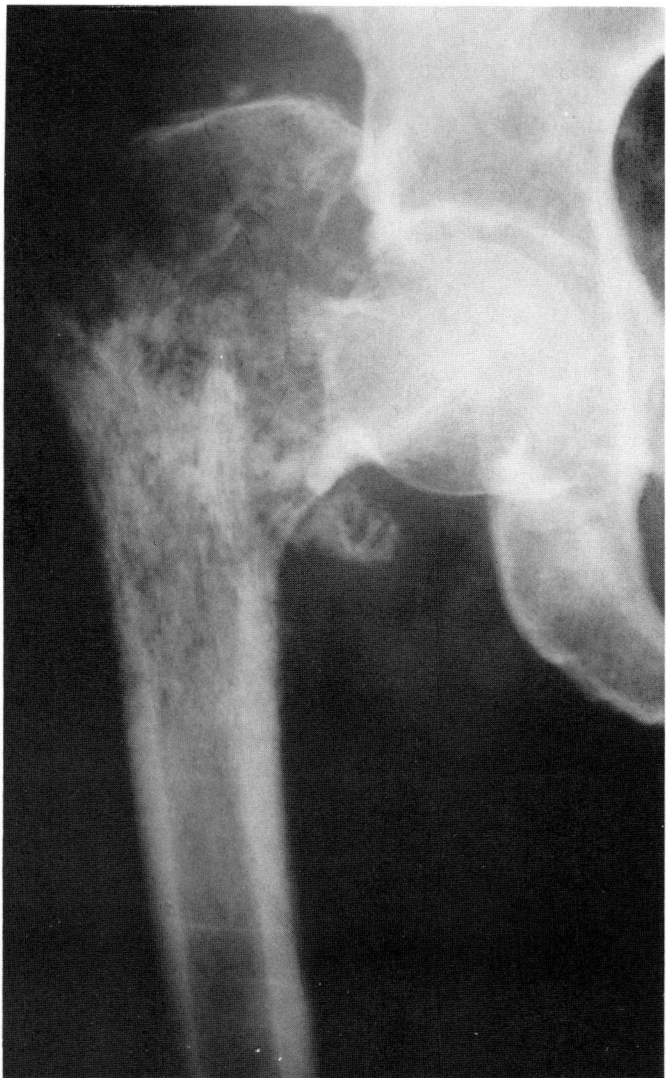

FIGURE 8-1 AP roentgenogram of the right hip in a 72-year-old woman with metastatic melanoma. Until this spontaneous fracture occurred, she had been apparently well for 18 years after enucleation of her right eye for a choroidal melanoma. Note the extensive destruction of cortical bone proximal and distal to the fracture site.

with a metastatic pathological fracture were excluded from consideration for internal fixation or prosthetic replacement because of the extent of bone destruction about the fracture site (Fig. 8-2). Among those actually undergoing operative fixation by conventional methods, the incidence of fixation failure was high (Fig. 8-3, *A* to *C*). Fewer than half regained an ambulatory status, and the great majority of these required external assistance. In the large series of Parrish and Murray,[42] only 11.4% of 70 patients who underwent open fracture fixation were restored to full weight-bearing ambulation and another 30% regained the ability to walk only with support. The results with prosthetic replacement for femoral neck fractures were somewhat better, with approximately 60% regaining at least a partial ambulatory status. However, the incidence of prosthetic loosening among patients who survived more than 6 months postoperatively was disturbingly high[42] (Fig. 8-3, *D*).

The mean survival for patients with a pathological single-bone fracture managed before

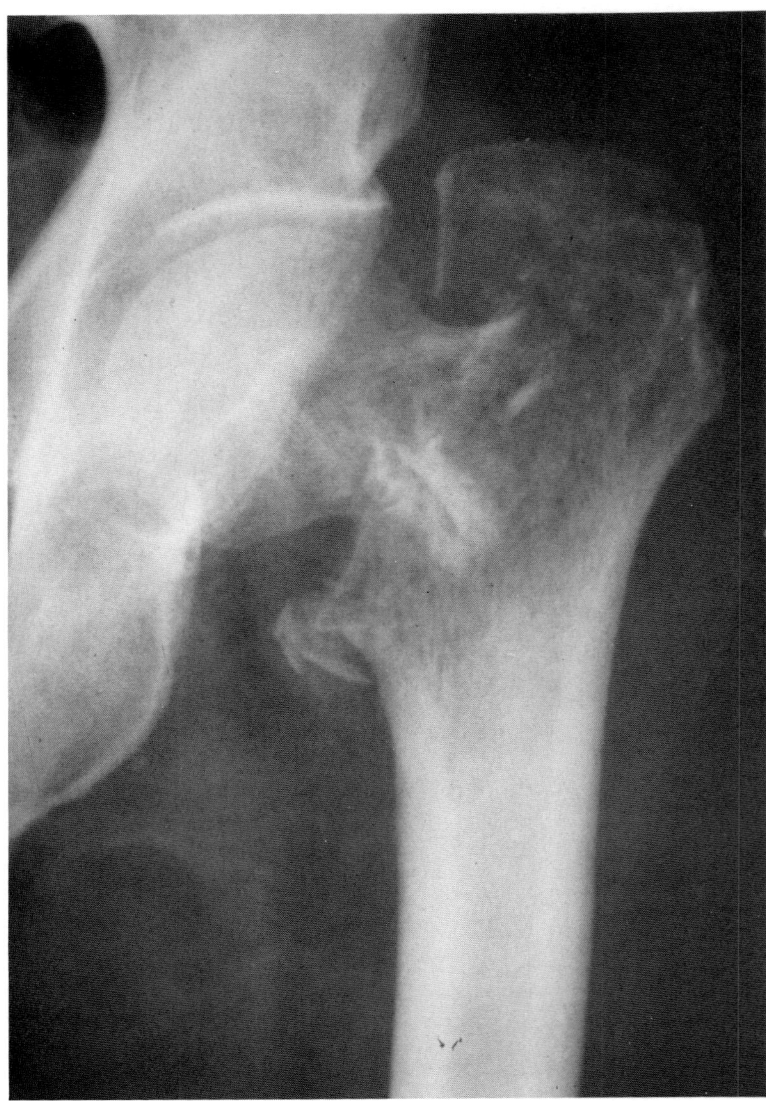

FIGURE 8-2 Pathological fracture of the left hip in a 61-year-old man with metastatic lung carcinoma. Note, again in this patient, the extensive bone lysis proximal and distal to the fracture.

1970 by conventional operative reduction and fixation or by prosthetic replacement was 7.2 months.[16,33,39,42] Approximately 60% survived 3 or more months postoperatively, 40% survived 6 or more months, and only 20% lived longer than a year. Patients with a pathological fracture secondary to metastatic breast carcinoma had a somewhat better prognosis, with a mean survival of 12.7 months in the series of Parrish and Murray[42] and Perez et al.[44]

In an effort to improve these statistics, Francis et al.[13] suggested in 1962 resecting the femoral head and neck as the most appropriate management of pathological fractures of the proximal femur in which the calcar femorale had been destroyed. For extensive cortical destruction around more distal fractures, Francis et al.[13] and Graham[17] both advocated amputation as the most conservative and successful approach to palliation of pain.

The reasons for the high incidence of fixation failure are complex but can be summarized by using a prototype subtrochanteric femur fracture as an example. A focus of metastatic malignancy progressively destroys cortical bone within the proximal femur, usually most actively within the richly vascularized areas of the greater and lesser trochanters. The area of major compressive trabeculae along the medial femoral cortex, centered at the lesser trochanter, eventually becomes sufficiently weakened that, from a structural

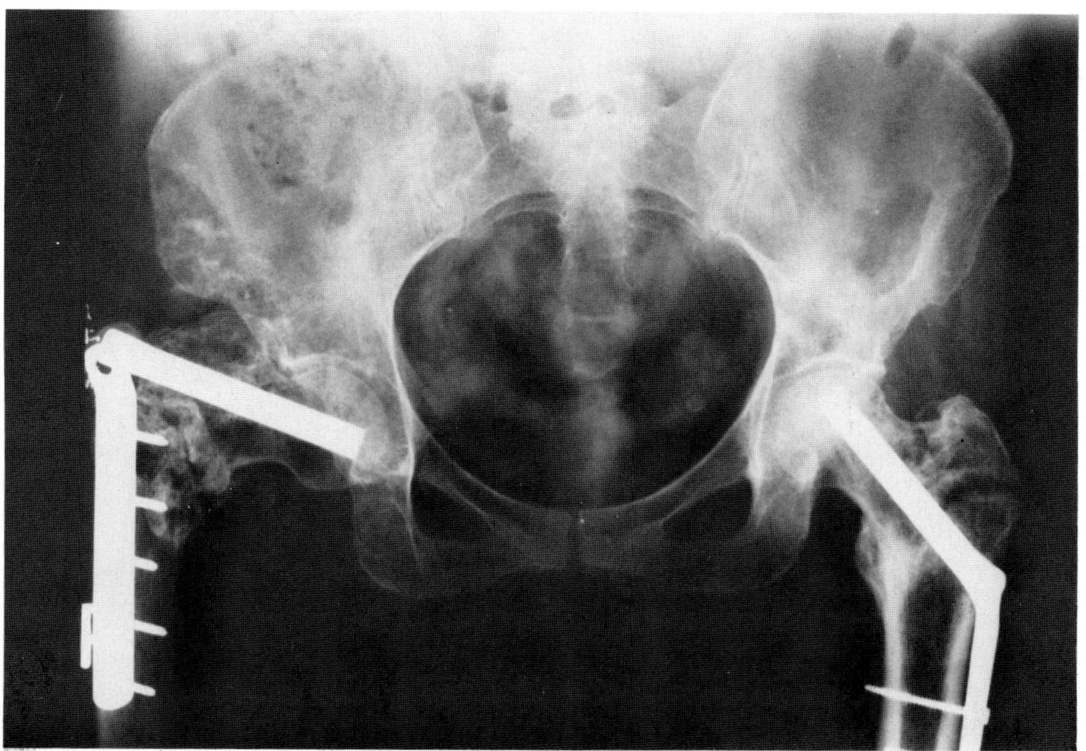

A

FIGURE 8-3 **A,** Bilateral pathological intertrochanteric fractures in a woman with extensive bone metastases from a breast carcinoma. Neither fracture was healed. Note, *on the left,* where the medial cortex remains intact, that mild varus angulation of the proximal fragment has occurred but fixation remains intact; *on the right,* however, where there is extensive destruction of the medial cortical bone, the fixation device has failed at the nail-plate junction and the proximal fragment is angulated into a varus malalignment. This is the most common type of failure for conventional fixation and occurs because of the loss of medial cortical stability. (**A** and **D** reprinted with permission from Parrish, F.F., and Murray, J.A.: J. Bone Joint Surg. **52A:**665, 1970.) *Continued.*

B

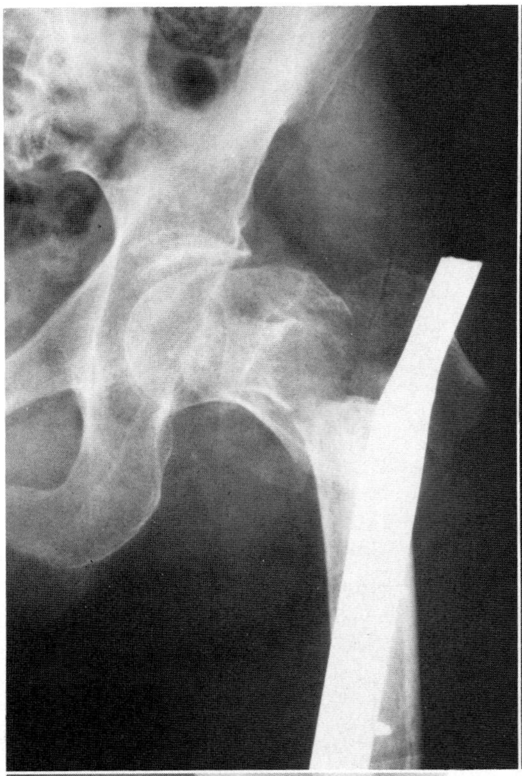

C

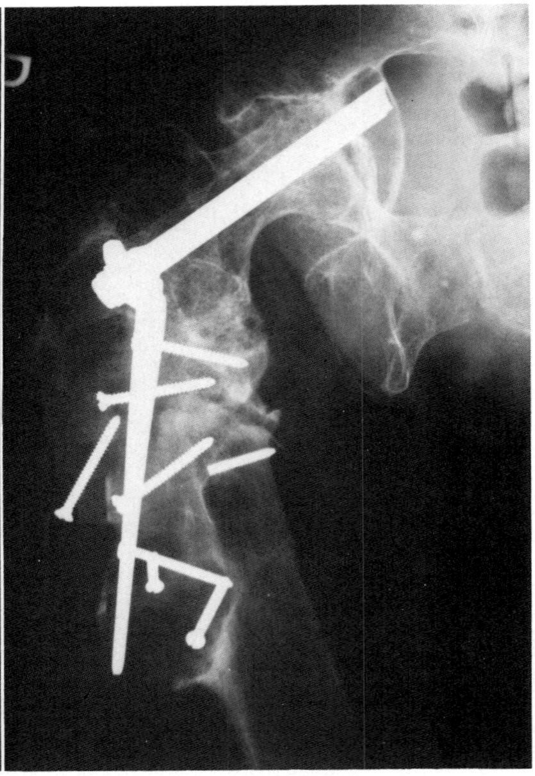

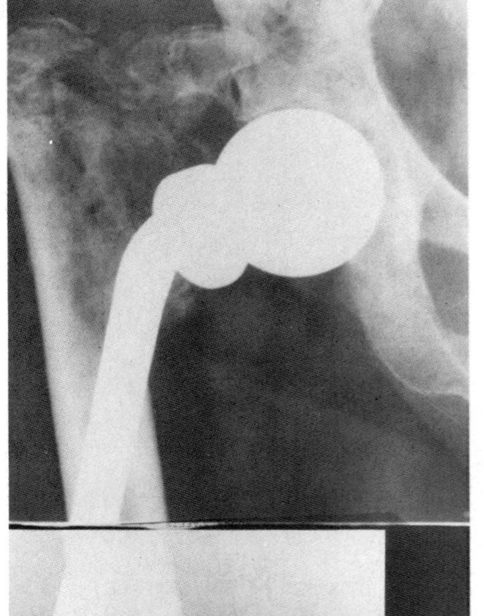

D

FIGURE 8-3, cont'd. **B,** Fixation failure in another patient with a similar fracture. In this case the second most common mode of failure is demonstrated: the nail has cut out of the tumor-weakened bone of the proximal fragment. **C,** Another intertrochanteric fracture actually has healed despite several modes of failure of the same type of fixation. However, in this case osteonecrosis of the femoral head and extensive destruction of the acetabular wall have resulted. **D,** Pathological fracture of the femoral neck in patient with breast carcinoma metastases. A prosthesis had been inserted but migrated distally and angulated into varus as its tip cut through the lateral cortex. This roentgenogram demonstrates vividly the type of complication predictable when an attempt is made to seat the prosthesis on medial cortical bone that has been destroyed by tumor lysis.

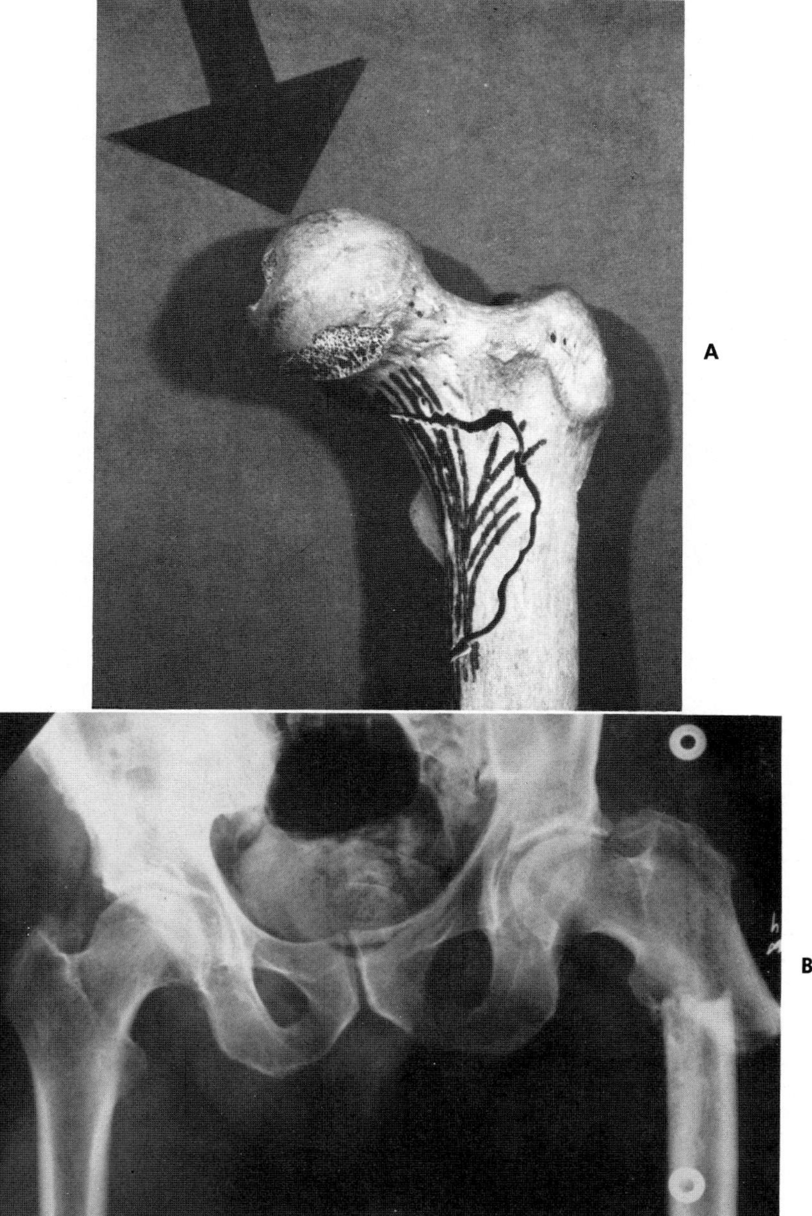

FIGURE 8-4 **A,** From a biomechanical viewpoint, almost all pathological fractures of the upper femur are alike, in that the medial cortical bone is weakened and becomes structurally insignificant while the proximal head-neck fragment tends to become displaced and angulated into a varus malalignment. **B,** Roentgenogram of a pathological fracture demonstrating the typical pattern of displacement and angulation encountered.

Continued.

viewpoint, the medial cortex ceases to exist (Fig. 8-4, *A*). The remaining tensile trabeculae, also weakened by the tumor process, have insufficient strength to resist the weight-bearing loads and a pathological fracture occurs. The proximal femur angulates into a varus position (Fig. 8-4, *B*), and it is this tendency that is the underlying cause of almost all fixation failures. Conventional fixation devices that impart stability well lateral to the fulcrum of such varus angulation cannot resist the inherent instability imparted by the loss of bone across that medial cortical gap. The fixation device either breaks or cuts out of the proximal femur, and in both instances the fracture fragment again settles into a position of varus malalignment.

Attempts have been made to frustrate this

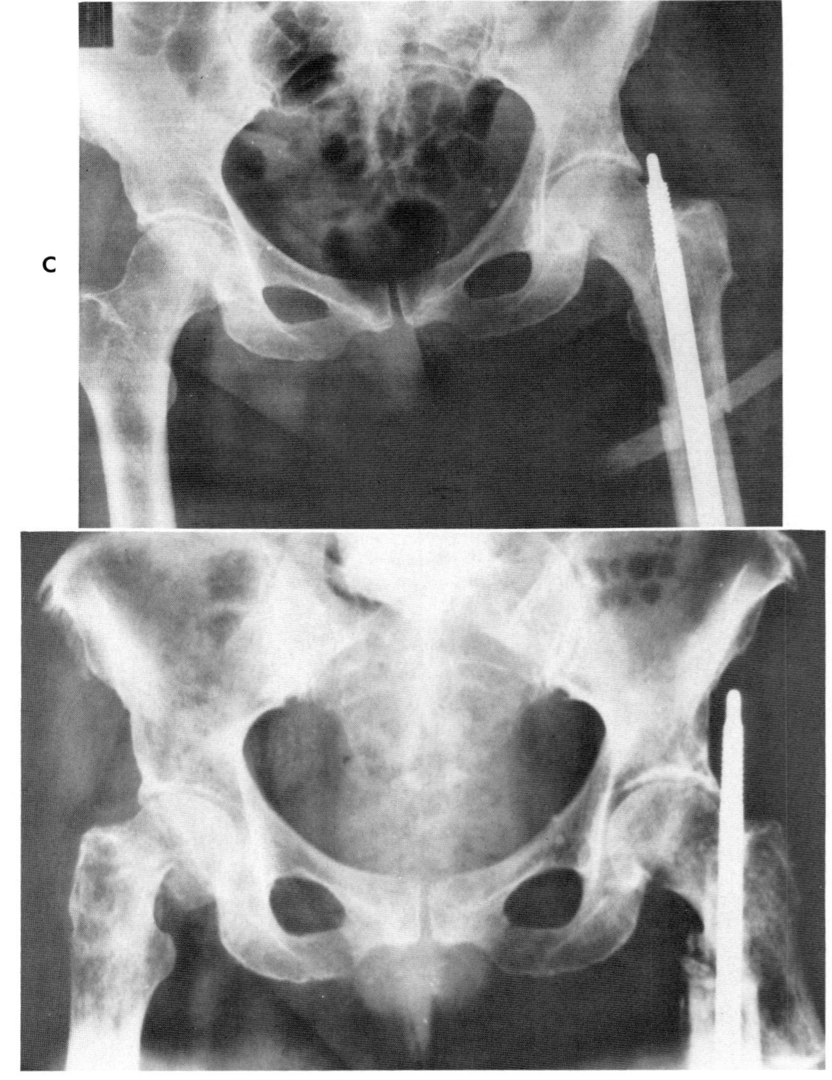

FIGURE 8-4, cont'd. **C,** Internal fixation has been accomplished with a Schneider intramedullary nail. **D,** Despite this method of fixation, the inadequacy of the medial cortical bone has resulted in a telescoping and angulation of the major fragments, a loss of fixation, and a painful protrusion of the nail proximally. Spontaneous fracture of the neck now has occurred, again resulting in varus malalignment of the proximal fragment. (**D** reprinted with permission from Parrish, F.F., and Murray, J.A.: J. Bone Joint Surg. **52A:**665, 1970.)

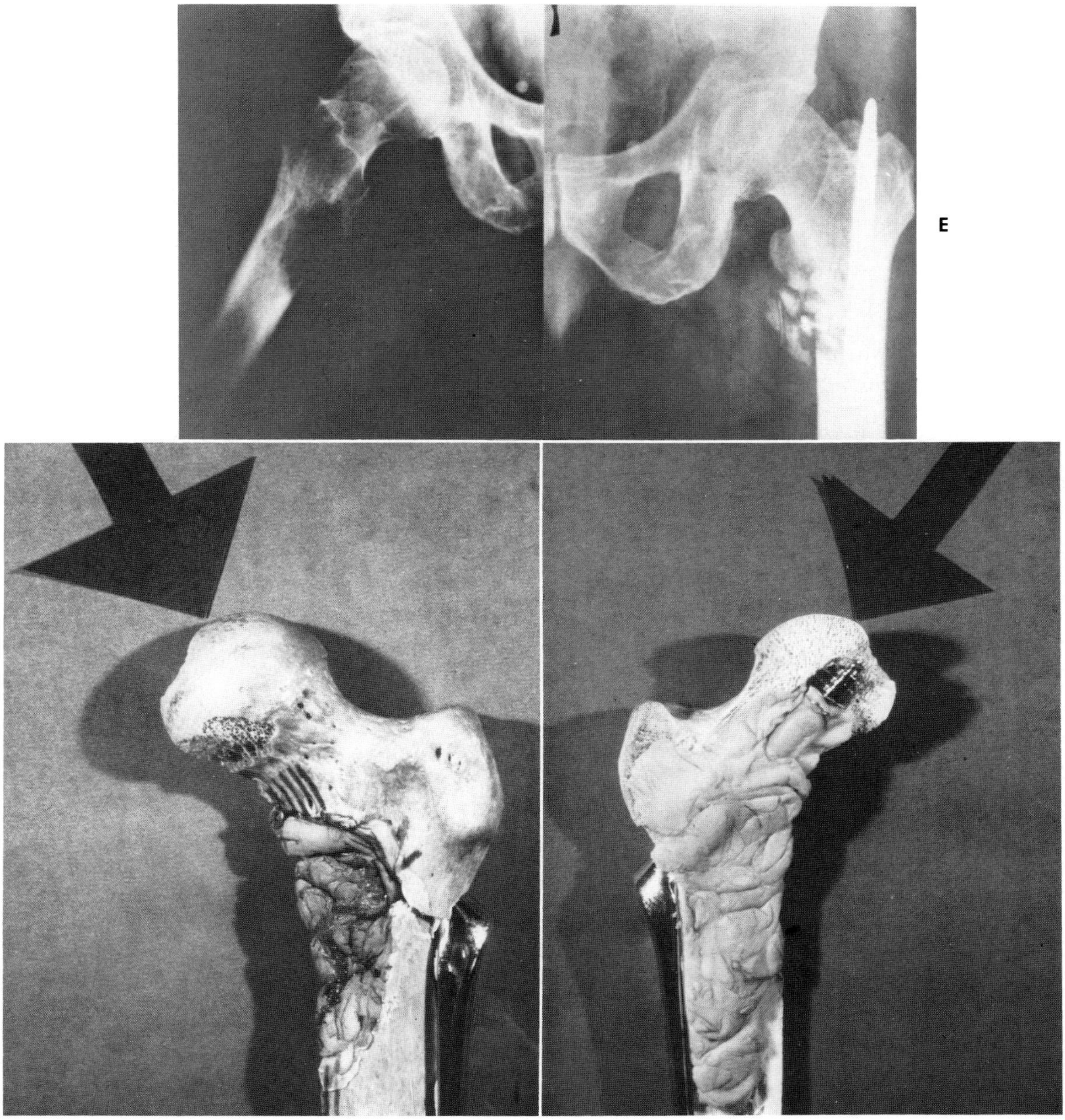

E

F

G

FIGURE 8-4, cont'd. **E,** Attempts to reconstruct the medial femoral cortex with cancellous grafts rarely are successful because postoperative radiation of the fracture site almost always frustrates or at least delays bone graft incorporation until after fixation failure has occurred. **F,** A much more secure and effective alternative to bone grafting the defect is to fill it with methylmethacrylate, a material that can be molded to expand into the defect completely and yet, once polymerized, enjoys excellent strength in resisting compressive loads. **G,** By filling the hollowed out proximal and distal fragments with methylmethacrylate, one also enhances the ability of a conventional fixation device to resist torque and shear forces and thereby prevents the major fragments from telescoping and shortening.

tendency by using intramedullary rods instead of nail-plate devices for fixation. An intramedullary device tends to center the focus of stability closer to the inadequate medial cortex (Fig. 8-4, *C*); but in the face of extensive destruction of cortical bone, the predisposition for telescoping of the major fragments and recurring loss of alignment in varus remains high (Fig. 8-4, *D*). Attempts to reconstruct the medial cortical deficit using cancellous bone grafts (Fig. 8-4, *E*) rarely are successful because postoperative irradiation of the fracture site almost always frustrates or at least delays bone graft incorporation until after fixation failure has occurred.

In approximately 1968 a technique was devised[22] whereby the structurally deficient medial cortex simply was replaced by methylmethacrylate polymerizing in situ and supplemented by a metal fixation device (Fig. 8-4, *F*). The acrylic cement could also be packed into the medullary canal to prevent telescoping of the fracture fragments and enhance the resistance to shear and torque stresses primarily afforded by the metal device (Fig. 8-4, *G*). This combination of materials was similar in concept to reinforced concrete, and it possessed the structural capacity to withstand the stresses of immediate weight-bearing. Moreover, the plasticity of the acrylic cement before polymerization allowed complete filling of any cavity with the irregular confines typical of tumor destruction.

Biomechanical Considerations. From a biomechanical viewpoint, methylmethacrylate is a brittle material that breaks easily and abruptly without bending under minimal shear or torque loads (500 to 1200 psi) (Fig. 8-5). When it is entirely encased within intact cortical bone, as in a conventional joint replacement arthroplasty, the ductility or pliability of the surrounding bone compensates somewhat for its brittleness. However, when used to replace large segments of bone destroyed by tumor metastases, it has little resistance to torque or shear stresses and must therefore always be

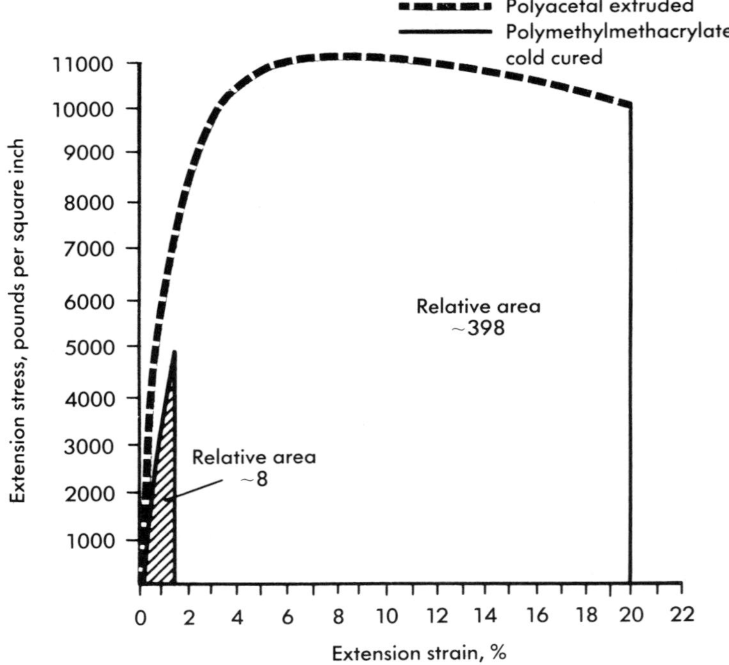

FIGURE 8-5 Methylmethacrylate is brittle and will fail abruptly if torque or shear stresses exceed its relatively low yield point. Unlike true plastic materials, when methylmethacrylate is loaded rapidly by torque or shear stress it will break without bending. *Relative areas* in this graph represents energy absorbed to failure. (Courtesy Jack Wickstrom, M.D.)

used with a metal fixation device that can effectively resist such loads. It should never be employed to span large bone defects where ancillary metal stabilization can be only tenuous at best (Fig. 8-6).

Conversely, the principal forces least well resisted by a conventional metal fixation device, particularly about the proximal femur, are those in which a compressive load is exerted across the tumor defect. The metal device, positioned lateral to this load, is unable to resist the inexorable deformation of the proximal femur into varus and ultimately breaks (Fig. 8-3, *A*), cuts out of the femoral head (Fig. 8-3, *B*), or tears loose from its fixation points on the femoral shaft (Fig. 8-3, *C*). Methylmethacrylate used to fill the tumor defect easily withstands such compression loads, its ability to do so falling into the area of 15,000 psi. Bartucci et al.[2] noted that compression hip screw and cement constructs could be subjected to repeated loads in excess of 300 pounds in the direction of normal weight-bearing and muscle forces on the femoral head and consistently withstand 100,000 repetitions of loading without cement failure; testing of similar specimens without cement resulted in failure of the fixation in six of seven specimens after fewer than 1000 repetitions.

The nature of the bond between the acrylic polymer and bone can be adversely affected by the following factors:

1. Residual tumor or reactive fibrous tissue interposed between bone and cement

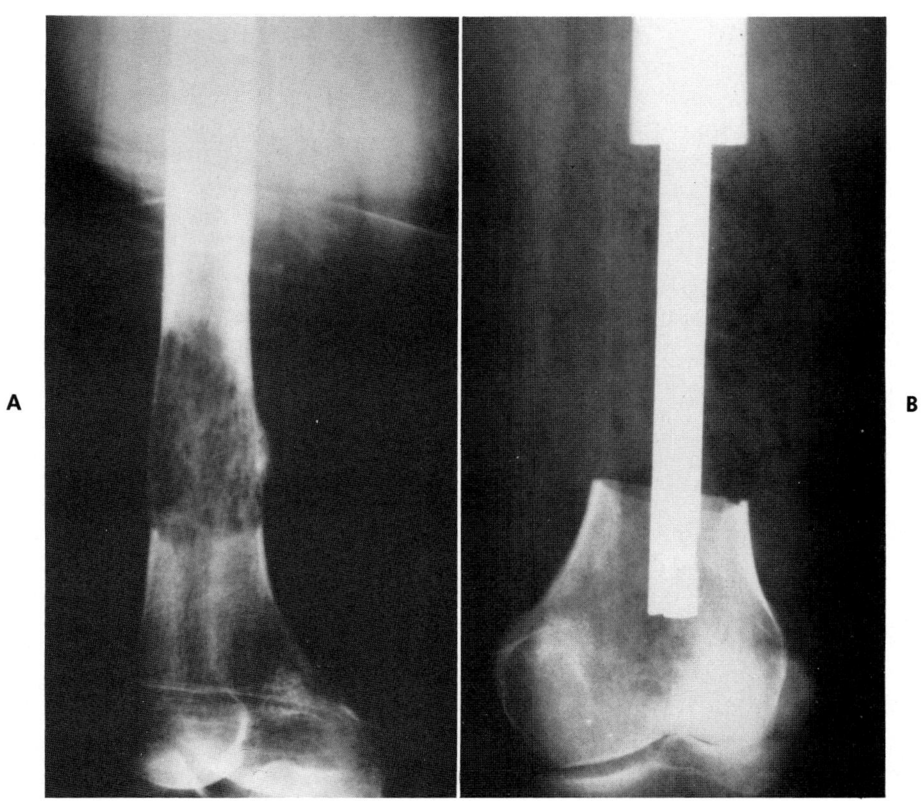

FIGURE 8-6 **A,** Anterior-oblique roentgenogram of the distal femur in a patient with a large destructive myeloma of the diaphysis. Shortly after this film was obtained, a fracture occurred through the markedly thinned cortices about the lesion. **B,** Fixation was accomplished with an intramedullary Kuntscher rod augmented by radiolucent methylmethacrylate across the resected tumor site. However, this means of fixing a fracture is biomechanically unsound: fixation of the distal fragment by the rod clearly is inadequate, and the ability of the large cement mass to resist torque stress is minimal.

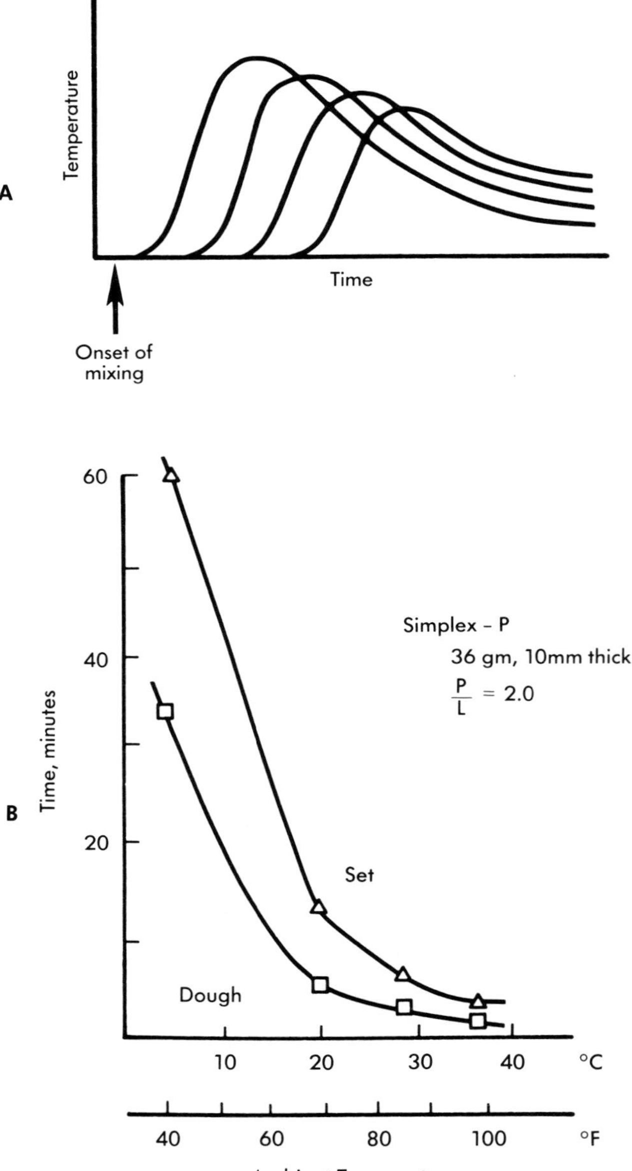

FIGURE 8-7 **A,** The polymerization time of methylmethacrylate can be controlled by varying the proportions of monomer and polymer. The faster the polymerization takes place, the faster heat will be generated and the higher the temperature will rise. The area under each curve represents total heat. The faster the cement hardens, the hotter it will become. **B,** The higher the operating room temperature, the faster polymerization will occur. Similarly, if methylmethacrylate is mixed in a bowl held in an ice water bath or is kept in a refrigerator for 24 hours before surgery, the time of polymerization can be slowed markedly. However, as soon as the material is placed in bone, its polymerization will accelerate again. (Courtesy Jack Wickstrom, M.D.)

In an effort to minimize this, we cleanse the bone cavity by brushing its surface with hydrogen peroxide and, on occasion, mechanically debride the cavity with a Water-Pik.

2. A tendency for some polymethlmethacrylate compounds to shrink slightly (up to 2%)

   Simplex P, the currently available cement used most widely in the United States, has the least tendency for such shrinkage. In fact, it expands (up to 5% in volume) during the final stages of polymerization rather than shrinks, thus forcing itself into the interstices of bone along its surface.

3. High curing temperature causing local thermal necrosis

   Potentially this is the most serious adverse interaction and thus warrants some expanded consideration. The polymerization process is an exothermic one. The faster it takes place, the faster heat will be generated and the higher the temperature will rise (Fig. 8-7, *A*). It is this peak temperature that is most responsible for local bone necrosis. The speed of polymerization can be reduced by using a slightly lower monomer-to-polymer dough ratio or, more practically, by reducing the ambient temperature where mixing takes place (Fig. 8-7, *B*). This can be accomplished[22] by storing both monomer and polymer in a refrigerator for 12 hours before use, by lowering the operating room temperature during mixing, or occasionally even by using an ice water bath around the bowl during the initial phases of mixing. The mass of methylmethacrylate needed to fill a defect also affects the peak heat of polymerization in situ. Thus, in general, the larger the defect to be filled and the more packages of cement required to fill it the greater will be the exothermic reaction that can be anticipated.

Certain methylmethacrylate compounds, particularly Palacos and Cranioplast, undergo polymerization more slowly than does Simplex P. The most commonly available compounds are quite similar, however (Fig. 8-8). In deciding which polymethylmethacrylate compound to use and at which temperature to mix it, the surgeon must take into account the practical disadvantages of a prolonged time to polymerization in situ versus the advantages of reducing the peak of the exothermic reaction and thereby decreasing the risk of local bone necrosis. After trying different combinations of these factors, we have settled on conventional Simplex P cement, prestored in a refrigerator, for all fixation procedures except when more than two packages of cement will be required. Under those circumstances we suspend the mixing bowel in an iced saline bath, allowing the material to remain in an almost liquid consistency for up to 7 minutes after combining the polymer with the monomer.

Despite the potential problems inherent in using methylmethacrylate to augment conventional fixation, the much improved stability and longevity of such fixation are indeed impressive. Among the first 399 patients we treated[27] there were only five failures of fixation and eight patients were given a functionally poor rating because of inadequate relief of pain or because stabilization of the fracture or prosthesis was insufficient to allow reasonable mobility. Thirty-four additional patients died within 2 months of surgery and thus failed to fulfill the criteria for proper preoperative selection. Ninety-four patients who were ambulatory prior to their fracture regained the ability to walk postoperatively. Pain relief was rated as excellent or good in 85% and poor in only 2%.

Survival statistics for these patients more than 2 years after operation were subdivided into those with primary carcinoma of the breast and those with a primary malignancy at other sites. In general, patients with a primary breast malignancy enjoyed a more than twofold improvement in their survival prognosis as compared to breast cancer patients treated by conventional fixation before the advent of methylmethacrylate. Similarly patients with lymphoma, myeloma, hypernephroma, prostatic cancer, or other primary malignancy also enjoyed an approximately twofold improvement in their survival prognosis. Only those with the most dismal overall outlook (e.g., patients with metastatic lung carcinoma) failed to survive for a longer period. In fairness, of course, it should be emphasized that advances in other palliative techniques, particularly in the field of chemotherapy, undoubtedly have contributed to this striking improvement in patient survival.

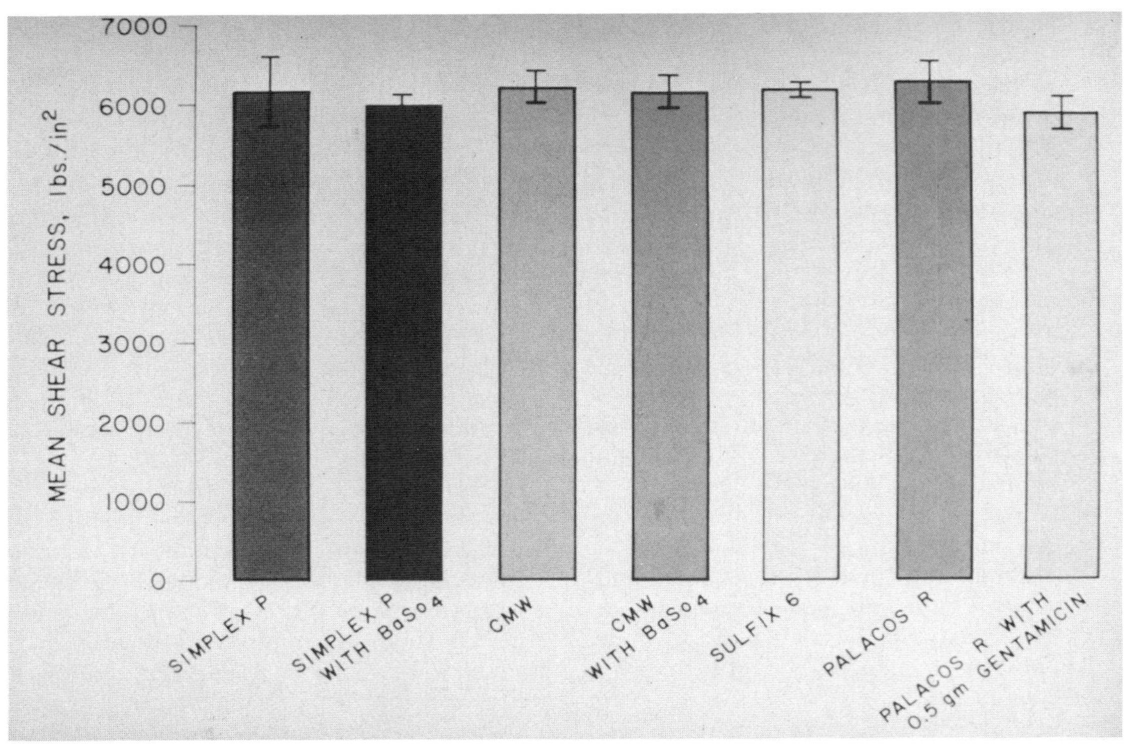

FIGURE 8-8 A variety of polymethylmethacrylate preparations is available, some combined with barium sulfate and some with antibiotics. They vary in fluidity and speed of polymerization. No significant differences exist, however, in the ability of each to resist shear stresses. (Courtesy Edward T. Habermann, M.D.)

Preoperative Preparation. As was noted earlier, patients with long bone fractures secondary to metastatic disease do not tolerate prolonged delays before stabilization or prosthetic replacement. However, it must be remembered that, with few exceptions, patients suffering pathological fractures are debilitated systemically and thus subject to a variety of complications not experienced with more elective orthopaedic procedures.

Hypercalcemia. Hypercalcemia has been discussed already in this chapter but warrants reemphasis. On all patients a baseline serum calcium, phosphorus, and total protein determination should be performed preoperatively, and they may also require evaluation of renal function at least on a superficial basis. These patients should remain well hydrated, usually by the intravenous route, during even minimal periods of enforced bedrest pre- or postoperatively. This is especially true for patients with breast carcinoma and those with myeloma. Furosemide diuresis may be required, and in extreme situations the use of mithramycin, steroids, oral or intravenous phosphates, or even diphosphenate therapy may have to be considered.

Pancytopenia. Most patients are chronically anemic from their systemic disease and have varying degrees of leukopenia and thrombocytopenia from receiving chemotherapeutic agents. Although the white blood cell and platelet counts will recover given a sufficient time off chemotherapy, rarely is it possible to delay operative intervention enough to allow recovery of any significance. As stated in Chapter 1, the nadir of cytopenia often is 2 to 3 weeks after the administration of a given chemotherapeutic agent. Consequently, at the time of suffering a pathological fracture, any given patient may still be on the downward slope of blood cell depression and exogenous replacement of blood elements may be essential before operative stabilization can be considered. Although the overall WBC count is important, it is the granulocyte level that is critical with regard to the prognosis of infection. Patients with granulocytopenia below 500 to 800 WBC/mm^3 are at high risk of postoperative infection. WBC transfusions have been used in patients with active sepsis but are inefficient as prophylaxis because of their short life-span (6 hours) and because of the rapid autoimmunization that occurs with such transfusions. Platelet transfusions should be given preoperatively to patients whose count is below 50,000 to 60,000 in whom an orthopaedic procedure is planned, although it is possible to perform an emergency splenectomy safely with a platelet count at the 40,000 level. When platelet transfusions are indicated, we administer 10 units of platelets preoperatively and usually repeat this transfusion 3 days postoperatively as necessary.

Nonspecific Coagulopathies. Although uncorrected thrombocytopenia is the most common cause of clotting problems intraoperatively, other coagulation parameters should be assessed as well. Patients with liver metastases, in particular, can be expected to demonstrate a prothrombin deficiency and may also suffer from a deficiency of other factors in the coagulation chain. We have found that both a prothrombin time and a partial thromboplastin time ordinarily are required to determine specific deficiencies in clotting. However, a bleeding time is the most accurate prognosticator of intraoperative hemorrhaging. Theoretically vitamin K can be used to enhance prothrombin production by the liver, but rarely is this of any practical benefit, both because of the delay in its effect and because the liver's inability to produce prothrombin in advanced cancer patients is not due to a vitamin K deficiency alone. Fresh frozen plasma effectively replaces clotting factors acutely necessary for operative intervention in most instances, although multiple such transfusions may be required. On occasion, intravascular coagulopathies develop in patients with metastatic cancer and a bleeding diathesis can be prevented only by the administration of anticoagulants. In these situations operative intervention may be precluded by the fact that such prothrombin antagonists severely interfere with clotting; and yet a failure to continue the patient on them makes the bleeding diathesis even worse.

MANAGEMENT OF SPECIFIC PATHOLOGICAL FRACTURES

Femoral Neck Fractures. Pathological fractures of the femoral neck almost never heal, even if undisplaced,[17,27] and should be managed by prosthetic replacement (Fig. 8-9). The inclination to attempt internal fixation of undisplaced fractures should be resisted, in part because of the abysmal rate of union and in part because there is no effective means of reinforcing fixation by methylmethacrylate when the fracture is so proximal in the femur. The incidence of femoral head osteonecrosis is high after metastatic pathological fracture of the femoral neck, again even if the fracture is nondisplaced, because the femoral head usually is extensively infiltrated by tumor tissue and its circulation already tenuous before the fracture occurred (Fig. 8-10). We have seen three cases of spontaneous femoral head osteonecrosis in patients without radiographically demonstrable fractures but with hip pain, proximal femoral metastases, and increased technetium-99 uptake in the femoral neck all suggesting the presence of an occult fracture.

Whether a total hip arthroplasty, femoral endoprosthesis, or bipolar femoral prosthesis is used, a long-stemmed femoral component (140 to 200 mm) should be used in most cases to prophylactically reinforce the remaining proximal femur, which almost invariably has also been weakened by lytic metastases. It should be remembered that the extent of metastatic tumor lysis is almost always considerably in excess of that appreciable from conventional roentgenograms. Moreover, reactive hyperemia typically occurring at the periphery of aggressive lytic lesions contributes a weakening of the bone even outside the area of immediate tumor destruction. Finally, patients recently subjected to local irradiation will have a temporary hyperemic softening of bone unrelated to the tumor process per se but contributing to the potential for fracture. Many patients who have one or more pathological fractures of the femoral neck also have acetabular lesions. Habermann et al.[19] reported that of 23 women with breast metastases involving the femoral head or neck and in whom there was no radiographic evidence of an acetabular lesion, 19 showed evidence of acetabular metastases at direct biopsy. On this basis they recommended replacement of both

A

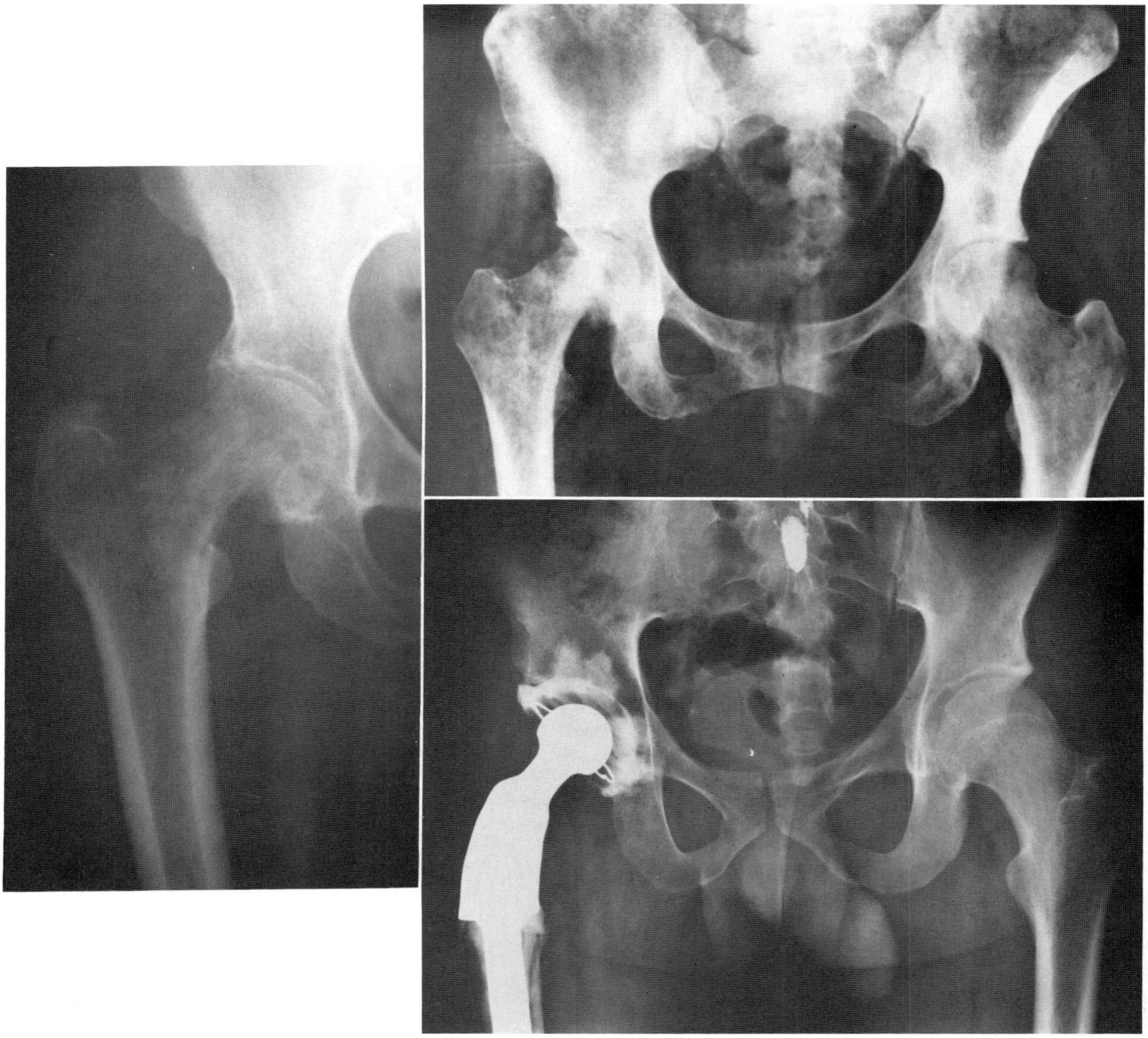

FIGURE 8-9 **A,** Pathological minimally displaced fracture of the femoral neck in a patient with metastatic breast carcinoma. The chances that such a fracture will heal after internal fixation are slight. Prosthetic replacement of the proximal femur is appropriate. **B,** Similar fracture of the right femoral neck in a patient with widespread bone metastases from a prostatic carcinoma. There is obvious and extensive involvement of the periacetabular bone, but no destructive changes have occurred to warrant a total hip replacement. Again, proximal femoral replacement alone is indicated. **C,** In this case a pathological fracture of the right femoral neck has been managed by total hip replacement because of lytic changes in the adjacent supraacetabular bone. Although the acetabular component appears to be well secured, it might have been advisable to anchor it more securely into strong unaffected ilial bone about the sacroiliac joint (see Chapter 9). (Courtesy Franklin H. Sim, M.D.)

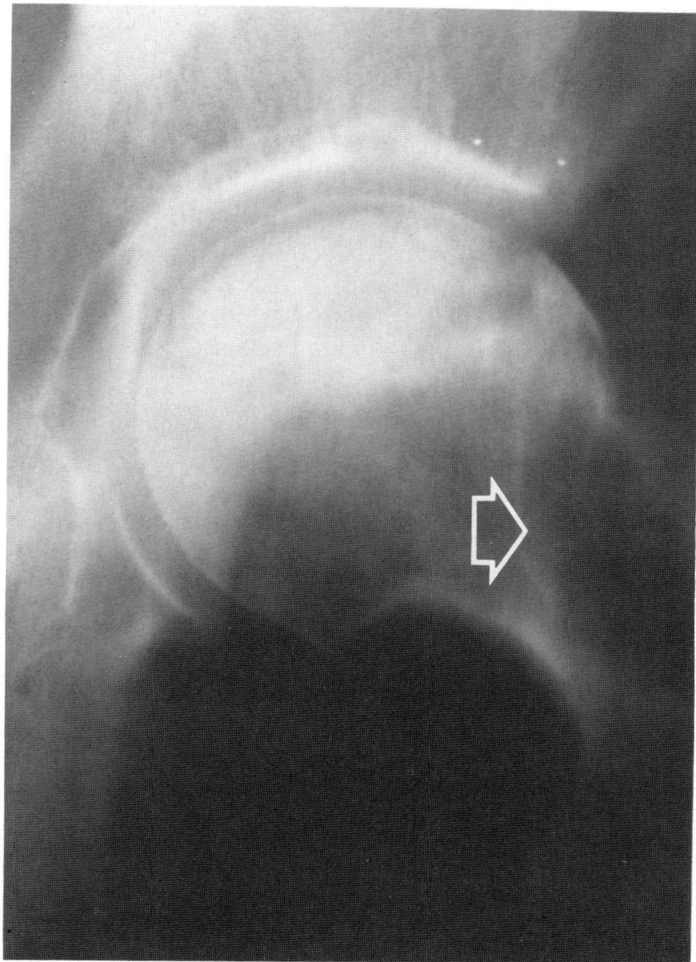

FIGURE 8-10 Roentgenogram of the femoral head and neck in a 64-year-old woman with multiple myeloma. During the previous month she had experienced progressively worsening pain in her hip. On a technetium-99 scan there was increased uptake in the femoral neck. Note the large lytic lesion *(arrow)* in the femoral neck without evidence of a fracture. An extensive area of osteonecrosis can be seen involving most of the weight-bearing dome of the femoral head.

sides of the hip joint if periactabular metastases are detected by bone scan (Fig. 8-11, *A*) of by direct biopsy at the time of operation, even with minimal evidence of disease there (Fig. 8-11, *B* and *C*). We have not found such an aggressive approach necessary, however. The presence of metastases in the acetabular region does not ensure that they will become symptomatic, particularly if the area is irradiated postoperatively. Of 52 patients with pathological fracture of the femoral neck treated by hemiarthroplasty, we have found only three in whom subsequent pain developed from an acetabular lesion or evidence of migration of the prosthesis because of weakened periacetabular bone. Routine replacement of the acetabular side of the joint subjects the patient to additional operative time and additional risks, including acetabular component loosening, hip dislocation, etc. These do not seem warranted simply because of the presence of acetabular metastases and in the absence of symptoms (Fig. 8-9, *B*).

Proximal femoral prosthetic replacement is

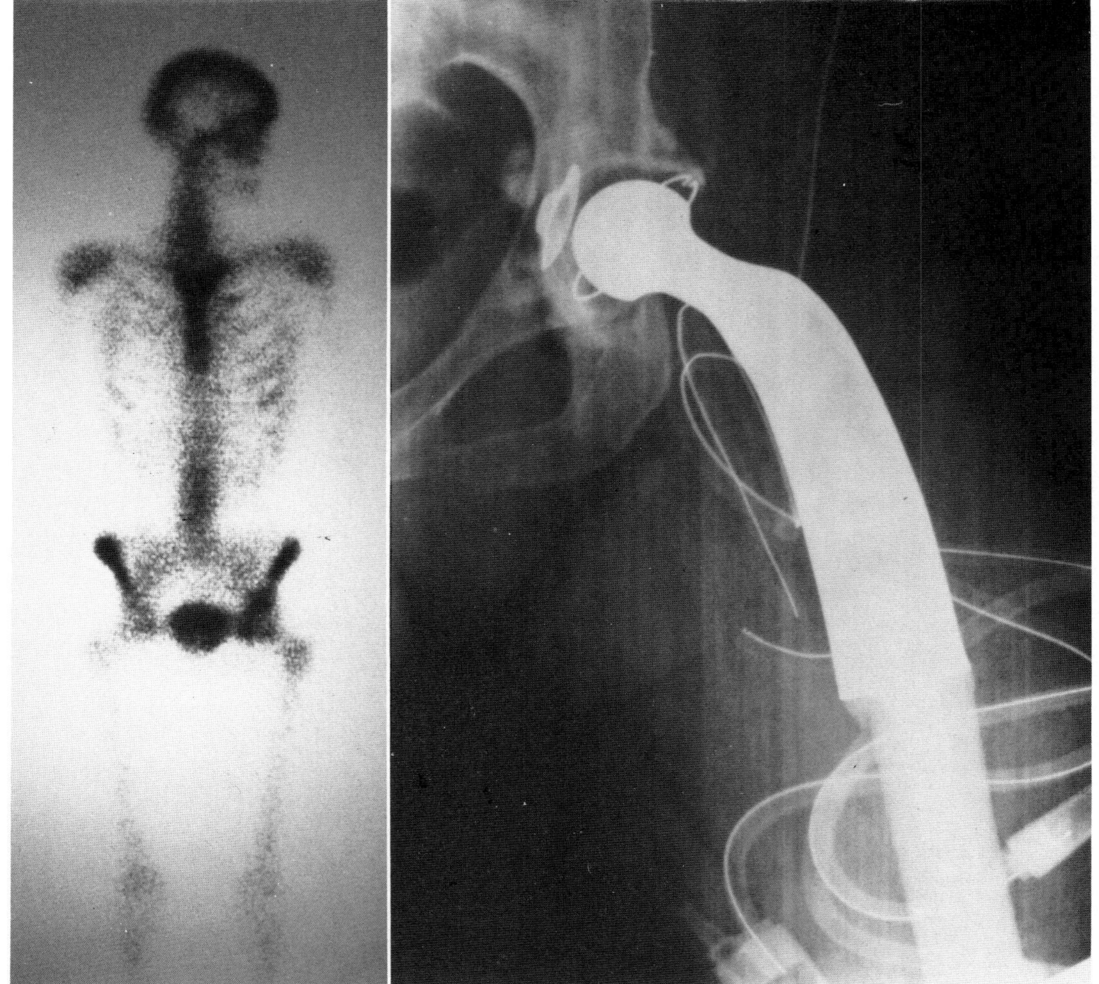

FIGURE 8-11 **A,** Technetium-99 bone scan of a patient with known rib metastases from a breast carcinoma in whom progressively increasing pain developed about the left hip on weight-bearing. No roentgenographic changes were apparent, but greater uptake is evident in both the proximal femur and the periacetabular bone. Shortly thereafter, an undisplaced intertrochanteric fracture became apparent. Because of the acetabular involvement, the decision was made to perform a total hip replacement with a custom proximal femoral prosthesis. **B,** A similar problem has been managed by a custom hip replacement arthroplasty. (Courtesy Franklin H. Sim, M.D.)

FIGURE 8-12 **A,** In this patient with femoral diaphyseal metastases, a long-stemmed proximal femoral replacement prosthesis has been used to manage a fracture low in the femoral neck. Methylmethacrylate was injected (and also sucked through a distal cortical vent) down the medullary canal well beyond the prosthesis tip. Note that the greater trochanter, reattached by wires, has failed to unite after irradiation. **B,** Intraoperative roentgenogram taken during prosthetic replacement of the left proximal femur. Tumor and structurally weak bone have been resected, and a Moore prosthesis inserted. Note the lack of a cortical margin upon which the prosthesis might seat. **C,** The prosthesis was removed, the medullary canal plugged, and methylmethacrylate injected therein. The prosthesis then was replaced and cement was molded about the upper stem to give axial and rotational stability.

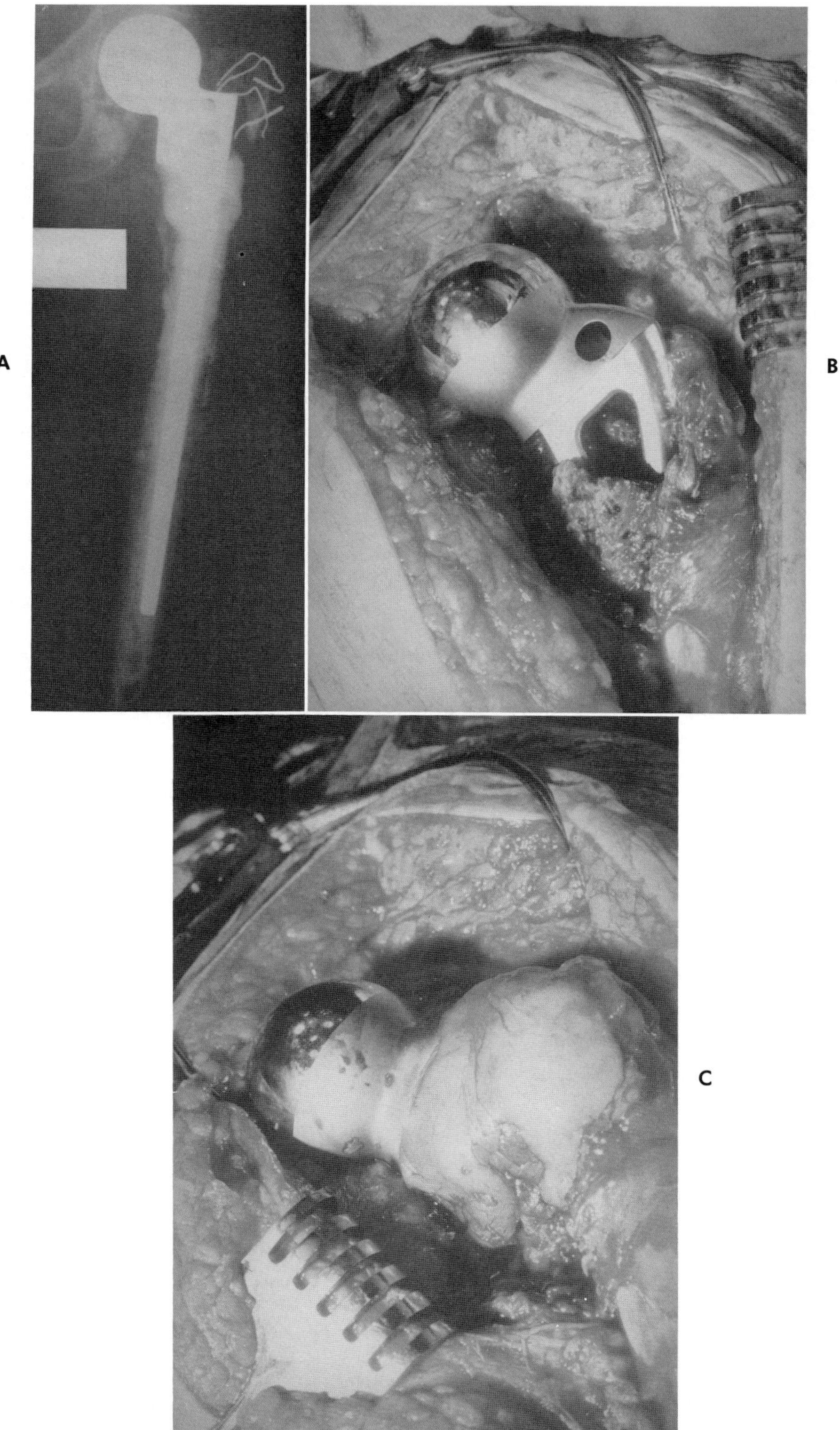

FIGURE 8-12 For legend see opposite page.

performed with the patient in a lateral decubitus position and from a posterolateral (Gibson) approach.

Transection of the greater trochanter should be avoided whenever possible to obviate the risk of subsequent trochanteric nonunion after irradiation (Fig. 8-12, *A*)

After the femoral canal has been rasped and curetted, the prosthesis is fitted into place and the hip reduced.

The correct seating of the prosthesis within the shaft is checked by direct vision for both limb length and joint stability. Thus the amount of methylmethacrylate that must be built up to attain the appropriate limb length is determined before fixation.

The prosthesis is removed and the canal thoroughly lavaged with hydrogen peroxide or a Water-Pik to remove as much intramedullary fat, residual tumor tissue, and other debris as possible before cementing the prosthesis in place.

Methylmethacrylate is mixed for only 80 seconds, poured into a cement gun, and injected as far as possible down the medullary canal in an effort to surround the prosthesis stem as far distally as possible (Fig. 8-12, *A*).

Occasionally a ¼-inch hole is drilled percutaneously through the distal femoral cortex and a vacuum created in the medullary canal by suction to encourage the cement to fill the canal fully. If this technique is used, however, the drill hole should be made well above the level where the prosthesis stem tip ultimately will rest so a stress riser will not be created below the level of the diaphyseal reinforcement.

Finally, the cement is molded about the flanged upper stem of the prosthesis by a malleable hard rubber dam wrapped around and above the proximal part of the femoral shaft to hold the acrylic in a form approximating the upper end of the femur (Fig. 8-12, *B* and *C*). The dam also protects adjacent soft tissues during the exothermic phase of polymerization.

Peritrochanteric Fractures. Pathological peritrochanteric fractures of the femur are difficult to manage operatively because, on the one hand, there usually are extensive lytic changes extending proximally into the femoral neck and yet, on the other hand, typically there is enough destruction of cortical bone distal to the intertrochanteric line to obviate proximal femoral replacement except by a custom prosthesis (Fig. 8-11, *B*). Many surgeons[19,36,54] have advocated using just such a custom prosthesis, believing that it allows the patient to regain the ability to walk more rapidly and also enhances nursing care in the more debilitated cancer patient who will never regain an ambulatory status. However, although the use of a custom prosthesis does obviate the risk of fixation-device failure it also introduces new variables and risks not encountered if the femoral head and neck are salvaged. At the simplest level such a policy necessitates stocking a wide variety of different-sized prostheses to allow accurate restoration of limb length depending on the amount of proximal femoral bone resected. Moreover, the technique introduces the necessity of reattaching the greater trochanter and its abductors to the prosthesis. Despite the use of heavy-gauge wire and reinforcing mesh, such

FIGURE 8-13 **A,** Pathological intertrochanteric fracture internally stabilized with a compression hip screw reinforced by methylmethacrylate *(stippled area)*. By extending from the level of the first screw thread proximally to the third side-plate screw distally, the acrylic cement effectively reinforces the thinned cortices. This degree of filling of the intramedullary and tumor space is ideal. **B,** Pathological fracture of the intertrochanteric femur fixed by a compression hip screw without an attempt to reinforce the deficient medial cortex by injecting methylmethacrylate. The proximal fragment angulated into a varus malalignment as the nail cut out of the femoral head. **C,** The fracture was restabilized with another compression hip screw augmented by cement. The methylmethacrylate, injected while liquid from a cement gun, has leaked through the previous defect created in the femoral neck by the migrating hip screw *(arrow)* and has entered the joint space. A cement arthrogram effect has been created. Surprisingly, the patient regained good hip motion and excellent relief of pain postoperatively; consequently no effort was made to retrieve the cement from within the hip joint.

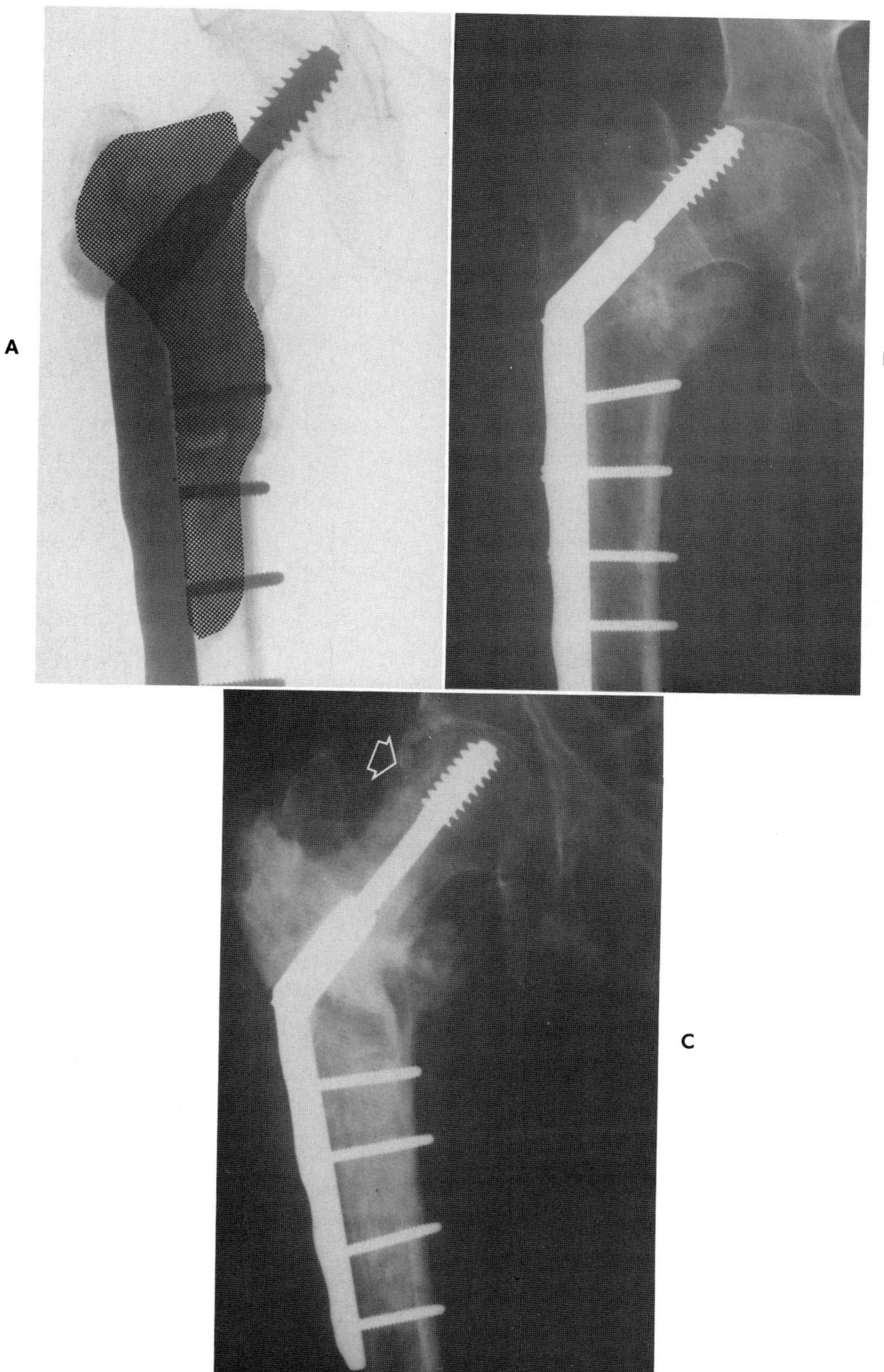

FIGURE 8-13 For legend see opposite page.

fixation is tenuous at best and in our experience often results in trochanteric detachment once the patient regains the ability to walk (Fig. 8-12, *A*). The use of a hip replacement arthroplasty to manage such a fracture also introduces the risks of dislocation, prosthesis loosening, and prosthetic stem failure, all of which are avoided if the fracture is internally fixed. For these reasons we avoid, whenever possible, discarding the proximal femur, preferring instead to internally stabilize the fracture by the combination of a compression hip screw and intramedullary methylmethacrylate (Fig. 8-13).

The technique for such fixation is similar to that used for conventional hip fracture fixation.

The patient is anesthetized and placed supine on a fracture table. A closed manipulative reduction of the fracture is accomplished using traction and image-intensifier control (Fig. 8-14, *A*).

An attempt is made to achieve an anatomical reduction, care being taken to ensure that the fracture fragments are not distracted since with distraction the cement could extrude between the fragments and hold them apart. Distraction can be avoided[2] by first manipulatively reducing the fracture and applying traction and then releasing the traction just enough to allow the reduction to be maintained while as much contact as possible occurs between the cortices of the major fragments.

A conventional lateral approach is used, and a 1.5 to 2 cm window is created in the lateral femoral cortex just distal to the greater trochanter (Fig. 8-14, *B*).

Resection of tumor tissue and structurally inadequate bone is accomplished with a rongeur and curet, any remaining cancellous bone within the distal femoral neck or trochanters being removed as well (Fig. 8-14, *C*).

Under image-intensifier control, a calibrated guide pin is inserted into the center of the femoral head and its position is confirmed by both anteroposterior and lateral views. Some surgeons prefer to place the guide wire tip, and thus the nail threads, into the inferior half of the femoral head, assuming that this will afford maximal bone superior to the nail tip and thereby reduce the risk that the nail will cut out of the femoral head. However, with the hip screw in the inferior part of the femoral head and neck, it is difficult to fill the entire medial cortical defect with methylmethacrylate and it is *by filling this void* with cement that the compression loads on the fracture leading to a progressive varus deformity can be resisted.

Once the guide pin is properly positioned, the femoral neck, head, and lateral cortex are reamed to accept the corkscrew portion of the fixation system as well as its side plate (Fig. 8-14, *D*). The compression hip screw then is twisted into place, its tip positioned as high as possible into the subchondral bone of the femoral head (Fig. 8-14, *E*).

Care should be taken to avoid penetrating the articular cartilage with either the guide pin or the hip screw because this would allow cement to enter the joint space (Fig. 8-13, *B* and *C*).

Once the hip screw is positioned properly, a long medium curet is used again to complete hollowing out of the femoral neck as far proximally as the first threads on the hip screw and as far distally in the femoral shaft as the level where the second screw will be used to affix the side plate (Fig. 8-14, *E*). It is this cavity that later will be filled completely with methylmethacrylate (Fig. 8-14, *F*).

A four-holed 130-degree side plate is fitted over the hip screw, positioned along the femoral shaft, and affixed with a Loman clamp to ensure that the fracture reduction is acceptable and the fixation components can be articulated easily even after the medullary canal is filled with cement.

When this process can be accomplished easily, the side plate is removed, the mixing of methylmethacrylate monomer and polymer is commenced, and after approximately 70 seconds of mixing the cement is injected into the defect with an Oh-Harris cement gun (Fig. 8-14, *F*). The long plastic tip of the cement gun is inserted as far proximally as possible into the femoral neck cavity and the cement is injected to fill the cavity from proximal to distal.

Hand pressure is exerted against the medial thigh by an assistant, allowing the adductor muscles to be pressed against the

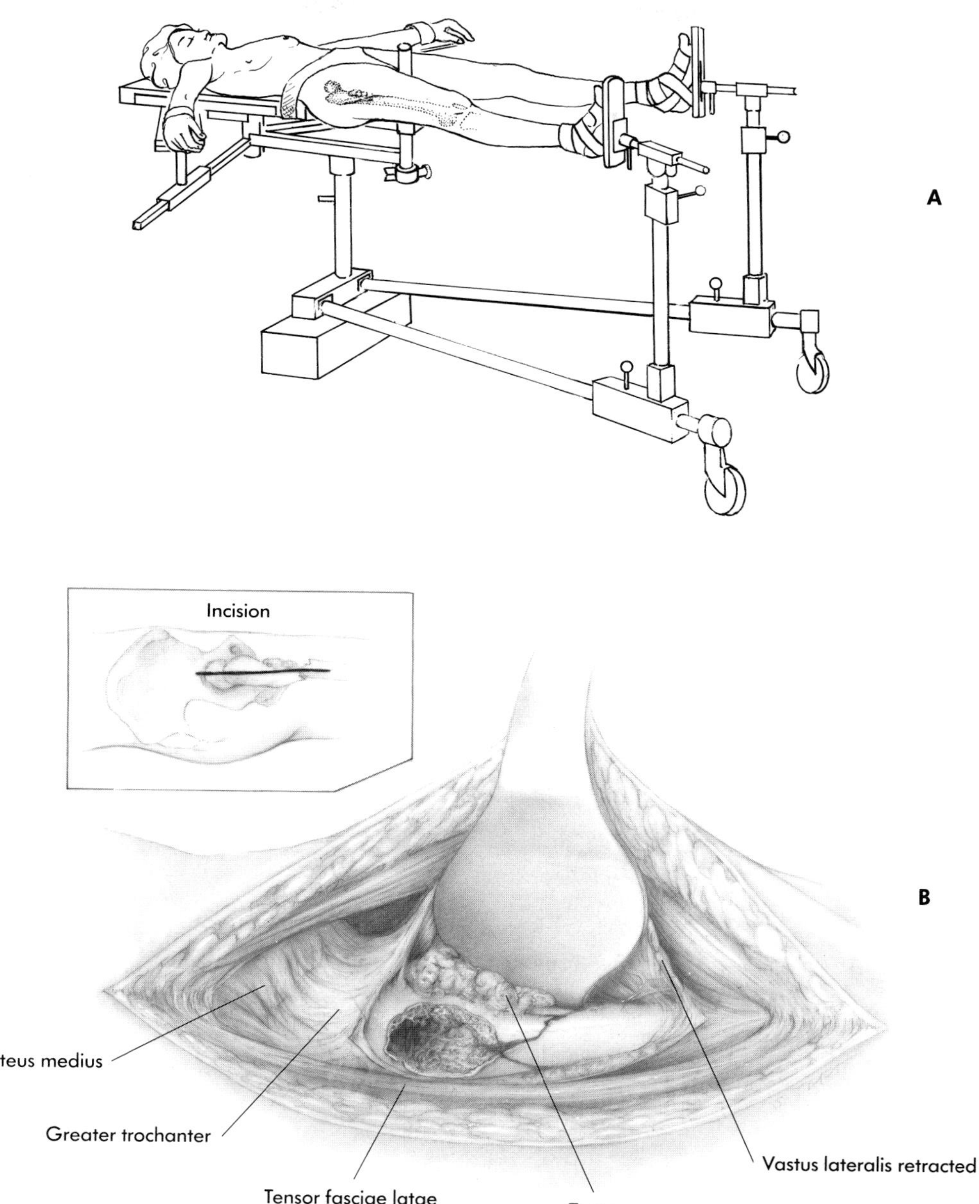

FIGURE 8-14 **A,** Pathological intertrochanteric femoral fractures are reduced as anatomically as possible by closed manipulation on a conventional fracture table under image-intensifier control. **B,** A standard straight lateral incision is made, centered over the greater trochanter, and the lateral femoral shaft is exposed (as for any hip fracture) by incising the vastus lateralis and reflecting its bulk anteriorly. Tumor tissue may be exposed as it escapes through the typical medial cortical defect. A 2 × 1.5 cm window is made in the lateral cortex for removal of the tumor and a fixation device may be inserted.

Continued.

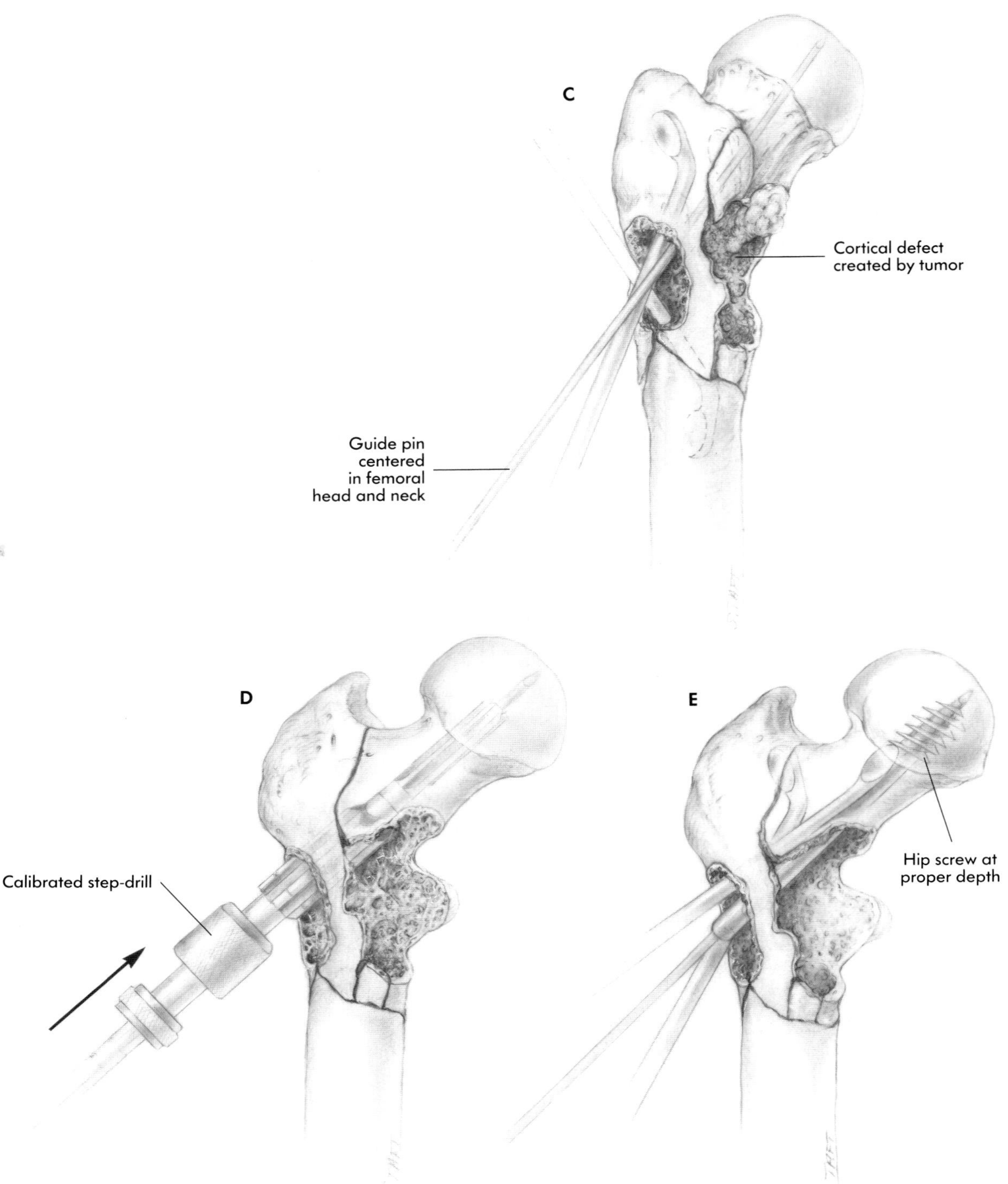

FIGURE 8-14, cont'd. **C,** Through this lateral cortical window a large angled curet is used to remove tissue as well as remnants of intramedullary fat and bone extending from the midfemoral neck and greater trochanter proximally to well below the fracture level distally. A calibrated guide pin is inserted under roentgenographic control into the center of the femoral head. **D,** A step-cut reamer is inserted over the guide pin to create channels for the compression hip screw proximally and its side-plate sleeve distally. **E,** The corkscrew portion of the compression hip screw is inserted over the guide pin until its threads come within about 1 mm of the femoral head cortical margin. Remaining intramedullary tumor and bone then are removed up to the level of the distalmost threads on the screw.

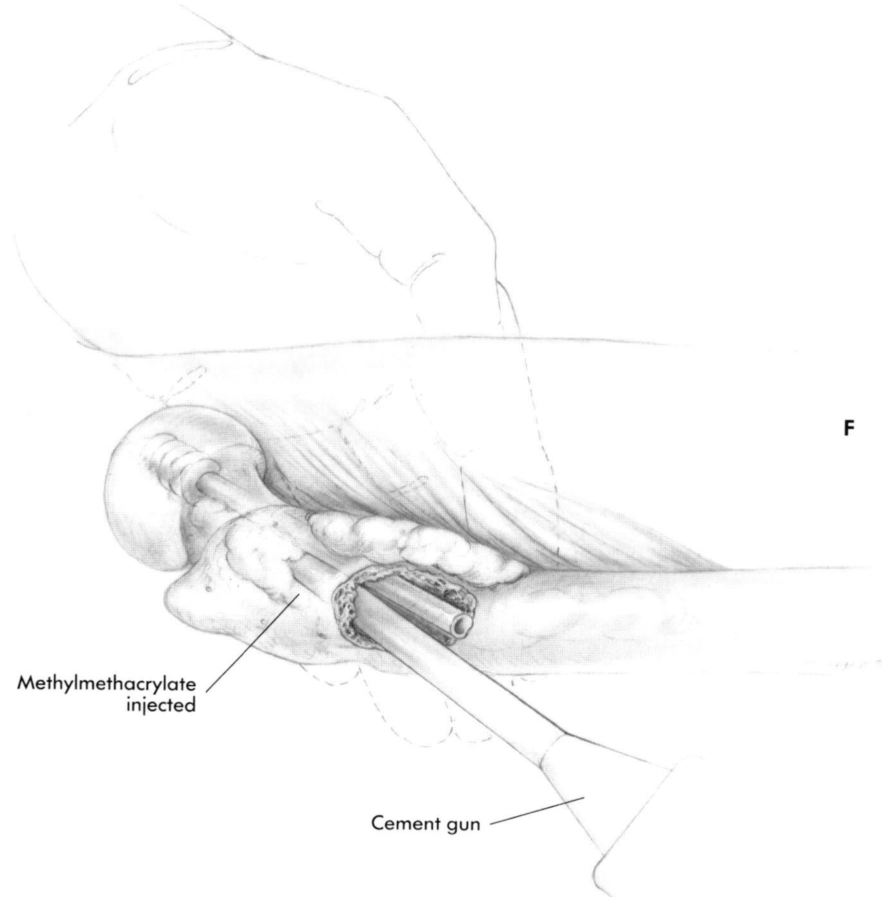

FIGURE 8-14, cont'd. **F,** The side plate is fitted over the hip screw to lie flush with the lateral femoral cortex and it is then removed. Methylmethacrylate then is injected into the space created by previous curettage and around the hip screw. The assistant should press firmly against the medial thigh as shown to force the adductor muscle against the medial cortical defect and thereby prevent liquid cement from escaping into the soft tissues. Ideally the methylmethacrylate will extend proximally on the hip screw threads and distally to the level of the first or second side-plate screw as shown in **A.**

Continued.

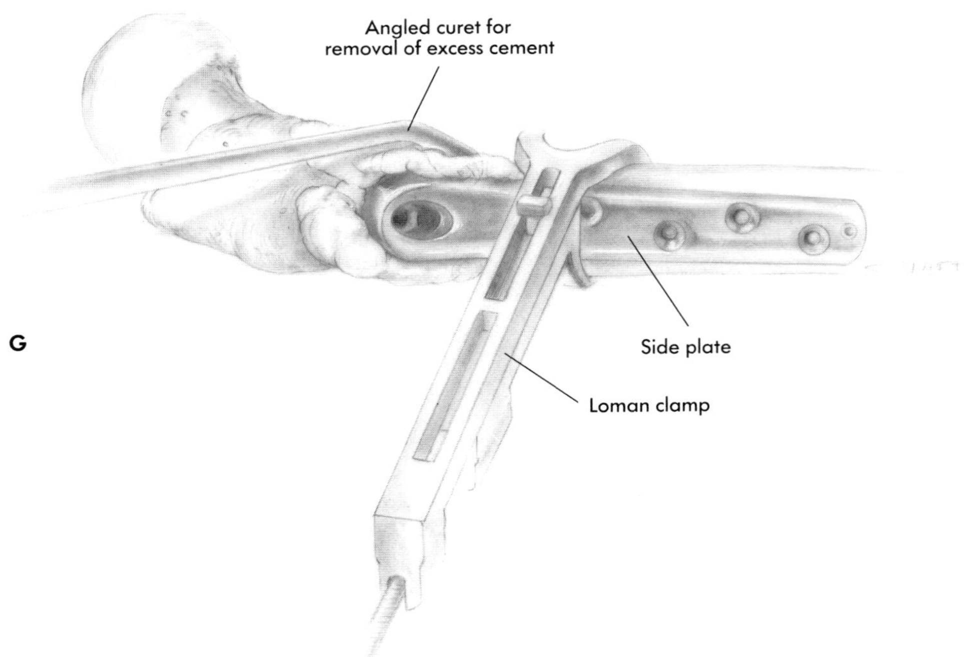

FIGURE 8-14, cont'd. **G,** The side plate then is replaced in its predetermined position and held with a Loman clamp until polymerization of the cement is complete. Any excess cement that escapes from the medullary canal should be removed by a curet before polymerization is complete. Once the cement has hardened, holes for the side-plate screws can be drilled and tapped and the screws inserted in a conventional manner.

medial cortical defect to prevent any extrusion of cement (Fig. 8-14, *F*). We have found this simple maneuver to be extremely effective in preventing escape of cement into the soft tissues of the thigh and thereby forming a palpable mass in the medial groin.

Once the cement has been injected and digitally packed into the cavity proximally and distally, the side plate again is repositioned over the hip screw and affixed loosely to the shaft with a Loman clamp (Fig. 8-14, *G*).

The traction is released, the femoral shaft is impacted proximally sufficiently to ensure maximal bony contact between the major fragments, and the side plate is clamped firmly against the femoral shaft.

In the remaining time until in situ polymerization is complete, any excess cement that has escaped through cortical defects is removed (Fig. 8-14, *G*).

It is important that every effort be made to ensure that the methylmethacrylate does not extrude outside the cortex or interfere with contact between the major fracture fragments. When bony union occurs, it is through the apposition of periosteal new bone; and this process can be adversely affected by the presence of cement extracortically.

Only after the intramedullary cement is solidly polymerized are drill holes made for fixation of the side plate. An impatient surgeon who attempts to drill such holes through unpolymerized cement will find that the drill bit binds in the cement mass and tends to break off. In contrast, holes can be drilled through hard cement without difficulty, the sensation being one of drilling through a mass of solid cortical bone.

The drill holes through both cortex and cement can be tapped in a conventional manner and the side plate affixed to the shaft by appropriately lengthened screws. Adjunctive methylmethacrylate will prevent the compression screw from sliding within the barrel of the plate because it surrounds both the threads and the shaft of the screw, blocking distal migration of the screw within the barrel. Since the device is no longer a sliding one, a strong reinforced fixation system (e.g., the Holt nail or a reinforced Jewett nail) can be used as effectively. However, such a one-piece device may complicate the injection of liquid cement and thus prevent the unhurried positioning of the components before cement injection as occurs with the two-piece compression hip screw and side plate.

Postoperatively the patient is encouraged in full unrestricted weight-bearing as soon as pain allows. There is no need to restrict stress across the fracture site until healing ensues. The few failures that have occurred with this technique did not become apparent for many months or years after operative fixation and then resulted only because of metal fatigue across a fracture defect where ultimate bony union had been prevented by postoperative irradiation (Fig. 8-15, *A* and *B*). However, we also have seen roentgenograms in which the nail-plate device broke prior to the completion of bone healing and yet the intramedullary cement prevented any loss of alignment until healing was complete (Fig. 8-15, *C*).

Some surgeons have chosen to hollow the femoral head and neck by drilling up to the subchondral bone with a ½-inch drill, filling the cavity thus created with methylmethacrylate of liquid consistency, and then twisting the hip screw into the bed of cement and bone before applying the side plate. The rationale for this variation is that the combination of screw threads and cement gives a greater surface area of contact for the fixation device in the femoral head and thus reduces the risk of the screw's cutting out of that head (Fig. 8-16, *A* and *B*). Bartucci et al.[2] prefer to use methylmethacrylate in this way rather than to fill the bone defect along the medial femoral cortex, because they believe it minimizes the risk that cement will escape extracortically into the soft tissues and perhaps interfere with ultimate bony union.

Although their reported results are good, we have preferred not to adopt this modification for the following reasons:

1. There is concern that hollowing out the femoral head and injecting cement well proximally into the subchondral bone may result in osteonecrosis of the head. They may also cause the release systemically of methylmethacrylate microemboli through the rich network of venous sinusoids there. In fact, Ewald et al.[12] demonstrated that the development of cartilage degeneration and osteoarthritis was accelerated in canine femoral heads in which the subchondral cancellous bone had been replaced by methylmethacrylate. Bartucci's group,[2] however, did not find evidence of this complication in 21 patients so treated but did find osteonecrosis in the contralateral femoral head in one patient.
2. The possibility seems great that cement injected under pressure will enter the joint through any small hole created by inadvertent penetration of the femoral cortex during guide pin placement. Bartucci's group[2] reported one such complication in their series, and we also have seen one (Fig. 8-13, *C*).
3. In more than 100 unstable intertrochanteric fractures in patients with severe osteoporosis managed by internal fixation and augmented by methylmethacrylate across the medial cortical defect, we have encountered only one nonunion.[22] In the series of Muhr et al.,[41] in which 231 comminuted intertrochanteric fractures in patients older than 75 years were treated with an angled bladeplate and acrylic cement, there were no nonunions. Consequently the concern that cement used in this manner will extrude outside the confines of the medullary canal and somehow interfere with healing of the fracture appears to be more theoretical than real.
4. When methylmethacrylate is confined entirely to the femoral head, in an effort to dissipate forces on the hip screw threads, overall fixation stability must depend entirely on the strength of the nail-plate junction to prevent varus angulation at the fracture. As has been demonstrated in Fig. 8-3, *A* and *C,* fixation may be lost because of failure of

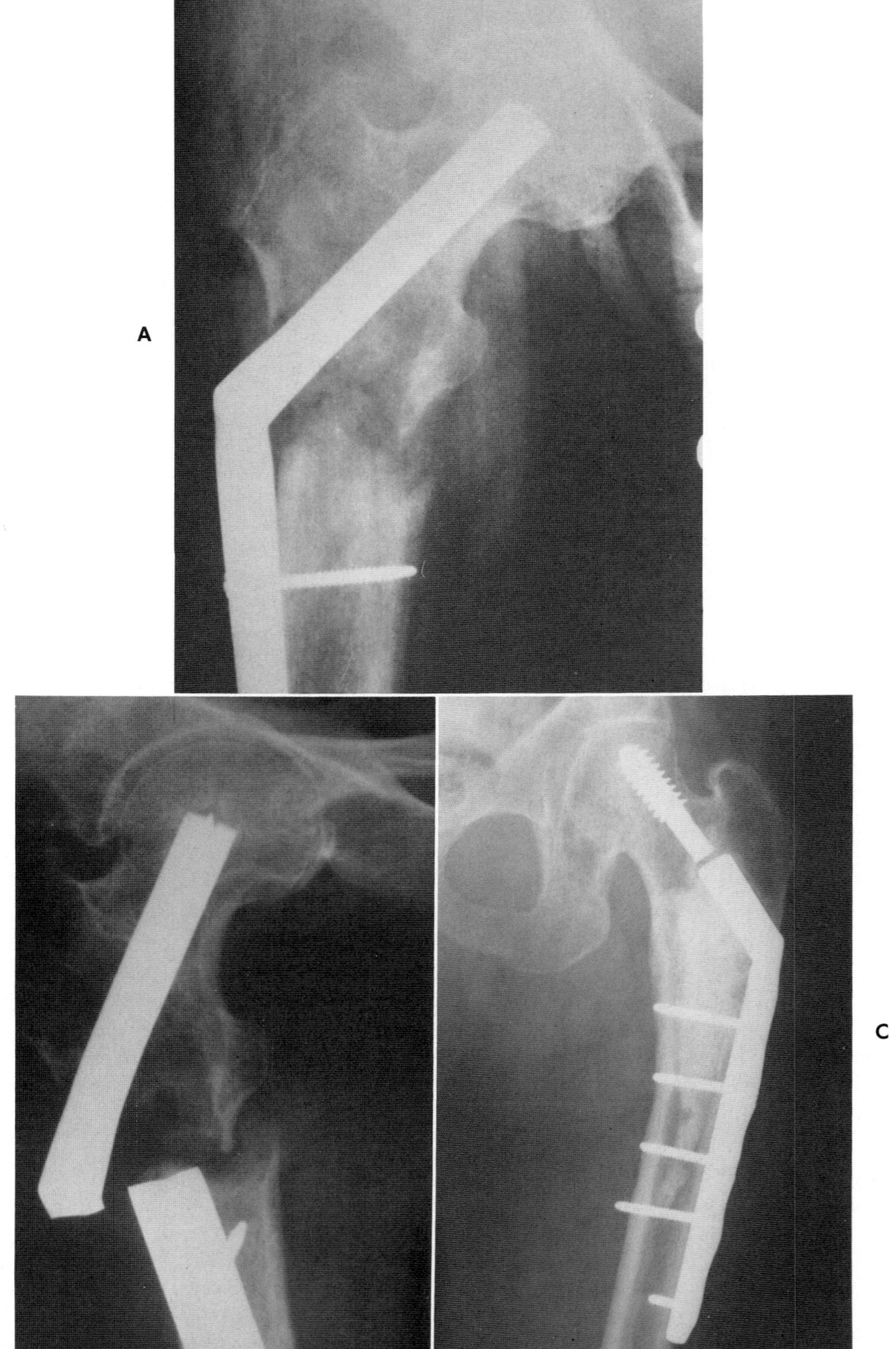

FIGURE 8-15 **A,** Pathological subtrochanteric fracture of the femur that had been internally fixed 8 months earlier with a Jewett nail augmented by radiolucent methylmethacrylate. The fracture did not unite, and bone resorption was evident. **B,** Eventually a fatigue fracture occurred at the nail-plate junction. **C,** Another example of fatigue failure at the nail-plate junction. In this instance the intramedullary cement afforded sufficient stability of the fracture fragments to maintain alignment until bony union occurred.

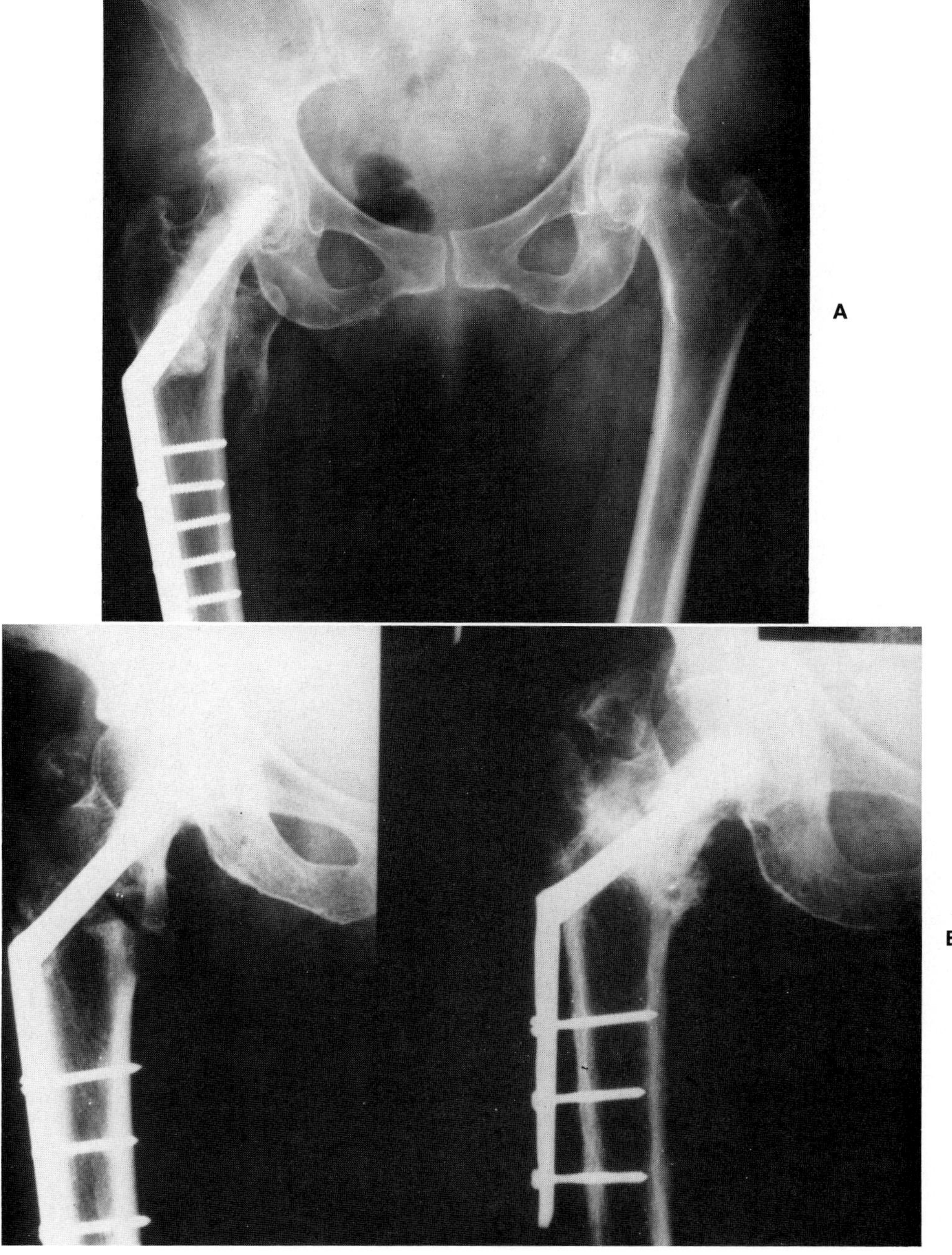

FIGURE 8-16 **A,** In an effort to minimize the risk that the nail tip may cut out of the proximal fragment, some surgeons have advocated using methylmethacrylate only around the nail shaft. However, despite the fact that this technique lessens the risk of nail tip migration, it does not decrease the tendency of unstable fractures to settle into varus with other types of hardware failure, **B.** Using intramedullary methylmethacrylate to fill the medial cortical defect and thereby reestablish medial continuity would have prevented this. (**A** courtesy Eugene Bartucci, M.D.) *Continued.*

C 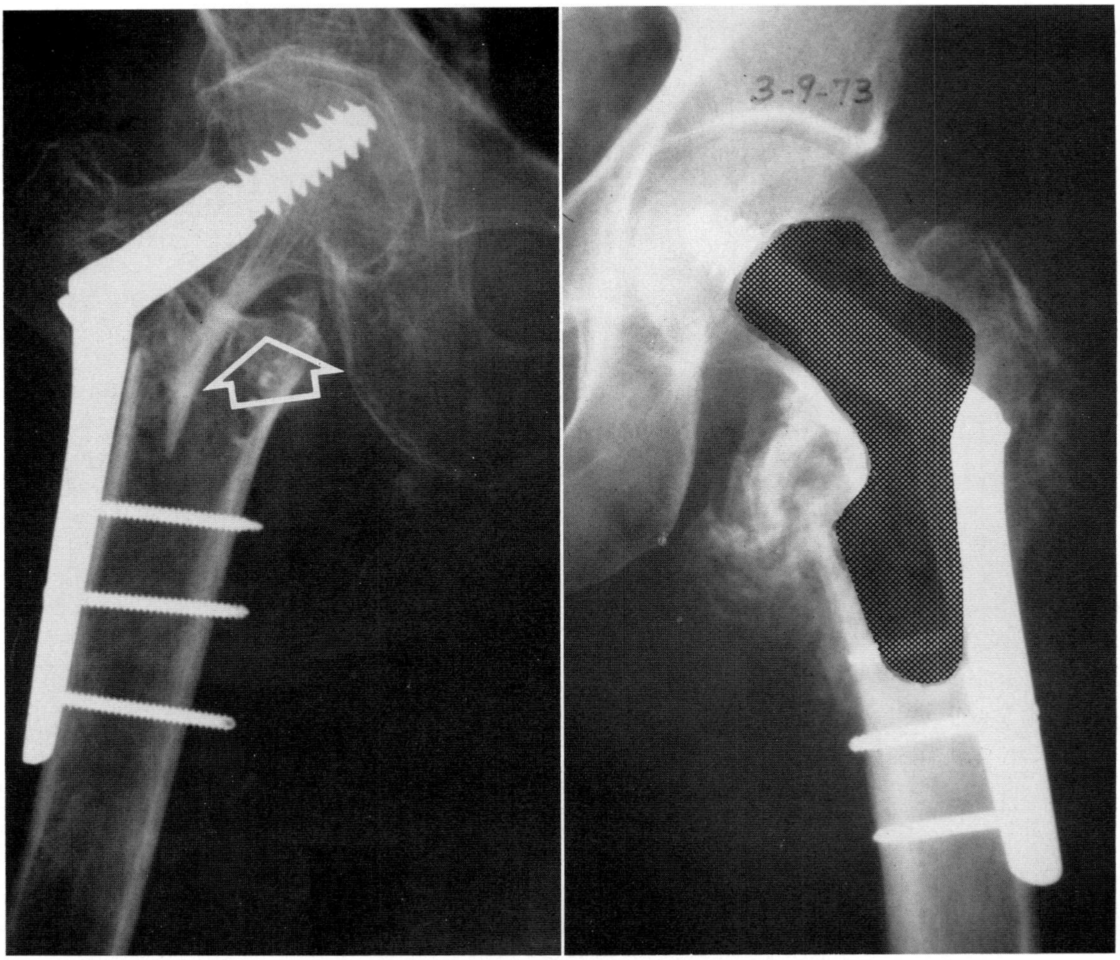 D

FIGURE 8-16, cont'd. **C,** Attempts to restore fracture stability by displacement of the femoral shaft medial to the proximal fragment spike will not be successful unless contact is first established between the cortices. In this instance a large gap exists between the cortices *(arrow)* and fixation is likely to fail. If a notch had been cut in the lateral cortex of the shaft and the nail plate seated distally, this gap could have been obviated albeit at the cost of marked shortening of the limb. **D,** Medial displacement also frustrates attempts to reinforce fixation by intramedullary methylmethacrylate *(stippled area)*. Here the narrow neck of the cement affords minimal resistance to varus angulation of the proximal fragment and loss of stabilization.

the fixation device even if the hip screw does not cut out of the femoral head. By filling the medial cortical defect with methylmethacrylate, one effectively resists the tendency toward varus angulation and nail-plate failure by using a material whose maximal strength against such compression loads has been amply shown.

We have chosen to reduce these fractures anatomically whenever possible for two primary reasons: First, several authors[2,29,48] have shown that no protection is afforded from the complications of fixation by the use of medial displacement. Roberts et al.[48] also demonstrated a significant functional loss resulting from a medial displacement osteotomy secondary to an average 1.8 cm limb shortening and to a functional weakening of abductor strength because the femoral head-neck lever arm was shortened. Second, if the proximal head-neck fragment is allowed to become displaced laterally relative to the femoral shaft, the medullary canal is proportionately narrowed. As a result the space available to be filled with cement, especially along the critically weak medial cortex, also is reduced and the efficacy of acrylic enhancement thereby impaired (Fig. 8-16, *C* and *D*).

The medial displacement osteotomy technique originally popularized by Dimon and Hughston[10] for the management of unstable comminuted intertrochanteric fractures has not proved to be effective for the management of such fractures in patients with severe osteoporosis or metastatic disease.[27,29,48] In such patients a complication rate between 20% and 68% has been reported, and Segal[53] found that less than half regained the ability to walk. In addition to limb shortening and abductor weakening, the major risk of the technique is that it will not establish the inherent stability it was designed to achieve. This failure usually occurs because the medial cortex of the proximal fragment is not impacted intraoperatively against the medial femoral cortex of the shaft (Fig. 8-17), which may result either from the surgeon's inattention to achieving a stable reduction or because the proximal fragment spike is left too thick to allow its effective impaction into the medullary canal.

An alternative method of achieving stability for such fractures was described by Sarmiento[51] in 1973. A valgus-producing osteotomy of the proximal fragment is performed, and the fracture reduced anatomically but with a high neck-shaft angle. Although this avoids some of the pitfalls of the medial displacement technique, it still fails to ensure a stable reduction for most pathological intertrochanteric fractures, because the large posteromedial cortical defect remains and the fracture fragments retain their inexorable tendency to angulate into varus. Gustilo[18] has advocated an anatomical reduction of the fracture fragments and the use of a high angled nail-plate combination for fixation. He notes that the major advantage of using such a device is that the impaction forces across the fracture closely parallel the long axis of the nail. However, when a cortical defect exists at the fracture site, such impaction may well encourage the nail to penetrate the femoral head as the proximal fragment telescopes distally. Again, by using methylmethacrylate to prevent such telescoping, it is possible to avoid this complication. The major disadvantage of the high-angled nail is that its displacement necessitates making a hole well below the level of the greater trochanter, thereby further weakening the lateral subtrochanteric femoral cortex, already almost invariably infiltrated by metastases. The use of this device, not surprisingly, has been complicated also by the development of a secondary subtrochanteric fracture.

Condylocephalic nails[21] for fixation of pathological fractures in the intertrochanteric area have been advocated because fixation can be achieved without opening the fracture site. However, in our experience and in that of others[6,30,38] the technique has been effective only rarely for such fractures. Its failure is due to the high incidence of loss of reduction, particularly with malrotation, and also to the consequent distal migration of the Ender pins toward the knee. Attempts to augment Ender pin fixation have been made by exposing the fracture site and injecting methylmethacrylate into the medullary canal through a lateral cortical window. By so doing, it was hoped that the inevitably present medial cortical defect could be reinforced, thereby obviating proximal fragment angulation, rotation, or impaction. Unfortunately, however, because the placement of Ender pins must be achieved in a stepwise fashion under image-intensifier con-

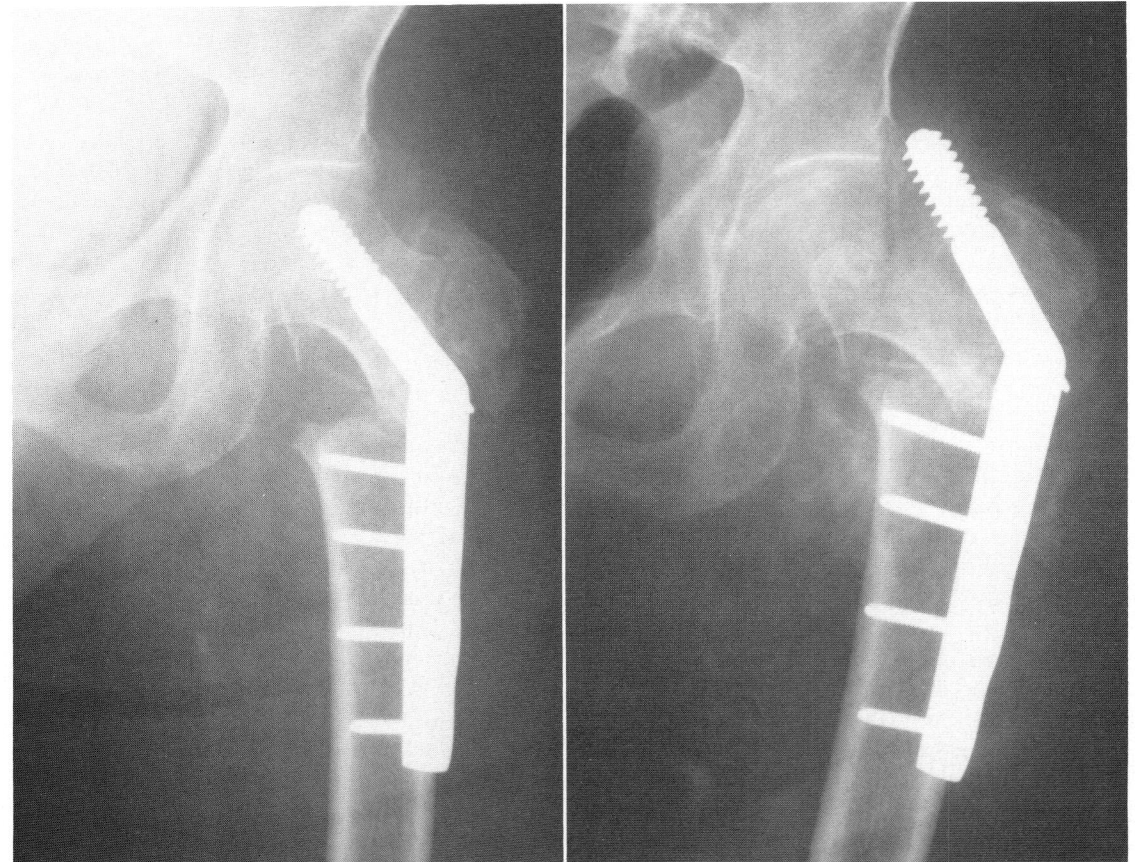

FIGURE 8-17 **A,** Another example of attempted fracture stabilization with the medial-displacement technique. A large gap persists between the medial cortices. **B,** Predictably, the proximal fragment has collapsed into enough varus to allow the medial cortices to meet.

trol, there is no time to inject the cement and effectively fill the medullary canal and then to advance the pins across the cemented defect before polymerization is complete. Consequently, the cement must be injected after all the pins have been placed and are effectively blocking the canal. In no way can the acrylic reach the medial cortical defect under these circumstances, and its placement lateral to the Ender pins offers nothing to enhance stability (Fig. 8-18).

On occasion, fractures that appear to be primarily in the intertrochanteric region will be seen to extend into bone where obvious lytic metastases already exist in the subtrochanteric region. Often such fractures are essentially undisplaced, and it is difficult to determine whether any fracture lines actually lie subtrochanterically or whether the bone there simply is osteopenic on the basis of tumor infiltration. If a displaced avulsion fracture of the lesser trochanter is apparent, this usually is a good indication that the fracture lines extend well into the subtrochanteric region. Such fractures should be internally fixed with a Zickel nail (Fig. 8-19). Details concerning the technique are presented in the following section (Fig. 8-24).

Subtrochanteric Fractures. Pathological fractures in the subtrochanteric area of the femur are the most difficult to manage because both the surface area of cortical contact and the vascularity of the bone are poorer than in the proximal intertrochanteric area. At the same time, however, the proximal fragment remains relatively small and difficult to

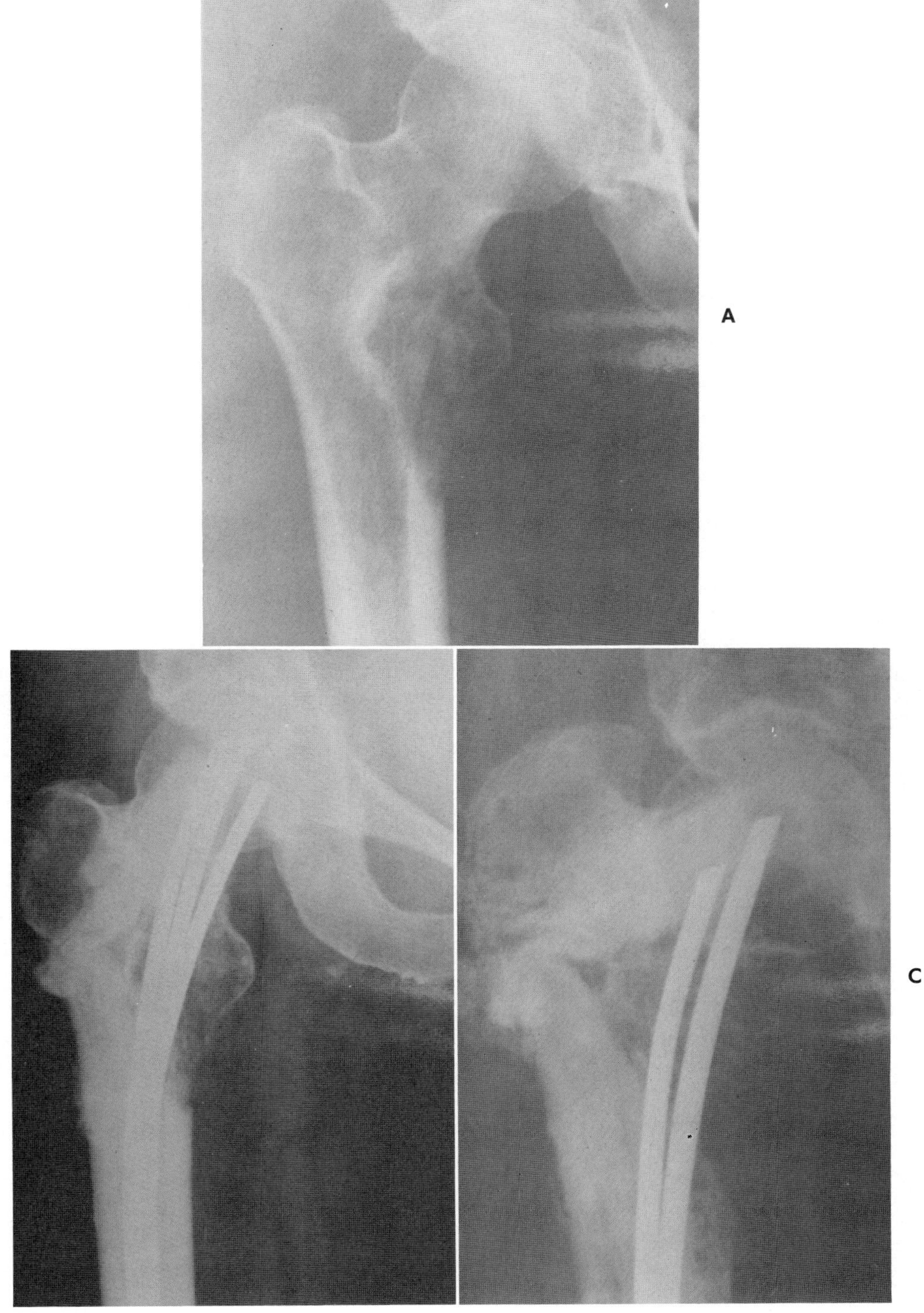

FIGURE 8-18 **A,** Large lytic metastasis that has destroyed most of the medial cortical bone of the proximal femur about the lesser trochanter. **B,** Fixation was attempted with three Ender nails augmented by methylmethacrylate injected through a lateral cortical window. No cement was packed into the medial cortical defect, and medial stability therefore depended almost entirely on the nails. **C,** Not surprisingly, the Ender nails became displaced as the fracture fragments angulated into varus malalignment.

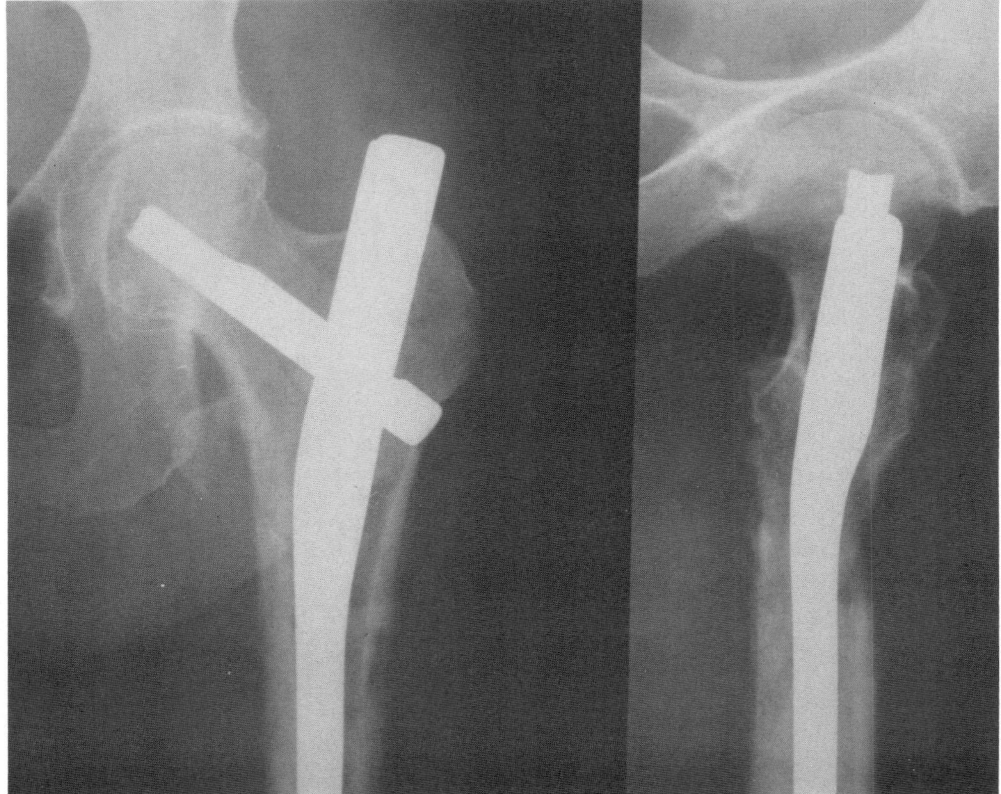

FIGURE 8-19 Fracture through the base of the femoral neck extending across the subtrochanteric femur and encompassing the lesser trochanter. Such a pattern usually suggests extensive cortical lysis, a condition more apparent on the lateral than on the AP film. This fracture is ideal for fixation by a Zickel nail.

control by conventional fixation techniques.

These fractures are not ideally suited for nail-plate fixation, even if the device is reinforced at the nail-plate junction by intramedullary cement. Rather than being concentrated at the reinforced nail-plate junction, as it is with an intertrochanteric fracture, maximal stress here is focused on the side plate at its weakest point, the position of the first screw hole. If such a fracture does not progress ultimately to bony union, and many do not in the face of perioperative irradiation, metal fatigue and plate failure will occur inevitably despite the presence of acrylic cement (Fig. 8-20).

Occasionally prosthetic replacement of the entire proximal femur[19,54] has been advocated in the management of pathological subtrochanteric fractures when there is evidence of metastatic disease in the femoral neck as well (Fig. 8-21, *A*). However, all the disadvantages previously mentioned for prosthetic replacement after intertrochanteric fractures still exist and, in fact, are magnified to some extent by the enlarged size of the prosthesis required.

From a biomechanical viewpoint the most practical position for a subtrochanteric fixation device is within the medullary canal of the femur. There is eccentric loading of the femur at the subtrochanteric level, with the magnitude of forces higher than at any other level. The medial cortex has been shown to be subjected to compressive forces in excess of 1200 psi, whereas the lateral cortex must resist tension stresses exceeding 900 psi. Intramedullary devices compensate to some extent for these eccentric loads by affording balanced resistance midway between the cortices.

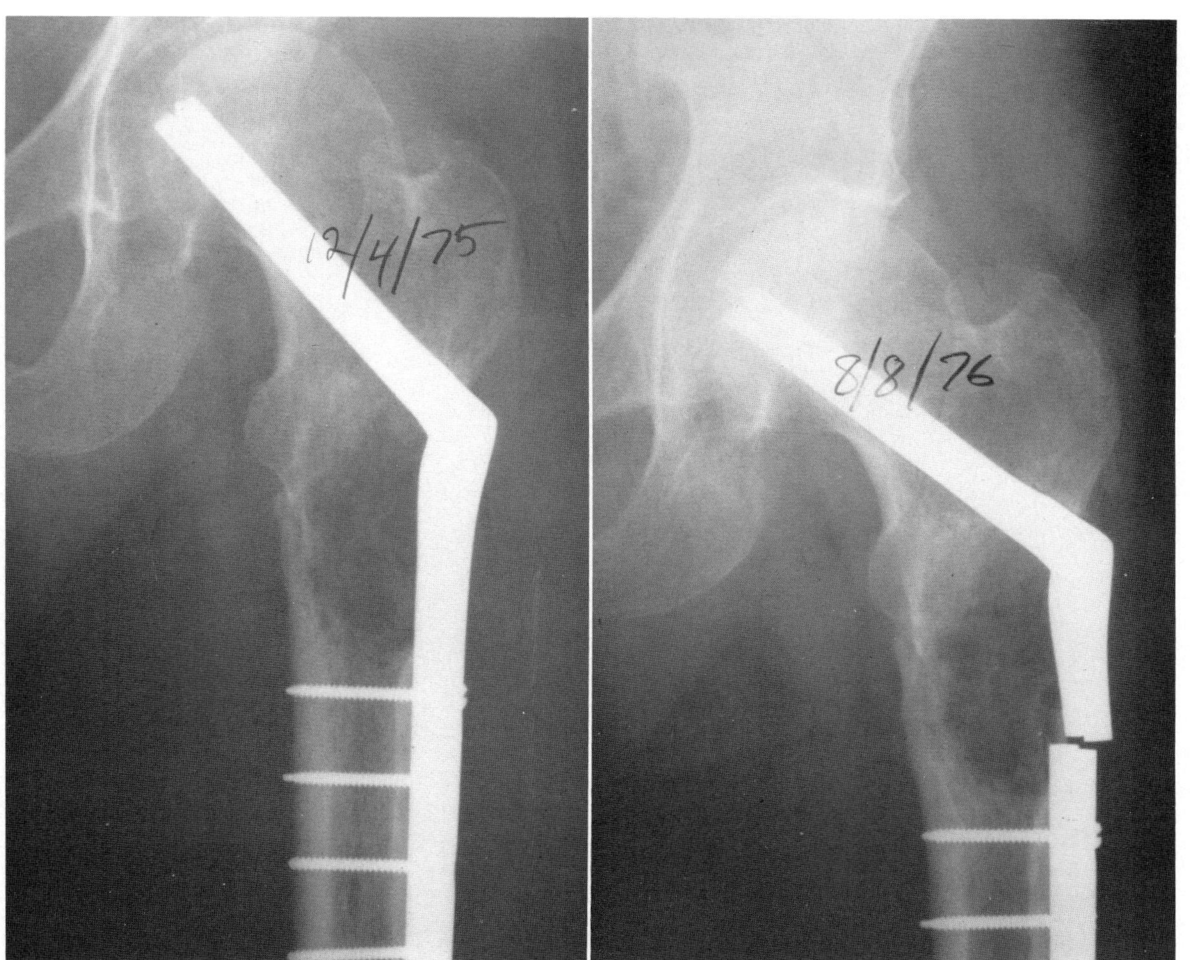

FIGURE 8-20 **A,** Large subtrochanteric lytic defect that resulted from growth of a solitary myelomatous focus. Prophylactic fixation was accomplished by means of a reinforced Jewett nail without cement. The lesion was irradiated. **B,** Eight months later, a fatigue fracture has occurred through the side plate. The size of the lesion remains unchanged.

Continued.

C 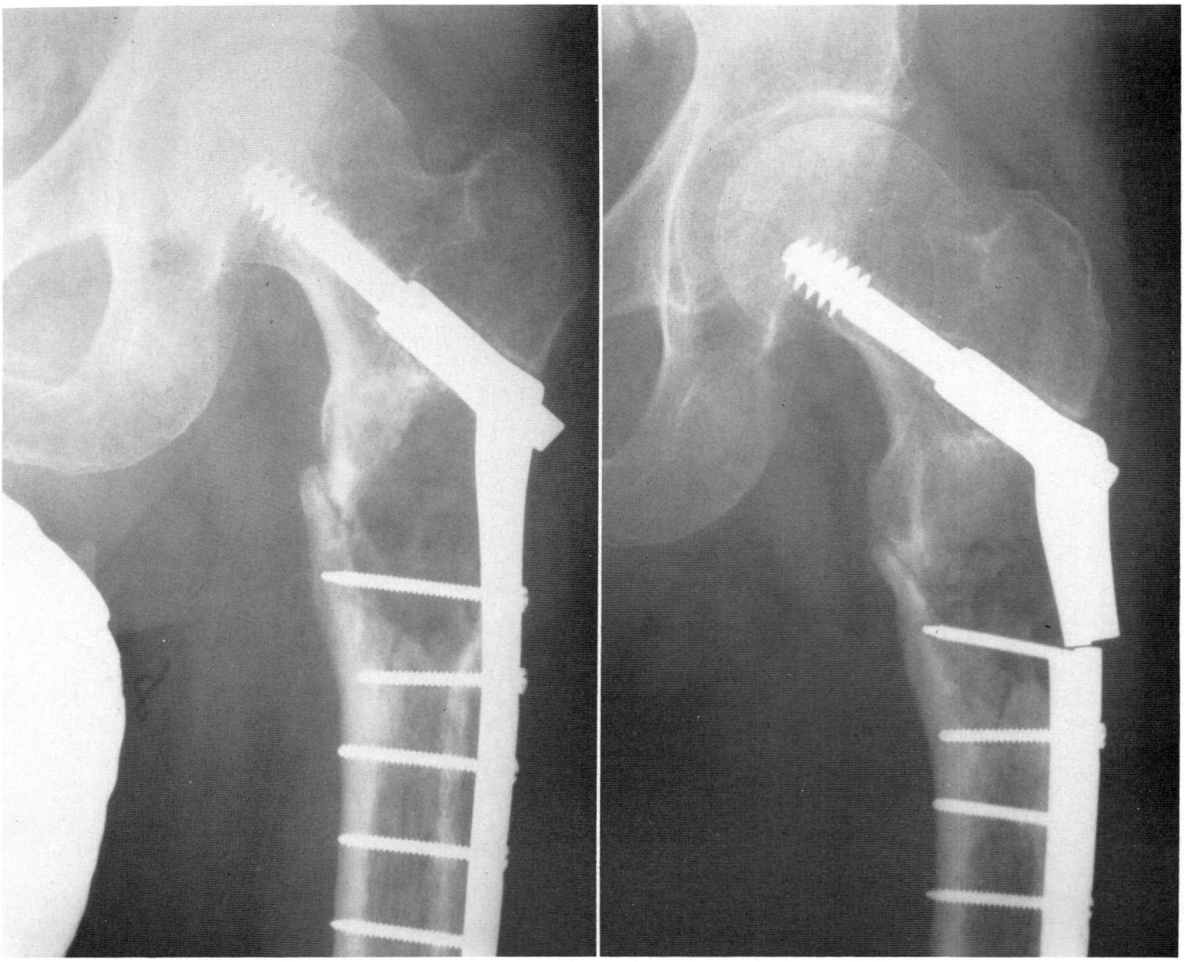 D

FIGURE 8-20, cont'd. **C,** Internal fixation was accomplished with a compression hip screw augmented by intramedullary radiolucent methylmethacrylate and an extracortical cancellous bone graft. **D,** Four years later the appearance of the lesion remains unchanged. No bone healing is apparent. Once again, stability has been lost because of a fatigue fracture through the side plate. The fracture was restabilized with a Zickel nail and cement and remained unhealed but stable until the patient's death 3½ years later.

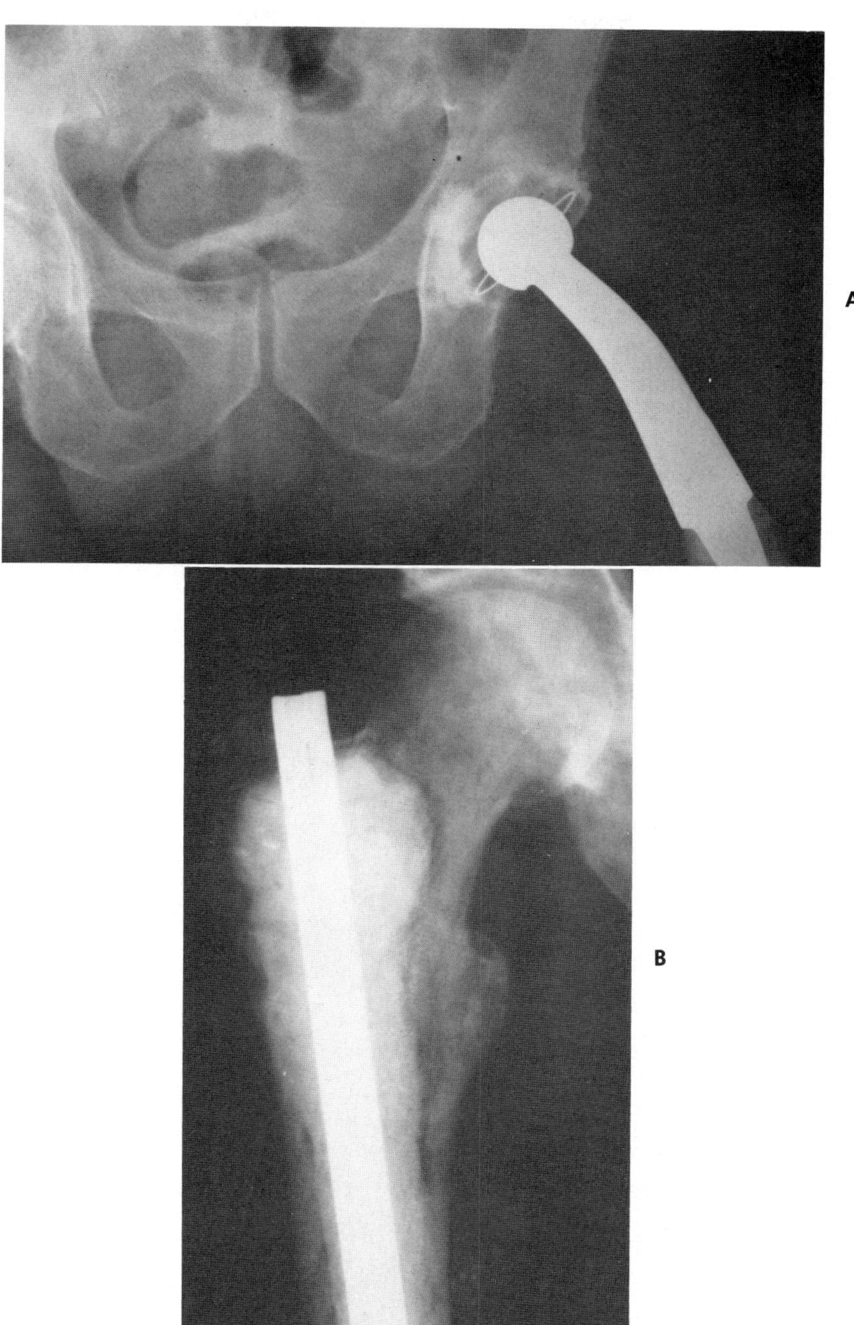

FIGURE 8-21 For legend see p. 179.

Continued.

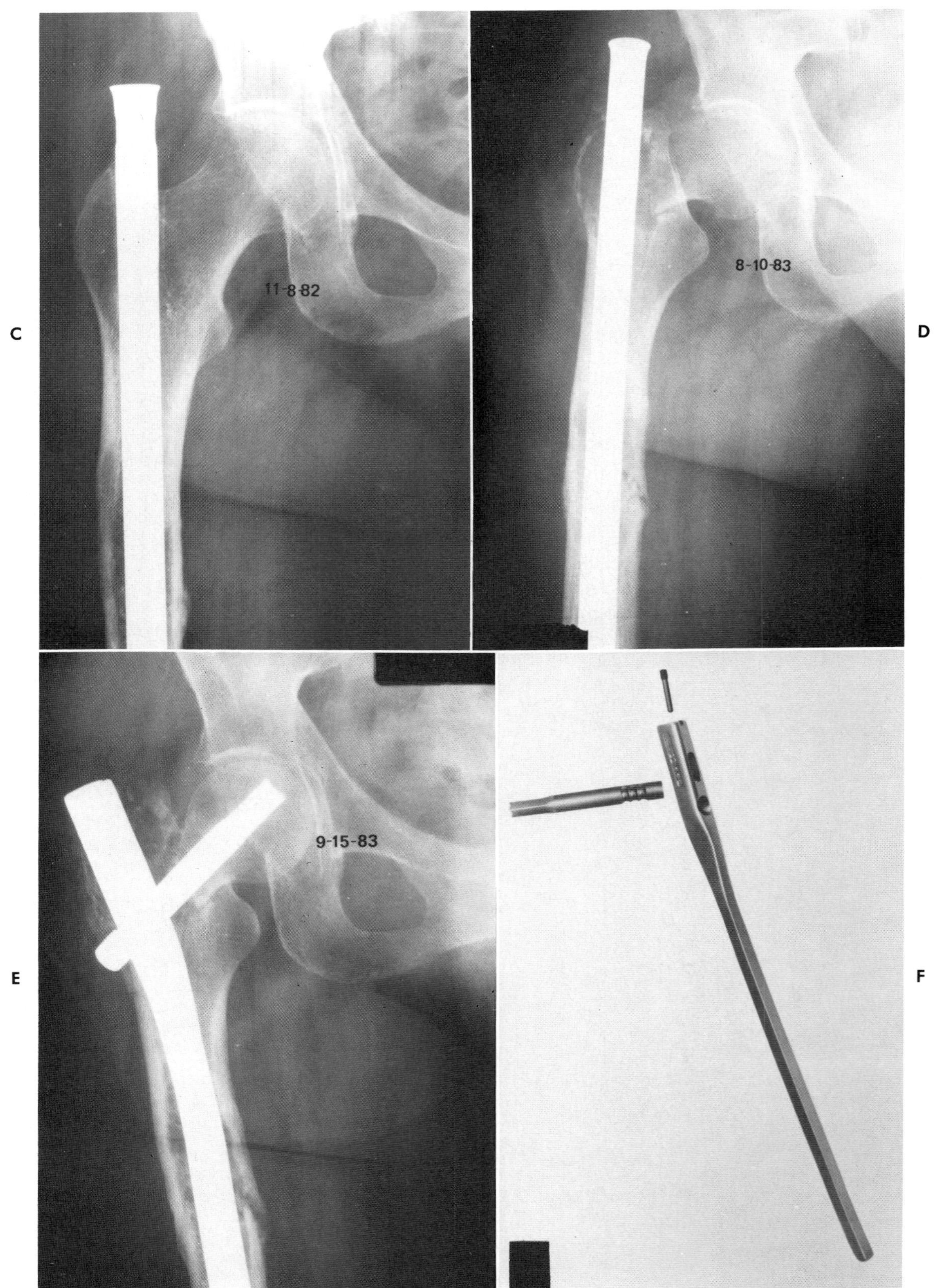

FIGURE 8-21, cont'd. For legend see opposite page.

FIGURE 8-21 To obviate the difficulties demonstrated in Fig. 8-20, some surgeons have advocated prosthetic replacement, **A,** as a means of managing all proximal femoral pathological fractures, even in the subtrochanteric region. Others, however, have advocated stabilization of subtrochanteric fractures with an intramedullary rod reinforced by methylmethacrylate, **B,** despite the fact that tumor has likely weakened the bone along the medial cortex extending into the femoral neck and such fixation does not stabilize these areas. **C,** A subtrochanteric fracture has been stabilized by an intramedullary rod. Although no lytic changes were apparent in the femoral neck, a technetium-99 scan demonstrated markedly increased uptake there and in the greater trochanter, suggesting metastatic disease. **D,** Nine months later these metastases are apparent roentgenographically, as is a displaced fracture at the base of the femoral neck. **E,** Both fractures were stabilized with a Zickel nail and remained stable until the patient's demise 19 months later. **F,** The Zickel nail and long intramedullary rod, the cross-nail pin guide for fixation of the femoral head and neck, and the small set screw. (**A** courtesy Franklin H. Sim, M.D.; **C** to **E** courtesy Bruce J. Sangeorzan, M.D.)

Bending forces on intramedullary devices are much lower than on laterally located plates. Moreover, axial impaction of the fragments is possible, with the load being transmitted through the bone as well as through the device. Thus intramedullary devices are load sharing, and that situation does not change if methylmethacrylate is used to augment fixation.

Conventional intramedullary Kuntscher nail fixation has been used for pathological subtrochanteric fractures, with stabilization of the proximal fragment enhanced by acrylic cement, when extensive cortical disruption exists (Fig. 8-21, *B*). This technique has the advantage of simplicity, but it suffers the major disadvantage of offering no reinforcement to the femoral neck. As has been emphasized already, the extent of tumor lysis proximal and distal to any given femoral fracture is almost always much more extensive than appreciable from conventional roentgenograms. Consequently a patient with a pathological fracture at the subtrochanteric level also will have weakened bone extending into the femoral neck. A failure to reinforce that area at the time of fracture fixation will concentrate stress at the base of the neck and encourage a secondary fracture there (Fig. 8-21, *C* and *D*).

In our experience the ideal device for fixation of a subtrochanteric fracture is the Zickel nail (Fig. 8-21, *E*). Its intramedullary portion is made of a chrome-cobalt alloy, it comes in diameters 11 to 17 mm, and it is designed with a bow approximating the normal curve of the femoral shaft. A cannulated triflanged nail, available in various lengths, is inserted across the upper end of the rod and very effectively reinforces the femoral head and neck as well as maintains proper rotational alignment of the proximal femur (Fig. 8-21, *F*). The device is quite strong, and the fixation afforded by it extremely secure. We have never seen a failure of either, even when there has been extensive lysis of bone about the fracture site and extending well into the proximal fragment (Figs. 8-22 and 8-23, *A* and *B*). However, in such situations we do advocate reinforcing the fixation by intramedullary methylmethacrylate for three reasons: (1) to prevent rotation of the distal femoral shaft fragment about the tapered and relatively short distal rod segment; (2) to reinforce fixation of the femoral head-neck fragment by the small (⅜ inch) triflanged cross-nail; the cement can be injected into the femoral neck to dissipate forces that would otherwise be exerted on the device and to resist compression varus, which would produce forces across the medial cortical defect; and (3) to prevent shortening of the femur caused by collapse of weakened bone on either or both sides of the fracture with subsequent progressive telescoping of the distal fragment proximally. Zickel and Mouradian[59] and Mickelson and Bonfiglio[40] reported a significant incidence of femoral shortening and loss of rotational alignment when pathological subtrochanteric fractures were internally fixed with the Zickel nail but without augmentation by acrylic cement. When

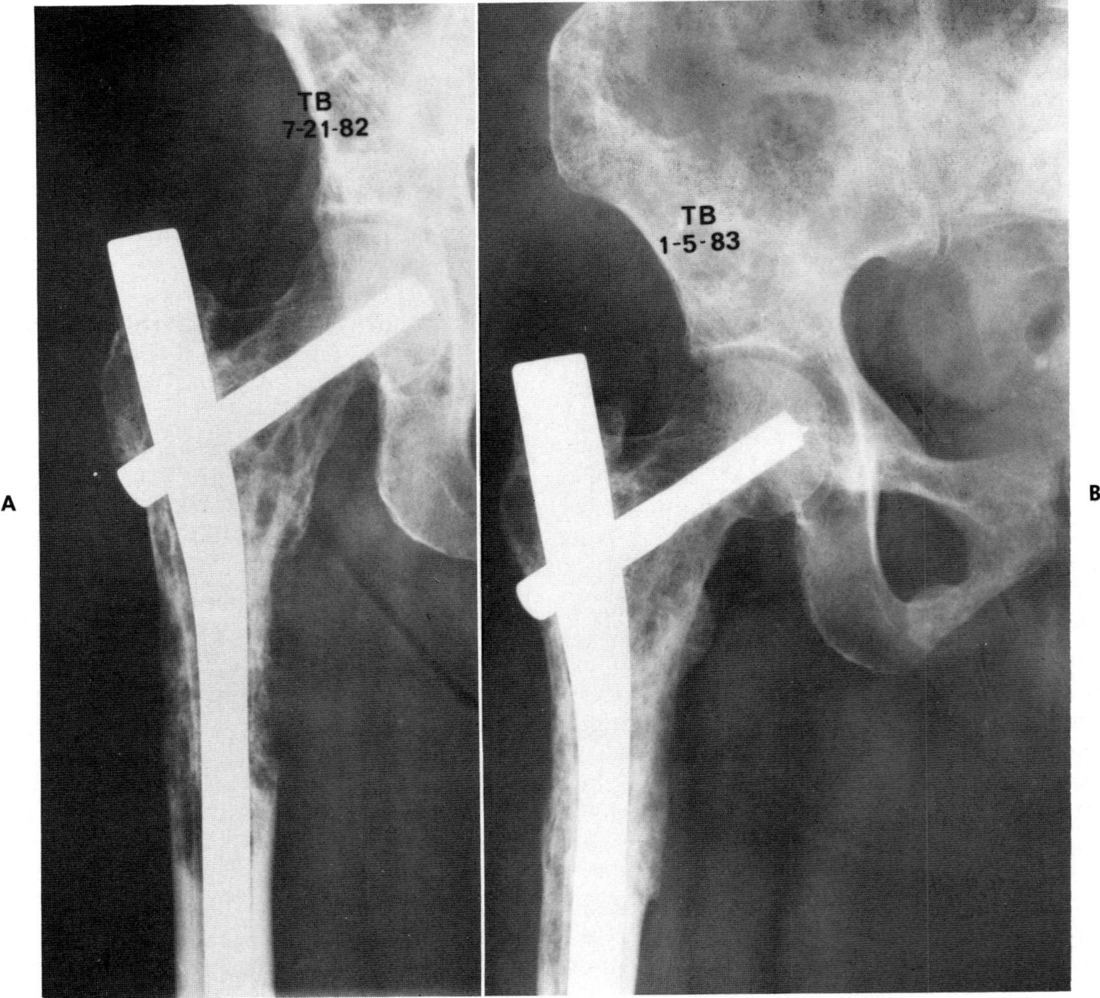

FIGURE 8-22 **A,** Extensive destructive changes involving most of the proximal half of the right femur. Prophylactic fixation has been accomplished with a Zickel nail. The femur was irradiated. **B,** Five months later the lytic metastases have healed and femoral stability remains secure. (Courtesy Bruce J. Sangeorzan, M.D.)

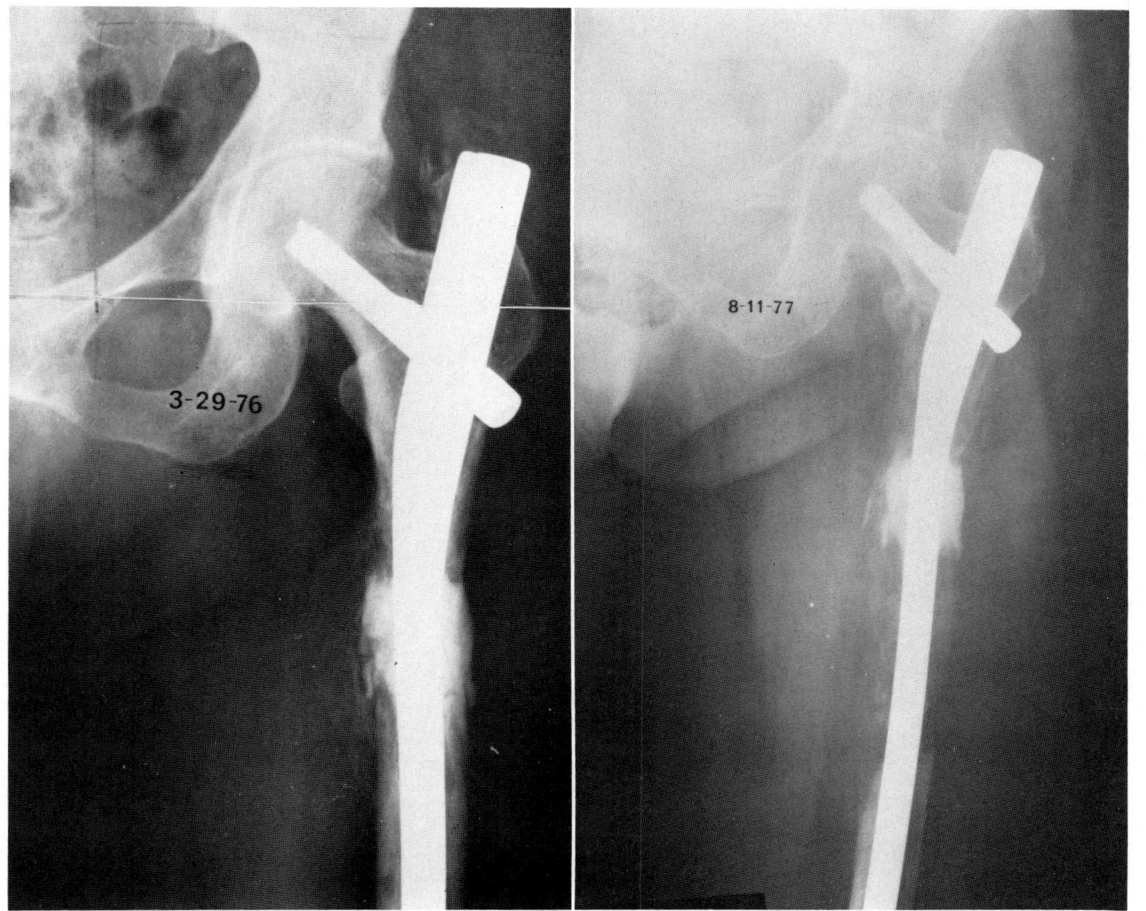

FIGURE 8-23 **A,** Pathological fracture through the subtrochanteric diaphysis of the femur stabilized with a Zickel nail augmented by methylmethacrylate. After irradiation there is some suggestion of healing along the medial cortex. **B,** Seventeen months later, however, much more extensive destruction of cortical bone is apparent. Despite this, fixation with the Zickel nail remained secure and the patient continued full weight-bearing on the affected extremity. (**A** and **B** courtesy Bruce J. Sangeorzan, M.D.) *Continued.*

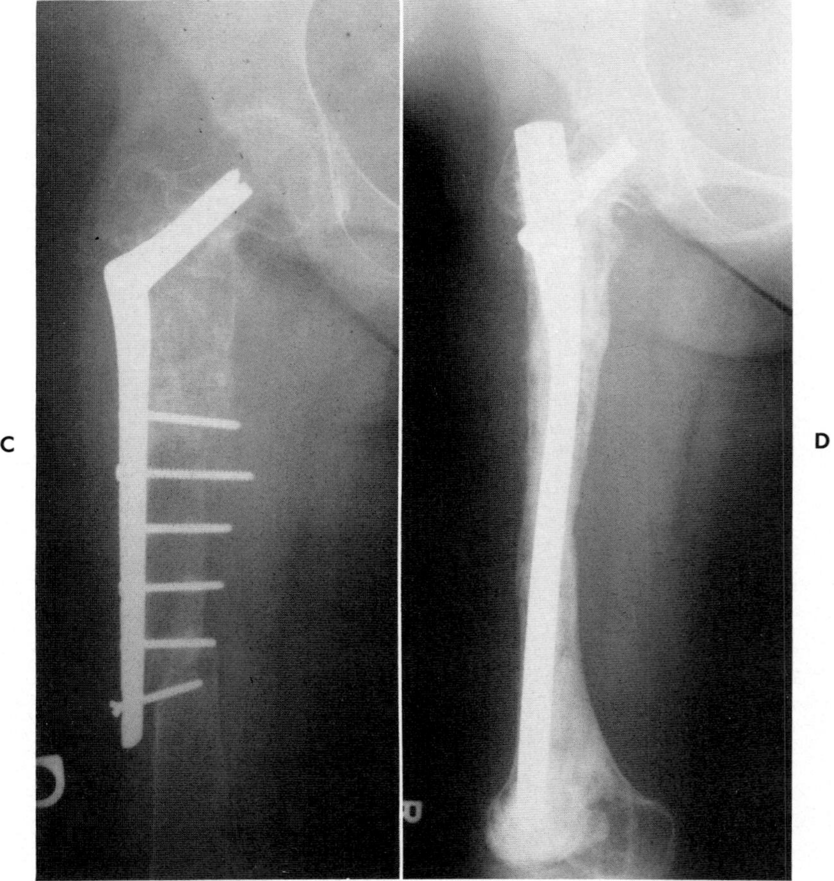

FIGURE 8-23, cont'd. **C,** Femur of a 14-year-old girl who 5 years earlier had received extensive irradiation and internal fixation of a pathological fracture caused by a Ewing sarcoma. A second pathological fracture occurred through an area of radiation osteitis near the end of the plate. **D,** Internal fixation was accomplished with a Zickel nail reinforced by methylmethacrylate. Because the entire femur was brittle following irradiation, the cement was used to fill much of the distal femoral condyles and to surround the nail well proximally. The upper end of the Zickel rod was cut off with an acetylene torch and rethreaded to accommodate the patient's short bone. The femur remains stable and pain free 4 years later.

methylmethacrylate has been used, we have not encountered such complications, and the reports of others[19,37,50] reflect a similar freedom from fixation failures.

The Zickel nail is not an easy device to use, however, and the surgeon must pay careful attention to the technical details of its insertion to avoid the pitfalls of malrotation[19,50,59]: penetration through the femoral cortex (Fig. 8-25, *B*), comminution of the greater trochanter, and malposition of the cross-nail. Some surgeons[50] prefer to do the procedure with the patient on a fracture table and under biplanar image-intensifier control so the fracture fragments will be brought into a position of stable approximate reduction before fixation is attempted. Zickel himself does the procedure on a standard operating table with the patient in a semisupine position and the ipsilateral buttock slightly elevated to enhance exposure of the greater trochanter. We prefer to use a standard operating table as well, but we place the patient in a lateral decubitus position so the cross-table roentgenogram will give a good anteroposterior view of the proximal femur and a vertical one will give a good lateral view (Fig. 8-24, *A*). Preoperative roentgenograms are obtained for selection of the proper size of device.

In small patients the standard Zickel nail may be too long and it may be necessary to shorten the device preoperatively. This requires the use of an acetylene torch and cannot be accomplished with a hacksaw in the operating room under sterile conditions. On two occasions, again in small patients, we have found it necessary to cut off 1 cm or more of the proximal nail end to prevent it from protruding markedly into the abductor musculature (Fig. 8-23, *C* and *D*). Again, this must be accomplished preoperatively with an acetylene torch. Under such circumstances retapping of the proximal end of the nail also may be necessary to allow secure positioning of the setscrew that holds the triflanged nail within the rod.

Our technique is as follows:

The leg is prepped and draped so it can be manipulated freely during the procedure.

The skin is incised along the posterior border of the greater trochanter and the incision extends approximately 6 cm proximal to its tip (Fig. 8-24, *B*). It is important that the incision curve slightly behind the trochanter so the trochanteric tip will be accessible with the femur flexed.

The fascia lata is incised and the vastus lateralis detached from its origin along the base of the trochanter. It is reflected anteriorly and distally to expose the fracture site (Fig. 8-24, *C*).

A 2 cm hole is created in the lateral femoral cortex and through it tumor tissue and bone debris are removed with an angled curet (Fig. 8-24, *C*). This must be accomplished to allow room for methylmethacrylate to be injected within the medullary canal.

If the fracture is undisplaced, the gluteus muscle fibers are split sufficiently to expose the tip of the greater trochanter, and a pointed awl is used to penetrate its tip (Fig. 8-24, *C*).

A small blunt-tipped guide pin is inserted, and reaming of the proximal fragment is begun with a 9 mm cannulated reamer (Fig. 8-24, *D*). Reaming of the distal femoral canal usually is necessary as well to achieve a proper snug fit of the nail. The proximal fragment must be reamed serially up to 17 mm, and the distal femur to between 11 and 15 mm depending on the size of the bone.

It is important to recognize that the upper end of the Zickel nail is angulated by design slightly laterally to allow the cannulated cross-nail to enter the femoral neck at an angle of 130 degrees. Although the tip of the nail must be inserted into the sulcus just medial to the greater trochanter to be directed down the medullary canal, the upper end must eventually reside more laterally within the tip of the greater trochanter so the tunnel locator guide can pass freely around the trochanter during impaction. Sangeorzan et al.[50] have developed a technique for accomplishing both aims during insertion of the nail. Rather than make a simple round hole into the tip of the trochanter, they create a slotted groove from posteromedial to anterolateral in the proximal femur (Fig. 8-25, *A*) using a drill and narrow osteotome (Fig. 8-24, *E*). Such a groove allows the nail to be initially inserted through the trochanteric sulcus yet allows the laterally

Text continued on p. 188.

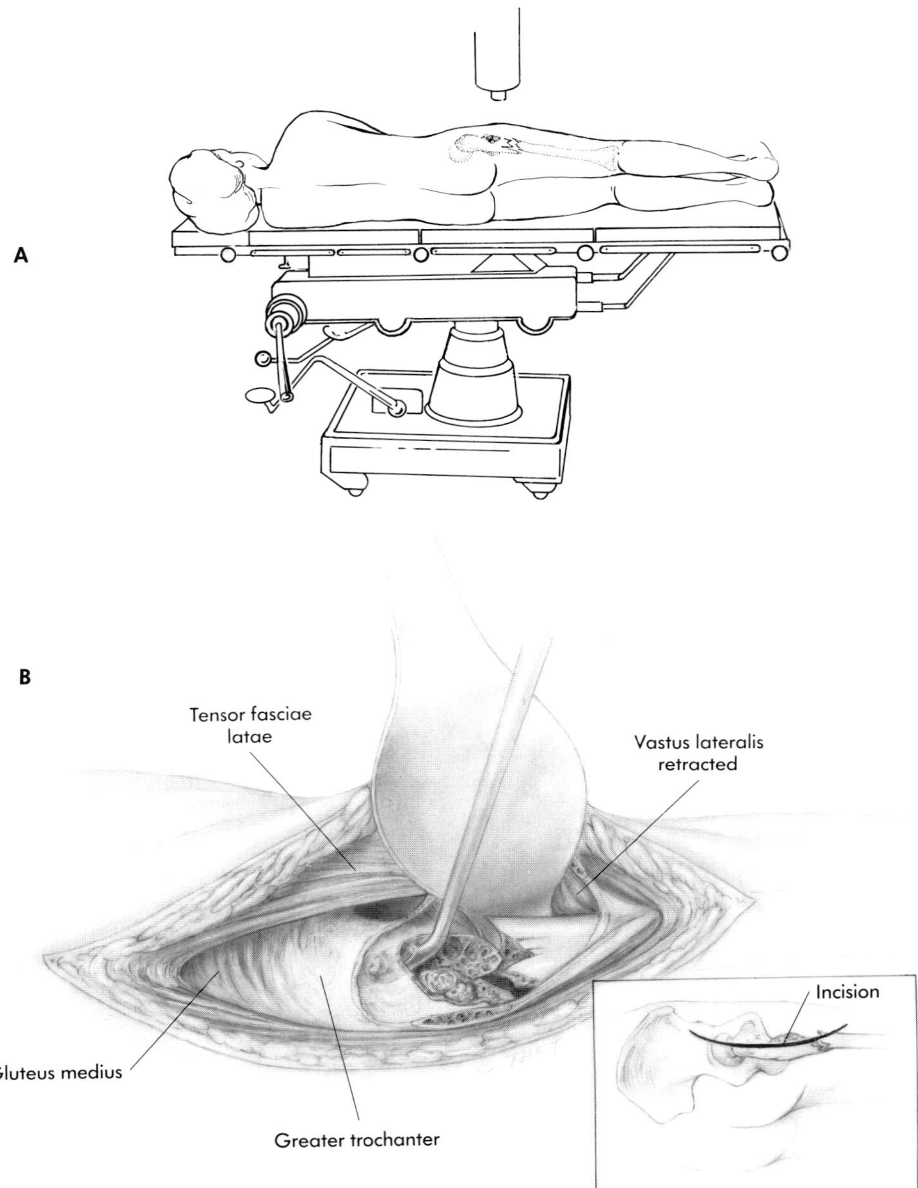

FIGURE 8-24 Operative technique for inserting the Zickel nail. **A,** We prefer to place the patient in a lateral decubitus position. Then with an image intensifier, acceptable AP and lateral films of the femoral neck are obtained simply by rotating the femur after the intramedullary portion of the nail has been inserted under direction vision. Some surgeons prefer to reduce the fracture on a conventional fracture table and to insert the nail under continuous fluoroscopic control. The only disadvantage of this technique is that the affected leg is difficult to adduct fully and thus exposure of the greater trochanteric tip is limited. **B,** A curved incision is made extending just posterior to the greater trochanter. The fracture is exposed by an incision through the forward displacement of the vastus lateralis. With curved curet the medullary canal is cleansed of gross tumor tissue, fat, and bone fragments.

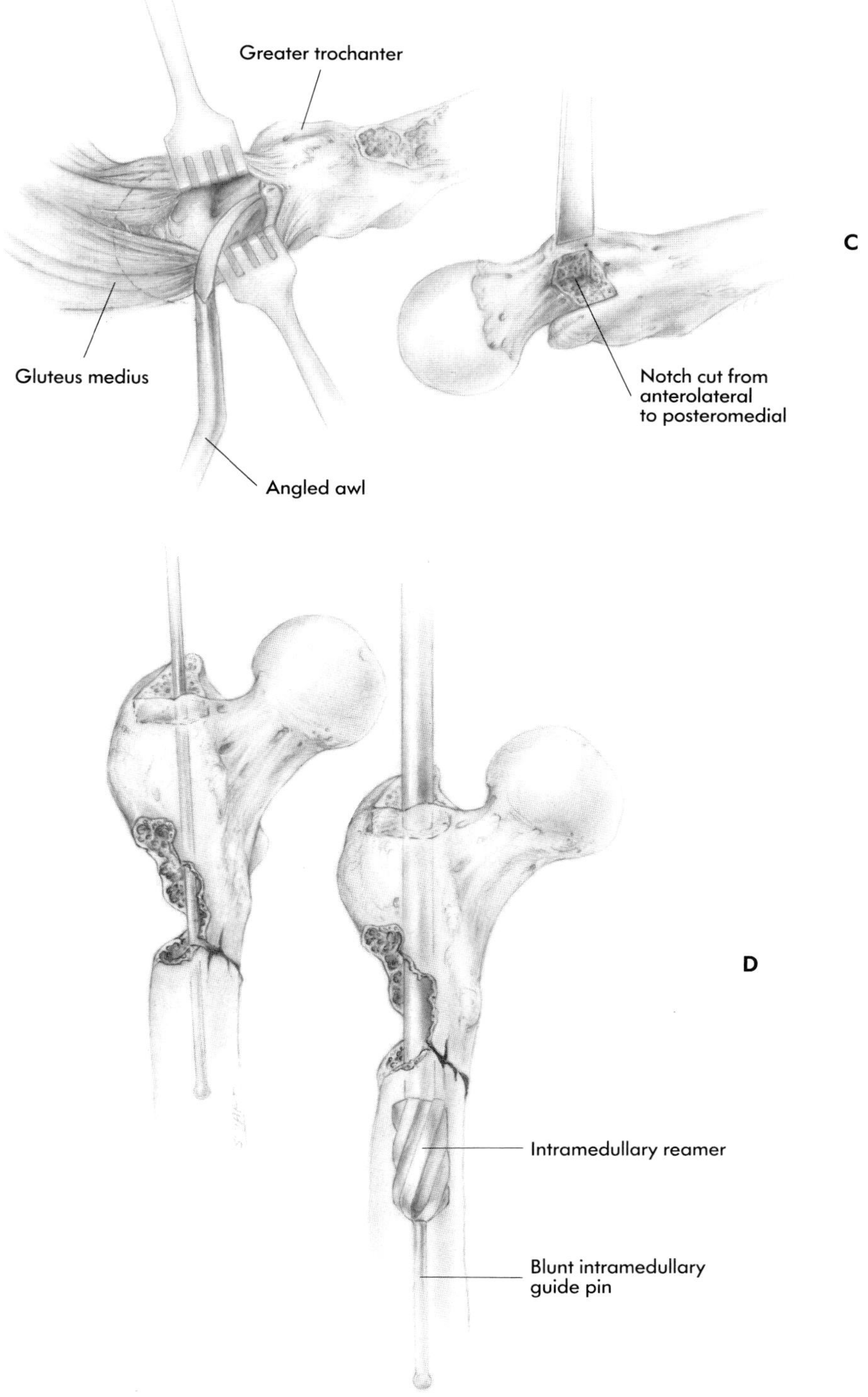

FIGURE 8-24, cont'd. **C,** The abductor tendon is split longitudinally. With an angled awl the sulcus just medial to the tip of the greater trochanter is located and broached. A notch is then cut in the superior and lateral aspect of the greater trochanter from anterolateral to posteromedial (see Fig. 8-25, *A*). **D,** A blunt-tipped guide pin is inserted down the medullary canal of the proximal fragment. The fracture is reduced under direct vision, and the guide pin then is pushed into the distal fragment canal. With serial reamers the medullary canal is enlarged to accept the appropriate-sized Zickel nail. The proximal fragment must be reamed to 17 mm. *Continued.*

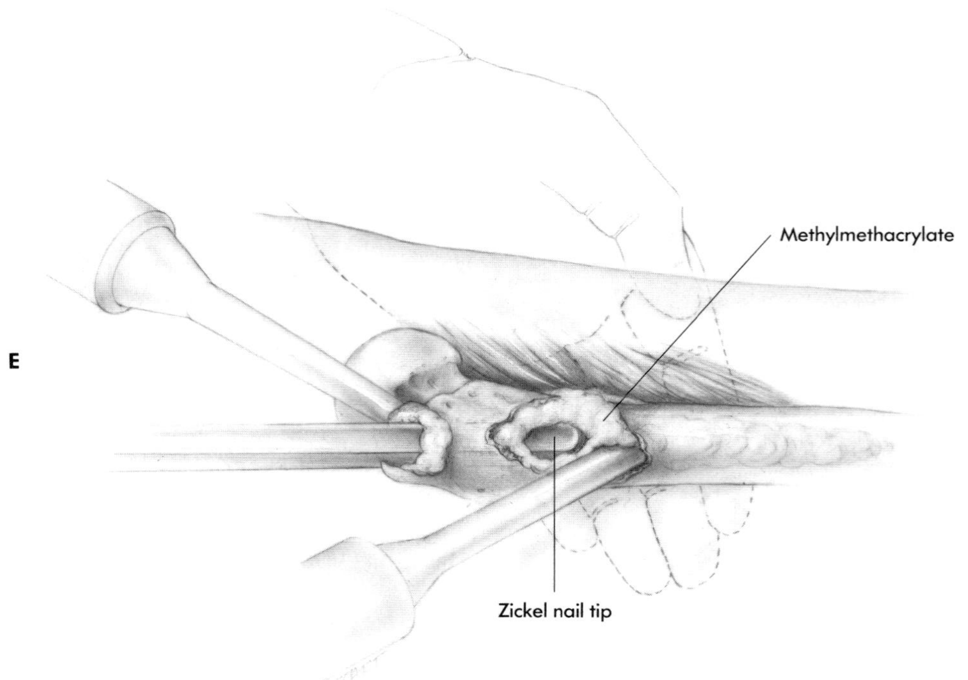

FIGURE 8-24, cont'd. **E,** The intramedullary portion of the Zickel nail is inserted and positioned as far distally as necessary, with approximately 12 degrees of anteversion, and is withdrawn until its tip is just visible through the lateral cortical defect. The proximal and distal canals are filled with methylmethacrylate of liquid consistency, and the nail is driven back into its final position. **F,** The Zickel cross-nail pin guide is fitted over the proximal tip of the nail and held firmly in place while a guide pin is inserted down the center of the femoral neck. If the cement still is soft, the guide pin may be inserted directly. If not, a $^{5}/_{64}$-inch drill can be used to create a track for the pin. **G,** A cannulated drill is inserted over the pin and drilled proximally into the center of the femoral head. The cross-nail then is inserted as shown and once in place is held firmly within the intramedullary nail by a friction-stabilized longitudinal pin.

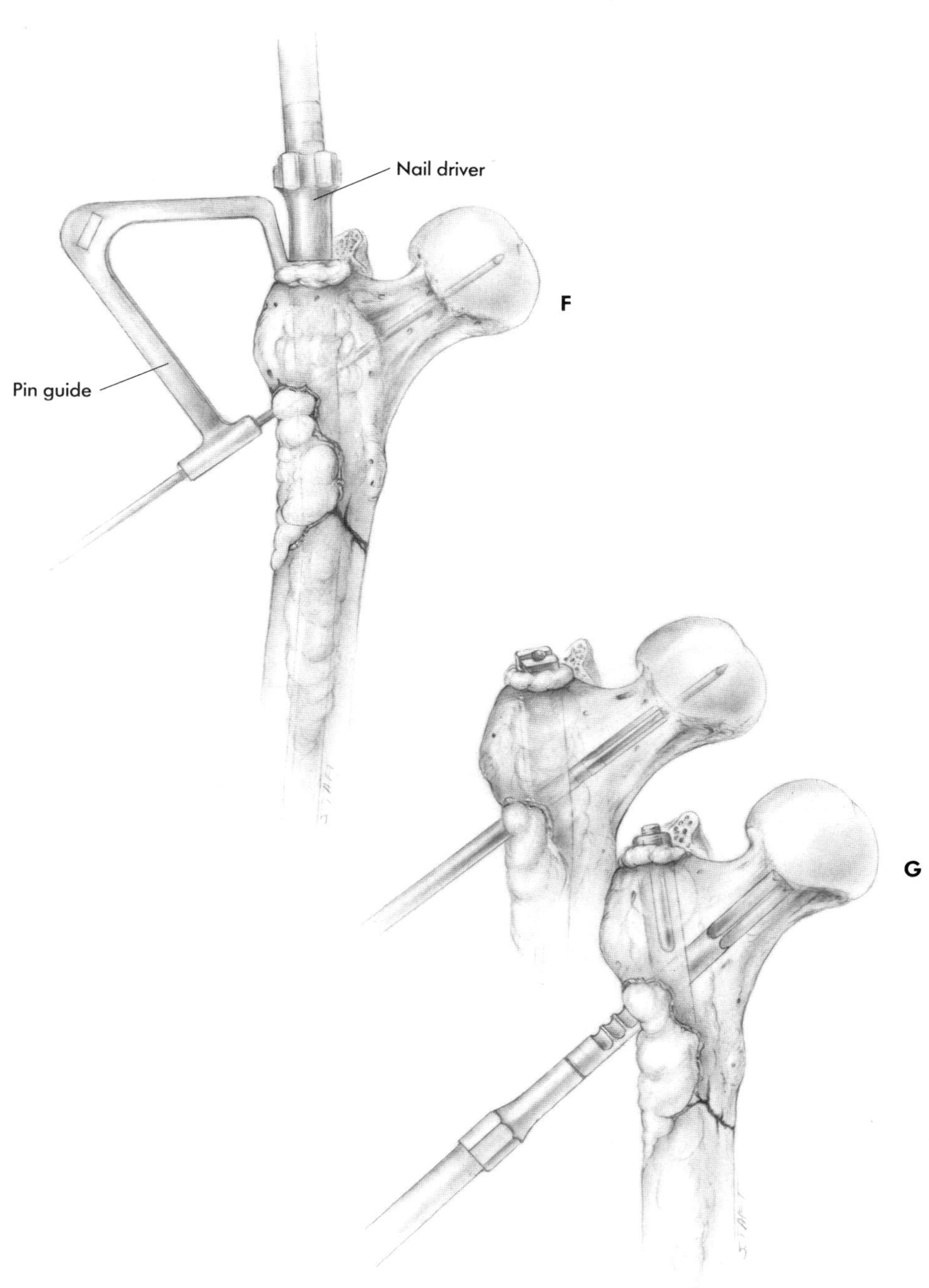

FIGURE 8-24, cont'd. For legend see opposite page.

angled and anteverted upper nail to pass through the trochanter laterally without comminuting the weakened bone. By creating such a groove, they avoid comminuting the trochanter as the proximal nail forces itself from a medial to a lateral position. In addition, they still can center the nail tip directly over the medullary canal during the initial phase of insertion and thereby avoid the complication of the nail tip's penetrating the weakened lateral cortex and missing that canal altogether (Fig. 8-25, *B*).

Because there is 6 degrees of anteversion built into each rod, a different-shaped nail must be used on the left from that used on the right. Once the nail has been inserted, the tunnel locator guide is assembled to it as shown in Fig. 8-14, *G*.

The tunnel locator is secured to the top of the rod by the threaded adapter connected to the driver-extractor. A guide pin should be passed through the arm of the tunnel locator to ensure a correct assembly. If alignment is proper, the pin will pass through the central axis of the round tunnel in the rod.

The guide pin is removed, the leg adducted, and the Zickel nail retracted until its tip is visible through the window just above the fracture site. If necessary, the fracture can be reduced over the tip of the nail under direct vision.

Methylmethacrylate is mixed and after approximately 75 seconds is poured into an Oh-Harris cement gun and injected under pressure well proximally into the hollowed-out cavity of the upper fragment and well distally into the intramedullary canal of the femoral shaft (Fig. 8-24, *F*).

Pressure is maintained over the medial groin to ensure that the adductor muscles are pushed into any defect in the medial femoral cortex to prevent the escape of cement extracortically.

The Zickel nail is driven down the cement-filled medullary canal of the distal femur, care being taken that its tip does not exit either medially or laterally through any cortical defects and that it is positioned in approximately 6 degrees of anteversion.

When the nail is properly positioned, the remaining minutes until polymerization is complete can be spent removing any cement that has escaped extracortically and roentgenographically checking the proper reduction of the fracture.

Once these steps have been completed, the tunnel locator guide is reassembled and a Steinmann pin is passed through the cortical window (if the cement is still soft) and through the nail hole into the central portion of the femoral head (Fig. 8-24, *G*). If the cement has already hardened, a 3/32-inch drill hole may be made in the same manner as for inserting the Steinmann pin.

A cannulated step drill (3/8 inch) is used to create a channel over the guide pin extending into the femoral head (Fig. 8-24, *H*). Generally this can be accomplished without difficulty despite the canal's being filled with hard acrylic cement.

Finally, the guide pin is removed and the triflanged nail of appropriate length is driven through the canal until it is properly seated in the femoral head (Fig. 8-24, *I*).

A small setscrew is inserted into the proximal nail tip and when tightened will firmly stabilize the triflanged nail within the Zickel rod.

Femoral Shaft Fractures. Closed management has no place in the treatment of pathological fractures of the femoral shaft because healing is unlikely in the face of irradiation, particularly if rigid internal fixation has not been accomplished.[4,7,15,19] The use of a cast brace[20] also is inadvisable because, even if healing occurs, there is a high likelihood of unacceptable shortening of the femur.

Intramedullary nail fixation of such fractures is most appropriate. In our opinion closed femoral nailing rarely is indicated because of the high likelihood that the fracture fragments will telescope together as tumor-destroyed bone on either or both sides of the fracture site collapses under the axial stress imposed by weight-bearing (Fig. 8-26, *A* and *B*). Even when preoperative roentgenograms suggest that cortical bone is well maintained (Fig. 8-26, *C*), there will likely be some collapse or resorption of that bone after closed rod fixation if the fracture has been irradiated perioperatively (Fig. 8-26, *D* and *E*). Consequently we strongly recommend that all pathological fractures of the femoral shaft be managed by open intramedullary rod fixation. At the time of open

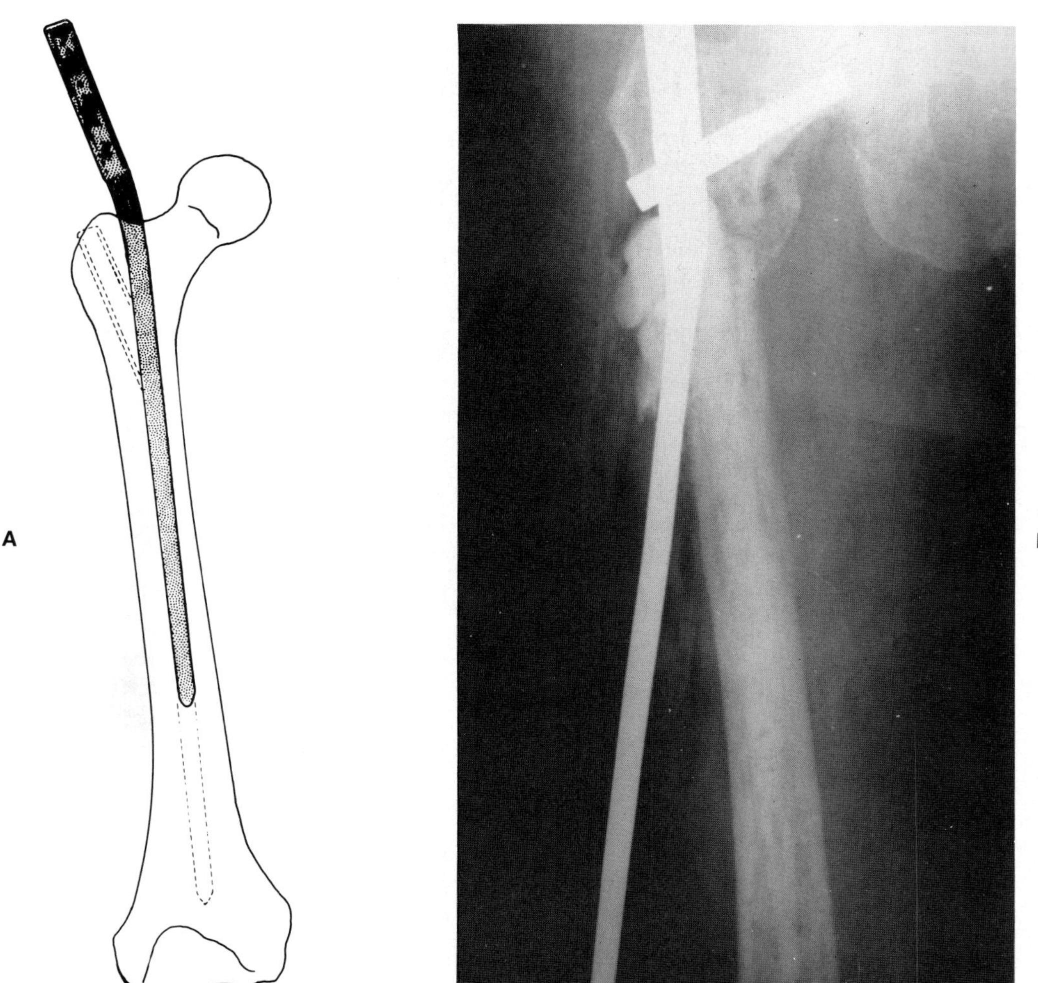

FIGURE 8-25 Sangeorzan et al. have emphasized that the upper end of the Zickel nail is by design angulated laterally and slightly anteriorly. Its tip should be inserted directly above the femoral canal (i.e., in the trochanteric sulcus), **A;** however, a trough also must be cut into the greater trochanter (Fig. 8-24, *C*) so the upper end of the nail will seat properly. If such a trough is not cut, the greater trochanter (usually weakened by metastatic tumor) is in danger of being split out laterally. In cases in which this trough has not been created before insertion of the Zickel nail, **B,** a common error is to direct the nail tip too far laterally. Then the nail must be reinserted after the medullary canal has been filled with cement, and the resulting fixation is somewhat less than ideal. (**A** courtesy Bruce J. Sangeorzan, M.D.; **B** courtesy Edward T. Habermann, M.D.)

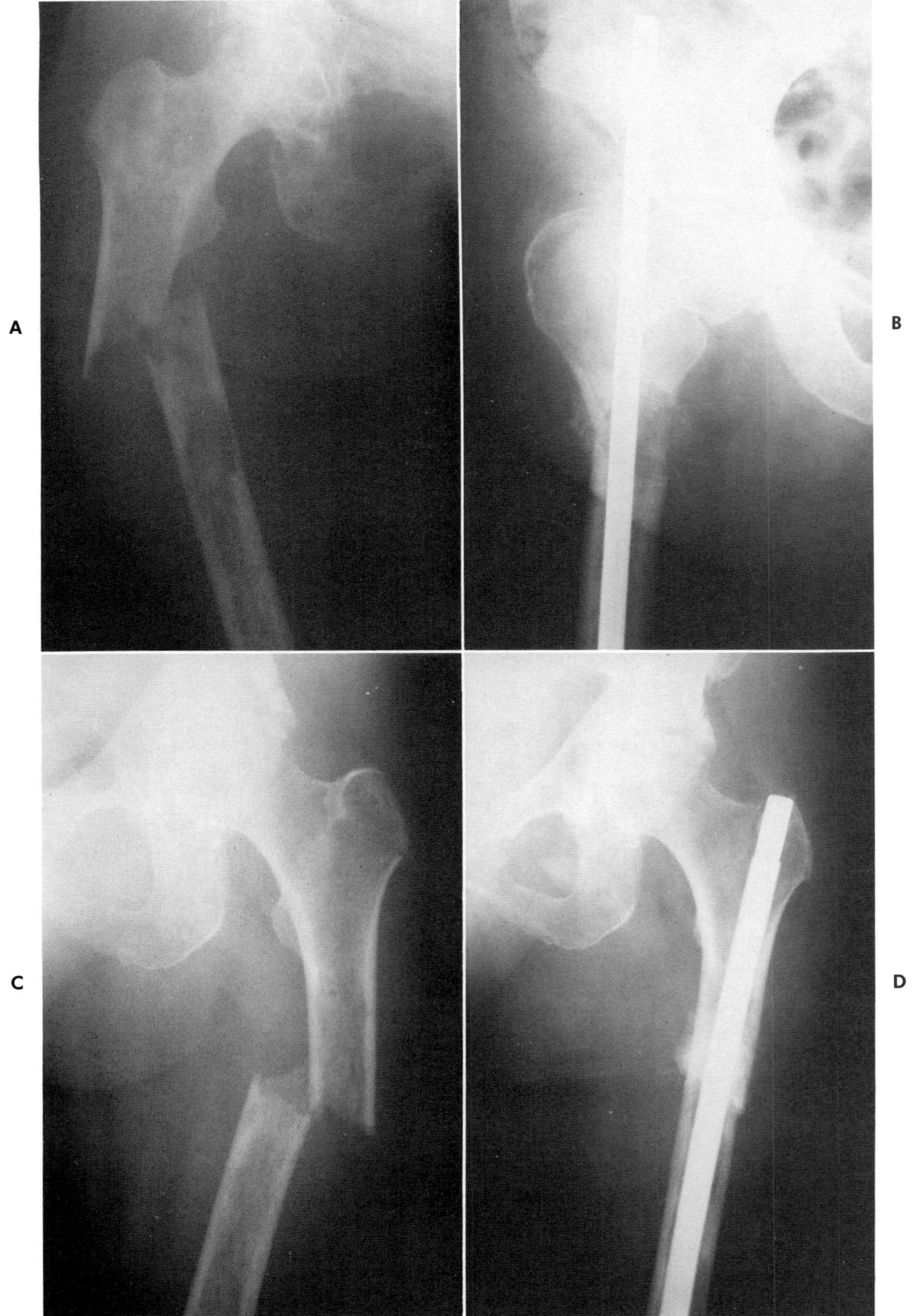

FIGURE 8-26 For legend see opposite page.

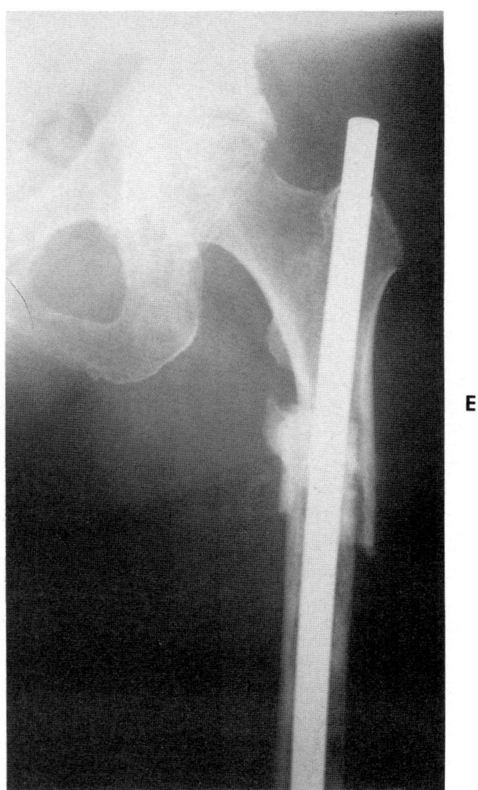

FIGURE 8-26 **A,** Pathological fracture of the proximal femoral diaphysis through an area of extensive cortical lysis. **B,** An attempt was made to stabilize the femur internally by means of a Kuntscher nail without methylmethacrylate, but it failed because the major fragments telescoped about the nail as the cortical bone crumbled. **C,** Similar fracture in another femur with extensive destructive changes throughout the diaphyseal cortex. **D,** In this case fixation has been accomplished by using a large Sampson intramedullary nail without cement augmentation. **E,** Within 3 months the major fragments telescoped about the nail. Despite the size and strength of the Sampson device this patient was left with a painful unstable femur.

Continued.

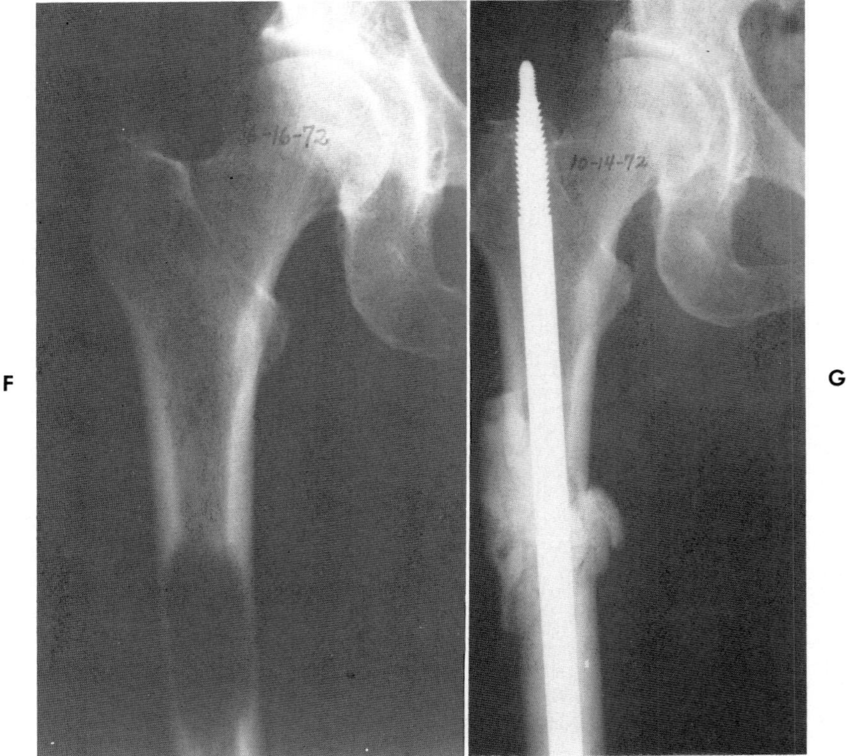

FIGURE 8-26, cont'd. **F,** Large myelomatous lesion of the femoral shaft. **G,** Fixation has been accomplished by a Schneider nail augmented with acrylic cement packed into the tumor cavity. Greater care should have been exercised, however, to keep the acrylic cement within the confines of the cortical defect. Nevertheless, the patient has a stable pain-free extremity despite the absence of bony union 14 years postoperative.

fracture reduction, gross tumor tissue and cortical bone obviously rendered structurally inadequate by tumor can be removed under direct vision. The cavity thus created then can be filled with methylmethacrylate before the rod is advanced into the distal fragment in a manner similar to that used with the Zickel nail. We have found that after using this technique progressive shortening of the femur does not occur, the fracture fragments do not telescope, and the nail does not migrate proximally (Fig. 8-26, *F* and *G*).

One disadvantage of using an intramedullary rod for fixation of a pathological femoral shaft fracture is that the distal nail tip, imbedded in the femoral metaphysis, acts as a stress-riser and may promote a secondary fracture when that area is also weakened by metastases (Fig. 8-27). If such a risk is suspected from preoperative roentgenograms or bone scans, the distal femoral canal should be curetted thoroughly and methylmethacrylate injected well distally into the subchondral bone of the condyles (Fig. 8-28, *B* and *C*). The cement then can dissipate the concentrated forces between the weakened cortical bone and the nail tip and prevent a secondary fracture.

An alternative method of managing a pathological fracture of the femur where there is extensive loss of bone stock about the fracture is to employ an interlocking nail for fixation[1,31,32] (Fig. 8-28). Developed by Grosse and Kempf, this involves the use of an intramedullary nail for axial alignment and for fixation of that nail by cross-bolts in the proximal and distal femur. The procedure is technically difficult because insertion of the distal

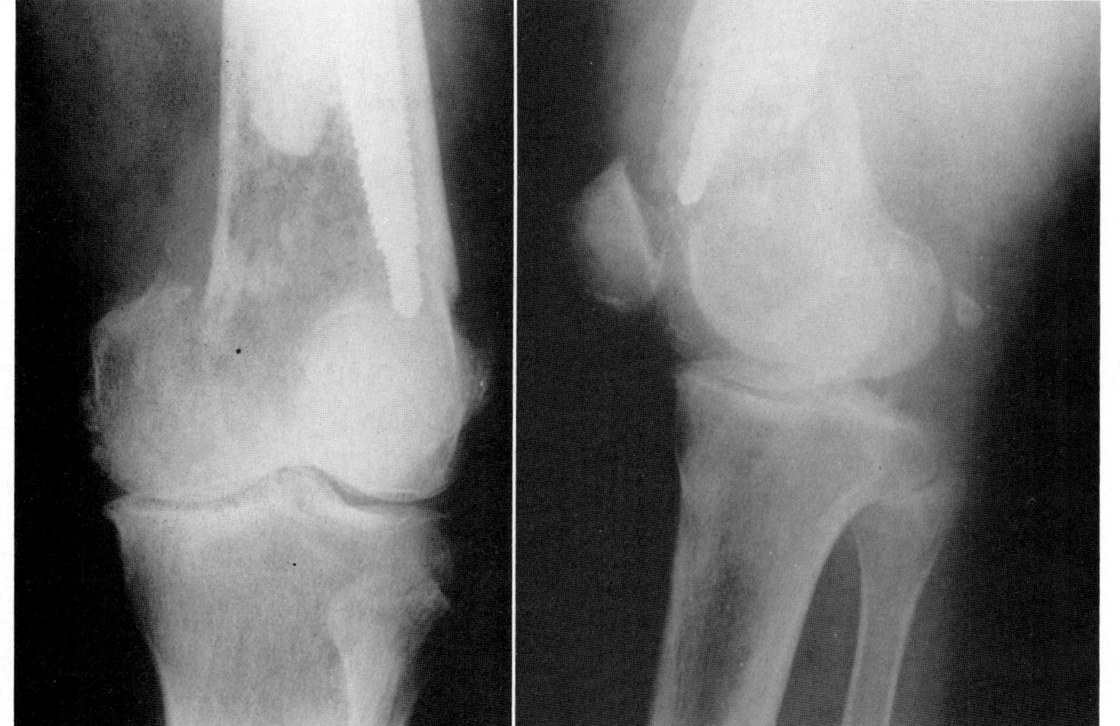

FIGURE 8-27 Every effort should be made to fill the medullary canal with cement well distal to the nail tip (see Fig. 8-23, *D*). Otherwise, a stress riser is created by the nail tip, **A,** that encourages secondary fracture to occur. A lateral roentgenogram, **B,** shows the femoropatellar articular surface disrupted by such a fracture.

cross-bolts must be performed under roentgenographic control, which is inaccurate at best. Furthermore, the cross-bolts are of limited strength and can be anticipated to break eventually in the face of weight-bearing and prolonged delay or failure in fracture union after irradiation. For this reason we advocate open resection of tumor and destroyed bone at the time of fixation followed by filling of the cavity with methylmethacrylate to discourage telescoping of the major fragments (Fig. 8-18, *A*).

Supracondylar Fractures. In our experience metastatic foci in the distal femoral metaphysis frequently will break through the cortical bone and form a palpable mass in the soft tissues (Figs. 8-29, *A* and *C*, and 8-30, *D* to *G*). Under such circumstances, and even in the absence of an extracortical mass, there usually is extensive destruction of cortical bone apparent before an actual fracture occurs.

The two alternatives for fixation include an intramedullary device and an angled blade plate. The former must incorporate the femoral condyles sufficiently to ensure stability of the distal femur against torque and shear stresses. The latter affords excellent resistance to such loads and, when augmented by methylmethacrylate in the defect created by tumor lysis, resists varus and valgus deforming loads as well (Fig. 8-29, *A, B,* and *D*).

However, a laterally applied blade plate in the supracondylar area is subject to the same accentuation of tension loads as is a compression hip screw and plate in the proximal femur and is just as apt to suffer fatigue failure if progression to bony union is frustrated by ir-

Text continued on p. 198.

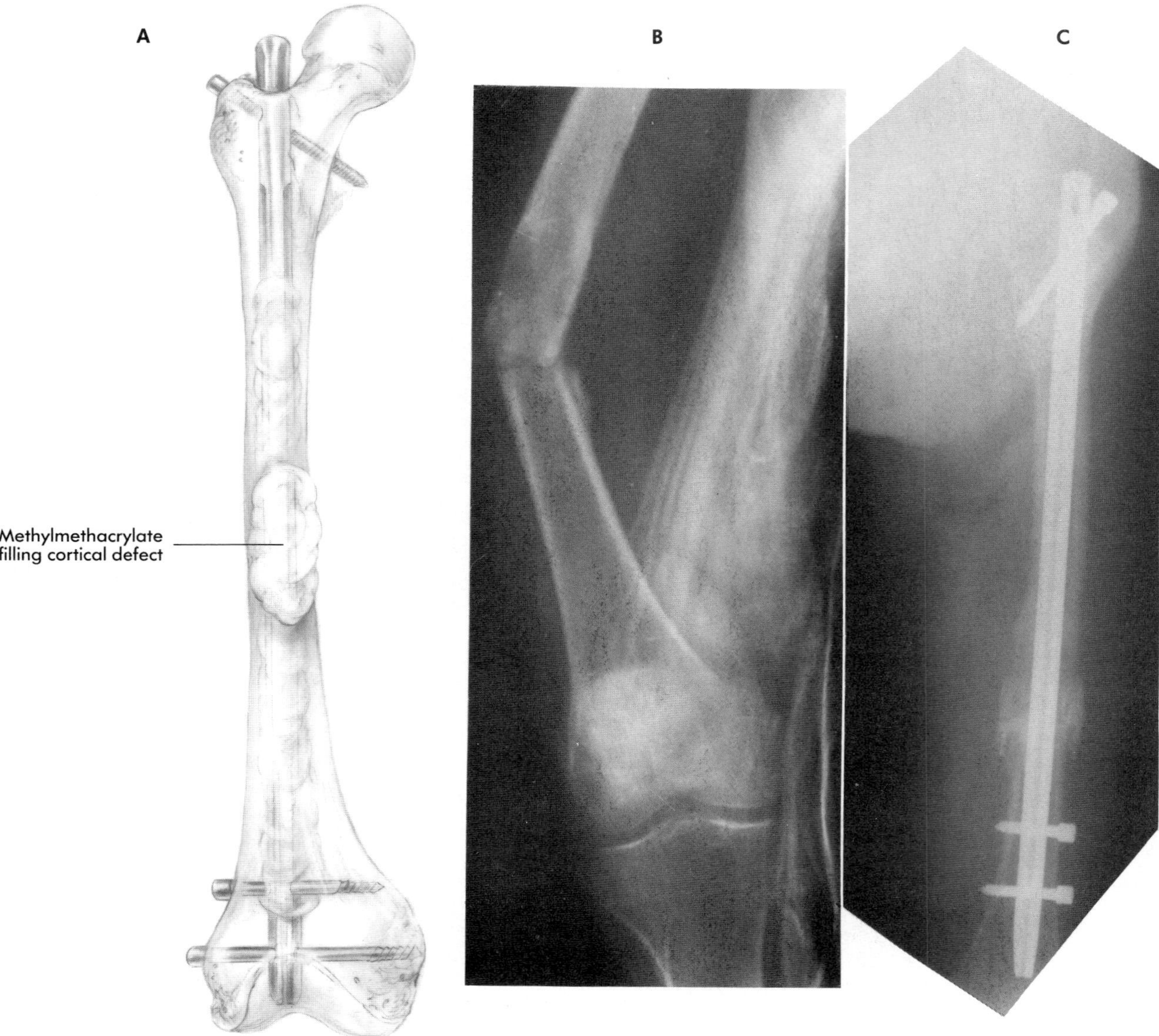

FIGURE 8-28 **A,** The Grosse-Kempf interlocking nail is an ideal means of fixing femoral diaphyseal fractures when there is extensive destruction of cortical bone (see Fig. 8-26,*A, C,* and *F*). Such stabilization may be accomplished by "closed nailing," **A,** without exposing the tumor site. However, the efficacy of subsequent irradiation is improved by debulking as much tumor tissue as possible. Consequently, in most instances, we advocate exposing the fracture, curetting out the tumor tissue, and filling the defect with methylmethacrylate. **B,** Pathological fracture in the diaphysis of a femur with a large lytic metastasis. **C,** Fixation has been accomplished with a Grosse-Kempf interlocking nail augmented by acrylic cement filling the curetted lesion. Although the cross screws above and below the lesion obviate the tendency toward femoral shortening, the cement also helps to reduce the stress on these screws and may help prevent their breaking if the patient survives the fracture for a long period. (**B** and **C** courtesy Kevin Louie, M.D.)

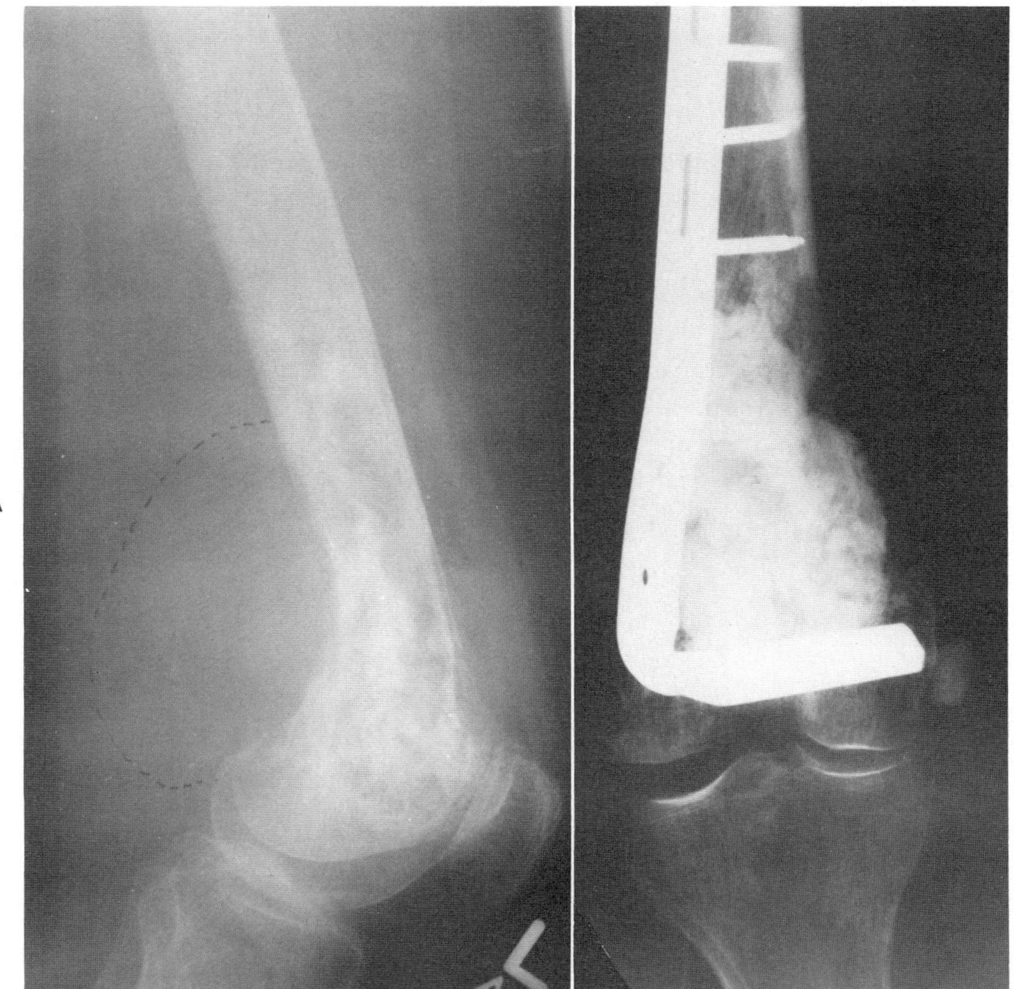

FIGURE 8-29 **A,** Lateral roentgenogram of the distal femur in a patient with metastatic colon carcinoma. A pathological fracture has occurred without displacement. In addition, there is a large exophytic tumor mass protruding posteriorly. **B,** Three years after resection of the tumor, curettage of the bony cavity, internal fixation with a blade plate augmented by methylmethacrylate, and postoperative irradiation. The patient has regained 90 degrees of painless knee motion. *Continued.*

C

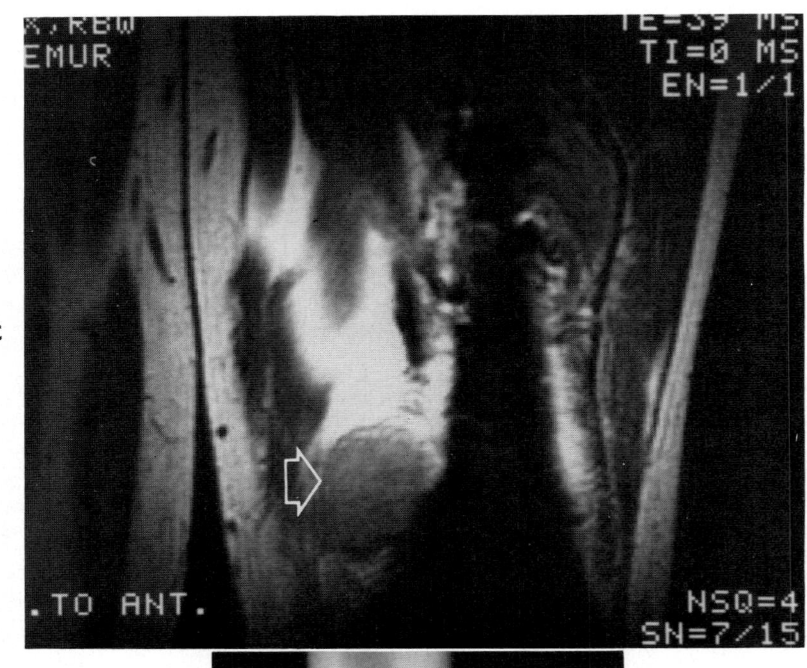

D

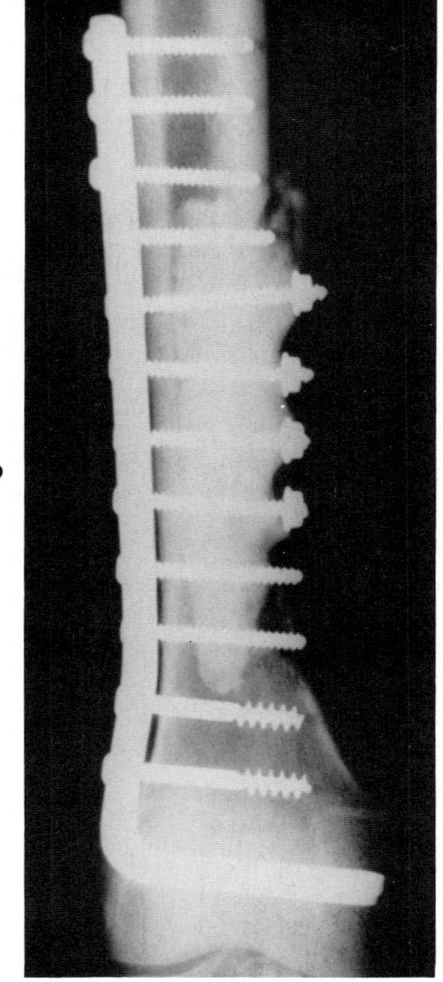

FIGURE 8-29, cont'd. For legend see opposite page.

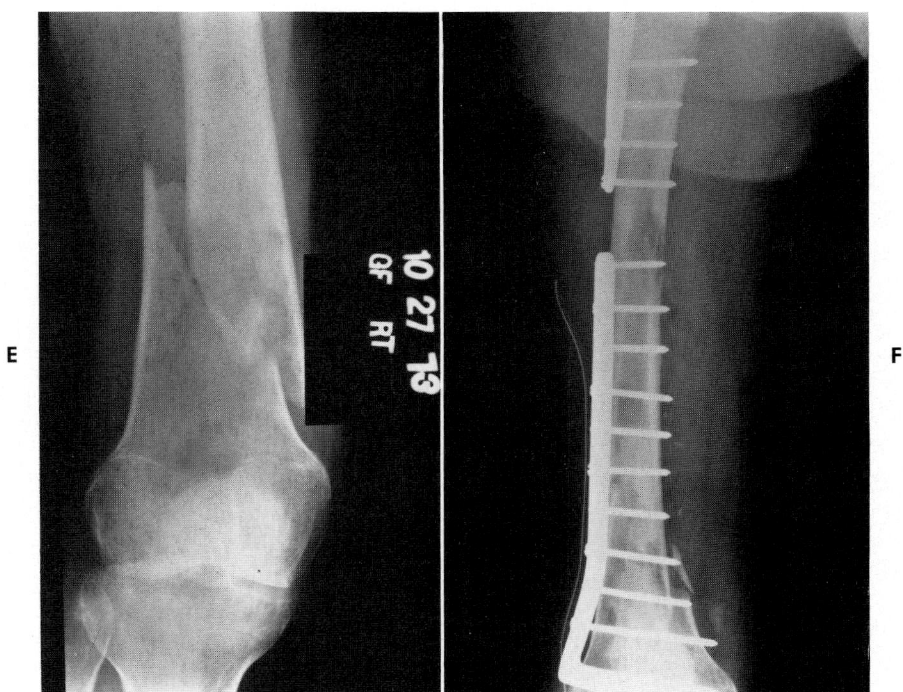

FIGURE 8-29, cont'd. **C,** An MR image of a similar femoral lesion demonstrates the large well-defined soft tissue mass that extends medially *(arrow)* from the distal femoral metaphyseal cortex. **D,** Internal fixation of a similar fracture of the distal femur has been accomplished with an angled blade plate augmented by methylmethacrylate. It would have been better if the cement had filled the distal femoral fragment to a greater extent, thereby more effectively reinforcing the medial cortical defect. **E,** Pathological fracture of the distal femur in a patient with extensive metastatic disease throughout the bone. **F,** The fracture has been internally fixed with an angled blade plate augmented by cement. The upper end of the plate extends proximally to a point only 4 cm distal from the tip of a previously applied proximal nail plate. The unprotected femoral diaphysis in between shows evidence of extensive cortical lysis and now is subjected to a greatly increased focal stress on weight-bearing. Not surprisingly, a pathological fracture occurred here. The distal femur would have been better managed by using intramedullary nails as demonstrated in Fig. 8-30, *H*.

radiation in patients who survive their fracture fixation for years. Moreover, a major stress riser is created just proximal to the tip of the side plate, which increases the likelihood of a secondary fracture there (Fig. 8-29, *E* and *F*). Conversely, the asymmetrical loads on an intramedullary device, which might ultimately lead to fatigue failure of fixation, are much less prominent than when a blade plate is used. For this reason, and because an intramedullary device encourages continuing impaction of the major fragments with weight-bearing, we prefer such fixation whenever possible.

There has been a tendency by some surgeons to encourage intramedullary fixation of such fractures by closed means, using multiple small rods (e.g., Rush) that do not effectively stabilize the distal fragment and do not resist torque or shear stresses well (Fig. 8-30, *A*). The intramedullary Kuntscher or reinforced Samson nail also has been advocated for strong

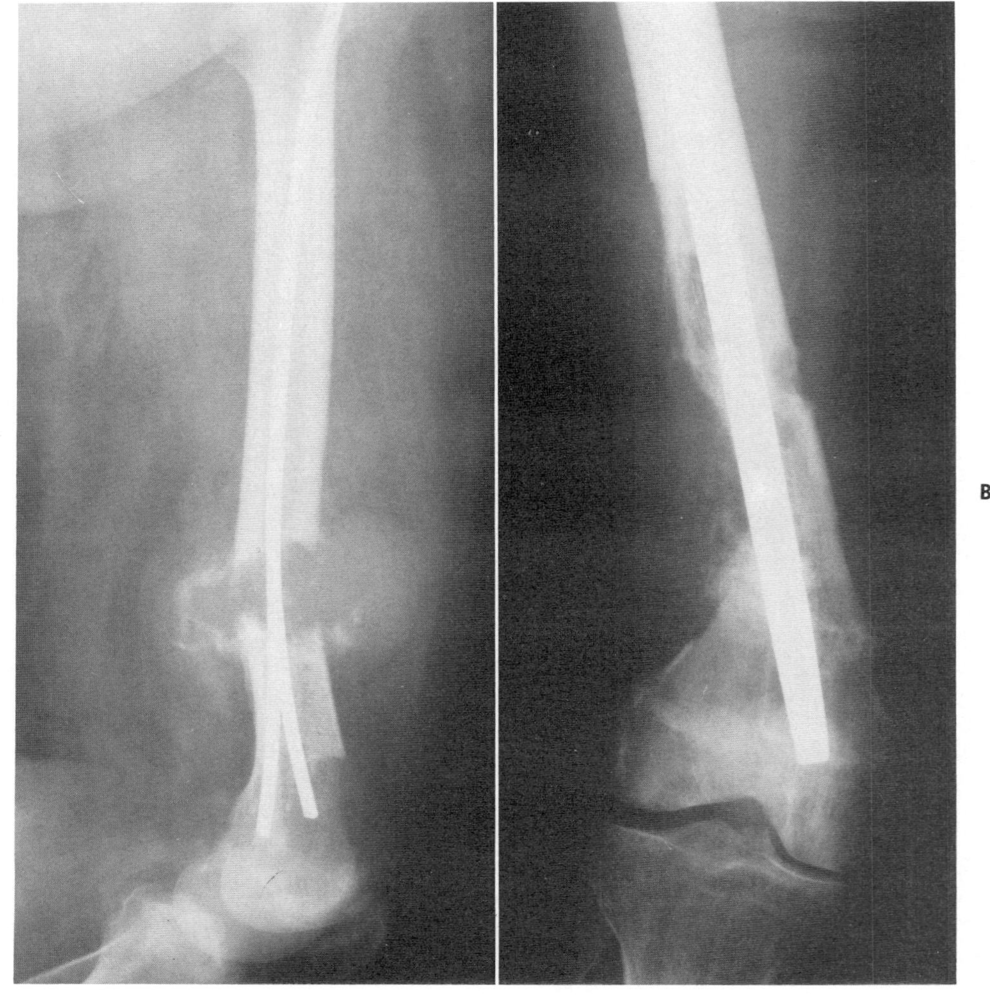

FIGURE 8-30 **A,** An attempt has been made to stabilize a pathological supracondylar femoral fracture by "closed" pin fixation. The fracture is inadequately stabilized, a large extracortical tumor mass has not been resected, and there is danger of the pin's migrating distally through the anterior condylar lytic focus. **B,** Pathological fracture of the distal femoral metaphysis internally stabilized with a Kuntscher nail. Fixation of the distal fragment clearly is inadequate, and an unstable nonunion has resulted with 20 degrees of valgus malalignment.

C

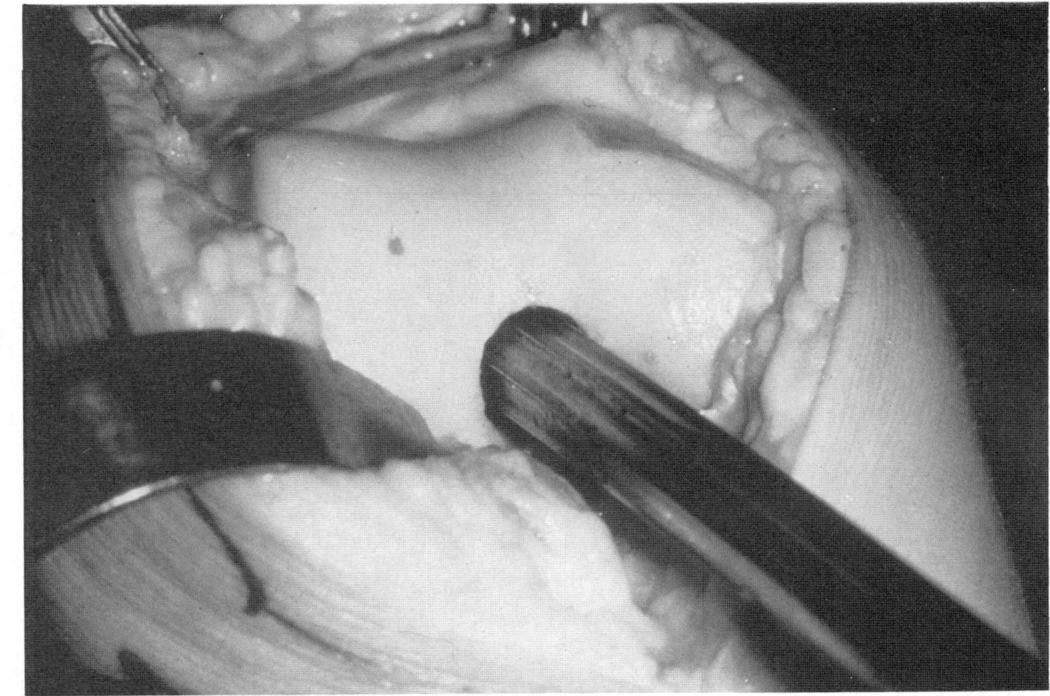

D

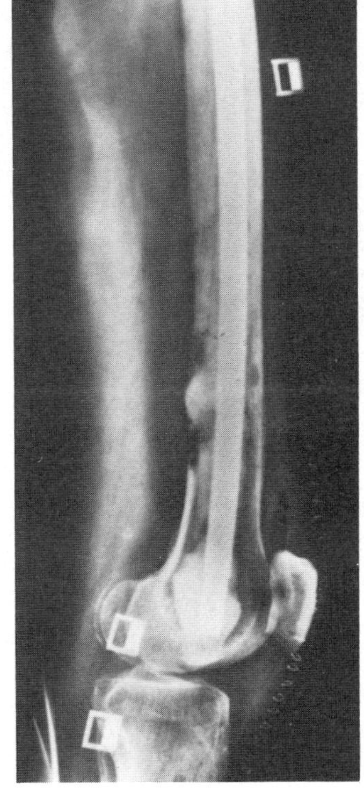

FIGURE 8-30, cont'd. **C,** Intraoperative view of the knee demonstrating a large fluted intramedullary rod inserted retrograde through the intercondylar notch for stabilization of the distal femoral fracture. To seal the intercondylar defect and, hopefully, also to prevent distal migration of the rod, methylmethacrylate should be injected around the tip of the nail. **D,** Postoperative roentgenogram of such fixation. (**C** and **D** reprinted with permission from Springfield, D.S., and Brower, T.D.: In Rockwood, C.A., and Green, D.P., editors: Fractures in adults, vol. 1, Philadelphia, 1984, J.B. Lippincott Co., p. 307.)

Continued.

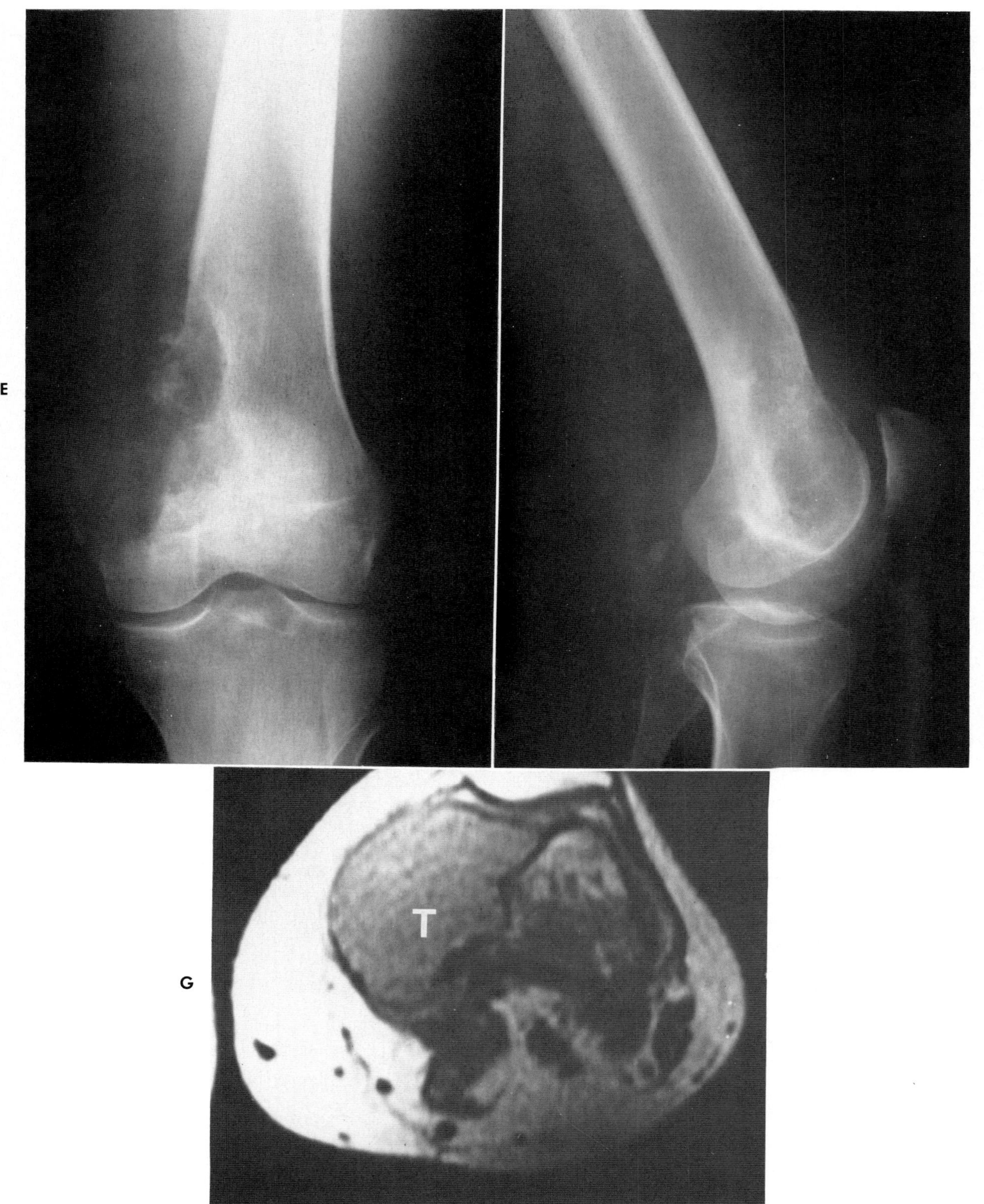

FIGURE 8-30, cont'd. For legend see opposite page.

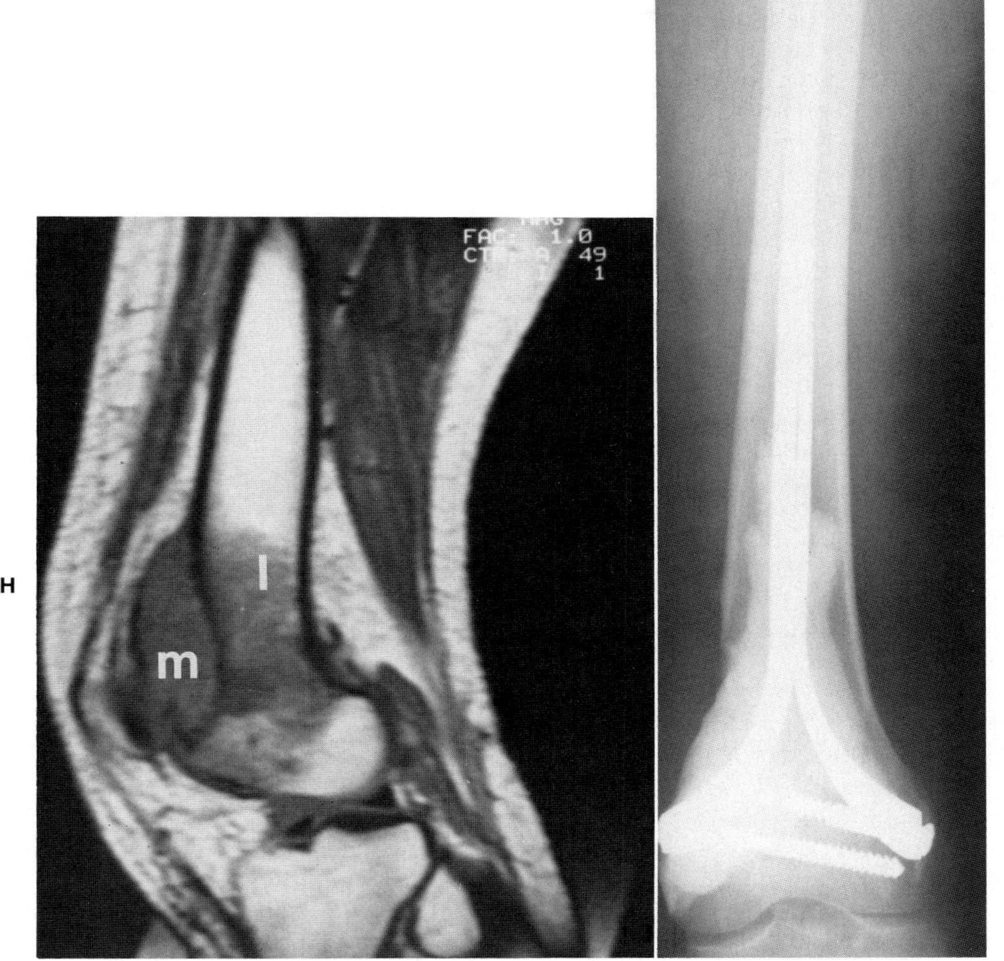

FIGURE 8-30, cont'd. **E,** Aneurysmal lytic metastasis from a cutaneous melanoma has created a large extracortical mass. **F,** On the lateral film it is apparent that the mass has eroded through the anterior femoral cortex and entered the knee. **G,** A CT scan of the distal femur demonstrates the extent of bone replacement by the mass *(T)*. **H,** An MR image lateral to the lesion shows that the mass extends well anteriorly and has broken through the femoral cortex *(m)*. The extent of the reticulated lysis also is apparent in the distal femur *(l)*. **I,** The tumor mass and structurally destroyed bone have been resected, and the distal femur is stabilized with two Zickel supracondylar nails augmented by methylmethacrylate.

fixation of supracondylar fractures. It is true that stabilization of the distal fragment can be enhanced by inserting the nail retrograde through the femoral intercondylar notch (Fig. 8-30, *C*) and injecting cement around the nail tip and into the cancellous framework of the condyles (Fig. 8-30, *D*). Nevertheless, the stability so created is tenuous if bony union does not occur ultimately. We have seen two late failures of such fixation, with the distal fragment angulating or rotating axially about the nail tip (Fig. 8-30, *B*).

The Zickel supracondylar nail[8,60] affords excellent intramedullary fixation yet, because it transfixes both femoral condyles by a combination of rods and screws, ensures secure resistance to rotational forces as well (Fig. 8-30, *E* to *I*). It can be inserted by a closed technique (without opening the fracture site) using small medial and small lateral epicondylar incisions. More commonly, however, we have chosen to use an anteromedial parapatellar incision, whereby the knee joint is opened and the fracture site exposed directly (Fig. 8-31, *A*). Obviously such an approach allows tumor cells to contaminate the joint even if the joint has not been invaded already, but we have never seen this result in metastatic implants within the joint or any other functional disability. The entire extent of the extracortical tumor mass can be exposed, and with the knee flexed both epicondyles are approached easily.

Our technique follows:

As much tumor as possible is removed together with bone obviously destroyed by the lytic process.

A ¼-inch drill hole is made through the anterior portion of the epicondylar prominence medially or laterally in line with the long axis of the femoral canal (Fig. 8-31, *B*).

We use the largest-diameter Zickel rods that will fit within the medullary canal and long enough that at least two thirds of their length will be above the proximal extent of obvious tumor lysis (Fig. 8-31, *D*).

The rods are advanced together. As they are impacted within the medullary canal, their ends are forced against the femoral cortex as they spring against each other.

Once positioned, an intraoperative roentgenogram should be obtained to ensure that neither rod has penetrated the cortex through a proximal and often occult metastatic focus.

The horizontal intercondylar screws are inserted after appropriate drilling of bone. Often the tip of one screw, the end of one nail, or both will not engage cortical bone because of the extent of tumor lysis; but all components of the fixation system should be of a length and in a position that would be appropriate if the cortex were intact (Fig. 8-31, *D* to *E*).

The bony defect is filled with methylmethacrylate injected from a cement gun while in a liquid consistency and then digitally packed to fill the confines of the tumor cavity and extend as far proximally as possible (Fig. 8-31, *F*).

It may be necessary to reattach a portion of the medial or lateral capsular complex to the cement mass with a barbed staple before polymerization is complete. The capsule then will scar down to adjacent soft tissues and restore amazingly good collateral stability even in the absence of actual attachment to bone.

The fixation and ligamentous stability achieved by this method allow immediate full and unrestricted weight-bearing and early resumption of knee range-of-motion exercises,

FIGURE 8-31 **A,** For stabilization of a supracondylar femoral fracture, the distal femur and knee can be approached by a median parapatellar incision with lateral displacement of the patella. It is worthwhile to open the knee in most instances to expose and resect as much tumor tissue as possible. In this illustration, as in Fig. 8-30, *G*, the large exophytic tumor mass has replaced much of the anterior femoral articular surface. **B,** Tumor resected and the remaining cavity curretted to enhance the efficacy of subsequent irradiation. **C,** A drill hole is made in each epicondyle and is enlarged to ⅜ inch to allow seating of the squared tip of the Zickel nail.

Continued.

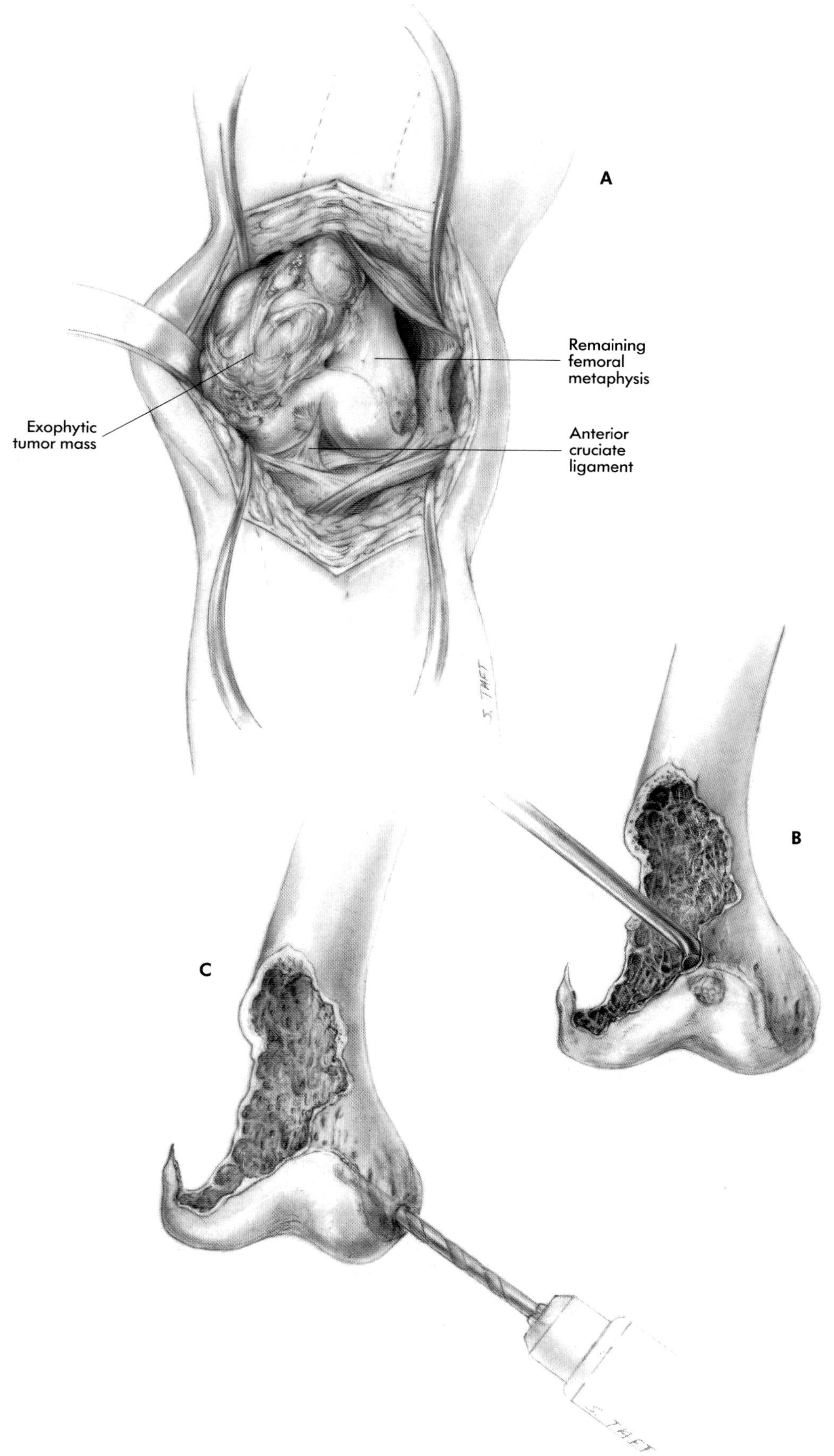

FIGURE 8-31 For legend see opposite page.

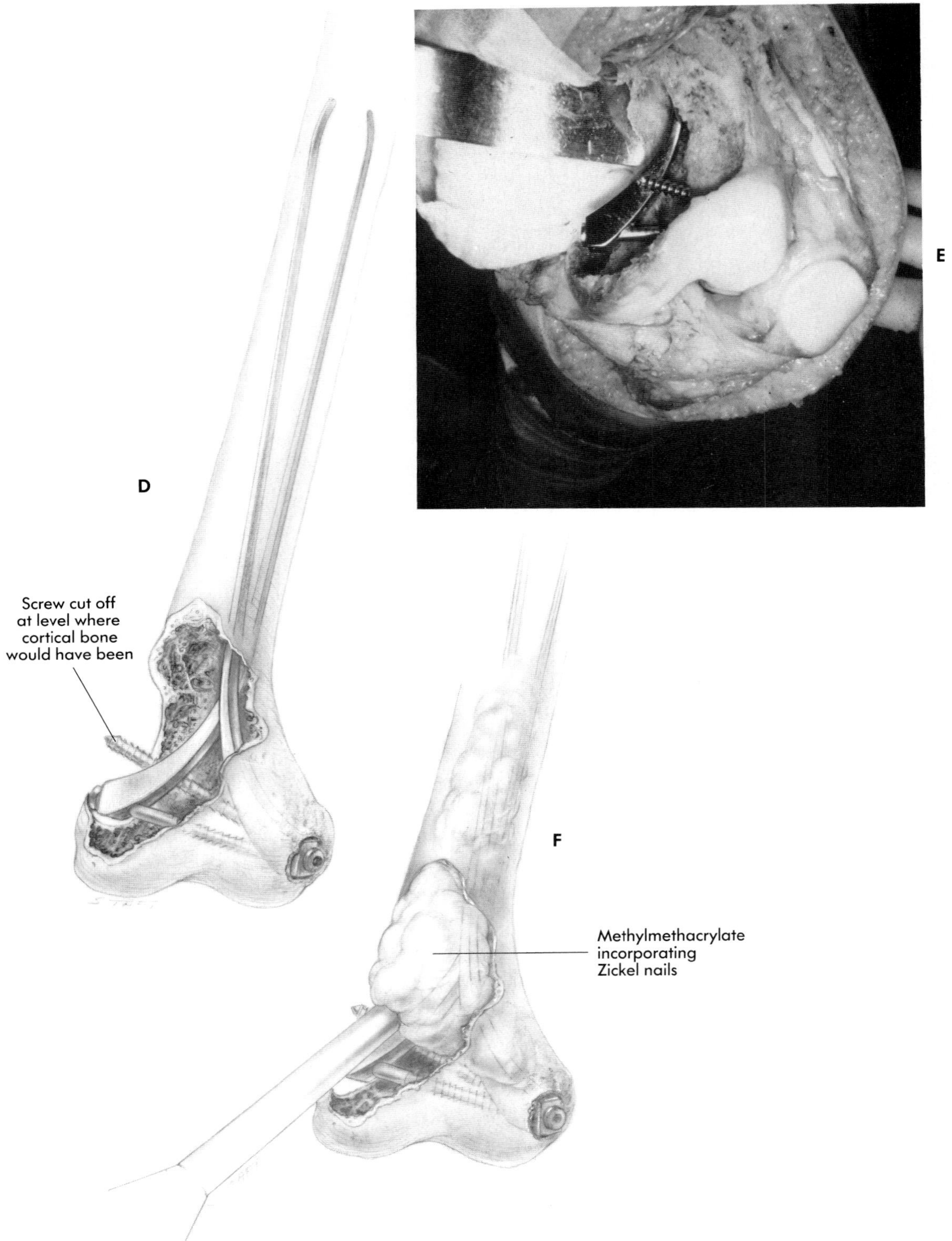

FIGURE 8-31, cont'd. **D** and **E,** After being bent to allow full seating of their squared tips flush with the epicondylar cortex, the Zickel supracondylar nails are inserted retrograde. The cross screws then are inserted as shown. The angles of insertion differ, so there is no interference between the nails and the screws. Note that the screws rarely are seated entirely in bone. However, because they have large cancellous threads throughout most of their length, fixation still can be achieved. **F,** Methylmethacrylate is injected while quite liquid to fill the curetted cavity and to reinforce the stability afforded by the Zickel nails.

exercises for strengthening of adjacent muscles, and general restoration of joint function.

Tibial Fractures. Metastatic pathological fractures of the tibia are uncommon, accounting for only 36 of 399 long-bone fractures in our series.[26]

The great majority of tibial metastatic foci likely to result in fractures involve the proximal tibial metaphysis. They usually occur either as minimally displaced "rotten wood" fractures through sclerotic and often irradiated bone (Fig. 8-32, *A*) or as fractures through thin tibial plateau cortices weakened by a vascularized lytic lesion (Fig. 8-32, *B*). In the former instance the Zickel supracondylar nails can be inserted effectively for fixation and often can be inserted by a closed technique (not requiring exposure of the fracture or augmentation by methylmethacrylate).

When a fracture of one or both plateaus has occurred, internal fixation usually is impossible because the remaining bone is too thin. Under such circumstances and when a patient has an acceptable prognosis for prolonged survival, the fracture is best managed by prosthetic knee replacement using a semiconstrained device with a long-stemmed tibial component.

OTHER CONSIDERATIONS IN PATHOLOGICAL FRACTURES

Fractures of the distal tibia often are difficult to stabilize if tumor lysis extends into the supramalleolar area. There is little bone available in the distal fragment for fixation. An

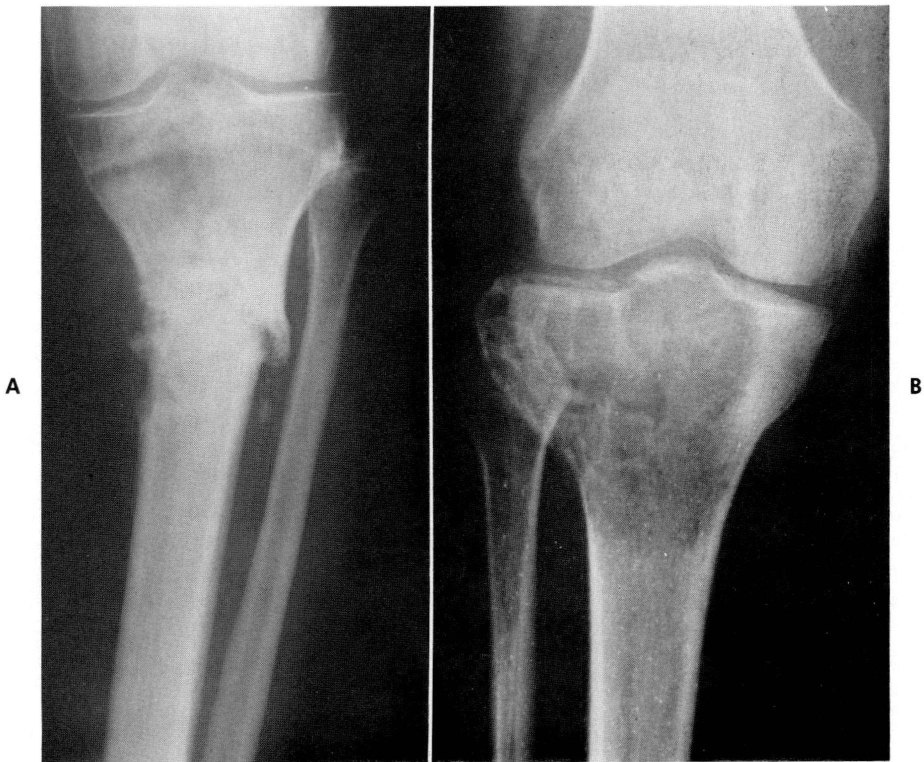

FIGURE 8-32 **A,** Pathological fracture through an irradiated focus of reticulum cell sarcoma. Despite the relatively normal overall appearance of the tibia, it is unlikely that this fracture will heal. Consequently, stabilization of the fracture (best accomplished with two reversed Zickel supracondylar nails and cement) must be secure and lasting. **B,** The more common roentgenographic pattern for proximal tibial metastases is that of poorly circumscribed bone lysis eventually resulting in pathological fracture of one or both plateaus. *Continued.*

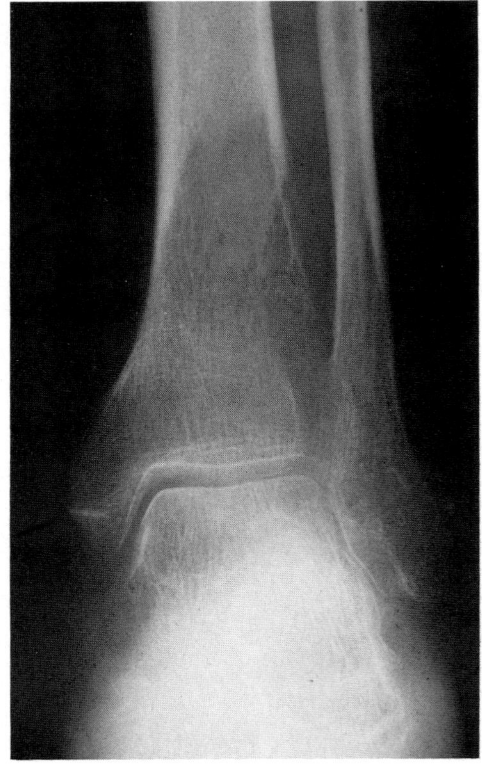

FIGURE 8-32, cont'd. **C,** A large lytic metastasis in the distal tibial metaphysis from a breast carcinoma has resulted in a pathologic fracture essentially without displacement. The lesion was curetted, and methylmethacrylate was injected without additional fixation. The fracture was stabilized by cement and partially splinted by the adjacent fibula, and the patient was able to bear full weight pain-free and to regain full ankle motion.

intramedullary rod augmented by methylmethacrylate may be required. However, in three instances with minimal deformity, we have been successful in stabilizing the tibia simply by filling the large lytic defect with cement alone and not using any ancillary fixation (Fig. 8-32, *C*).

Limb Preservation in the Face of Solitary Metastases. On rare occasion, solitary metastases may appear in bone long after ablation of the original primary tumor and in the absence of any evidence of other metastatic foci. The most common tumor to behave so is the renal carcinoma (hypernephroma), but we have also seen this occur with carcinomas of the colon, prostate, and thyroid.

Under such circumstances it may be appropriate to consider resection of the metastasis as if it were a primary malignancy, obtaining sufficiently wide margins to afford a reasonable chance for cure. Obviously, such lesions should be staged just as if they were primary tumors and the alternatives of amputation versus wide resection weighed in light of the curature potential of each under the circumstances.

If a wide resection is performed, limb reconstruction can be accomplished by autogenous grafts, allografts, custom prostheses, or a combination of these techniques. Except in young people, we generally favor the use of a custom prosthesis, which affords the best prognosis for rapid resumption of walking.

Healing of Pathological Fractures. This topic has been discussed already in Chapter 1, but warrants at least brief coverage again.

As already described, Pugh et al.[46] demonstrated experimentally that when conventional internal fixation of a pathological long-bone fracture is augmented by intramedullary methylmethacrylate the repetitive loads required for failure of the construct are much higher and more numerous than when the cement is not used. Moreover, if failure ultimately does occur, the fixation assembly of a metal splint augmented by acrylic cement can continue to withstand a surprisingly large load with only minimal deformation. Nevertheless, if true bony union does not occur, eventually complete loss of stability and a return of the patient's prefixation pain and inability to walk can be anticipated.

As also noted in Chapter 1, the overall reported incidence of bony union of metastatic pathological fractures in long bones varies between 7.5% and 60% depending on the efficacy of internal fixation.* After rigid fixation augmented by methylmethacrylate and with the techniques described in this chapter,[25] the anticipated rate of bony union is about 30% to 40%. Preoperative or postoperative chemotherapy has been implicated as a factor both predisposing to fracture and interfering with healing once a fracture has occurred. Friedlaender et al.[14] have demonstrated experimentally that both methotrexate and doxorubicin (Adriamycin), even after short-term administration, markedly reduce the trabecular bone volume and thereby increase the risk of fracture. Furthermore, both exert a profoundly toxic effect on osteoblasts that is reflected in reduced bone-formation rates by almost 60% and reduced volume, thickness, and strength of the osteoid formed. Buchardt et al.[5] have reported similar results. In a statistical analysis of the incidence of pathological fractures among bone tumor patients, Rosenstock et al.[49] showed the risk to be significantly higher in patients receiving adjuvant chemotherapy than in those treated by irradiation alone.

The prognosis for union also depends on the primary tumor type. Gainor and Buchert[15] reported bone healing in 67% of 129 pathological long-bone fractures secondary to multiple myeloma, 44% from metastatic hypernephroma and 37% from breast carcinoma. However, not a single fracture in their series caused by lung cancer was seen to demonstrate such union. They further noted, however, that the single most significant determinant of osseus healing appeared to be patient survival. In patients who lived more than 6 months following their fractures, 79% showed evidence of bony union. Not surprisingly, hardly any patients with metastatic lung cancer were alive then.

In our experience the single most important factor affecting the prognosis for bone healing is radiation therapy, its timing and dosage. Patients who receive local irradiation to the fracture site within 4 to 6 months either pre- or postoperatively have a much poorer prognosis for bony union than do those who have not been irradiated during that time. The physiological factors responsible for this effect have been discussed fully in Chapter 1.

The adverse effect on healng extends as well to the incorporation of cancellous bone grafts. Consequently, in our opinion, it is not worthwhile to augment pathological fracture fixation by bone grafting under such circumstances. However, in patients whose fractures have occurred more than 6 months after local irradiation or in whom no irradiation is contemplated postoperatively, we recommend packing cancellous iliac grafts about the fracture site and along the extent of all cortical defects whenever possible. Although it is impossible to document this impression when so many other factors affect healing, we believe that the incidence of bony union is significantly higher in such patients. A similar conclusion was reached by Parrish and Murray[42] with regard to the efficacy of bone grafting these fractures. After histological examination of several long bones more than 6 months after fracture fixation (without methylmethacrylate and without local irradiation) they were impressed by the "extraordinary ability of [such] bone to heal and regain its original integrity by remodelling." The original metastatic focus was found to be an acellular nidus within the haversian canals composed of calcium and phosphorus salts intermingled with irregular spicules of bone but with no evidence of osteogenic activity. Surrounding this and overlying the original fracture line was a mass of osteoid in which the stimulus toward osteogenic proliferation and reorganization obviously still was present as long as 10 months postoperative.

When methylmethacrylate first was used to augment internal fixation of such fractures, it was suggested[11] that its presence within the intramedullary canal would interfere with bone healing by blocking normal endosteal bone circulation. Subsequent investigations,[22,28,58] however, have revealed that a thin fibrous layer actually forms between the cement and bone and acts as a scaffold for further vascular ingrowth. Rhinelander et al.[47] demonstrated that when cement is used the loss of intramedullary blood supply is insignificant, at least in the trochanteric region, because of the availability and subsequent hy-

*References 3, 9, 15, 25, 42, 44.

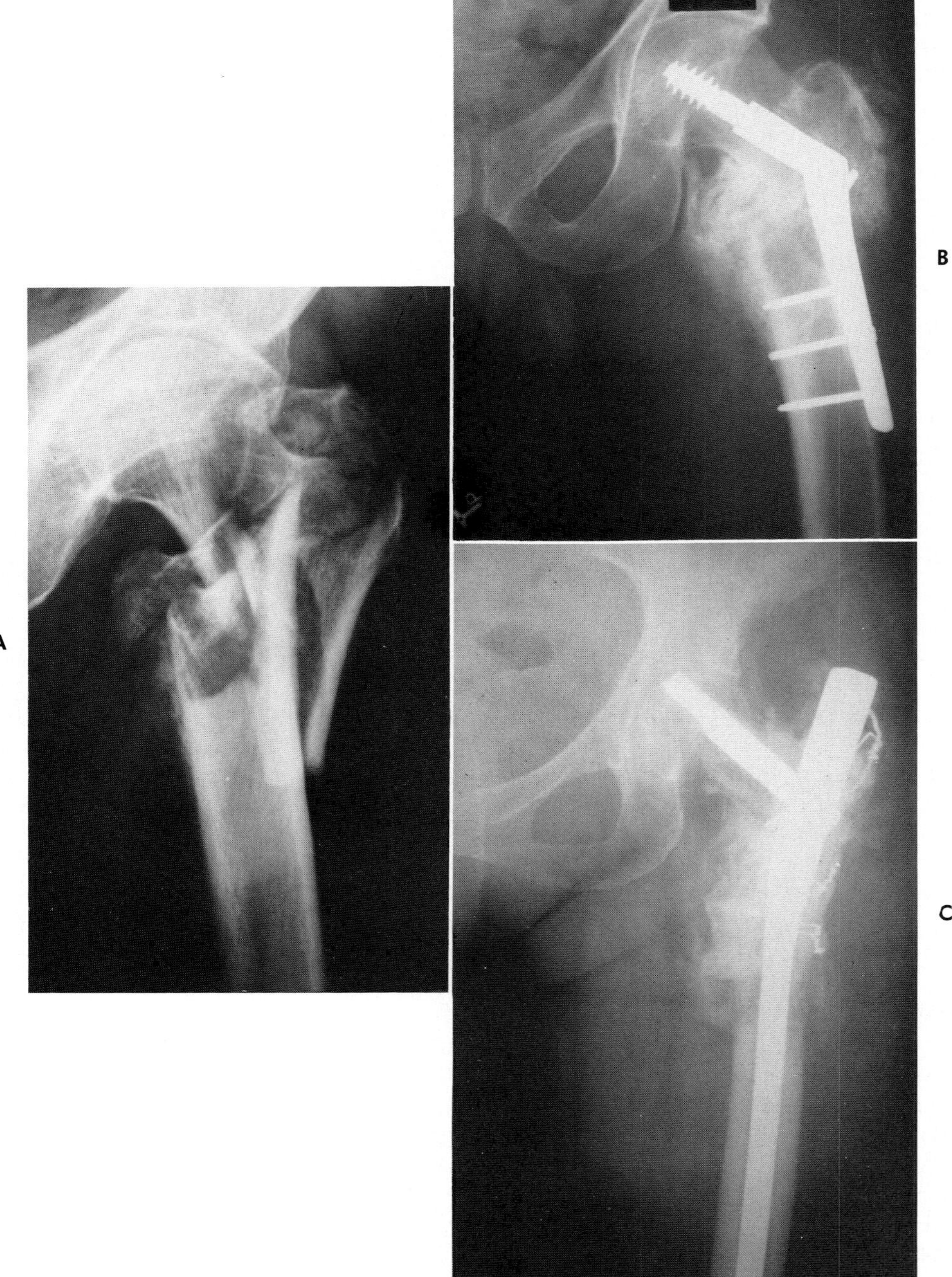

FIGURE 8-33 **A,** Markedly comminuted, very unstable, pathological fracture of the proximal femur. **B,** Five months after internal stabilization with a compression hip screw augmented by methylmethacrylate. The fracture has healed through formation of abundant periosteal new bone. The patient received 2000 cGy of postoperative irradiation. **C,** Similarly comminuted pathological fracture extending from the femoral neck well distally into the subtrochanteric area. Stabilization is by a Zickel nail augmented with methylmethacrylate. The fracture has healed through formation of extensive periosteal new bone. The patient received 2500 cGy of postoperative irradiation.

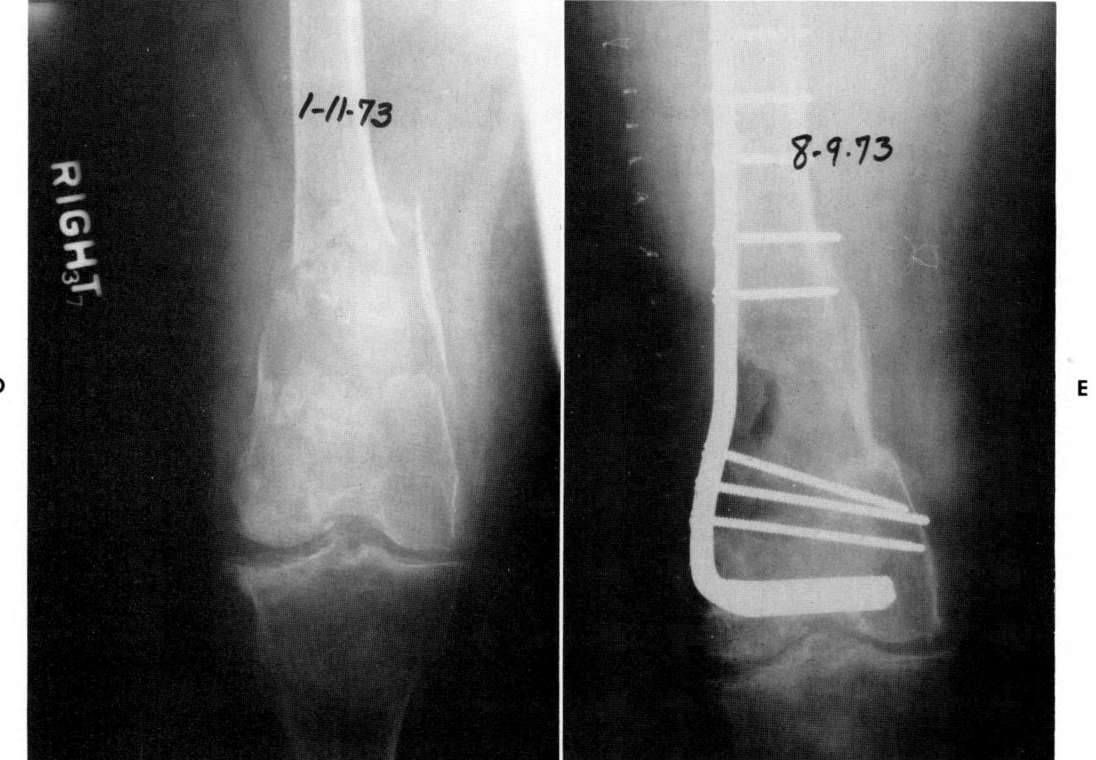

FIGURE 8-33, cont'd. **D,** Another highly comminuted pathological femur fracture, this time in the supracondylar region. **E,** Seven months after internal fixation with an angled blade plate augmented by intramedullary cement. The fracture has healed through formation of a neocortex of periosteal bone circumferentially except in the area immediately beneath the plate.

pertrophy of a large extraosseous vascular network. Paul and Yablon[43] have shown experimentally in dogs that healing new bone can be deposited on both the periosteal and the endosteal cortical surfaces surrounding such a fracture and the presence of methylmethacrylate within the canal does not significantly interfere with this process or with the bony union that it promotes.

Several authors[2,22,34,55] have noted that the presence of acrylic cement within the medullary canal, rather than interfering with bony healing, actually appears to stimulate the production of a thick mantle of periosteal new bone about the fracture site. This gradually matures into a strong and thick neocortex capable of withstanding stresses much greater than those that the original cortex could resist (Fig. 8-33, *A* and *B*). In fact, we have observed the production of an abundant mass of periosteal new bone about fractures fixed with intramedullary devices and augmented by methylmethacrylate in which preoperatively there was such extensive cortical lysis that it was feared no means of fixation would be effective (Fig. 8-33, *C*). However, it is only in areas where the periosteum has been stripped extensively (e.g., directly beneath a side plate used as part of the fixation system) that this constructive periosteal response is frustrated (Fig. 8-33, *D* and *E*). This therefore is another reason why we prefer to use intramedullary fixation devices whenever possible in preference to nail-plate fixation.

Complications. The management of pathological long-bone fractures is subject to two general types of complications: (1) those promoted by peculiarities of the tumor itself and its vascularity or to the debility of any given patient with metastatic bone disease and (2) those created by the surgeon in his attempts at fracture fixation.

With regard to the *first* category, we have always been concerned about the risk of infection in patients with multiple metastases in whom immunological competence is perpetually diminished by both the systemic nature of the disease and the chemotherapeutic agents used in its management. Surprisingly enough, this rarely has been a problem. In our series of 399 patients reported in 1976,[27] there was only one deep wound infection and this cleared after appropriate debridement and antibiotic coverage despite the presence of intramedullary cement and despite extensive irradiation of adjacent soft tissues. All patients are administered prophylactic antibiotics (cephalosporins) beginning immediately preoperatively and continuing for 24 to 48 hours thereafter.

Similarly, hyper- or hypocoagulation states rarely have been a source of complications. In view of the potential for postoperative bleeding, we do not anticoagulate prophylactically; yet we have had only three fatal pulmonary emboli in more than 500 patients. One of these occurred after fixation of a long-bone fracture. Despite the risks of clotting deficiencies caused by liver disease or platelet suppression, massive intraoperative bleeding has occurred in only three patients. In one, complications of prolonged hypotension developed and the patient ultimately died. In the other two the rapidly bleeding tumor cavity was packed with methylmethacrylate and, as the cement expanded, it effectively occluded the tumor vessels. The cement was then removed piecemeal with an osteotome and the process of fixation was continued in a dry field. Obviously it is preferable to avoid hemorrhage rather than be forced to manage it intraoperatively, and we now attempt to identify any lesion that is likely to cause excessive bleeding and to control it preoperatively. Tumors that are aneurysmal, aggressively lytic in appearance, or with minimal or no blastic response in surrounding bone are most likely to be highly vascular. The usual primary lesions responsible for such metastases are renal and colonic carcinomas and occasionally multiple myelomas. When such a lesion is apparent on conventional roentgenograms,[23,24] it should be evaluated further by arteriography (Fig. 8-34, *A* and *C*). Usually one or two primary feeder vessels can be identified, selectively cauterized, and then embolized with Gelfoam or free fat or other material.[25,27] This technique effectively devascularizes much of the tumor focus (Fig. 8-24, *B* and *D*), following which elective tumor resection and fracture fixation can proceed at any time without risk of major hemorrhage.

With regard to the *second* category, potential iatrogenic complications, the one most commonly feared by the general surgeon who resected the original tumor focus is a local recurrence and/or tumor implantation along the skin incision. Suffice to say, this problem almost never occurs with metastatic disease. In more than 500 metastatic bone lesions managed operatively we have had only one such local recurrence and this in a patient who had widely disseminated lung carcinoma.

The complication of a fracture occurring through a recently biopsied lesion also is rarely encountered, although there is no doubt that a surgical cortical defect created by such a biopsy weakens a long bone and reduces the local stress that it can withstand.[46] Based on biomechanical observations, Pomeroy and Johnson[45] warn against the danger of removing cortical bone when doing such a biopsy although they provide no data to support their impression that weakening of the cortex predisposes the patient to actual fracture. Springfield and Pagliarulo[56] have postulated that pathological fractures rarely occur through the actual sites of previous cortical biopsy. In only one of their 18 patients from whom tissue had been biopsied and who then suffered a pathological fracture did the fracture occur through the biopsy site.

The most common iatrogenic complication that definitely can be allied to fracture fixation is the development of a pathological fracture just distal or proximal to the end of the fixation device (Fig. 8-27). The more rigid the fixation construct and the more diffuse the metastatic involvement of the long bone, the more likely is this complication to occur. The most common location of such a fracture is in the femoral diaphysis just distal to the tip of a proximal femoral endoprosthesis. Wang et al.[57] have developed a technique for effective stabilization of such fractures using a compression plate screwed to the femoral shaft below the

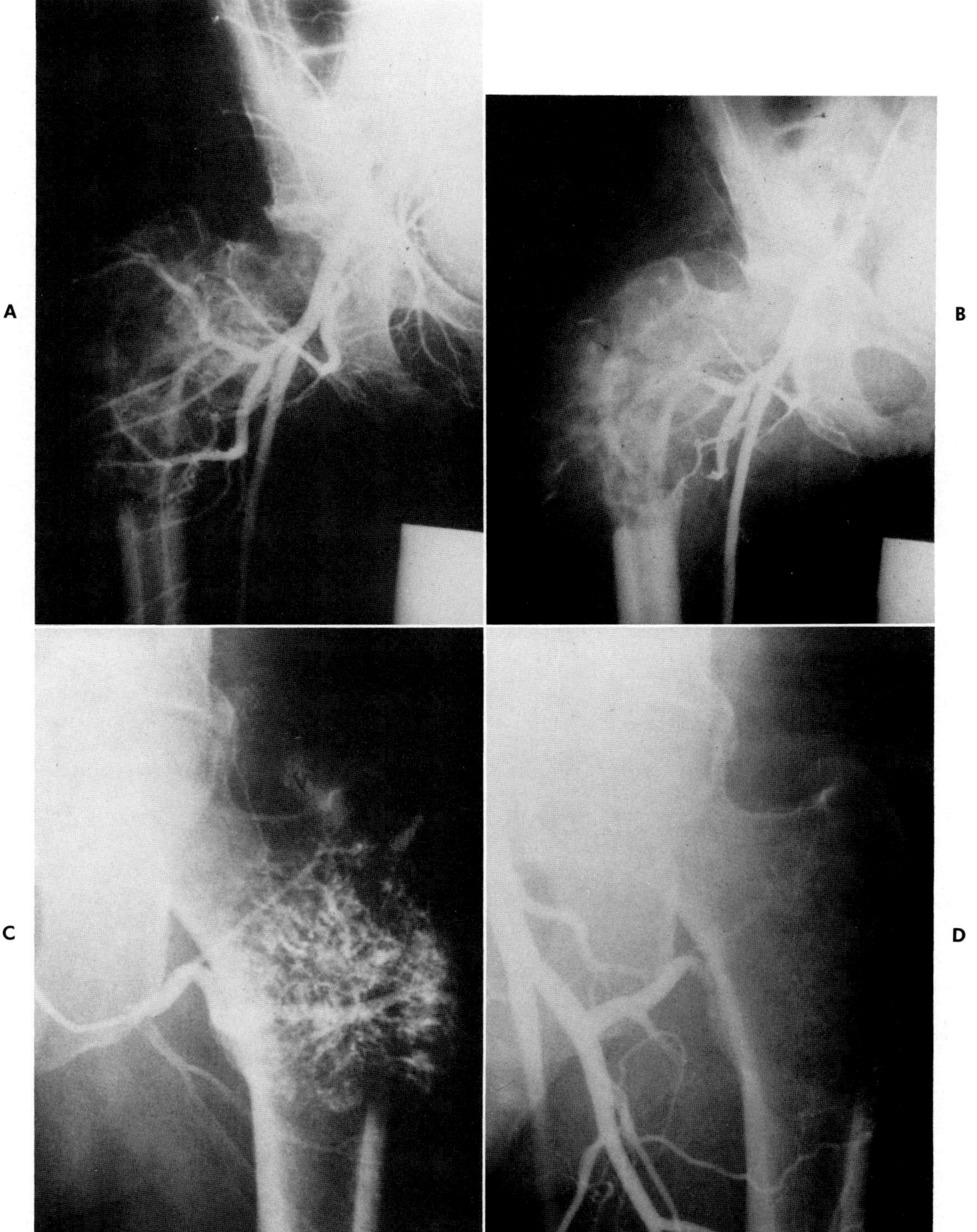

FIGURE 8-34 **A,** The abundant vascularity of a metastasis from a hypernephroma to the proximal femur is demonstrated by this arteriogram. The arterial supply to the tumor mass appears to originate from both the medial and the lateral circumflex vessels. An attempt to biopsy this lesion before arterial embolization had resulted in a six-unit blood loss. **B,** The circumflex arteries have been occluded by selective catherization and embolization with lyophilized Gelfoam. Subsequent resection of the proximal femur and replacement by a custom prosthetic hip were accomplished with minimum blood loss. **C,** Another large lytic and vascular lesion of the proximal femur, this time principally by the posterior circumflex artery. **D,** After embolization of the vessel at the tumor site, the lesion has been essentially devascularized. (**A** and **B** courtesy William H. Harris, M.D.)

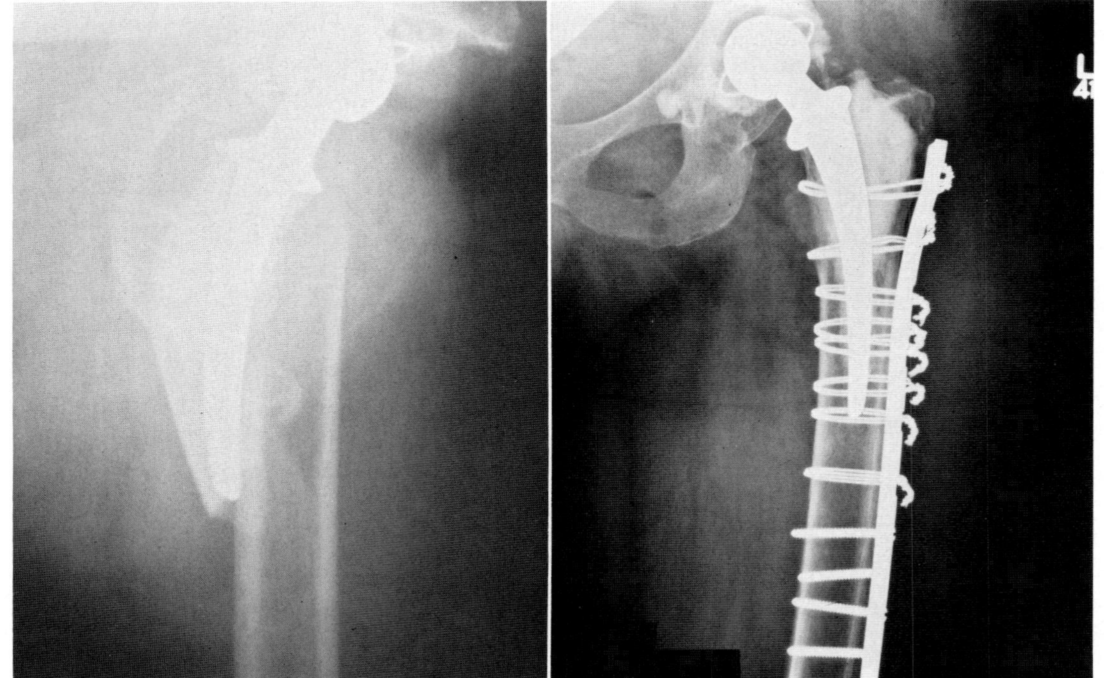

FIGURE 8-35 **A,** Pathological fracture immediately distal to the tip of a proximal femoral prosthesis. **B,** It has been stabilized by the application of a contoured side plate across both major fragments. Fixation was accomplished distally by conventional screws and proximally by cerclage wires. In a patient who will not be receiving further irradiation and in whom bony union therefore can be anticipated, this is an ideal method of fixing such a difficult fracture. (Courtesy Gwo-Jaw Wang, M.D.)

prosthesis tip and wired circumferentially above (Fig. 8-35). Such a construct is best augmented by cancellous bone grafts in the hope of achieving eventual bony union, particularly in individuals who have already received a maximal course of local irradiation.

In summary, the pathological lower-extremity fracture must by evaluated individually, with particular consideration given to the biomechanics of fixation in the face of often extensive local cortical destruction. Intramedullary fixation augmented by methylmethacrylate is ideal for most of these, except ones in the most proximal femur. When a patient has a prolonged life expectancy and will not be undergoing local irradiation, the fracture should be bone grafted at the time of initial fixation. Every effort should be made to create fixation constructs that will minimize transferance of stress proximally or distally into another region of bone that may already be weakened by metastatic disease.

REFERENCES

1. Acker, J.H., et al.: Treatment of fractures of the femur with the Grosse-Kempf rod, Orthopedics **8:** 1393, 1985.
2. Bartucci, E.J., et al.: The effect of adjunctive methylmethacrylate on failures of fixation and function in patients with intertrochanteric fractures and osteoporosis, J. Bone Joint Surg. **67A:**1094, 1985.
3. Blake, D.D.: Radiation treatment of metastatic bone disease, Clin. Orthop. **73:**89, 1970.
4. Bonarigo, B.C., and Rubin, P.: Non-union of pathologic fracture after radiation therapy, Radiology **88:**889, 1967.
5. Buchardt, H., et al.: The effect of Adriamycin and methotrexate on the repair of segmental cortical autografts in dogs, J. Bone Joint Surg. **65A:**103, 1983.
6. Chapman, M.W., et al.: The use of Ender's pins in extracapsular fractures of the hip, J. Bone Joint Surg. **63A:**14, 1981.
7. Cheng, D.S., et al.: Nonoperative management of femoral, humeral, and acetabular metastases in patients with breast carcinoma, Cancer **48:**1533, 1980.
8. Clancey, G.J., et al.: Fractures of the distal end of the femur below hip implants in elderly patients. Treat-

ment with the Zickel supracondylar device, J. Bone Joint Surg. **65A:**491, 1983.

9. Coran, A.G., et al.: The management of pathologic fractures in patients with metastatic carcinoma of the breast, Surg. Gynecol. Obstet. **127:**1225, 1968.
10. Dimon, J.H., III, and Hughston, J.C.: Unstable intertrochanteric fractures of the hip, J. Bone Joint Surg. **49A:**440, 1967.
11. Enis, J.E., et al.: Methylmethacrylate in neoplastic bone destruction. In The hip. Proceedings of the first open scientific meeting of The Hip Society, St. Louis, 1973, The C.V. Mosby Co.
12. Ewald, F.C., et al.: Hip cartilage supported by methacrylate in canine arthroplasty, Clin. Orthop. **171:** 273, 1982.
13. Francis, K.C., et al.: The treatment of pathological fractures of the femoral neck by resection, J. Trauma **2:**465, 1962.
14. Friedlaender, G.E., et al.: Effects of chemotherapeutic agents on bone, J. Bone Joint Surg. **66A:**602, 1984.
15. Gainor, B.J., and Buchert, P.: Fracture healing in metastatic bone disease, Clin. Orthop. **178:**297, 1983.
16. Galasko, C.S.B.: Pathological fractures secondary to metastatic cancer, J. R. Coll. Surg. [Edinb.] **19:**351, 1974.
17. Graham, W.D.: Pathological fractures secondary to metastatic cancer, J. Bone Joint Surg. **45B:**617, 1963.
18. Gustilo, R.B.: Management of open fractures and their complications, Philadelphia, 1982, W.B. Saunders Co.
19. Habermann, E.T., et al.: The pathology and treatment of metastatic disease of the femur, Clin. Orthop. **169:**70, 1982.
20. Hardy, A.E.: The treatment of femoral fractures by cast-brace application and early ambulation, J. Bone Joint Surg. **65A:**56, 1983.
21. Harper, M.C., and Walsh, T.: Ender nailing for peritrochanteric fractures of the femur, J. Bone Joint Surg. **67A:**79, 1985.
22. Harrington, K.D.: The use of methylmethacrylate as an adjunct in the internal fixation of unstable comminuted intertrochanteric fractures in osteoporotic patients, J. Bone Joint Surg. **57A:**744, 1975.
23. Harrington, K.D.: Management of unstable pathologic fracture-dislocations of the spine and acetabulum secondary to metastatic malignancy. In American Academy of Orthopaedic Surgeons: Instructional course lectures. Vol. 29, St. Louis, 1980, The C.V. Mosby Co.
24. Harrington, K.D.: The management of acetabular insufficiency secondary to metastatic malignant disease, J. Bone Joint Surg. **63A:**653, 1981.
25. Harrington, K.D.: New trends in the management of lower extremity metastases, Clin. Orthop. **169:**53, 1982.
26. Harrington, K.D., et al.: The use of methylmethacrylate as an adjunct in the internal fixation of malignant neoplastic fractures, J. Bone Joint Surg. **54A:**1665, 1972.
27. Harrington, K.D., et al.: Methylmethacrylate as an adjunct in internal fixation of pathological fractures, J. Bone Joint Surg. **58A:**1047, 1976.
28. Homsy, C.A., et al.: Some physiological aspects of prosthesis stabilization with acrylic polymer, Clin. Orthop. **83:**317, 1972.
29. Hunter, G.A., and Krajbich, I.J.: The results of medial displacement osteotomy for unstable intertrochanteric fractures of the femur, Clin. Orthop. **137:**140, 1978.
30. Jensen, J.S., and Sonne-Holm, S.: Critical analysis of Ender nailing in the treatment of trochanteric fractures, Acta Orthop. Scand. **51:**817, 1980.
31. Johnson, K.D., et al.: Comminuted femoral shaft fractures: treatment by roller traction, cerclage wires with an intramedullary nail, or an interlocking nail, J. Bone Joint Surg. **66A:**1222, 1984.
32. Kempf, I., et al.: L'apport du verrouillage dans l'enclouage centro-médullaire des os longs, Rev. Chir. Orthop. **64:**635, 1978.
33. Koskinen, E.V.S., and Nieminen, R.A.: Surgical treatment of metastatic pathological fracture of major long bones, Acta Orthop. Scand. **44:**539, 1973.
34. Kuntscher, G., and Jaumann, A.: Ein Hochfrequenzverfahren zum Auffinden von Metallfremdkörpern, Zentralbl. Chir. **67:**2338, 1940.
35. Lafferty, F.W.: Pseudohyperparathyroidism, Medicine **45:**247, 1966.
36. Lane, J., et al.: Treatment of pathological fractures of the hip by endoprosthetic replacement, J. Bone Joint Surg. **62A:**954, 1980.
37. Levy, R.N., et al.: Surgical management of metastatic disease of bone at the hip, Clin. Orthop. **169:**62, 1982.
38. Levy, R.N., et al.: Complications of Ender pin fixation in basicervical, intertrochanteric, and subtrochanteric fractures of the hip, J. Bone Joint Surg. **65A:**66, 1983.
39. Marcove, R.C., and Yang, D.J.: Survival times after treatment of pathologic fractures, Cancer **20:**2154, 1967.
40. Mickelson, M.R., and Bonfiglio, M.: Pathological fractures in the proximal part of the femur treated by Zickel-nail fixation, J. Bone Joint Surg. **58A:**1067, 1976.
41. Muhr, G., et al.: Comminuted trochanteric femoral fractures in geriatric patients: the results of 231 cases treated with internal fixation and acrylic cement, Clin. Orthop. **138:**41, 1979.
42. Parrish, F.F., and Murray, J.A.: Surgical treatment of secondary neoplastic fractures; a retrospective study of ninety-six patients, J. Bone Joint Surg. **52A:**665, 1970.
43. Paul, G.R., and Yablon, I.G.: Malignant pathologic fracture heals with methylmethacrylate, Orthop. Rev. **7:**73, 1979.
44. Perez, C.A., et al.: Management of pathologic fractures, Cancer **29:**684, 1972.
45. Pomeroy, T.C., and Johnson, R.E.: Integrated therapy for Ewing's sarcoma, Front. Radiat. Ther. Oncol. **10:**152, 1975.
46. Pugh, J., et al.: Biomechanics of pathologic fractures, Clin. Orthop. **169:**109, 1982.
47. Rhinelander, F.W., et al.: Experimental reaming of the proximal femur and acrylic cement implantation. Vascular and histologic effects, Clin. Orthop. **141:**75, 1979.

48. Roberts, A., et al.: A comparison of the functional results of anatomic and medial displacement valgus nailing of intertrochanteric fractures of the femur, J. Trauma **12:**341, 1972.
49. Rosenstock, J.G., et al.: Ewing's sarcoma, adjunct chemotherapy and pathologic fracture, Eur. J. Cancer **14:**799, 1978.
50. Sangeorzan, B.J., et al.: Prophylactic internal fixation of the femur with the Zickel nail: a retrospective analysis and recommendation for modification of the described technique, J. Bone Joint Surg. **68A:** 991, 1986.
51. Sarmiento, A.: Unstable intertrochanteric fractures of the femur, Clin. Orthop. **92:**77, 1973.
52. Scholz, D.A., et al.: Hypercalcemia and cancer, CA **25:**27, 1975.
53. Segal, G.K.: Management of comminuted intertrochanteric fractures of the femur. Presented at the A.A.O.S. Course: Update management of trauma problems around the hip joint, New York, May 1985.
54. Sim, F.H., et al.: Total hip arthroplasty for tumors of the hip. In The hip: Proceedings of the fourth open scientific meeting of The Hip Society, St. Louis, 1976, The C.V. Mosby Co.
55. Slooff, T.J.J.H.: The influence of acrylic cement, an experimental study, Acta Orthop. Scand. **42:**465, 1971.
56. Springfield, D.S., and Pagliarulo, C.: Fractures of long bones previously treated for Ewing's sarcoma, J. Bone Joint Surg. **67A:**477, 1985.
57. Wang, G., et al.: Treatment of proximal femur fractures in joint replacement patients using the Ogden Method. Unpublished data, 1986.
58. Wiltse, L.L., et al.: Experimental studies regarding the possible use of self-curing acrylic in orthopaedic surgery, J. Bone Joint Surg. **39A:**961, 1957.
59. Zickel, R.F., and Mouradian, W.H.: Intramedullary fixation of pathological fractures and lesions of the subtrochanteric region of the femur, J. Bone Joint Surg. **58A:**1061, 1976.
60. Zickel, R.E., et al.: A new intramedullary fixation device for the distal third of the femur, Clin. Orthop. **125:**185, 1977.

CHAPTER 9

PATHOLOGICAL FRACTURES OF THE ACETABULUM AND PELVIS

Metastatic disease involving the pelvic bones is common, being demonstrable roentgenographically in approximately 35% and scintigraphically in 55% of patients with advanced cancer. One would expect that primary carcinomas of the prostate, uterus, ovaries, and lower colon would have the highest incidence of such metastases in view of their proximity to the pelvic bones and the relative ease of spread directly through Batson's venous plexuses. In fact, such is not the case. Although prostatic cancer metastasizes to bone in 60% to 80% of advanced cases, it involves the lumbar spine more commonly than the pelvis. Moreover, prostatic-pelvic metastases are not commonly symptomatic because they tend to be blastic, with a low predilection for bone destruction or subsequent fracture. Colonic, ovarian, and uterine cancers metastasize to pelvic bones relatively infrequently, their reported incidence being less than 10% in most series. In contrast, carcinomas of the breast spread commonly to the pelvis and certainly are the most common source of pelvic metastases requiring treatment.

Patients who manifest solitary blastic lesions in the pelvic bones recognizable roentgenographically, or who show increased uptake in the pelvis on bone scintigraphy, should not necessarily be assumed to harbor metastases. The pelvis is a frequent location of benign bone islands or bone infarcts of longstanding duration and with no malignant potential (Fig. 9-1, *A*). Before treatment is considered for demonstrable pelvic lesions in patients with symptoms compatible with pelvic metastases, efforts should be made to confirm that the suspicious focus is indeed malignant. Fortunately, the pelvic bones are easily accessible to trocar biopsy, which can be performed with minimal risk under local anesthesia and, if necessary, CT control.

The confirmed presence of a pelvic bone metastasis is not necessarily an indication for treatment. The presence of an enlarging blastic lesion or lesions, for example, in a patient with known breast or prostatic malignancy may serve as an indication for more aggressive hormonal manipulation or chemotherapy but only because of being an indicator of uncontrolled systemic disease. Aggressive and expanding lytic lesions in the pelvis, however, do warrant prophylactic irradiation, occasionally even before they become symptomatic. Otherwise, there is a significant risk of eventual pathological fracture if the process is not controlled. Happily, fractures that do develop through the thin iliac wing or through the ischial or pubic rami rarely require more than brief treatment of symptoms. Even in the occasional instance when a pathological fracture of one or more rami fails to unite after local

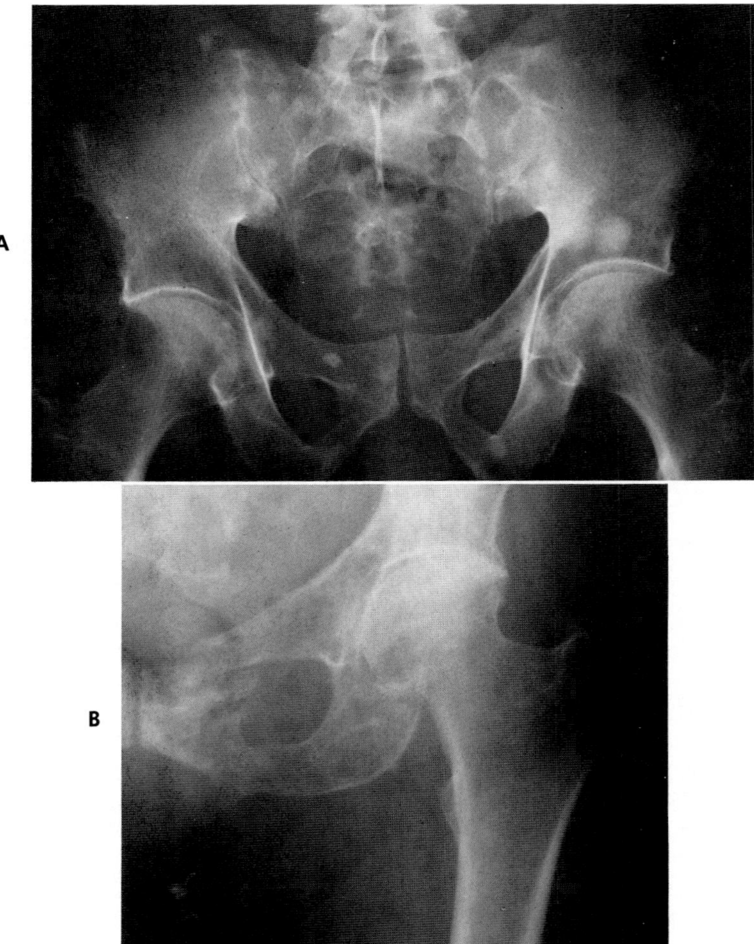

FIGURE 9-1 **A,** Roentgenogram of the pelvis in a 57-year-old woman who had undergone a mastectomy 8 years earlier for breast carcinoma. Although she had no symptoms and her bone scan was negative, this film was interpreted as demonstrating probable blastic bone metastases. Chemotherapy was considered until trocar biopsy of two such foci in the left ilium revealed them to be benign bone islands. **B,** Pathological fractures of the pubic rami in a patient with breast metastases. The fractures failed to unite after 1 year. Although mildly tender, they were otherwise asymptomatic after 6 weeks.

irradiation, the nonunion usually becomes minimally symptomatic with time (Fig. 9-1,*B*).

When a pathological fracture occurs in the pelvis of a patient with known metastatic disease who has received local irradiation, the possibility must be considered that it is the result of irradiation rather than of ongoing tumor lysis. This is particularly true when a fracture occurs through the pubic or ischial rami or through bone to either side of the sacroiliac joint. Such so-called insufficiency fractures develop because of the loss of normal elasticity of the bone and the subsequent inability of that bone to withstand the stresses of normal activity. Often these fractures occur at several sites about the irradiated pelvis, appearing almost simultaneously in both the anterior and the posterior portions of the pelvic ring (Fig. 9-1, *C*). Insufficiency fractures are typically not apparent roentgenographically or even scintigraphically for several weeks after their occurrence. When they do become apparent on roentgenograms, it is often in association with sclerotic changes

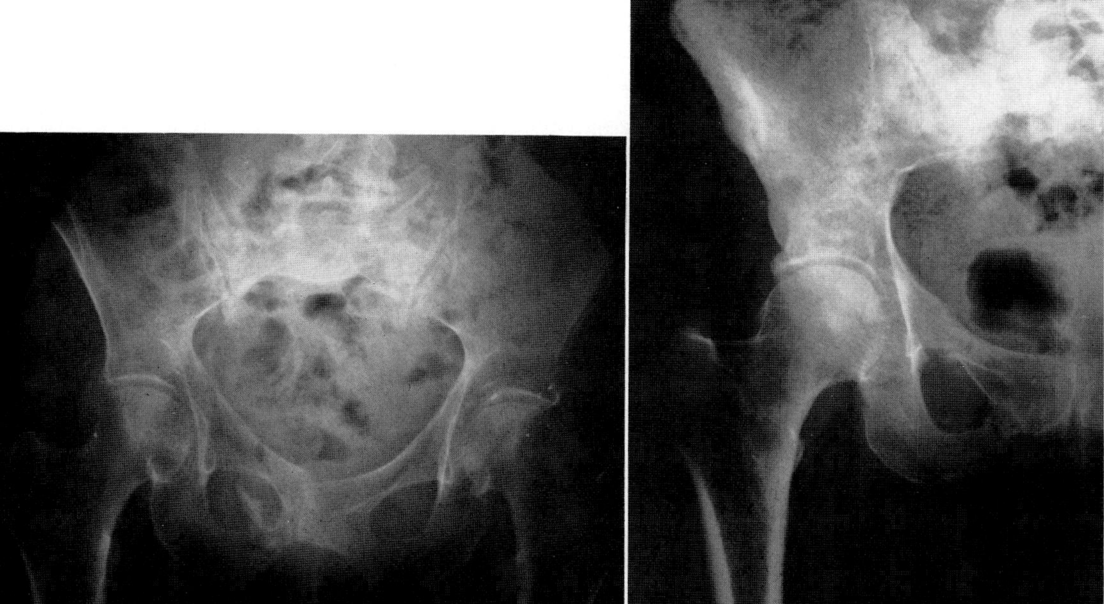

FIGURE 9-1, cont'd. **C,** So-called insufficiency fractures of the pubis and sacrum (the latter difficult to see on this roentgenogram). They resulted from radiation osteitis and were not indicative of active metastatic disease. Obviously further radiation would have increased this patient's disability. **D,** Osteoblastic and osteolytic destruction of bone in the sacrum and ilium has resulted in destruction of the sacroiliac joint. Although the joint did not become unstable or displaced, the patient continued to have pain there on sitting or standing until her death 9 months later.

about the fracture line, easily mistaken for a blastic metastasis.[1,14] Obviously it is essential to differentiate this process from a pathological fracture secondary to a recurrent metastatic malignancy. Whereas the latter is best managed by local irradiation, further irradiation of the insufficiency fracture will only increase the patient's disability and encourage the development of further fractures. Again, trocar biopsy of such lesions can be accomplished in most instances with relative ease.

• • •

In two areas of the pelvis metastatic pathological fractures usually will not respond to simple treatment of symptoms but require some type of operative stabilization or arthroplasty. These areas are the sacral wing or the ilium adjacent to the sacroiliac joint and the periacetabular bone (particularly the medial and superior walls of the acetabulum).

SACROILIAC JOINT DISRUPTION

Pathological fractures about the sacroiliac joint of sufficient severity to require internal fixation are uncommon, because the bone in that region is thick and strong and must be destroyed almost entirely before a significant instability or displacement will occur. When such does occur, stabilization becomes exceedingly difficult. Conventional fixation by contoured bone plates, as is effective in traumatic sacroiliac disruptions, rarely is effective here because of the extent of bone lysis (Figs. 9-1, *D,* and 9-2, *A*). The almost vertical alignment of both the joint and the fracture encourages superior displacement of the iliac wing with attempted weight-bearing and renders fixation by devices crossing the joint in a horizontal plane minimally effective. However, if fixation can be accomplished in a plane paralleling the weight-bearing stresses across the joint (approximately 15 degrees medial to horizontal) the likelihood of failure is reduced

A

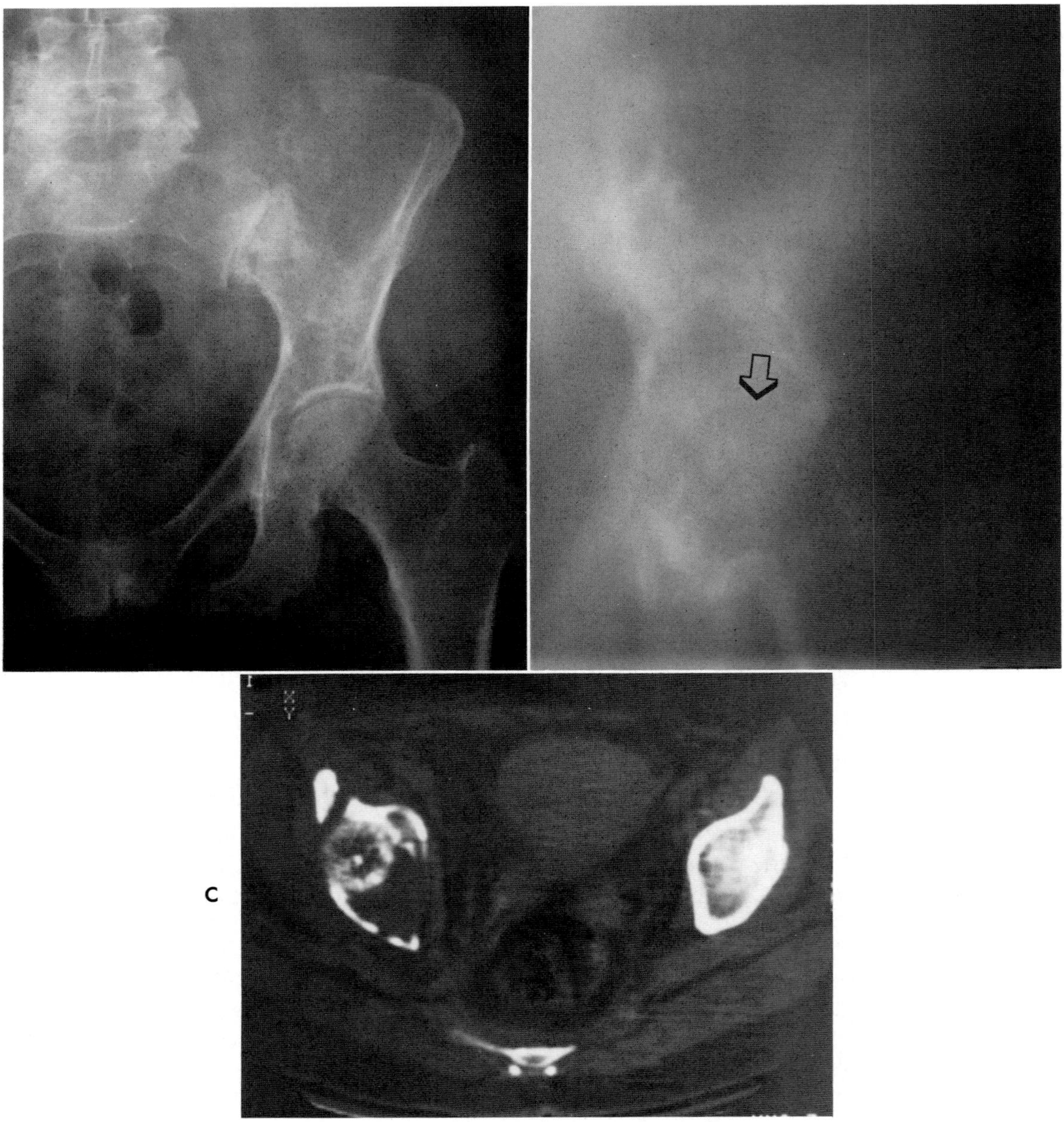

B

C

FIGURE 9-2 **A,** Left hemipelvis in a patient who had a metastatic breast carcinoma with obvious lytic and blastic changes throughout the ilium and with partial destruction of the sacroiliac joint. The supraacetabular bone appears intact, although the patient consistently complained of hip pain on weight-bearing. **B,** An AP tomogram of the hip reveals lytic destruction of the supraacetabular bone and much of the acetabular roof *(arrow)*. **C,** This finding was confirmed by CT scan, which also demonstrated extensive destruction of the medial wall of the acetabulum. The lesion fell into the Class III category for reconstruction.

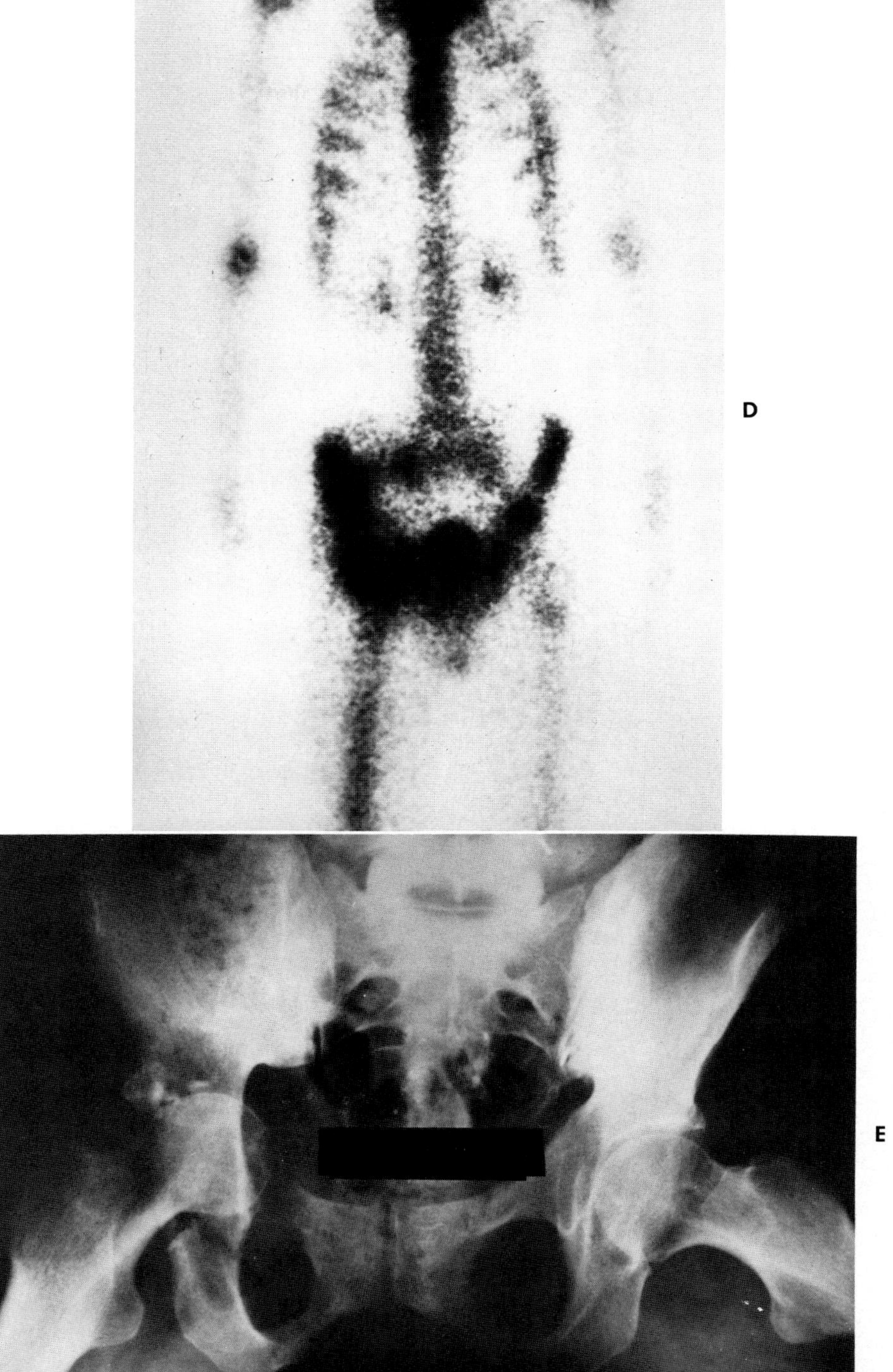

FIGURE 9-2, cont'd. **D,** Technetium-99 scan of another patient with persistent weight-bearing pain in the hip, this time on the right. Note the markedly increased uptake throughout the right hemipelvis. Because conventional films were interpreted as showing only diffuse metastatic changes, no specialized diagnostic roentgenograms were obtained and no treatment was rendered. **E,** Three months later a spontaneous central acetabular fracture occurred. This lesion is a Class III reconstruction problem.

greatly. We have found that large threaded Steinmann pins can be drilled across the joint in this plane with little difficulty in situations in which periacetabular fractures also warrant joint arthroplasty (Fig. 9-10, *E* to *H*). When exposure of the acetabulum is not warranted, the pins must be inserted through the ilial cortex just above the acetabular rim at an angle of approximately 45 degrees. We have used 45-degree pin fixation on only two occasions, and fracture-joint stability remained effective until the patients' demises 11 and 37 months postoperatively.

ACETABULAR FRACTURES

In contrast to sacral joint disruptions, pathological fracture-dislocations about the acetabulum are relatively common. The blood supply to the supraacetabular ilium is rich, and there are abundant venous sinusoids that allow easy escape of malignant cells from the circulation. It is not uncommon for periacetabular metastases to remain symptomatically quiet until just before a major fracture occurs. This is because the acetabular articular cartilage offers an effective barrier to tumor invasion of the joint. Consequently the joint space usually appears to be deceptively normal until massive mechanical collapse finally occurs (Fig. 9-2, *D* and *E*).

Displaced pathological acetabular fractures challenge the orthopaedic surgeon because they reflect the culmination of two simultaneously destructive processes leading to joint instability. The first is the phenomenon of gradual softening of the periacetabular bone, from the tumor process and also (often) from the superimposed irradiation osteolysis, both

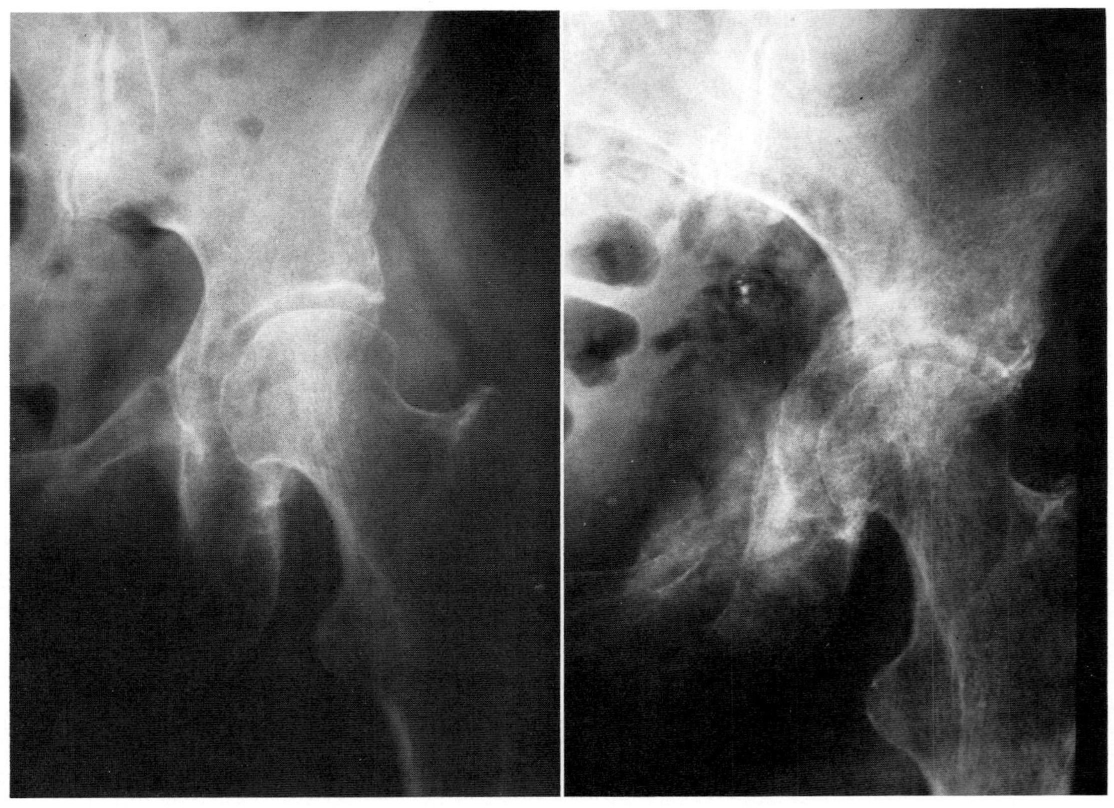

FIGURE 9-3 **A,** An AP roentgenogram of the left hip in a 52-year-old woman with metastatic carcinoma of the rectum shows lytic infiltration of the medial acetabular wall with a minimally displaced fracture. **B,** Six weeks later, after the completion of local irradiation (4000 cGy), more extensive lysis and softening of the bone are apparent, with displacement of the femoral head. Protrusio has resulted from softening of the bone caused by a combination of tumor lysis and postirradiation hyperemia.

conditions resulting in progressive deformity of the acetabular walls (Fig. 9-3). The second process is the ablation of subchondral blood circulation by the gradually expanding tumor focus, which eventually results in frank disruption of the joint surface (Fig. 9-4, *A*). The loss of periacetabular bone in both conditions seriously interferes with attempts at joint stabilization or reconstruction.

Biomechanical Considerations

The progression of acetabular deformity (Fig. 9-3) is comparable to benign protrusio acetabuli as encountered with inflammatory or osteolytic processes unrelated to metastatic disease.[5,13,18] The femoral head tends to migrate medially and superiorly in accordance with the normal stress forces acting across the hip joint. Conventional efforts to arrest this process have included bone grafting of the medial acetabular wall,[13] valgus osteotomy of the femur, and total hip replacement with a specialized prosthesis augmented by bone graft reinforcement or methylmethacrylate.[18]

However, because of the necessity to irradiate the tumor site to control progressive bone destruction, acetabular protrusion secondary to metastatic disease differs from the

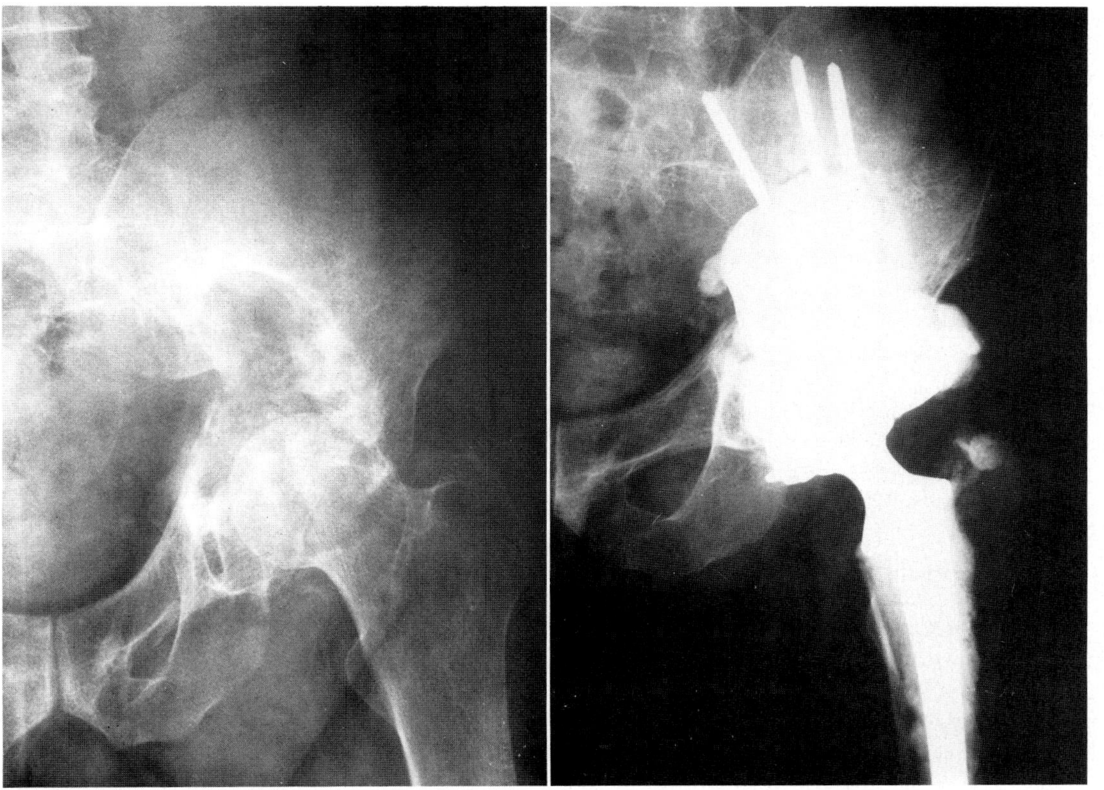

FIGURE 9-4 **A,** Class III involvement of the hip in a 51-year-old man who has metastatic carcinoma of the adrenal cortex. Extensive lytic destruction of the supraacetabular bone is apparent, with migration of the femoral head proximally. Although no other metastatic foci were evident, the patient had been confined to a wheelchair a year earlier after being advised that the hip joint was not reconstructable. **B,** Twenty-eight months after resection of the destroyed bone and tumor and reconstruction of the hip joint, the acetabular component remains securely fixed to the pelvis by a combination of threaded Steinmann pins, wire mesh, a protrusio acetabuli shell, and methylmethacrylate. The lucent halo above the cement mass was apparent from the time of operation and has not increased in width. Absence of apparent loosening of the fixation pins attests to the stability of the prosthetic reconstruction.

more benign condition. Radiation, in conventional doses of 4000 to 6000 cGy,* seriously reduces the likelihood that bone grafted for reinforcement of the acetabular wall will ever be incorporated. The healing of an osteotomy of the adjacent proximal femur also will be endangered. The protrusio often accelerates dramatically[8] as a result of the hyperemia and osteitis caused by irradiation itself (Fig. 9-3, *B*).

Loss of articular congruity as a result of direct tumor lysis (Fig. 9-4, *A*) or of disruption by a fracture-dislocation prevents the attaining of a pain-free hip except by resection of the femoral head, amputation of the limb or a portion of the pelvis, or incorporation of a specialized prosthetic replacement. Ablation of the joint by resecting the femoral head or hemipelvis has been advocated by many,[4,11] particularly where extensive tumor osteolysis exists. Enneking and Durham[4] recommended that hip fusion be attempted even after wide resection of the acetabular bone for primary malignancy but emphasized that a successful pain-free fusion occurred in less than half their cases when it was attempted. In any event, prosthetic reconstruction of a stable hip generally is considered to be preferable to ablation or fusion, particularly in patients with a limited life expectancy.

In most cases when no significant displacement of the femoral head has occurred, total hip replacement arthroplasty can be performed with the anticipation of achieving a stable and pain-free joint. Sim et al.[17] reporting on 35 hip replacements after pathological fracture of the proximal femur in patients with minimal involvement of the periacetabular bone, encountered no difficulties in securing the acetabular component, and their results were excellent with regard to joint stability and relief of pain.

However, when major displacement of the femoral head has occurred, conventional total hip replacement is likely to fail because there is insufficient structurally adequate bone around the acetabular component to prevent its loosening and migration. Simply removing gross tumor tissue and filling the resultant cavity with excess cement will not prevent medial and superior migration of the acetabular component (Fig. 9-5, *A*). The cement is much harder than the surrounding tumor-infiltrated bone, and the prosthetic component with its attached acrylic will loosen as soon as weight-bearing is attempted. Meshes of various materials do not enhance acetabular component stability or limit this tendency toward migration (Fig. 9-5, *B*). Attempts to attach the acetabular component to the lateral pelvic wall in the absence of an intact roof are equally ineffective and will result in rapid component loosening and migration (Fig. 9-5, *C*). In patients with a congenitally deficient acetabular roof, the superior acetabular bone stock can be enhanced by splitting the ilium, by using acetabuloplasty of the shelf or Chiari type, or by bolting the resected femoral head to the acetabular rim as a graft and then reaming it inferiorly to form part of the acetabular roof. These measures are ineffective in the management of metastatic pathological fractures, however, because in the face of postoperative irradiation, all such techniques that depend on healing of osteotomized or grafted bone must be anticipated to fail. Finally, any attempt to suspend the acetabular component by creating a bridge of methylmethacrylate spanning the gap of destroyed bone also is doomed to failure (Fig. 9-5, *D*). Methylmethacrylate possesses little ability to resist the shear stresses that inevitably are concentrated on such a construct with even minimal weight bearing.

The solution to insufficiency of bone stock in the acetabular rim or roof lies in transmitting the weight-bearing forces away from the periacetabular bone destroyed by tumor and into the bone of the ilium and sacrum still structurally intact. It may be possible to accomplish this in patients with a major bone deficiency that involves only the medial wall of the acetabulum by transmitting weight-bearing stresses onto the intact acetabular rim. When both the rim and the medial wall are deficient, however, it is necessary to devise some means of transmitting the weight-bearing load onto structurally intact bone, often at some distance from the acetabulum itself.

Classification of Acetabular Insufficiencies

In an effort to establish guidelines for effective acetabular reconstruction and, in particular, to avoid the complications illustrated

---

*Centigray (cGy) is the currently accepted designation for rad.

in Fig. 9-5, we have established[9,10] a classification system for acetabular insufficiency secondary to metastatic disease. It is based on the location of the fracture within the periacetabular bone, the extent of tumor or radiation osteolysis, and the specialized technical requirements needed to accomplish a secure arthroplasty.

Class I. The lateral cortices and superior and medial parts of the walls are structurally intact.

Class II. The medial part of the wall is deficient.

Class III. The lateral cortices and superior part of the wall are deficient.

Class IV. Resection is required for cure.

Operative Techniques

Class I. Patients in the Class I category, although often showing extensive invasion of bone by metastases (Fig. 9-6, *A* and *B*), have sufficient unaffected periacetabular bone that conventional fixation of the acetabular component can result in an incidence of loosening or migration not exceeding that likely with routine total hip replacement

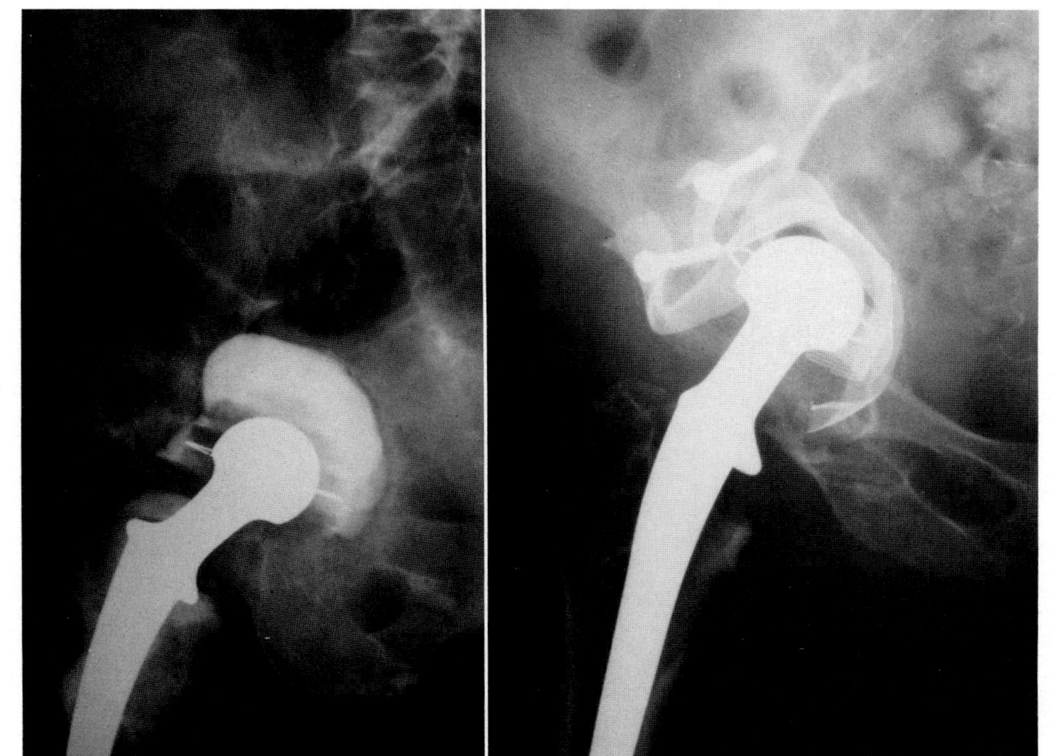

FIGURE 9-5 **A,** Conventional hip replacement arthroplasty was attempted on this 62-year-old man with metastatic carcinoma of the prostate. The acetabular rim was intact but the medial wall had been destroyed by tumor (Class II). The acetabular component loosened rapidly and migrated medially. This case demonstrates that simply using an abundance of methylmethacrylate to secure the acetabular component does little to enhance its stability under such circumstances. **B,** An AP roentgenogram of the right hip in a patient who underwent hip replacement arthroplasty for a Class II pathological fracture through the medial acetabular wall. The surgeon erroneously attempted to achieve fixation of the acetabular component by a combination of mesh and methylmethacrylate alone. Medial and superior migration of the acetabular component has occurred. Acetabular mesh may be effective in minimizing the amount of cement escaping intrapelvically through the acetabular defect, but it adds little to component fixation strength. *Continued.*

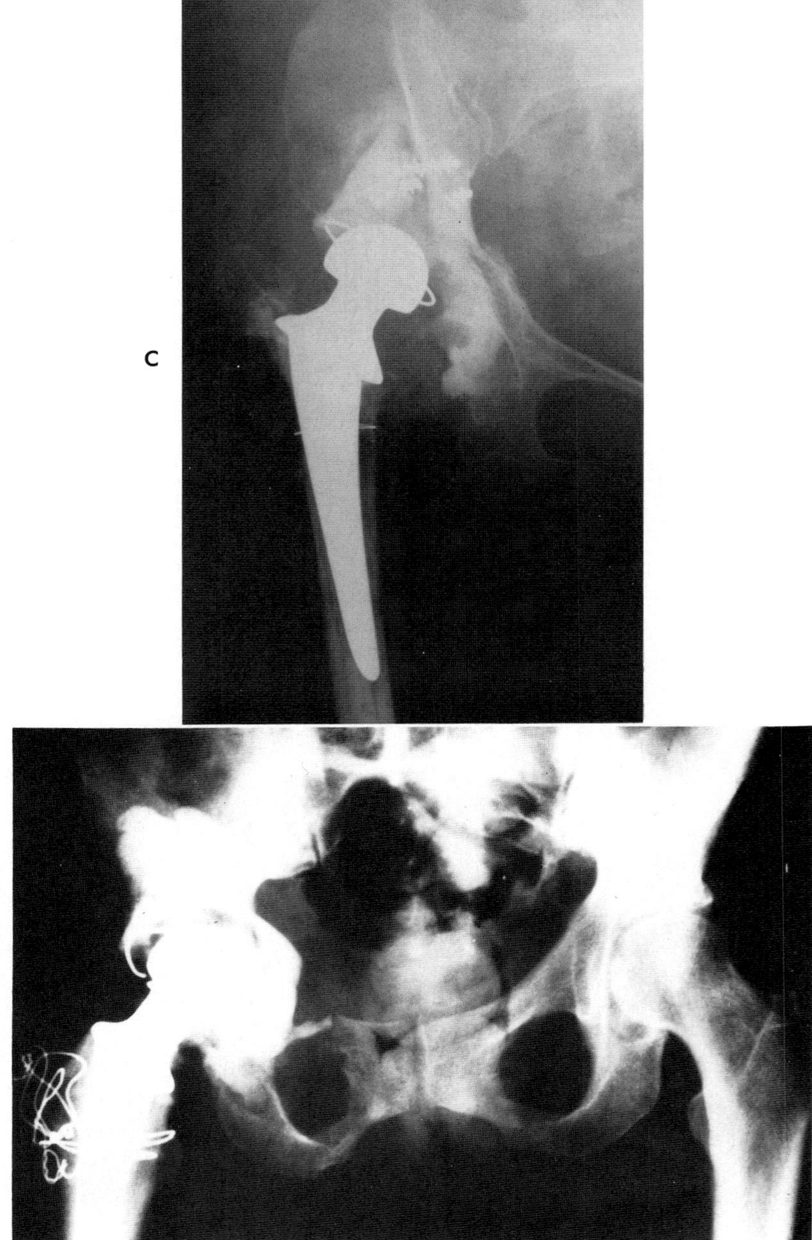

FIGURE 9-5, cont'd. **C,** Another example of failure to stabilize the acetabular component adequately. Cancellous screws were employed in an effort to secure the prosthesis-cement complex to the ilium. However, the acetabular component promptly migrated proximally into a large supraacetabular metastatic defect. **D,** In this case fixation of the acetabular component has been attempted by spanning a large bone defect with methylmethacrylate alone. Weight-bearing forces are being concentrated at a right angle to the long axis of the cement mass, thereby exerting maximum shear stresses on the construct. Failure of the fixation is inevitable.

arthroplasty. Although all patients in this group typically have severe and progressive hip pain on weight-bearing, the extent of their joint damage often is not appreciable by plain roentgenography because of the irregular patterns of bone sclerosis in reaction to the metastases (Fig. 9-6, *A*). However, defects in the subchondral bone, often of surprising size, are readily demonstrable by plain films or computed tomography (Fig. 9-6, *B* and *C*); and the patients in this group also have disruptions in the normal congruity of their acetabular surfaces evident at operation.

Conventional total hip arthroplasty is performed with the patient in the lateral decubitus position.

- A modified Gibson posterolateral approach is used, without trochanteric osteotomy.
- Chromium-cobalt mesh frequently is placed along the medial part of the acetabular wall in an effort to perhaps reinforce its strength, but primarily to minimize the escape of cement into the pelvis through bone defects created by tumor lysis (Fig. 9-6, *D*).
- No other specialized techniques are considered necessary to secure the acetabular component in these hips.

On the second or third postoperative day patients are allowed out of bed to begin walking with full weight-bearing on the affected extremity and are progressed through the same program of motion and strengthening exercises as used by patients with a conventional hip replacement.

Class II. Patients in the Class II category have in common a loss of structural continuity of the medial wall of the acetabulum (Fig. 9-7, *A, C,* and *D*). However, the superior part of the wall (roof) of the acetabulum and the lateral cortices of the ilium, ischium, and pubis adjacent to the acetabulum (acetabular rim) remain intact.

As demonstrated in Fig. 9-5, *A,* conventional seating of a prosthetic acetabular component usually will fail because the combination of prosthesis and its attached cement migrates through the medial wall defect. The use of mesh reinforcement along the medial wall is not an effective deterrent to such migration (Fig. 9-5, *B*). However, if the stresses of weight-bearing can be transferred away from the deficient and out onto the intact acetabular rim, migration failure will not occur.

We have found[9,10] that the Oh-Harris protrusio shell is the most effective and versa-

A

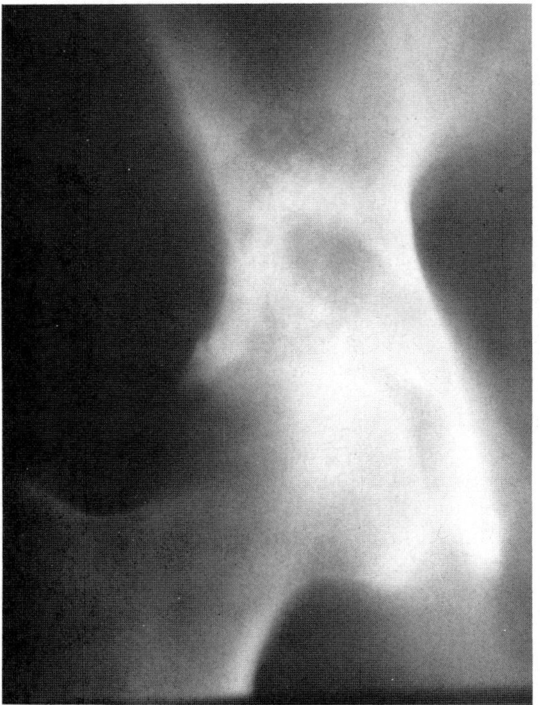

FIGURE 9-6 **A,** An AP tomogram of the right hip in a patient who complained of progressively increasing pain on weight-bearing but had minimal changes apparent by conventional plain roentgenography. The medial wall and the acetabular rim are intact, but an area of the acetabular roof has been destroyed. This is a Class I fracture.

Continued.

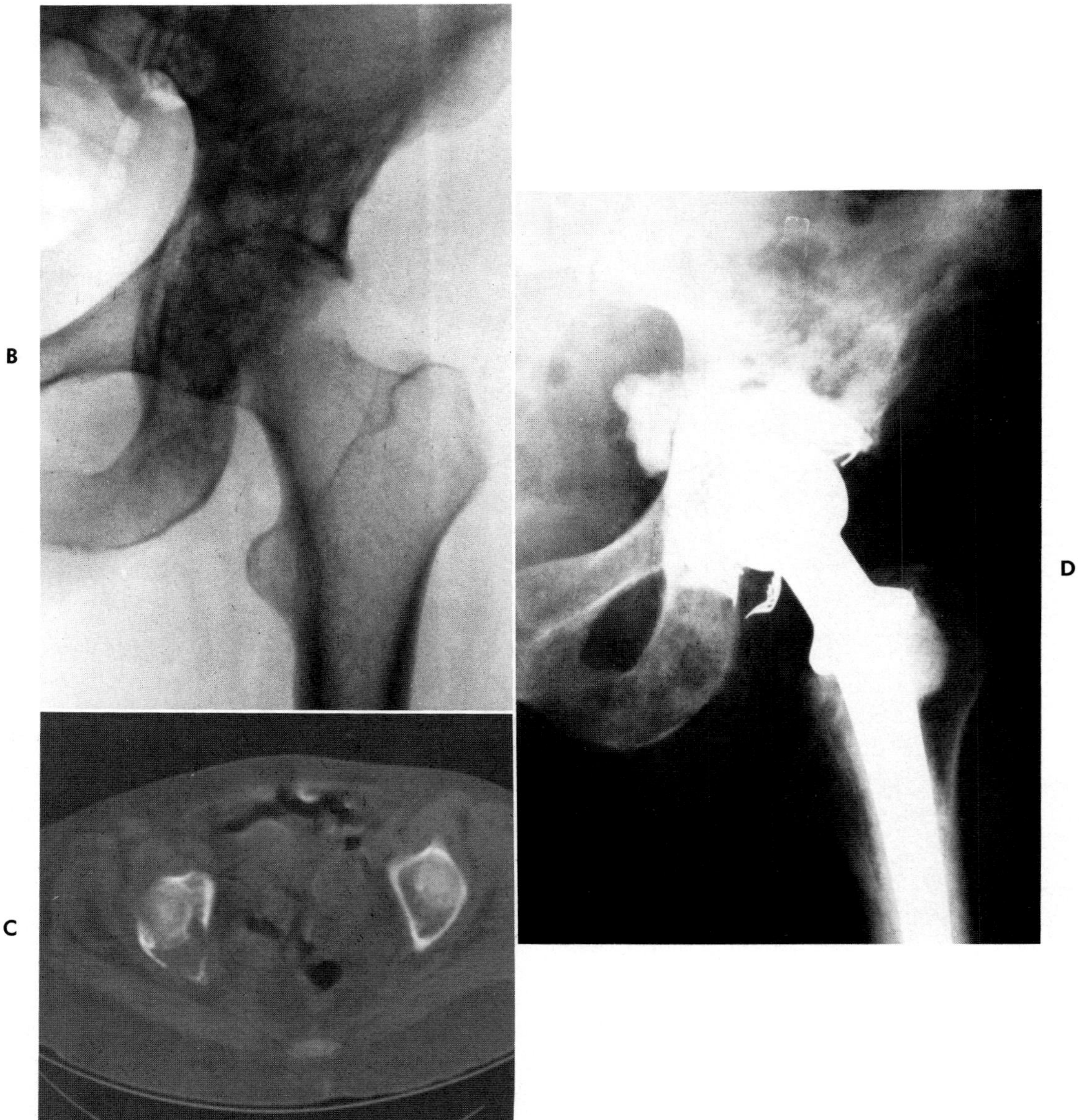

FIGURE 9-6, cont'd. **B,** Minimally impressive changes in the supraacetabular ilium of another patient. **C,** The CT scan shows destruction of the posterior acetabulum but preservation of the rim. Other tomographic cuts confirmed that the acetabular roof was intact. This also is a Class I metastatic lesion. **D,** Reconstruction has been completed—replacement arthroplasty with acetabular mesh to minimize escape of methylmethacrylate into the pelvis.

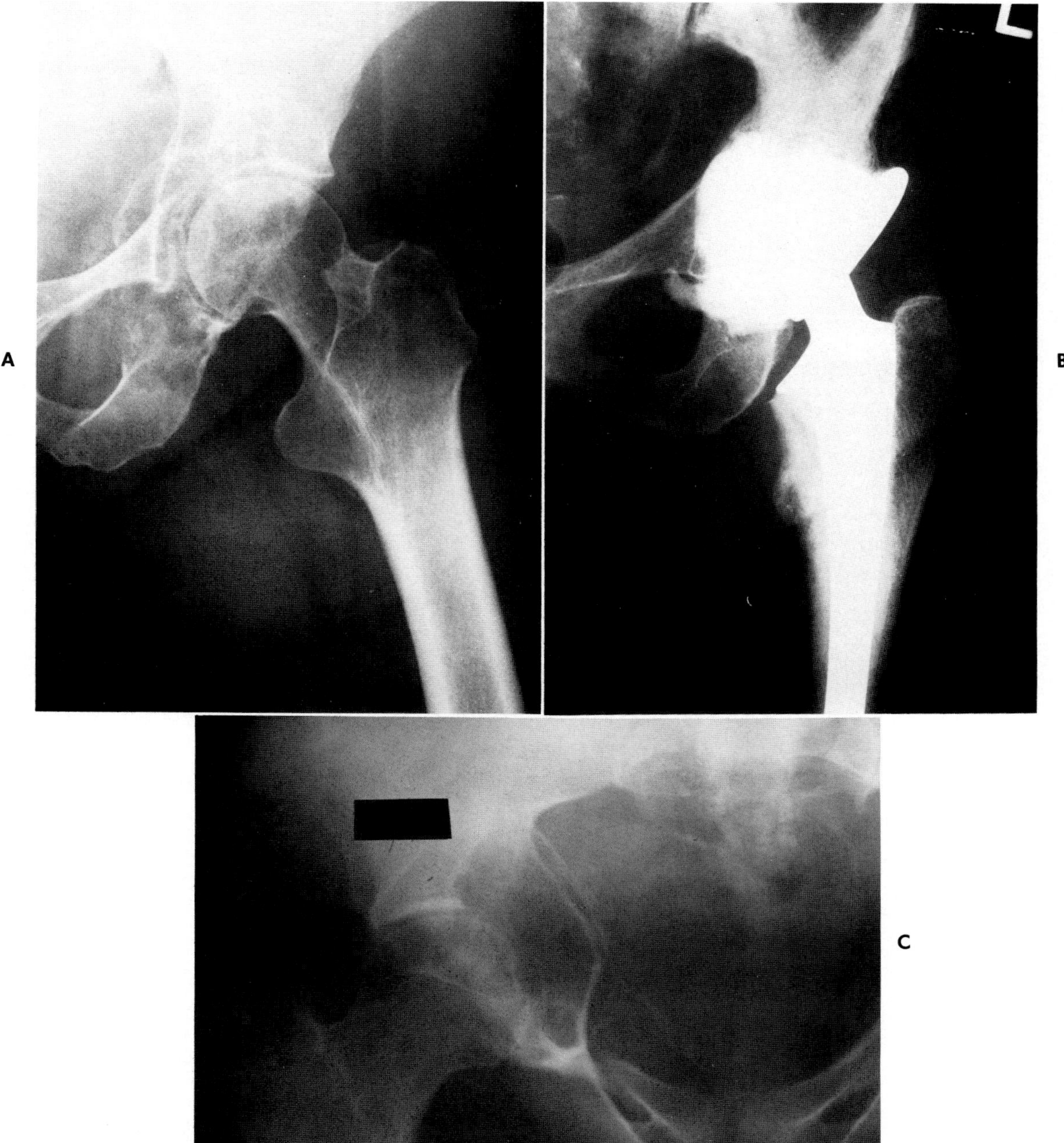

FIGURE 9-7 **A,** Class II osteolytic destruction of the medial part of the acetabular wall leaving the acetabular roof and rim structurally intact. The patient had metastatic carcinoma of the breast. **B,** Thirteen months after reconstruction of the hip and postoperative irradiation. The protrusio acetabuli ring effectively transfers weight-bearing stresses onto the intact acetabular rim. **C,** Another Class II fracture of the medial wall with a large aneurysmal metastasis having destroyed the medial wall of the acetabulum.

Continued.

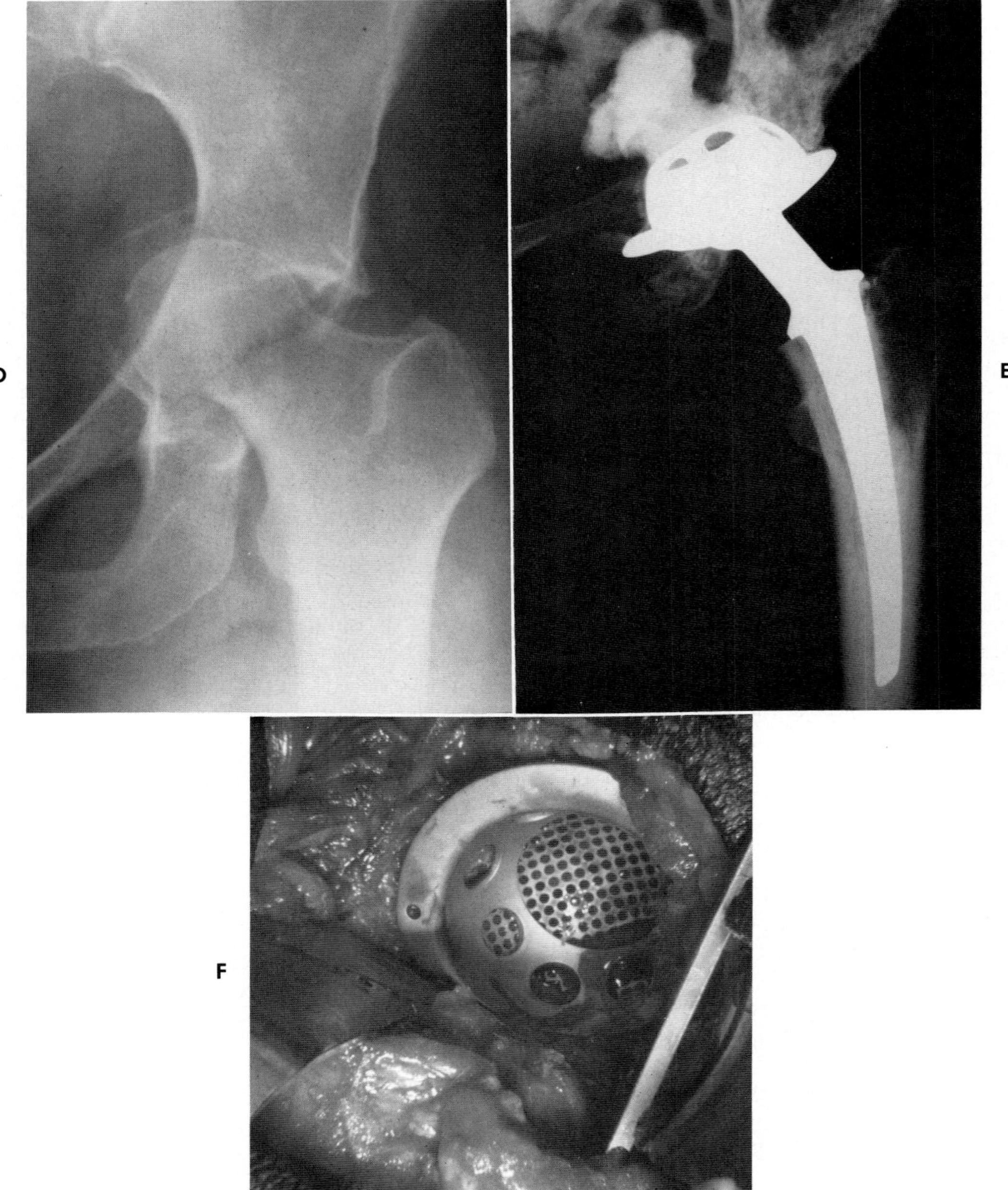

FIGURE 9-7, cont'd. **D,** Pathological central acetabular fracture in a 55-year-old patient with metastatic breast cancer. Most of the superior dome of the acetabulum is intact, as is the acetabular rim. **E,** The acetabulum has been reconstructed with an Oh-Harris protrusio cup. Escape of cement into the pelvis could have been prevented, or at least minimized, by lining the acetabulum with mesh. **F,** Intraoperative view of a Class II reconstruction showing proper lining of the acetabular cavity by mesh and subsequent positioning of the protrusio shell.

tile example of the many protrusio cups now available (Fig. 9-7, *B, E,* and *F*). It comes in three sizes, which correspond to the various available sizes of conventional acetabular prostheses. When the Oh-Harris shell is used, it is necessary either to overream the bony acetabulum or to use a smaller than usual acetabular component. The latter alternative is preferable. Bone stock deficiency already is a problem in these patients because of tumor lysis, and further acetabular reaming and consequent thinning of the remaining socket walls are likely to endanger the stability of the acetabular rim. In small women it is often necessary to use the smallest available protrusio shell and then the smallest (42 mm) acetabular component that will fit within it. However, we have encountered no evidence of loosening, instability, polyethylene wear, or other problems that we thought were attributable to the use of such a small component.

The rim of the protrusio shell must rest firmly on the superior and the anteroinferior margins of the bony acetabulum (Fig. 9-8, *E*) to be stable. If bone along these margins is deficient, it still may be possible to obtain secure seating of the shell by rotating it slightly. However, if there is extensive bone loss, particularly along the inferior rim, use of the shell alone will not be sufficient and more extensive measures must be undertaken to transmit weight-bearing loads into an area of intact bone (Fig. 9-8, *C*).

Whenever the protrusio shell is used in reconstructions for medial wall insufficiency, acetabular mesh should be placed along that wall before the shell is inserted, not in an effort to reinforce fixation but simply to minimize the amount of liquid cement escaping through the defect and into the pelvis. It is important to remember that if the rim extensions of the protrusio shell are properly in contact with the acetabular rim the shell will be aligned in approximately 65 degrees of valgus. If the acetabular component of the hip prosthesis also is aligned at this high oblique angle, hip instability will ensue. Consequently it is important to align and cement the high-density polyethylene socket independently within the shell at approximately 45 degrees of abduction and 20 degrees of anteversion.

Many patients with medial wall insufficiency and ultimate Class II acetabular fractures will have experienced a gradual medial and superior migration of the femoral head within the acetabulum for some months preoperatively. In these instances the affected extremity may well have become shortened slightly, and every effort should be made to restore leg length at the time of hip reconstruction. When such patients have not received irradiation preoperatively, it is rarely difficult to restore leg length intraoperatively. In the face of recent irradiation, however, great care must be taken to avoid excessive traction on the affected extremity lest the sciatic or femoral nerve, often trapped within dense fibrous scarring, be damaged. With this caveat in mind, the surgeon should attempt to use a femoral prosthesis having as long a neck as possible in an effort to minimize the risk of femoral neck or trochanteric impingement against the prominent rim of the protrusio shell.

The femoral intramedullary canal is prepared as for a conventional hip replacement prosthesis, unless there is roentgenographic or scintigraphic evidence of tumor lysis within the femoral cortices.

In this instance the femur should be prepared for prophylactic internal fixation as described in the previous chapter.

Levy et al.[12] have used a gynecological uterine suction-curet machine for rapid evacuation of tumor from the medullary canal or acetabular cavity, which effectively minimizes bleeding during that phase of the procedure. A no. 8 or 10 oblique tip is most efficient.

Whenever possible, a long-stemmed femoral prosthesis should be used because of its prophylactic value against fractures that might occur later within occult femoral metastases.

Trochanteric osteotomy is to be avoided because, in the face of perioperative irradiation, subsequent bony union would be unlikely.

Class III. This is the largest and most challenging group of candidates for reconstruction. Such patients have in common a loss of structural continuity not only of the medial part of the acetabular wall but also of the acetabular roof and rim (Figs. 9-2, 9-4, *A,* and 9-9).

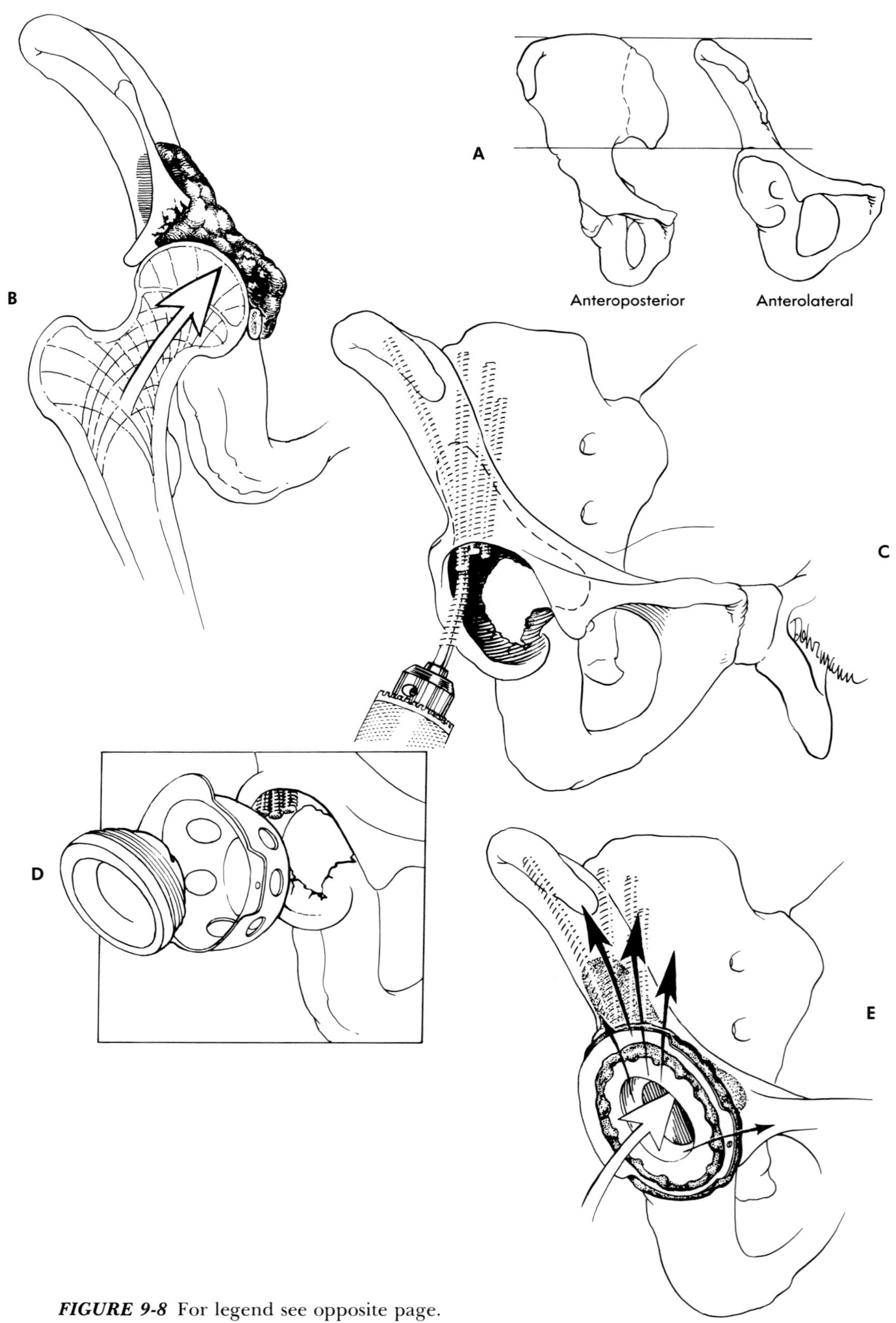

FIGURE 9-8 For legend see opposite page.

FIGURE 9-8 Schematic for reconstruction of Class III acetabular deficiency. **A,** Anteroposterior and anterolateral views of the pelvis demonstrate thinness of the ilium above the acetabulum. Attempting to anchor the acetabular prosthetic component higher than its normal position would provide poor fixation because of the thinness of the ilium there. **B,** Tumor has destroyed the superior and medial areas of acetabular bone, leaving minimal intact cortex for fixation of the acetabular component. **C,** After resection of the tumor a large cavity is apparent, as is destruction of the acetabular roof, medial part of the wall, and most of the rim. Steinmann pins can be drilled into structurally sound bone of the superior part of the ilium and across the sacroiliac joint. **D,** The acetabular component as it is positioned in the protrusio acetabuli shell. **E,** The combination of acetabular cup, protrusio shell, and Steinmann pins, all incorporated into methylmethacrylate, effectively transmits weight-bearing stresses into strong bone of the iliac wing and sacrum.

In most patients there is extensive lysis of either the ischium or the pubis, or both, so the inferior part of the acetabular rim is functionally nonexistent. Effective fixation of the acetabular prosthetic component in its normal location is impossible even with the Oh-Harris protrusio acetabuli ring.

Many surgeons[7,12] have chosen to treat these patients by Girdlestone resection arthroplasties instead of attempting a prosthetic replacement. Attempts at acetabular reconstruction by bridging the large tumor defect with rods or pins placed horizontally have failed because of the deficiency of strong bone lateral, inferior, or medial to the acetabulum. However, if the weight-bearing loads can be transmitted along a line 15 degrees medial to the true vertical[5] (the line of normal weight-bearing stress across the pelvis), the likelihood of fixation failure will be reduced markedly. This cannot be accomplished simply by attempting to secure the prosthetic acetabulum to intact bone higher in the ilium, because the iliac wing narrows markedly just above the normal acetabular roof, leaving an inadequate surface to withstand such loads (Fig. 9-8, *A*). As already mentioned, attempts at acetabuloplasty by various osteotomies or attempts to recreate the acetabular roof by bone grafting can be expected to fail in the face of irradiation.

We have found[9,10] that the most effective means of transmitting stresses along the medial vertical line and into intact strong bone not weakened by tumor is to drill several large threaded Steinmann pins from above the acetabular roof through the superomedial ilium and across and sacroiliac joint (Figs. 9-4, *B,* and 9-9, *F* to *H*). Despite the theoretical objections to concentrating the forces of weight-bearing on the small surface area of the threaded pins and to crossing the sacroiliac joint, in fact no instance of pin loosening or breakage or of sacroiliac pain has become apparent. Because the acetabular rim remains important,[6,15] we continue to use the protrusio shell, attempting to seat it as securely as possible on whatever bone there still is around the rim (Fig. 9-10, *I*).

The patient is placed on a conventional operating table in the lateral decubitus position, and a conventional posterolateral (Gibson or Moore) incision is used.

With the femur internally rotated, the piriformis tendon can be located, tagged, and transected (Fig. 9-10, *A*).

The remaining external rotators are transected as necessary to expose the joint capsule.

The hip joint capsule is excised, the femoral head dislocated, and the femoral neck transected at an angle appropriate to the femoral prosthesis chosen (Fig. 9-10, *B*). A large defect usually is apparent involving much of the medial and superior walls of the acetabulum and much of the acetabular rim as well.

All gross tumor tissue and loose bone fragments are removed (Fig. 9-10, *C*) until intact bone can be visualized and felt superiorly. This creates a large cavity usually extending well superiorly into the ilium.

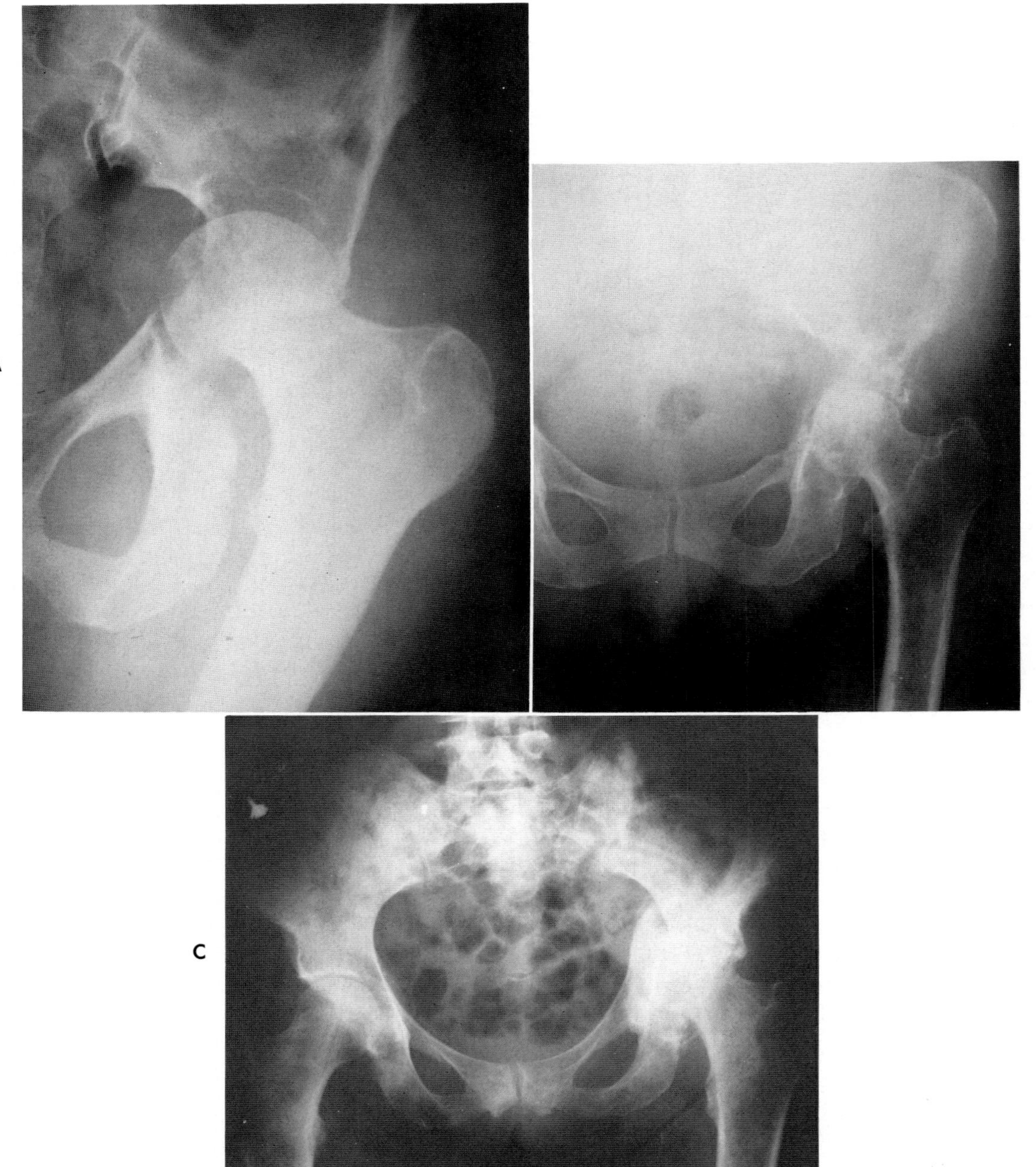

FIGURE 9-9 **A,** Class III acetabular fracture from lung cancer metastases. The medial wall, superior dome, and much of the acetabular rim have been destroyed, but the femoral bone appears unaffected. **B,** Class III acetabular insufficiency from metastatic breast cancer. There is destruction of the medial wall, superior dome, and acetabular rim. The femoral head has migrated superiorly and medially. **C,** Another Class III acetabular fracture, again secondary to a metastatic breast cancer. The femoral head has migrated proximally and medially.

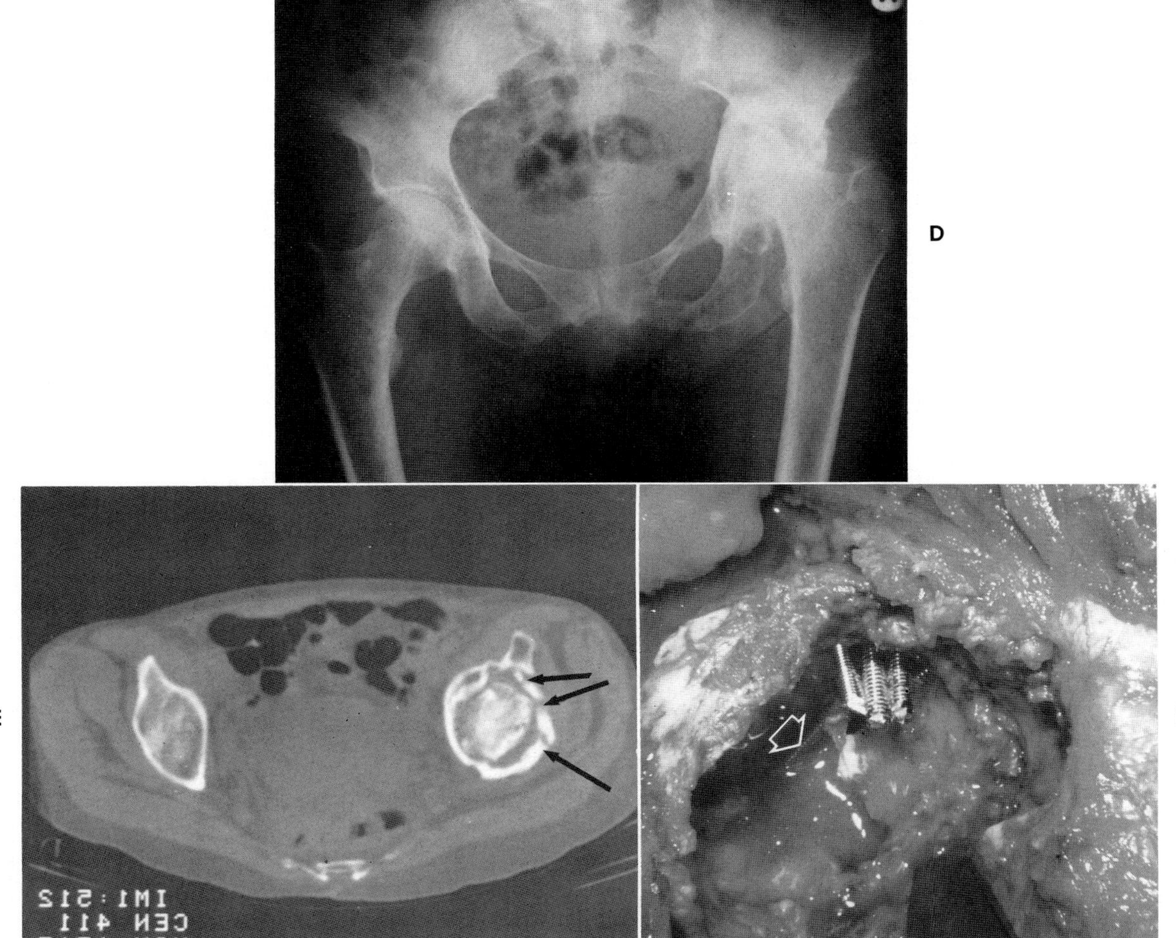

FIGURE 9-9, cont'd. **D,** After irradiation of the hip the medial wall fracture appeared to heal and the patient enjoyed several months of improved mobility and diminished pain. Eventually, however, she again began to experience progressively increasing joint pain and gradually lost the ability to walk. **E,** A CT scan revealed three fatigue fractures through the acetabular dome *(arrows)*. **F,** Intraoperative view of the acetabulum during joint reconstruction. Three large Steinmann pins have been drilled from the acetabulum superiorly across the sacroiliac joint. Also visible *(arrow)* is one of the three additional pins inserted from the anterosuperior iliac crest obliquely across the deficient acetabular roof.

Continued.

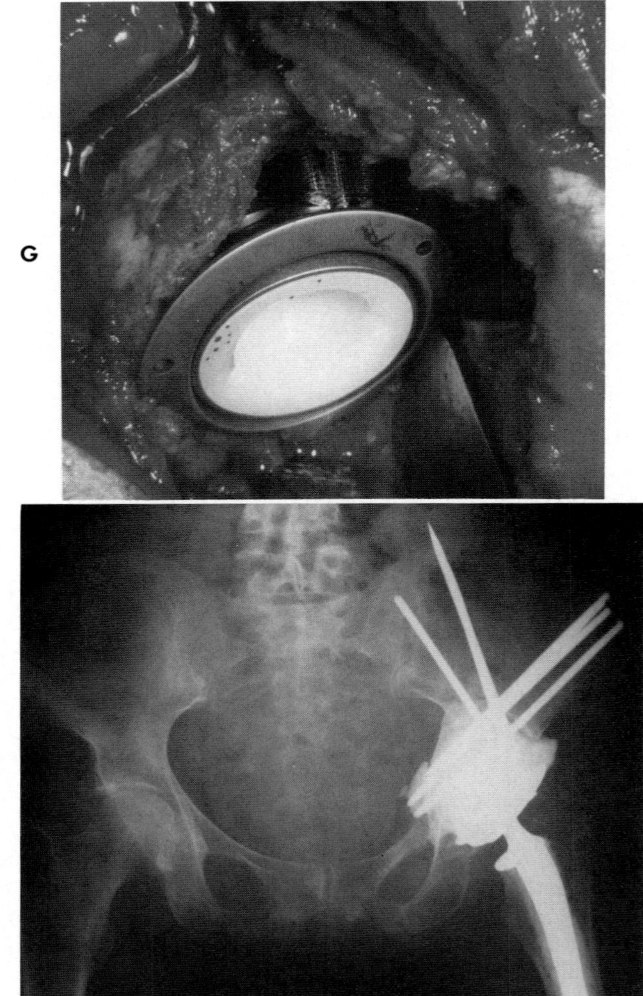

FIGURE 9-9, cont'd. **G,** With the pins properly positioned, the rim of the protrusio shell rests against and is partially supported by them. **H,** A postoperative roentgenogram shows the interrelationships of the protrusio shell, pins, and cement. The patient presently is 2½ years postoperative and enjoying a virtually pain-free hip with 100 degrees of hip flexion, full extension, and no evidence of component loosening.

A large hole in the medial wall is also apparent in most cases with the soft muscle mass of the iliacus palpable as it lies within the pelvis (Fig. 9-10, *D*).

By probing with the index finger along the course of the piriformis and behind the gluteus minimus, it is possible to feel the entire wall of the posterior ilium up to the sacroiliac joint (Fig. 9-10, *E* and *F*).

By palpating through the greater sciatic notch, just superior to the belly of the piriformis and beneath the broad surface of the iliacus within the pelvis, one easily can palpate the anterior wall of the inferior ilium as well as the anterior edge of the sacroiliac joint (Fig. 9-10, *G* and *H*).

Then by moving the finger inside and then outside the notch, it is possible to continuously monitor the course of the pins as they are drilled superiorly from the acetabulum toward and eventually through the sacroiliac joint.

An effort is made to drill at least two pins across the sacroiliac joint, one from the lower acetabulum along a line just above the greater sciatic notch and the other from the superior acetabulum.

A third and sometimes a fourth pin are drilled into the thick dense bone of the superomedial ilium just lateral to the sacroiliac joint (Fig. 9-10, *I*).

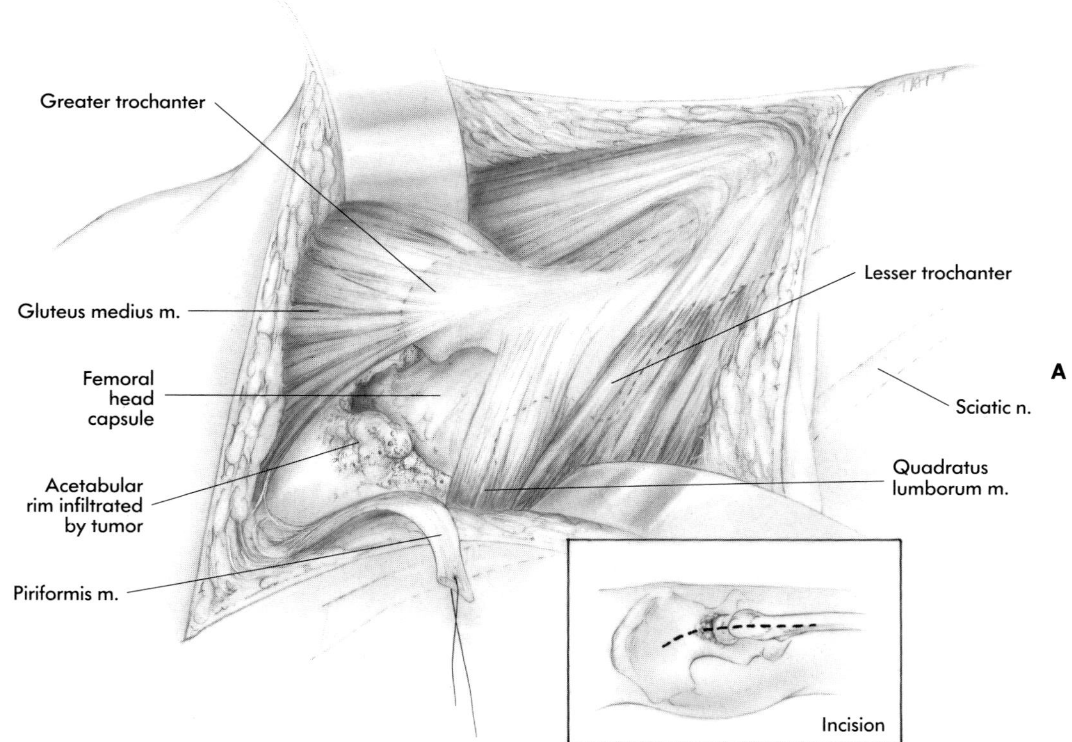

FIGURE 9-10 Class III operative repair. **A,** The patient is placed in the lateral decubitus position, and a modified Gibson incision is made centered over the greater trochanter. With the hip internally rotated, the external rotators can be tagged and detached. To protect the sciatic nerve, the tendon of the piriformis is transfixed by a suture and retracted. Even before the hip is dislocated, metastatic disease of the acetabular rim is apparent.

Continued.

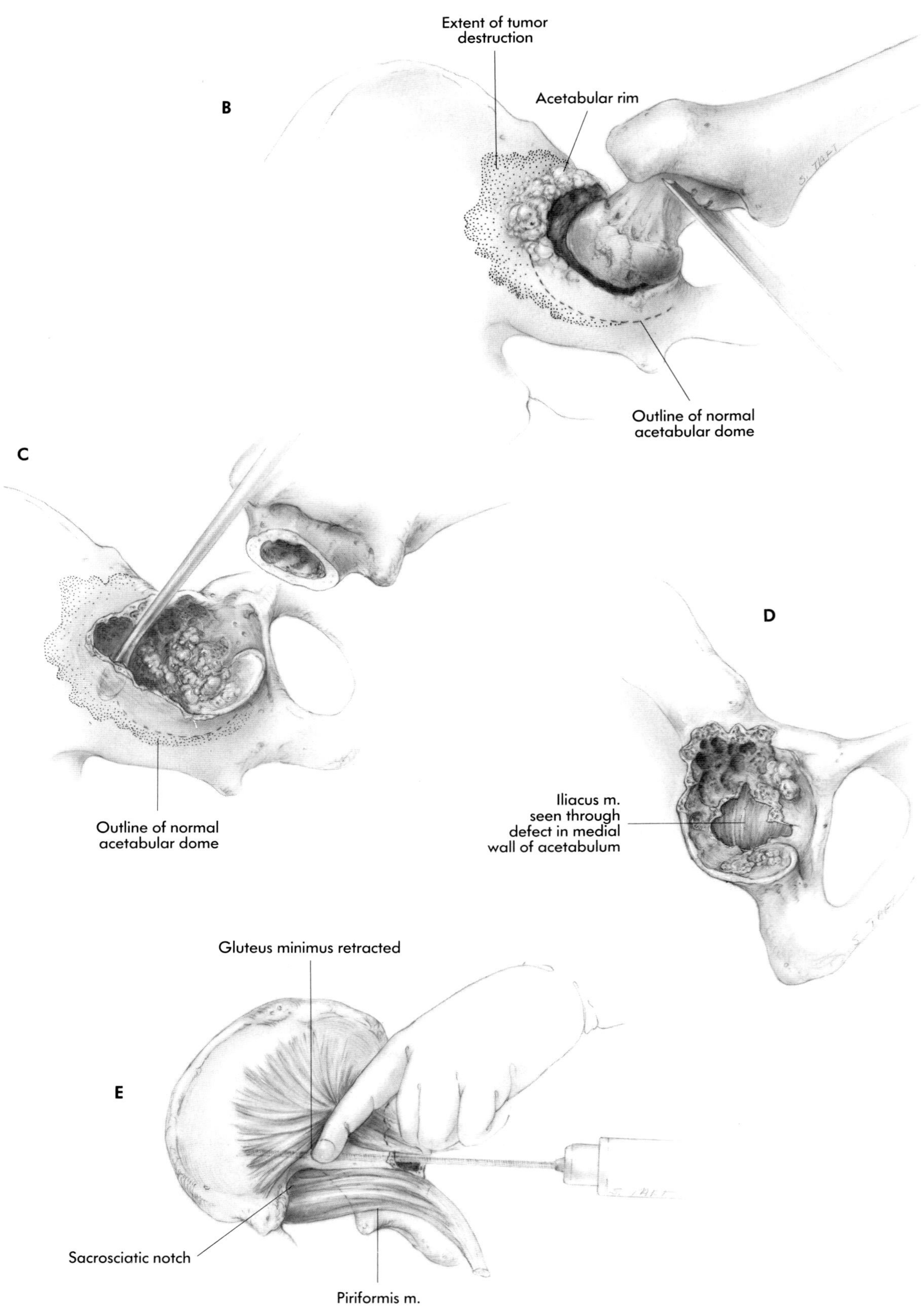

FIGURE 9-10, cont'd. For legend see opposite page.

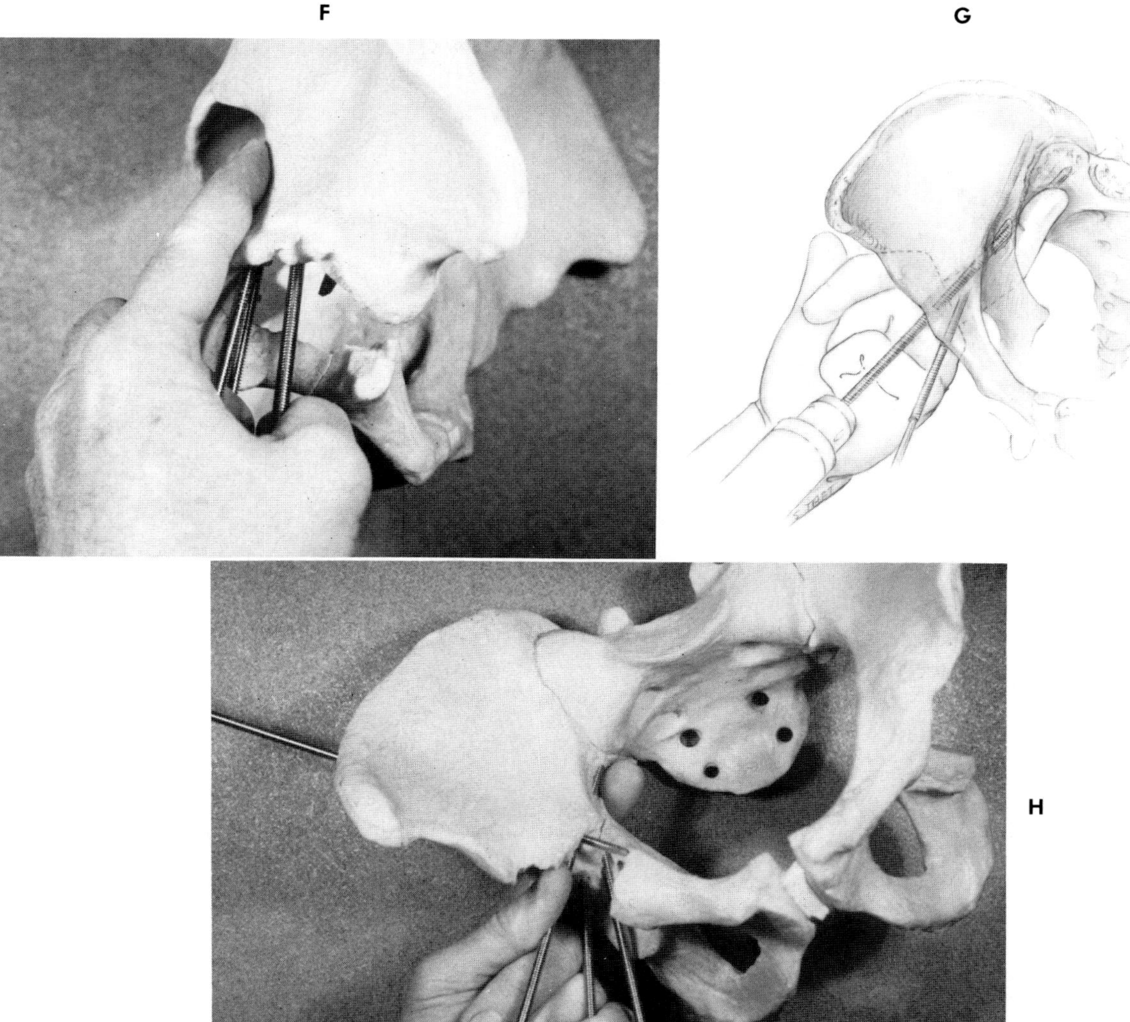

FIGURE 9-10, cont'd. **B,** Although exophytic tumor changes involving the rim may be obvious even before the capsule has been incised, the extent of acetabular roof destruction *(stippled area)* is never fully apparent until the hip is dislocated. The femoral neck is osteotomized along a line dictated by the collar of the femoral prosthesis to be used. **C,** Once the femoral head has been dislocated, extensive destruction of the acetabular walls, roof, and rim is apparent. Gross tumor tissue is removed by curettage until structurally intact bone is reached circumferentially. **D,** Typically, once the tumor tissue has been resected a large defect in the medial wall is apparent with the iliacus visualized in the pelvis. **E,** By blunt finger dissection along the posterior wall of the acetabulum, it is possible to find the interval between the extrapelvic gluteus minimus and the piriformis exiting the sacrosciatic notch. A finger positioned here ensures that a Steinmann pin drilled from below will not inadvertently become misdirected extracortically. **F,** By rotating one's hand, it is possible to insert the index finger into the notch and palpate the sciatic nerve. **G** and **H,** By further supination, it is possible then to palpate both the anterior surface of the sacrum and the sacroiliac joint to ensure that the Steinmann pin does not penetrate the cortex.

Continued.

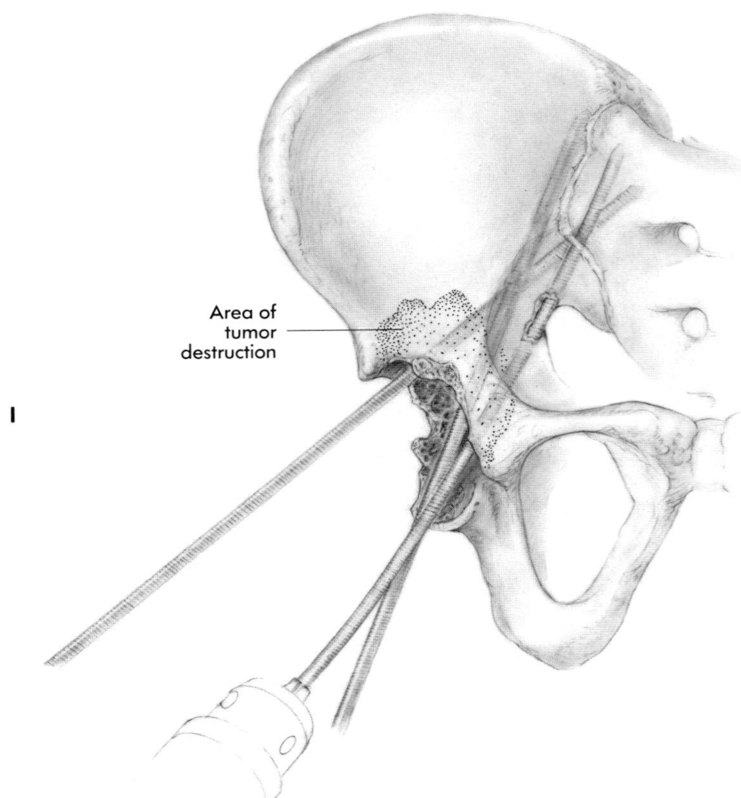

FIGURE 9-10, cont'd. **I,** Using continuous finger palpation along the inner and outer pelvis to protect the neurovascular structures as just described, the surgeon drills three large threaded Steinmann pins retrograde from the acetabular dome into the strong bone of the superomedial ilium or across the sacroiliac joint.

Early in our experience with this technique we used only three or four pins drilled along this medial-horizontal axis of weight-bearing. However, in 1980 we operated on a patient who had had such an acetabular reconstruction performed 3 years earlier and who had suffered subsequently from loosening of the acetabular component (Fig. 9-11, *C* and *D*). At reoperation it was found that the acetabular prosthesis and cement still were attached to the vertical pins but were tending to rotate around those pins, resulting in loss of fixation at the periphery of the construct. The acetabular component and cement were removed but the pins were left in place. Additional pins were drilled down into the joint from the anterosuperior iliac crest through a small 2 cm incision. They crossed the vertical pins obliquely at an angle of 30 degrees; and when the protrusio shell and acetabular component again were cemented in place, the tendency toward torquing of these components around the long axis of the pins had effectively been eliminated (Fig. 9-11, *E*).

Since that time, we have routinely inserted two or three pins downward into the acetabulum from the anterosuperior crest (Fig. 9-10, *J*). Ideally these pins from the anterior crest are drilled across the open acetabular defect and into the ischial bone below (Fig. 9-9, *F* and *G*). This allows rigid pin fixation in bone above and below the tumor defect and minimizes the risk of their loosening. Obviously, if acetabular mesh is to be placed against the deficient medial wall, it should be positioned before the transverse

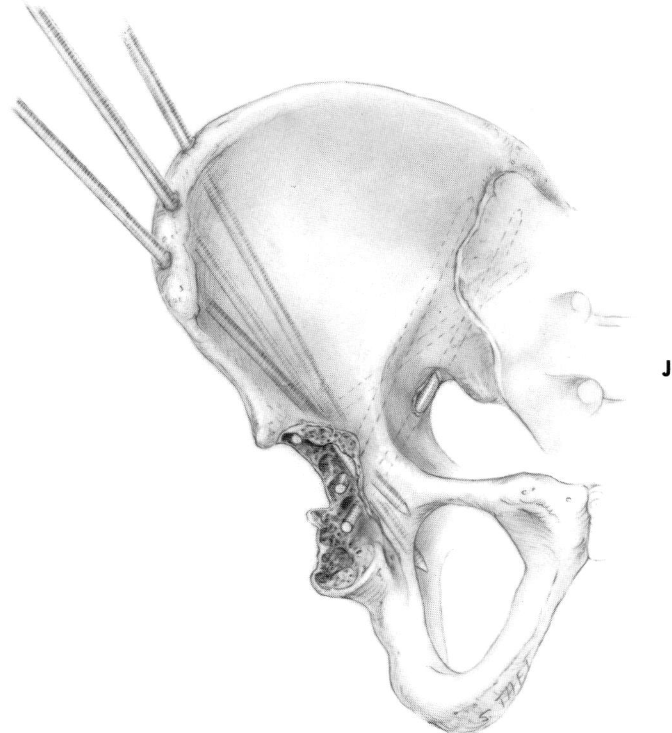

FIGURE 9-10, cont'd. **J,** The retrograde pins are cut off within the resected tumor bed. A 3 cm incision is made over the anterosuperior iliac crest and three additional large Steinmann pins are drilled antegrade through the ilium into the acetabular cavity. An attempt is made to bury their tips in the ischium and pubis. So positioned, these six pins create an excellent latticework for support of the Oh-Harris protrusio shell (see Fig. 9-9, *F*).
Continued.

pins are drilled from the iliac crest. During the drilling of all these pins, the index finger moves in and out of the pelvis through the greater sciatic notch, guarding against inadvertent penetration of the cortex and potential injury to soft tissue structures (Fig. 9-10, *E* to *H*).

Once the pins are positioned properly, they are cut off within the acetabular defect just deep enough to allow secure seating of the protrusio ring. Ideally, the rim flanges on the ring will seat firmly against the remaining intact bone of the acetabular rim and the deepest portion of the ring will rest against the pins crossing the acetabular defect from the anterosuperior iliac spine (Fig. 9-10, *K*).

The acetabular bed then is thoroughly cleansed first with hydrogen peroxide and then with a pulsating water lavage (Water-Pik) in an effort to expose the cancellous bone surfaces and enhance the contact between bone and cement.

Methylmethacrylate is injected from a gun into the exposed bony interstices while a finger is pressed from within the pelvis against the medial wall defect to minimize cement extrusion intrapelvically. Generally, two and occasionally three packages of methylmethacrylate are required.

The protrusio ring and the acetabular component are pressed firmly into position, care being taken that the acetabular component is at a less oblique angle than the protrusio ring so joint instability will be minimized (Fig. 9-10, *I*).

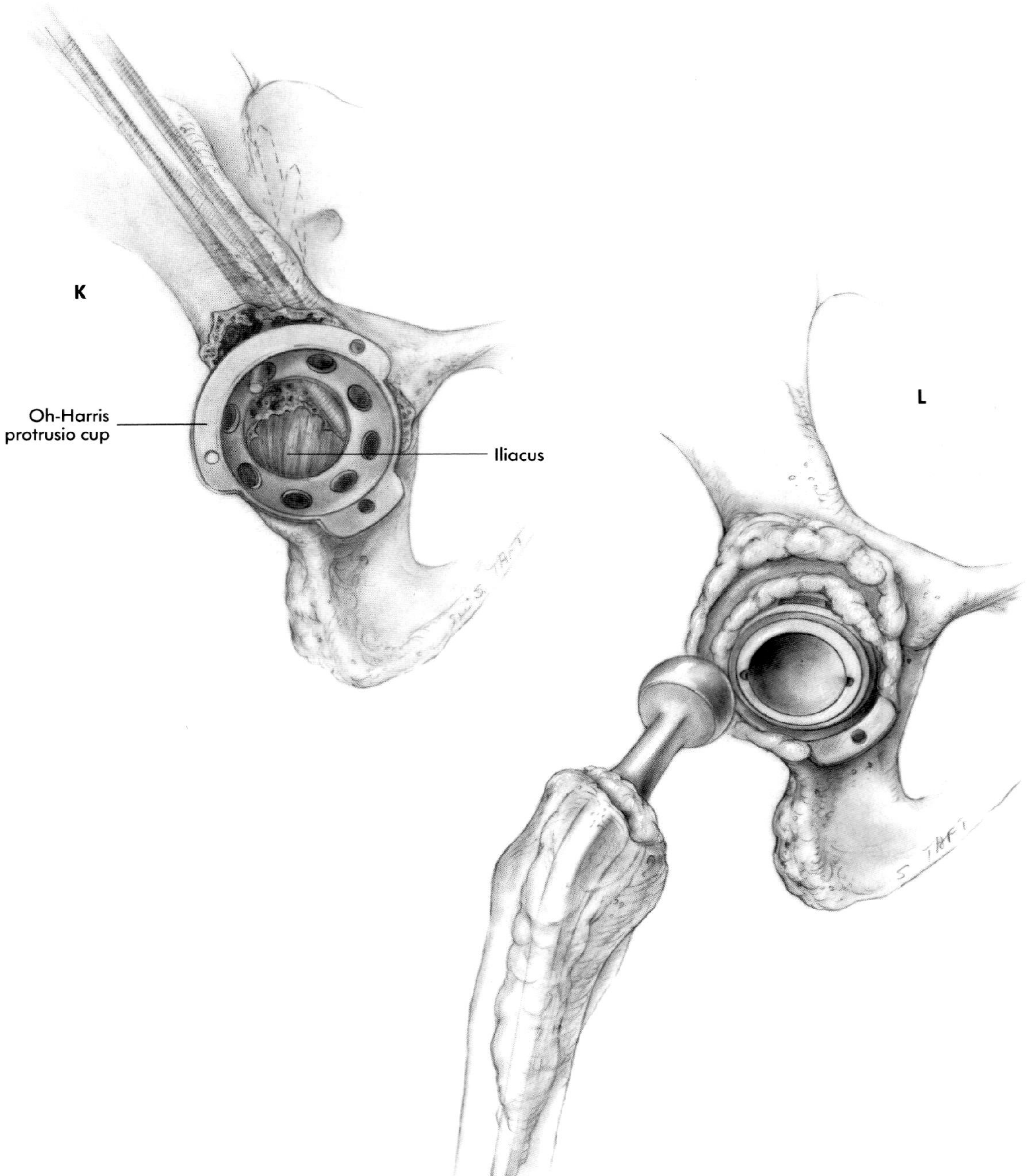

FIGURE 9-10, cont'd. **K,** The protrusio shell is seated. Its rim flanges should rest on whatever bone remains of the acetabular rim. The depth of the cup should rest against the latticework of crossed Steinmann pins (see Fig. 9-9, *G*). **L,** The acetabular bed is cleansed with a Water-Pik or hydrogen peroxide and is dried. Then the prosthetic acetabular component, protrusio shell, and pins are imbedded in methylmethacrylate injected conventionally and packed into the defect. For stability of the total hip replacement, it is important to align the acetabular component at 45 degrees of abduction and to antevert it approximately 20 degrees rather than in the 60-degree abduction of the protrusio shell. A standard femoral component is used unless prophylactic stabilization of the femoral shaft is required. In these cases a 10- or 12-inch stemmed prosthesis may be used.

After polymerization of the cement is complete, the femur is prepared and the femoral component cemented in place.

On occasion, it may appear roentgenographically that although both the acetabular roof and the medial wall have been destroyed by tumor there is minimal destruction of bone superiorly in the iliac wing (Figs. 9-11, *A*, and 9-12, *A*). Almost invariably this impression will prove to be erroneous when the ilium is further evaluated by computed tomography (Fig. 9-11, *B*). Even if the supraacetabular bone is not clearly destroyed, one should assume the high probability that it is infiltrated by metastatic tumor and there is a significant reduction in its ability to resist transmitted weight-bearing loads. For this reason we do not advocate using short cancellous screws extending only into the supraacetabular bone as a means of dissipating vertical stress away from the cement bone junction (Fig. 9-12, *B*). Instead, long large threaded Steinmann pins are much more reliable for transmitting such loads into clearly intact (and inherently stronger) bone around and across the sacroiliac joint.

Tumor Embolization. Some metastatic lesions in the pelvis, particularly those from myeloma and from carcinomas of the colon, pancreas, and kidney, tend to be highly vascular. Blood loss at attempted fixation or even at biopsy may be prohibitive. The technetium-99 bone scan is not a reliable means of attempting to quantitate the vascularity of these lesions at a fracture site. The roentgenographic appearance of the lesions, however, may be helpful. Where a sharp sclerotic reactive rim is apparent on the film (Fig. 9-9, *B*), the likelihood of excessive intraoperative blood loss is minimal; but where extensive reticulated osteolysis exists and extends irregularly and vaguely into the iliac

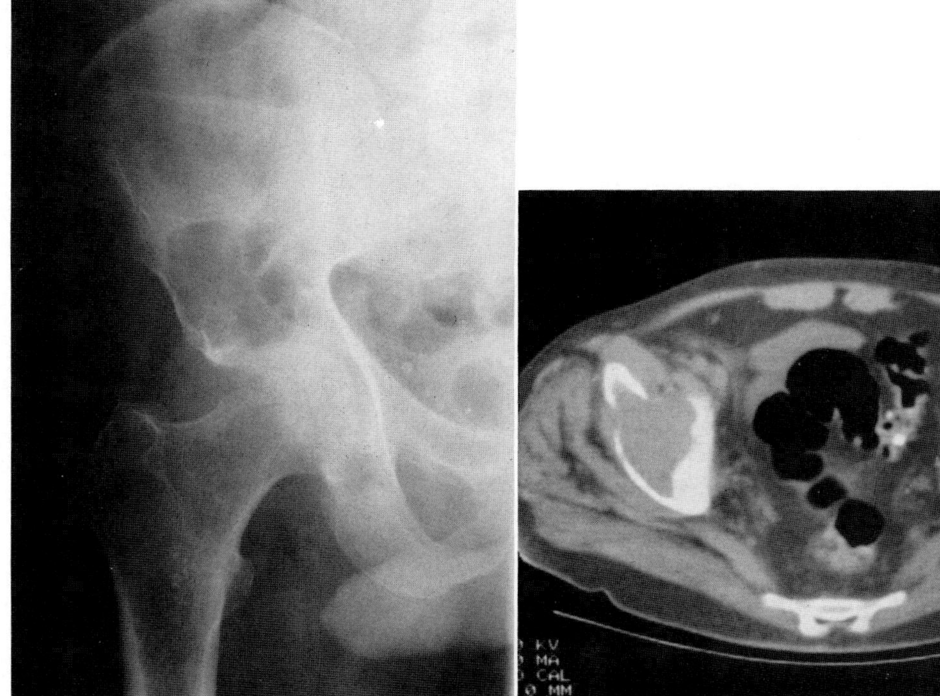

FIGURE 9-11 **A,** Roentgenogram showing a metastatic hypernephroma that has destroyed the weight-bearing dome of the acetabulum. **B,** A CT scan demonstrates the extent of acetabular roof and iliac cortical destruction. *Continued.*

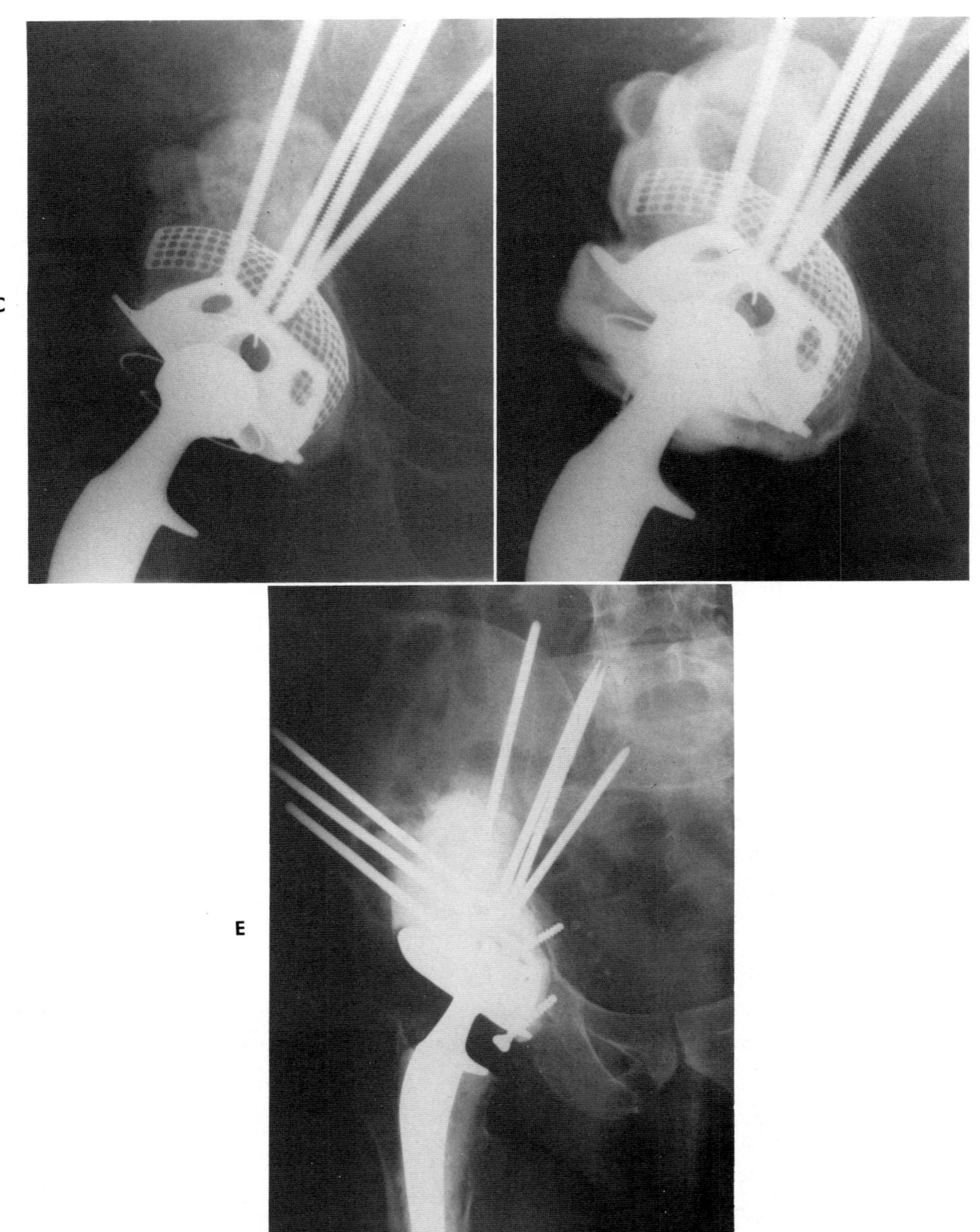

FIGURE 9-11, cont'd. Two years after joint reconstruction, **C,** although there is no appreciable abnormality notable on this roentgenogram, the patient complained of hip pain on weight-bearing. (The Steinmann pins remained intact.) The thin radiolucent space along the medial wall had not widened since the operation. An arthrogram, **D,** however, revealed dye surrounding the construct everywhere except along its medial wall. At revision the cement-cup combination was found to be easily rotatable around the long axes of the parallel Steinmann pins, the pins themselves remaining secure within the bone. The arthroplasty was revised by removing the cement and acetabular components but leaving the pins in place. Three additional large threaded Steinmann pins, **E,** were inserted anterograde from the anterior iliac crest (see Fig. 9-10). This created a scaffolding that prevented further acetabular component rotation. The acetabular prosthesis and protrusio cup then were cemented within the scaffolding. Five years postoperative the patient is alive and without symptoms, and there is no evidence of further loosening.

wing (Figs. 9-12, *A,* and 9-13, *A*) or there is evidence of a soft tissue mass extracortically (particularly with myeloma) (Fig. 9-14, *A*), then one should consider preoperative arteriographic evaluation of the area to assess its vascularity and possible embolization of the tumor bed to minimize operative blood loss.

When the arteriogram demonstrates excessive vascularity of the tumor bed, one should selectively catheterize the major arterial trunk from which the tumor vessels arise. Small strips of Gelfoam (2 × 2 mm) then are cut and morcellized in sterile saline into a syrup of such consistency that it can just be forced through the catheter by injection. When thus selectively injected, the Gelfoam occludes only the tumor vessels (Figs. 9-13, *A,* and 9-14, *D*), sufficiently devascularizing the operative site to minimize blood replacement requirements. There is no urgency in proceeding with operative intervention after embolization. Although much of the tumor tissue presumably becomes necrotic, we have seen no evidence of late ill effects of this phenomenon even when the subsequent tumor resection and joint reconstruction were delayed for more than a week after embolization.

When an excessively vascular lesion has not been anticipated or controlled preoperatively, blood loss at the time of operation may be difficult to control. In the majority of instances, this bleeding occurs from tumor vessels within the bone. Such bleeding is minimally controllable by local pressure or electrocoagulation and rarely can be brought under control by synthetic clotting substrates such as fibrinogen soaked Gelfoam or tribromoethanol (Avitene). However, otherwise uncontrollable hemorrhage from within the confines of a bony tumor focus can be controlled very effectively by packing the site with methylmethacrylate in its doughy pre-

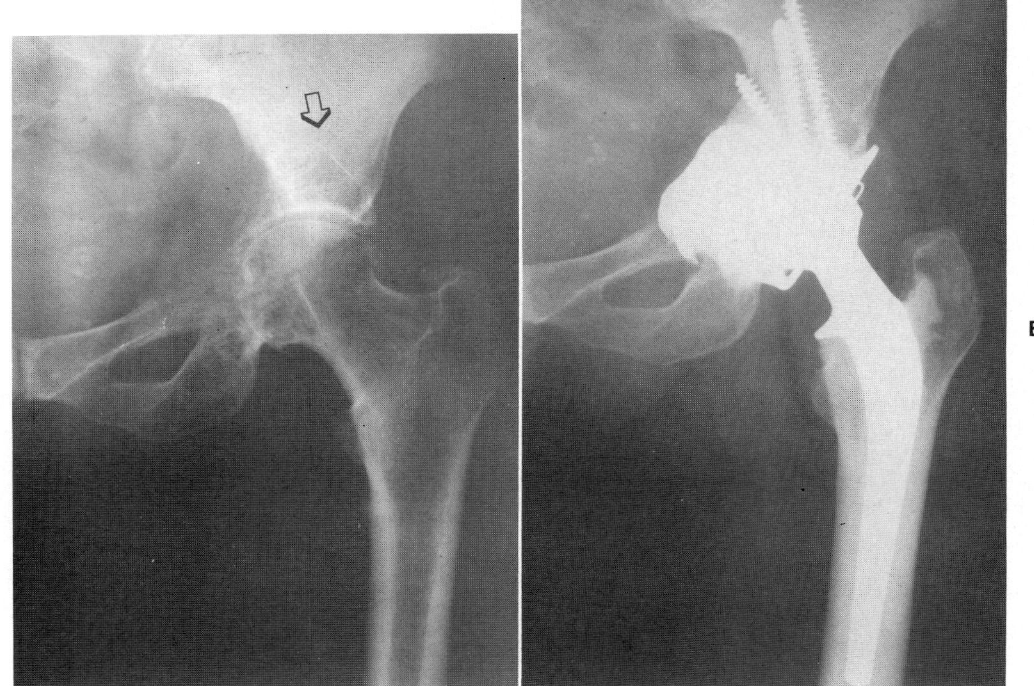

FIGURE 9-12 **A,** Class III acetabular fracture involving primarily the medial wall and inferior rim but with extensive lytic changes apparent superiorly as far proximally as the arrow. **B,** Rather than use large Steinmann pins anchored in strong bone across the sacroiliac joint, the surgeon chose to secure the acetabular prosthesis with short cancellous screws. The tips of these screws barely extended outside the area of tumor lysis, and prosthetic loosening followed rapidly.

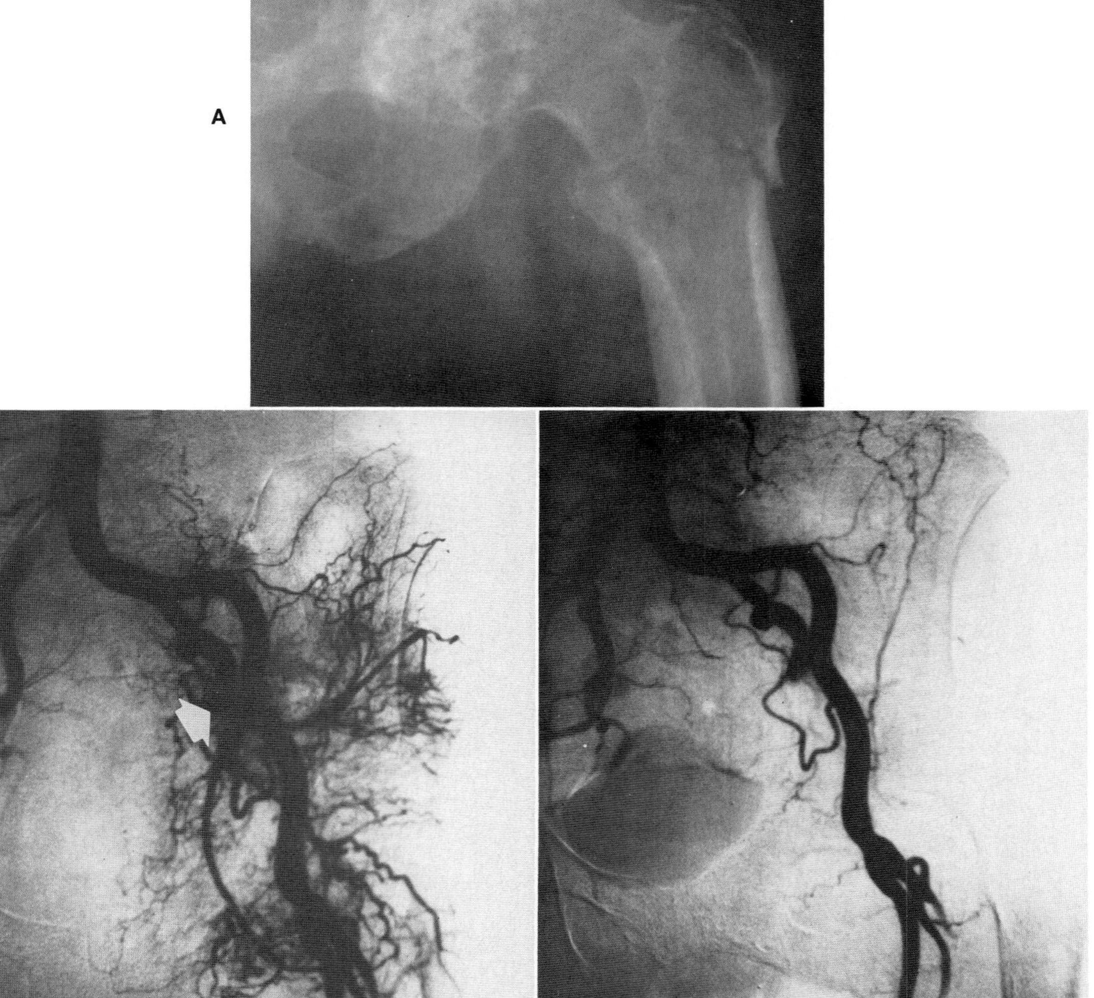

FIGURE 9-13 **A,** Roentgenogram of the left hip in a 66-year-old woman with metastatic colon carcinoma and pathological fractures of the proximal femur and acetabular walls. The extensiveness and the poorly circumscribed pattern of tumor lysis, particularly in a patient with metastases from a retroperitoneal cancer, suggest that the lesion will be highly vascular. **B,** An arteriogram demonstrates hypervascularization of the metastatic focus from multiple tumor vessels all originating from the hypogastric (terminal branch of the internal iliac) artery *(arrow)*. **C,** Arteriographic appearance after selective embolization of the hypogastric artery with Gelfoam. Joint reconstruction incorporating pins and methylmethacrylate was accomplished, with minimal blood loss.

polymerized consistency. As the acrylic gradually hardens, it also expands, thereby compressing the bleeding surfaces. The heat of polymerization may also assist by cauterizing exposed tumor vessels. After 15 minutes the methylmethacrylate can be removed piecemeal with a small straight osteotome, and the reconstruction can proceed in a blood-free field. Note that this technique is not an appropriate alternative to preoperative embolization. Before methylmethacrylate can control hemorrhage effectively, most or all of the gross tumor tissue present must have been removed. Blood loss during this procedure may become extreme, and by the time effective packing of the lesion with cement can be performed the technique may become a lifesaving effort to abate exsanguination.

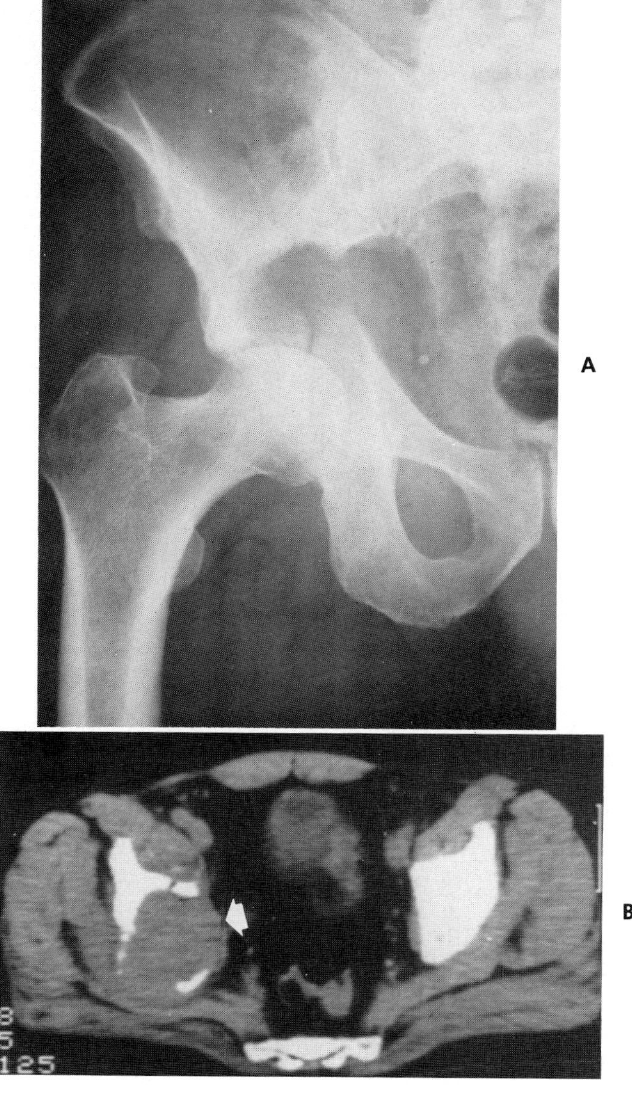

FIGURE 9-14 A roentgenogram of the pelvis in a 58-year-old man, **A,** shows a solitary metastasis from a renal carcinoma. Nephrectomy had been performed 6 years earlier, and careful screening had failed to reveal any other evidence of metastatic disease. The patient, therefore, was a candidate for a Class IV resection and reconstruction. A preoperative CT scan, **B,** however, revealed an extensive tumor mass *(arrow)* that had broken through the medial acetabular wall.

Continued.

Class IV. On rare occasion solitary metastases may be resected locally en bloc, with a reasonable anticipation of cure (Figs. 9-14 to 9-16). For example, the patient with solitary metastases from a hypernephroma or a thyroid carcinoma who is more than 4 years after resection of the primary lesion has a good prognosis for cure if the metastasis can be resected completely with good tumor margins. Although such solitary metastases can appear in any part of the skeleton, they seem to occur most commonly in the proximal humerus and in the supraacetabular portion of the pelvis. Before a resection for cure can be considered, extensive preoperative evaluation is necessary to rule out evidence of other bone, lung, or liver metastases in particular and to assess for any potential extraosseous extension of the tumor process. Computed tomography has been particularly helpful in evaluating the shape and extension of the metastatic process (Fig. 9-14, *B*).

At the time of resection the adequacy of tumor margins should not be compromised in an effort to allow pelvic reconstruction. If the procedure is appropriate in the first place, it is appropriate primarily as an attempt to cure the patient of his cancer. The extent of pelvic resection required may eliminate all possibility of subsequent reconstruction, and patients who are unwilling to allow this should be encouraged to undergo a palliative procedure as illustrated in Fig. 9-10. When the possibility of acetabular reconstruction does not exist, an internal hemipelvectomy should be considered (Fig. 9-14, *E*). We recommend that such patients receive local irradiation postoperatively, not only in an effort to improve the likelihood of complete tumor ablation but also for the positive effect of soft tissue scarring within the operative site. This scarring tends to stabilize the proximal femur within the soft tissues of the pelvic defect and thereby to minimize pistoning of the femoral shaft with weight-bearing. After internal hemipelvectomy *with* irradiation, most patients are able to regain approximately 90% of pseudo-hip motion and have sufficient limb stability to allow them to walk using a cane for support and to participate in a variety of recreational activities that would be impossible after a hip disarticulation amputation (Fig. 9-14, *F*). If good limb stability does not develop, either because irradiation of the postoperative bed is impossible or because excessive pistoning of the femur occurs despite irradiation, the patient is left with a minimally functional extremity. Pain relief usually is only partial, and walking can be accomplished only for short distances and with the assistance of a walker.[12]

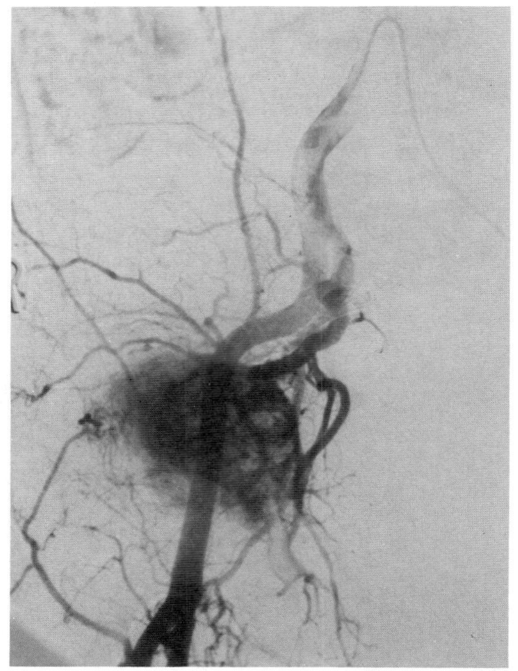

FIGURE 9-14, cont'd. For legend see opposite page.

When a solitary metastasis within the resected pelvic segment has not weakened the segment so much as to render it incapable of weight-bearing, it is possible to autoclave the segment and use it to reconstitute the pelvic ring as a prelude to hip joint arthroplasty (Figs. 9-15 and 9-16). The tumor-bearing segment of ilium is resected with wide bony and soft tissue margins, preserving the structural integrity of the acetabulum itself. Great care is taken to avoid violating the tumor margins, and intraoperative examination of frozen histological sections is performed if necessary to ensure that tumor tissue has not been transected. If the specimen's margins are clear, autoclaving proceeds at 135° C and 6.8 kg of pressure for 10 minutes. Once sterilized, the specimen can be

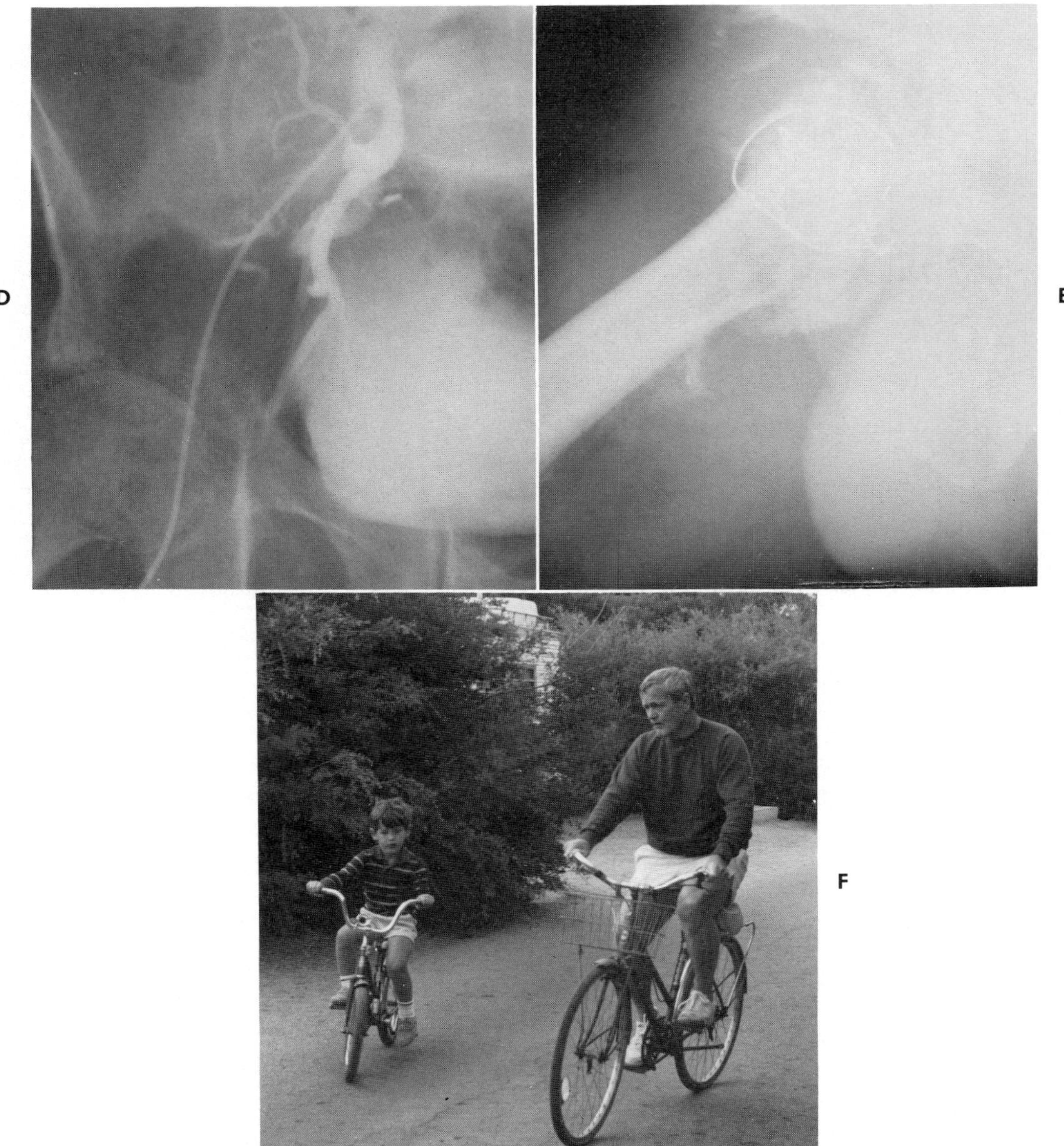

FIGURE 9-14, cont'd. An arteriogram, **C,** revealed abundant vascularity of the tumor originating from the internal iliac artery. **D,** After embolization the metastatic focus has been effectively devascularized, making it possible to proceed with wide resection of the tumor. **E,** One year later, following internal hemipelvectomy and irradiation. A stable pseudoarticulation has been created that allows the patient to walk bearing full weight with a cane. **F,** The patient, 6 months postoperatively, bicycling with his grandson.

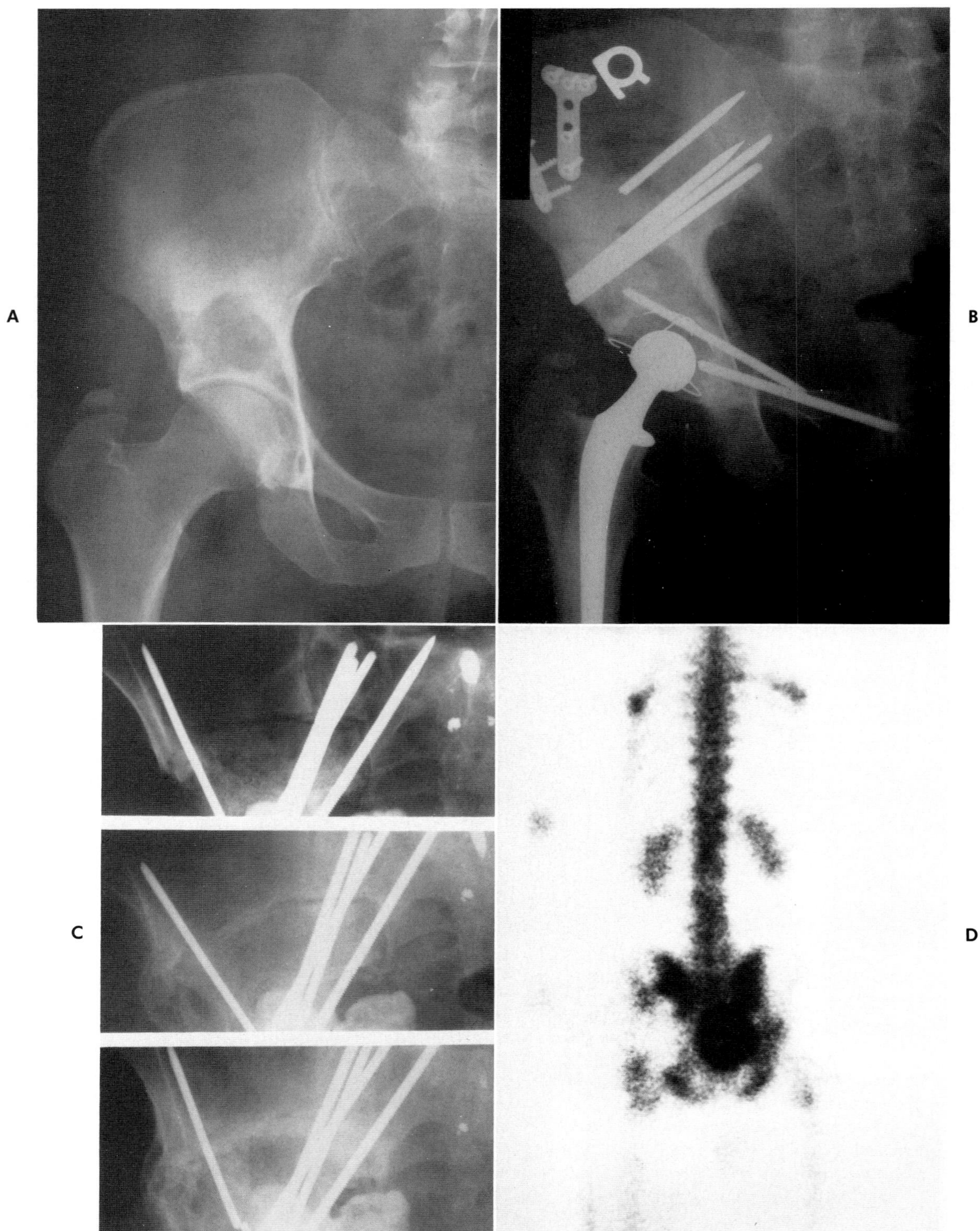

FIGURE 9-15. For legend see opposite page.

FIGURE 9-15 **A,** Class IV supraacetabular lesion similar to that shown in Fig. 9-14, *A,* but without a fracture through the involved segment. **B,** Five years after resection of the involved ilium with wide margins, autoclaving of the segment, and reconstruction of the pelvis with a total hip arthroplasty. **C,** Serial roentgenograms of a similar pelvic resection, autoclaving, and reconstruction for the management of a Class IV metastatic submaxillary cylindroma showing, *top,* the osteotomy line immediately postoperative, *middle,* 6 months later, and, *bottom,* 2 years postoperative after mature bony union of the graft. **D,** Three months postoperative, despite union at the graft-host junctions, the center of the autoclaved segment remains avascular (as demonstrated by a technetium-99 bone scan).

easily cleaned of extraneous soft tissues and remaining intraosseous tumor, leaving a bony model that obviously will fit exactly back into the pelvic defect. The implant then is affixed to the adjacent viable ischium, ilium, and pubis by a combination of threaded pins, cancellous bone screws, and bone plates (Fig. 9-15, *B*). Reaming and drilling of the acetabulum and cement fixation of an acetabular component are completed as for a conventional hip replacement arthroplasty.

Healing across the bone interspaces occurs rapidly and can be assessed roentgenographically (Fig. 9-15, *C*). However, because the nonviable segment of bone appears on roentgenograms to be no different from the adjacent viable bone, creeping replacement of the autoclaved segment by bone ingrowth must be evaluated with serial bone scans (Fig. 9-15, *D*). In the initial postoperative period these demonstrate a complete absence of blood supply to the central hemipelvic segment and no evidence of osteoblastic activity. Over the next 6 to 18 months creeping substitution of the segment can be documented. Once this appears to be well established (usually about 2 months postoperatively), full weight-bearing is allowed on the affected side.

We have performed seven such pelvic resections and replacements for carefully selected patients with solitary metastases. There have been no instances of local recurrence after follow-ups of between 18 months and 8 years. One patient evidenced pulmonary metastases 4½ years postoperatively and eventually died 1 year later of systemic carcinomatosis. However, during the first 5 postoperative years he was able to participate in a variety of recreational activities, including hiking and tennis, and enjoyed a pain-free range of hip motion from full extension to 100 degrees of flexion despite the formation of heterotopic bone about the implant. One other patient enjoyed an excellent return of function, resuming work as a carpenter (Fig. 9-16, *A*), until 2½ years postoperatively, when he experienced the sudden onset of pain and instability in the hip. Roentgenograms revealed that the implant had fractured through its central avascular portion despite bony union to the host pelvis at its periphery. The prosthetic acetabular component had become loosened and displaced as a result of the fracture (Fig. 9-16, *B*). At reoperation the autoclaved implant was found to be viable except for a distance of 1 to 2 cm on each side of the fatigue fracture. The prosthetic components were removed and the segment bone-grafted with cancellous allograft. During the succeeding 6 months the fracture healed. The hip arthroplasty components then were reinserted and the patient has had no further complications since.

RESULTS

The reconstructive procedures just described are extensive, the postoperative rehabilitation is lengthy, and the perioperative risks (at least potentially) are major. Obviously, only individuals with a projected life expectancy in excess of 18 to 24 months should be considered reasonable candidates. Patients with a poorer prognosis who suffer unstable acetabular fractures usually are better treated by a classical Girdlestone resection of the femoral head and neck despite the fact that such a procedure usually excludes the possibility of ever resuming unaided ambulation.

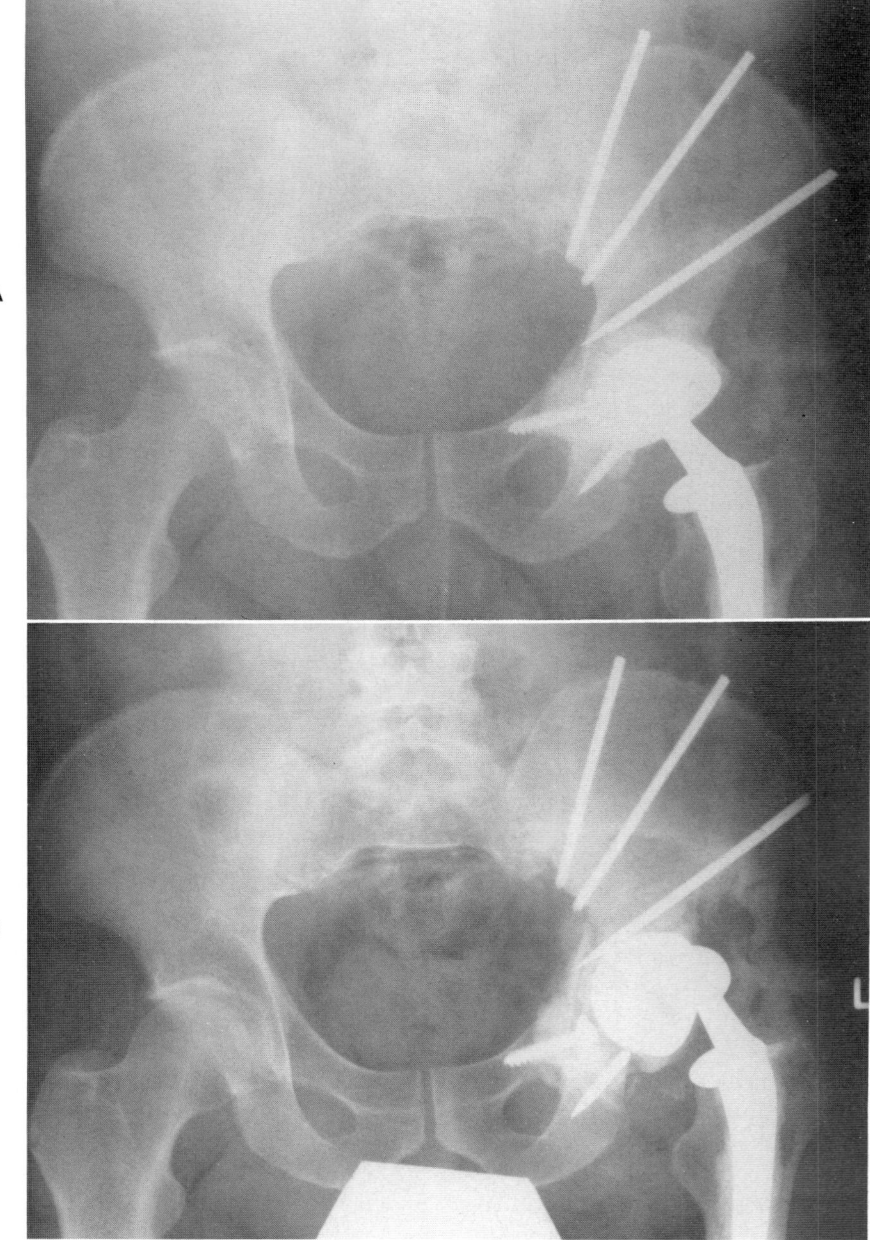

FIGURE 9-16 **A,** One year after resection and reconstruction of the right pelvis and hip in a 54-year-old man with primary chondrosarcoma of the ilium. The patient had returned to work as a carpenter and was without symptoms. **B,** Six months later he suffered a spontaneous fatigue fracture through the midportion of the still avascular graft. The acetabular prosthesis became displaced. The prosthetic components were removed, and the pelvis was bone grafted. Seven months later the graft had healed and the hip replacement was restored successfully.

To assess the applicability of prosthetic reconstruction in appropriate patients, it is necessary to analyze retrospectively the success of the procedure in affording lasting relief from hip pain and allowing resumption of independent walking. In addition, the incidence of prosthetic component loosening must be analyzed. Finally, survival statistics must be evaluated in an effort to ensure that the magnitude of the operation does not hasten the patient's ultimate demise. Fifty-eight patients with metastatic pathological fractures of the acetabulum, Classes I through III, who underwent prosthetic hip replacement were analyzed retrospectively with regard to these parameters. The results have been reported in detail previously.[10] The distribution of the primary sources of the 58 metastases is summarized in Table 9-1.

TABLE 9-1 **Distribution of 58 Primary Cancers**

Site	Number
Breast	22 (38%)
Other	36 (62%)
Colon	9
Prostate	5
Kidney	5
Thyroid	3
Lung	1
Miscellaneous	7
Unknown	3
Myeloma (multiple)	3

Pain Relief. The efficacy of affording relief from pain was considered to be the most important criterion of success for the procedure. Nine patients had experienced only minimal pain preoperatively and underwent tumor resection and hip replacement principally as prophylaxis against an impending fracture. Seven of these patients were in Class II. Thirty-one patients had had moderate pain preoperatively and required regular narcotic medications. They were unable to walk without external aids, and then only for short distances. Eighteen had had severe pain preoperatively, in most instances secondary to an acute fracture.

TABLE 9-2 **Pain***

	Minimum	Moderate	Severe
Preoperatively (58 patients)	9	31	18
Six months postoperative (51 patients)	37	10	4
Two years postoperative (30 patients)	24	0	6

*Minimum: used either no analgesics or non-narcotic analgesics. Moderate: used regular narcotic analgesics, not exceeding 30 mg of codeine. Severe: used regular, strong narcotic analgesics.

Postoperative pain was classified as minimum, moderate, or severe depending on the frequency and type of analgesics required. The results with regard to pain relief are summarized in Table 9-2. Not surprisingly, resolution of preoperative pain was significantly slower in these patients than is noted generally in patients undergoing conventional hip replacement arthroplasty for arthritis. This fact explains, at least in part, the much larger percentage of excellent results obtained in patients who were followed for 2 years as compared to those followed 6 months postoperatively.

At 6 months postoperative, the pain in 10 patients was rated as moderate and in 4 as severe. In 7 of the 10 who had a moderate rating, good or excellent pain relief was achieved later. The other three rated as moderate showed no evidence of recurrence of tumor, nerve invasion, or prosthetic loosening that could have explained the symptoms, although two of the three died shortly thereafter from systemic malignant disease. Of the four patients with results rated as poor (severe pain), two showed prosthetic loosening secondary to tumor recurrence locally and two showed intrapelvic invasion by tumor without evidence of prosthetic loosening.

At 2 years postoperative six patients had pain rated as severe. In two it was intractable hip and thigh pain that was thought to be secondary to intrapelvic invasion of the sacral plexus by tumor but was also aggravated by hip motion. Neither patient showed roent-

TABLE 9-3 **Ambulatory Status**

	Ambulatory			
	No Aids	**Cane or One Crutch**	**Crutches or Walker**	**Nonambulatory**
Six months postoperative (51 patients)	20	19	6	6
Two years postoperative (30 patients)	16	8	2	4

genographic evidence of loosening of the prosthetic components, however. In two patients there was definite loosening of the prosthetic components secondary to tumor recurrence and further osteolysis. The final two patients had resumed taking narcotics regularly in large doses as prescribed by the oncologists for a recurrence of "hip pain" that was considered to be probably secondary to tumor recurrence or prosthetic failure. However, an orthopaedic examination of both revealed evidence of simple trochanteric bursitis, which was successfully relieved after a single injection of triamcinolone acetate with lidocaine.

Ambulation. Of the 58 patients, 40 had been ambulatory (34 without external aids) until at least 3 weeks before hospitalization. Eighteen had been nonambulatory because of hip pain for more than 3 weeks preoperatively; six of these had been confined to a wheelchair for more than a year.

Postoperatively 54 patients regained the ability to walk with or without external aids. The four who did not walk postoperatively all had excellent relief from pain. The ambulatory status of the patients 6 and 24 months after arthroplasty is summarized in Table 9-3. Of the six who could not walk at 6 months, only two were so restricted because of hip pain. Two of the four who were nonambulatory 2 years postoperatively were so restricted by hip pain.

Solidity of Fixation. Postoperatively all patients received local irradiation if it had not been completed preoperatively. Despite this, in five patients there was evidence of local recurrence of tumor sufficiently large to result in loosening of the prosthetic acetabular component. There were no instances of loosening of either the femoral or the acetabular component for reasons other than recurrent tumor osteolysis. Although the patients with Class III disease had the most extensive evidence of bone destruction, none had prosthetic loosening or migration. There were no instances in which osteolysis became roentgenographically demonstrable about the threaded Steinmann pins. No symptoms were encountered that could be attributed to the pins' crossing the sacroiliac joint.

Survival. Of the 58 patients studied, two died in the early postoperative period. One patient with a highly vascular myeloma that had not been arterially embolized preoperatively died from the sequelae of extensive blood loss during tumor resection. The second patient died following a myocardial infarction 24 hours postoperative. Four patients were lost to follow-up between 8 and 39 months postoperatively but were doing well when last seen. Among the remaining 52 patients, the mean length of survival postoperatively is 29 months. This includes 20 patients still alive at more than 4 years postoperative.

When survival statistics for the 22 patients with metastatic carcinoma of the breast were analyzed separately, the mean length of survival was 36 months, with 10 patients still alive at the time of this writing. The mean survival for the remaining 36 patients with assorted primary tumors was 19 months, and 10 are still alive. Thirty of the fifty-eight patients have been followed for a minimum of 4 years postoperatively.

COMPLICATIONS

Prophylactic cephalothin was administered to every patient in a dose of 1 g intravenously just before the operation and then every 6 hours

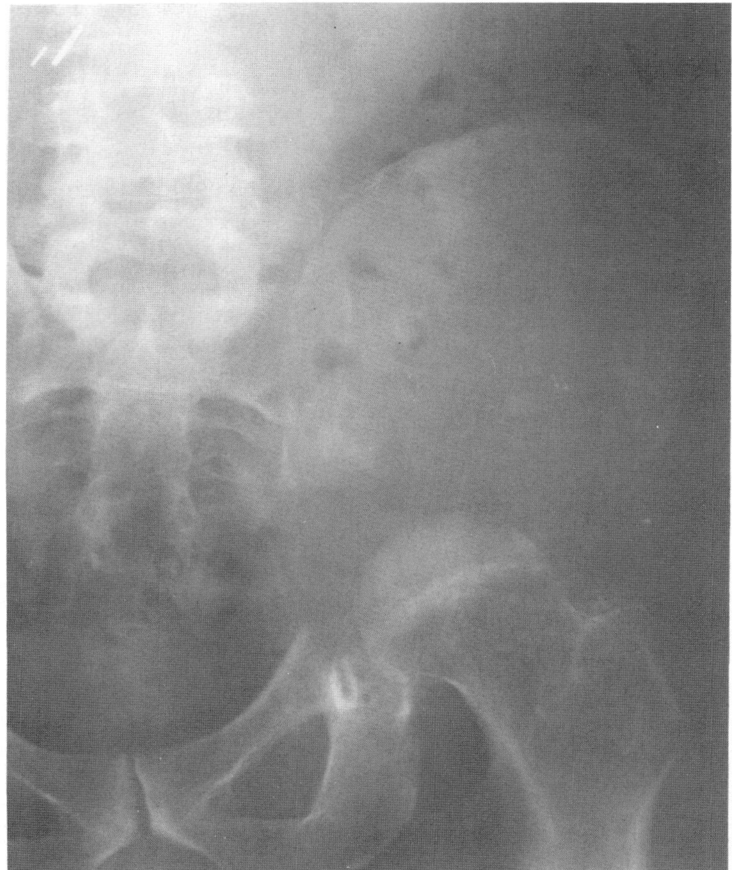

FIGURE 9-17 Extensive destruction of the left ilium from a metastatic lung cancer. This patient should not have been considered for any type of reconstruction, both because of the poor prognosis of the primary tumor and because the extent of destruction of the hemipelvis would have interfered with any reasonable attempt at reconstruction.

for the next 48 hours. There were no deep wound infections. Prophylactic anticoagulation was not used. One nonfatal pulmonary embolism occurred. One patient with Class III involvement had a complete femoral nerve palsy when a threaded Steinmann pin that was being inserted for prosthetic fixation penetrated the inner wall of the pelvis and "wound up" the nerve. No such soft tissue complications have occurred since we began using the technique of finger palpation along the inner and outer pelvic walls as demonstrated in Fig. 9-10, *E* and *F*. Cotler et al.[2] reported the development of an enteric fistula as the result of a medial wall acetabular fracture, but we have had no such direct complications of the fracture itself.

There is abundant clinical and experimental evidence[3,16] demonstrating that the presence of methylmethacrylate with metal prostheses or fixation devices neither is affected by nor interferes with the efficacy of postoperative irradiation.

SUMMARY

When considering whether to attempt reconstruction of the hip that has been destroyed by metastatic malignant disease, it is necessary to set up a hierarchy of surgical aims and to balance these against the risks of the specific procedure selected. In descending order of importance, these aims would be (1) to achieve lasting relief from hip pain, (2) to provide adequate stability of the hip for weight-bearing ambulation, (3) to regain sufficient hip motion for easy resumption of the activities of daily living, (4) to position and stabilize the hip for effective functioning of the normal surrounding muscles, (5) to restore equal limb lengths, and (6) to create a biomechanically sound joint system that is unlikely to collapse in the face of prolonged and repeated stresses. There certainly are situations in which tumor destruction is so extensive that joint stabilization or reconstruction by any technique cannot achieve a single one of these aims (Fig. 9-17). The surgeon also must be careful that his innate enthusiasm for mechanical hip reconstruction does not interfere with his ability to recognize a preterminal patient whose overall condition precludes any attempt at operative intervention.

Nevertheless, in all but the most severely affected patient, the techniques outlined here will successfully fulfill the criteria described and the reconstructed hip may be expected to function during follow-up periods that in our experience now extend for as long as 10 years postoperatively.

REFERENCES

1. Cooper, K.L., et al.: Insufficiency fractures of the sacrum, Radiology **156:**15, 1985.
2. Cotler, H.B., et al.: Enteric fistula as a complication of a pelvic fracture, J. Bone Joint Surg. **65A:**854, 1983.
3. Eftekhar, N.S., and Thurston, C.W.: Effect of irradiation on acrylic cement with special reference to fixation of pathological fractures, J. Biomech. **8:**53, 1975.
4. Enneking, W.F., and Durham, W.K.: Resection and reconstruction for primary neoplasms involving the innominate bone, J.Bone Joint Surg. **60A:**731, 1978.
5. Frankel, V.H., and Burstein, A.H.: Orthopedic biomechanics, Philadelphia, 1976, Lea & Febiger.
6. Greenwald, A.S., and Haynes, D.W.: Weight bearing areas in the human hip joint, J. Bone Joint Surg. **54B:**157, 1972.
7. Habermann, E.T., et al.: The pathology and treatment of metastatic disease of the femur, Clin. Orthop. **169:**70, 1982.
8. Hall, F.M., et al.: Protrusio acetabuli following pelvic irradiation, Am. J. Radiol. **132:**291, 1979.
9. Harrington, K.D.: The management of unstable pathologic fracture-dislocations of the spine and acetabulum secondary to metastatic malignancy. In American Academy of Orthopaedic Surgeons: Instructional course lectures, Vol. 24, St. Louis, 1980, The C.V. Mosby Co.
10. Harrington, K.D.: The management of acetabular insufficiency secondary to metastatic malignant disease, J. Bone Joint Surg. **63A:**653, 1981.
11. Harrington, K.D., et al.: The use of methylmethacrylate as an adjunct in the internal fixation of malignant neoplastic fractures, J. Bone Joint Surg. **54A:**1665, 1972.
12. Levy, R.N., et al.: Surgical management of metastatic disease of bone at the hip, Clin. Orthop. **169:**62, 1982.
13. McCollum, D.E., and Nunley, J.A.: Bone grafting in acetabular protrusio: a biologic buttress. In The hip. Proceedings of the sixth open scientific meeting of The Hip Society, St. Louis, 1978, The C.V. Mosby Co.
14. McGuigan, L.E., et al: Pubic osteolysis, J. Bone Joint Surg. **66A:**127, 1984.
15. Mizrahi, J., et al.: An experimental method for investigating load distribution in the cadaveric human hip, J. Bone Joint Surg. **63B:**610, 1981.
16. Murray, J.A., et al.: Irradiation of polymethylmethacrylate. *In vitro* gamma radiation effect, J. Bone Joint Surg. **56A:**311, 1974.
17. Sim, F.H., et al.: Total hip arthroplasty for tumors of the hip. In The hip. Proceedings of the fourth open scientific meeting of The Hip Society, St. Louis, 1976, The C.V. Mosby Co.
18. Sotelo-Garza, A., and Charnley, J.: The results of Charnley arthroplasty of the hip performed for protrusio acetabuli, Clin. Orthop. **132:**12, 1978.

CHAPTER 10

UPPER-EXTREMITY PATHOLOGICAL FRACTURES

The management of upper-extremity metastases has changed remarkably in recent years primarily because of the great improvement in survival statistics for patients with disseminated cancer. Twenty years ago pathological fracture of the humerus, by far the most commonly involved upper-extremity bone, was managed simply by external splintage and sling immobilization. Because upper-extremity stability was considered unimportant in a patient's ability to move in bed and/or walk, and because few patients survived long enough to warrant internal fixation of their fracture, the philosophy of management was one of benign neglect. However, as survival statistics have improved and techniques for irradiating metastases have changed, a complete reversal in the orthopaedist's attitude toward these fractures has occurred. This change principally has evolved from a gradual recognition of seven essential principles of upper-extremity pathological fracture management:

1. Once a displaced fracture occurs, healing rarely follows in the absence of internal fixation; and in the absence of healing, pain relief is difficult to obtain. Douglass et al.[5] reviewed a series of 29 pathological humeral fractures only eight of which were managed by internal fixation. Among the eight patients, seven enjoyed good relief from pain and restoration of arm function. However, of the 21 patients treated without internal fixation, only seven enjoyed relief from pain (five after irradiation) and the remaining 14 continued to be plagued by local fracture discomfort and instability, only minimally controlled by external immobilization. In essence, all fourteen were left with a functionally useless extremity.
2. The type of internal fixation required varies markedly depending on bone stability and the extent of tumor lysis. At one extreme is the patient with a localized lytic focus in whom a fracture appears likely but has not as yet occurred. This situation can be managed effectively by simple percutaneous intramedullary Rush rod splinting of the affected bone, local irradiation, and temporary limitation of activity until reossification of the lesion occurs. At the other extreme, and unfortunately much more commonly, an actual pathological fracture-displacement occurs, usually through a humerus diffusely weakened by metastatic disease (Figs. 10-1, *A*, and 10-2, *A*). In this situation attempts at simple percutaneous fixation by a small intramedullary device will not achieve effective limb stability or allow bony union even in the face of only minimal irradiation. Consequently internal fixation is required for most pathological upper-extremity fractures—including formal exposure of the fracture site, re-

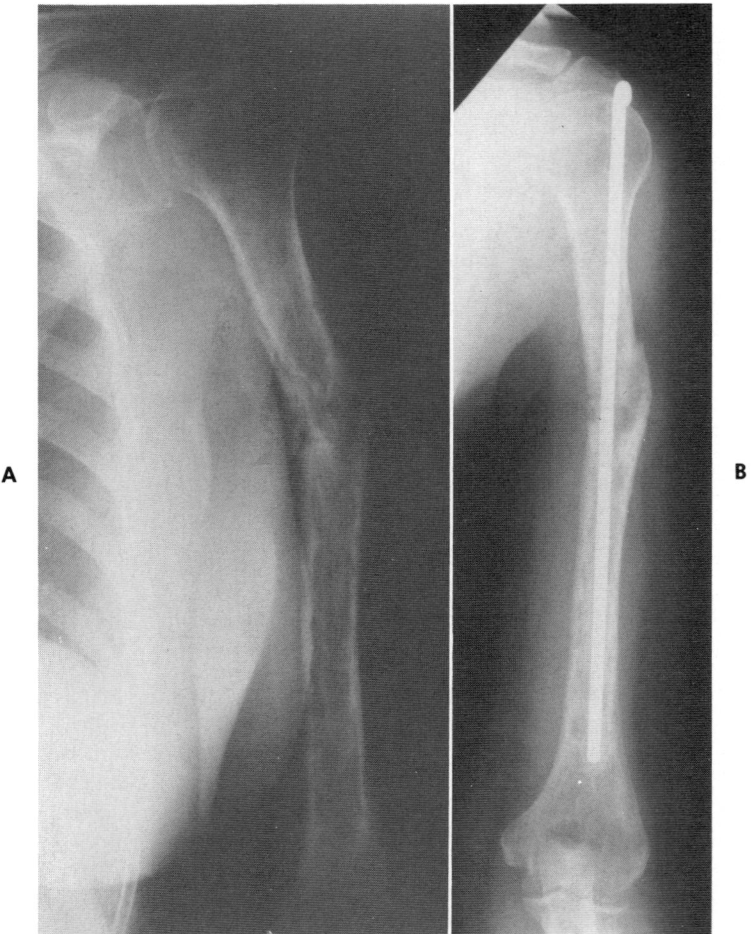

FIGURE 10-1 **A,** An AP roentgenogram of the left humerus in a 51-year-old woman with metastatic carcinoma of the breast. There is obvious involvement of the entire humeral diaphysis with marked cortical narrowing and a pathological fracture. **B,** Eight months after attempted internal stabilization by a Rush rod inserted without exposing the fracture site. The rod protrudes proximally and has caused shoulder pain and limitation of abduction. Painful motion of the unhealed fracture site has rendered the arm useless.

FIGURE 10-2 **A,** Left humerus of a 63-year-old physician with multiple myeloma. A large lytic lesion of the middiaphysis has progressed to a comminuted pathological fracture. **B,** Eleven months after attempted stabilization with a Rush rod inserted retrograde from the olecranon fossa. The fracture site was not exposed. The rod is much too small to fill the medullary canal. An obviously unstable nonunion of the fracture is apparent, resulting in a useless extremity. **C,** Two years 6 months after internal stabilization with a heavy compression plate augmented by methylmethacrylate. The patient has regained full shoulder motion and all but 15 degrees of elbow extension, and he has no residual pain at the fracture site. **D,** Pathological fracture of the right humerus initially stabilized internally with a small Rush rod inserted retrograde and augmented by intramedullary methylmethacrylate. Despite this fixation, the fracture became distracted, resulting in arm pain and instability. A secondary procedure was performed whereby further stabilization was attempted using a small bone plate. Five months later the plate broke and the pain and instability persisted. This case demonstrates the futility of attempting humeral stabilization with small intramedullary or extramedullary devices even when augmented by methylmethacrylate.

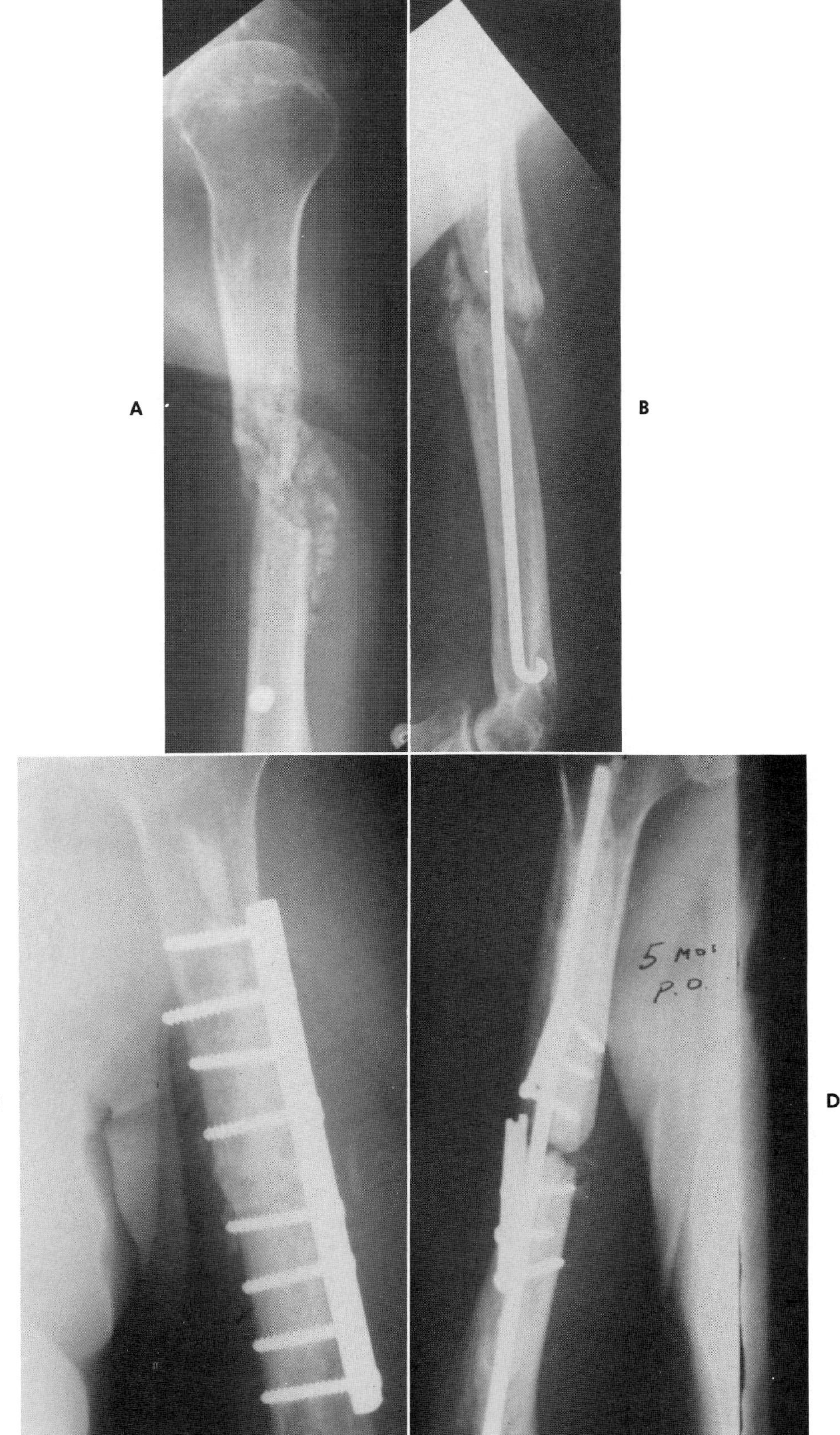

FIGURE 10-2 For legend see opposite page.

section of tumor tissue, and rigid fixation with strong devices augmented by methylmethacrylate to achieve bony union and lasting pain relief (Figs. 10-1, *B*, and 10-2, *B* and *C*).

3. As can be recognized from the two maxims just stated, the basic philosophy for managing fractures of the humerus secondary to metastatic disease is totally different from that applicable to the management of conventional humeral fractures. It is generally agreed[9,11,13,15] that most nonpathological fractures of the humeral shaft are best treated nonoperatively. However, occasionally indications exist for primary or secondary operative management. Stern et al.[18] have demonstrated that when open stabilization is called for percutaneous Rush rod fixation is preferable. They report a 9% incidence of nonunion among humeral shaft fractures managed thus as compared to a 39% incidence following open exposure of the fracture site for fixation, and they cite disruption of the intramedullary blood supply as the most likely cause of the higher nonunion rate.

   When a fracture results from tumor destruction of bone, one can assume that the intramedullary and often the periosteal vascular supply to any bone remaining locally already has been destroyed. The adverse effects on bone healing imposed by this local circulatory compromise, combined with the delays in bony union expected in the face of (often large) cortical gaps and after (even minimal) irradiation, renders the unstable intramedullary spintage advocated by Stern's group[18] for conventional fractures ineffective for pathological fractures.

4. As patients survive for longer and longer periods after the development of bone metastases, they are likely to become more and more dependent on their upper extremities to transfer in and out of bed, ambulate, or participate in even minimal activities of daily living. Once an individual suffers a pathological fracture of a lower-extremity long bone, the pelvis, or even a vertebra, it is likely that he will be forced to depend on some type of walking aid, at least intermittently, during the remainder of his life. If the use of such assistance is denied him by the inability to use his arms for partial weight-bearing, walking may become impossible even if the lower-extremity fracture is effectively stabilized.
5. Cancer patients who do become bedridden or confined to a chair eventually have little to look forward to during their remaining days if they are also denied the use of one or both arms. Most who have widespread metastases are able to adjust psychologically to the restrictions imposed by a chair- or bedbound existence. If, in addition, however, they are no longer able to use their arms to assist in daily hygiene, eating, reading, etc., they usually become severely depressed and lose the desire to live even in the absence of pain or mental deterioration.
6. Unlike the femur and the tibia, the humerus is a bone subjected to distractive forces at least as often as to compressive forces. Thus external functional braces of various sorts are less effective on the upper than on the lower extremity and, in fact, appear to afford little stability or pain relief for activities such as lifting, reaching, or even walking with the arm extended.
7. To achieve lasting relief from fracture pain, most patients require not only secure internal fixation but also subsequent postoperative irradiation. Modern radiation protocols that necessitate the use of more than a single portal to achieve maximal tumor control usually are impossible in the face of an unstable extremity where pain relief can be approached only by extensive external immobilization.

For all of these reasons most orthopaedic surgeons have become much more aggressive in advocating internal fixation for upper-extremity pathological fractures. At the same time they have been forced to develop fixation techniques that are quite different in concept from those usually applicable to lower-extremity fractures.

PATHOGENESIS

In Clain's series[4] of 2000 patients with metastatic bone disease, only approximately 20% had metastatic lesions of the upper extremity.

In Jaffe's study[10] of terminal cancer patients evaluated by meticulous postmortem examination, over 85% were noted to have bone metastases but less than 20% had demonstrable upper-extremity metastases. The usual sites were the vertebrae (69%), pelvis (41%), femur (25%), and ribs (25%). Among metastases to the upper extremities, by far most appeared in the humerus and that bone accounted for 94% of fractures requiring internal fixation. However, humeral lesions represented only 10% of the overall total of metastases. The scapula accounted for 6%, the clavicle 4%, and the bones distal to the elbow less than 1%. The majority of lesions distal to the elbow were from primary tumors of the lung, despite the fact[6,12,17] that only 6% of all metastatic pathological fractures come from lung metastases. This seeming paradox probably is explainable if one recalls that lung metastases to bone generally are seeded by direct arterial embolization whereas most other metastases spread through venous plexuses that rarely extend into the distal extremities.

The most frequent primary tumors responsible for metastases to the upper extremity are the same as those responsible for metastases elsewhere in the body—breast, prostatic, and kidney carcinomas and multicentric myelomas and lymphomas. In our series of 70 upper-extremity fractures (out of a total 399 long-bone pathological fractures) reported in 1976,[7] breast carcinoma accounted for 41%, myeloma for 29%, hypernephroma for 11%, prostatic carcinoma for 5%, and all other primary malignancies together for 14%.

PREOPERATIVE EVALUATION

Probably because the long bones of the upper extremities are subjected to less frequent and less intensive compressive and torque stresses than are those of the lower extremities, pathological fractures there usually occur relatively late in a patient's disease course. Almost invariably, when such fractures occur, a technetium-99 bone scan or even a roentgenographic bone survey will demonstrate multiple other metastatic foci throughout the body. The only exception to this rule is renal carcinoma, whose initial and often solitary bone metastasis may be to the proximal humerus. Renal carcinoma metastasis often produces a highly vascularized aneurysmal and expansile lesion of the proximal humerus (Fig. 10-5, *A* and *B*), occasionally produced by thyroid metastases as well. Such a single and aggressive-appearing metastatic lesion may be difficult to distinguish from a primary malignant sarcoma of bone, although in a patient over 50 years of age and with a history of another earlier malignancy, one should consider metastatic disease as the most likely diagnosis. Every such patient should receive at least an intravenous pyelogram and on occasion also a renal arteriogram even in the absence of a recognized primary tumor of the kidney.

When a primary carcinoma can be demonstrated elsewhere (unless its relationship with the osseus lesion is obvious), a biopsy specimen should be obtained before treatment is initiated. A needle or trocar biopsy of the lesion is easily accomplished, often aided by computed tomography. Among the diagnoses to be considered, but usually excludable after trocar biopsy, are Paget's disease, radiation osteitis, postirradiation sarcoma, infection, and even mastocytosis. *Paget's disease* of the upper extremity is uncommon, usually affects the bone with a diffuse and sclerotic roentgenographic picture dissimilar to that of metastatic disease, and rarely produces lytic cortical changes. However, at times it may closely mimic breast metastases. Moreover, when it occasionally does progress to a pagetoid sarcoma, the roentgenographic and scintigraphic appearance may be indistinguishable. *Radiation osteitis* usually appears as a diffuse process consisting of patchy sclerotic and lytic changes in a bone included in a previously irradiated field. Because many patients with breast and lung carcinomas have received chest wall irradiation following initial operative tumor resection, the scapula, clavicle, and proximal humerus not infrequently are affected by this process. Differentiation of the roentgenographic changes of radiation osteitis from those of metastatic carcinoma often can be made only by trocar biopsy. The differentiation is critical, however, lest there be the tragic consequences of further irradiation to a patient with radiation osteitis in the mistaken belief that he is suffering from metastatic cancer. *Sarcomas* arising in the proximal humerus and shoulder girdle following irradiation for breast carcinoma are uncommon, but again these must be distinguished from metastatic disease. Sim et al.[17] reported 34 cases of postirradiation sarcoma collected at the Mayo Clinic. Of these, nine involved the upper extremity. *Mastocytosis,* an obscure condition typically involving the upper-extremity long bones by sclerotic foci, often is confused with metastases. In the series of Barer et al.[1] there were four such upper-extremity lesions reported that originally had been suspected of being metastases. However, typically mastocytosis[17] appears roentgenographically with a uniform medullary distribution in the humerus and without obvious lytic destructive changes.

OPERATIVE MANAGEMENT

Fractures of the Humerus

As already noted, metastatic lesions of the humerus have a good prognosis for bone healing after irradiation so long as no actual fracture has supervened. Once a fracture occurs, the likelihood of eventual bony union is significantly poorer than for lower-extremity long bone fractures, probably because of the forces that tend to pull the major fracture fragments apart even after internal fixation (Fig. 10-2). Consequently the orthopaedic surgeon is faced with a difficult dilemma, trying to decide among three alternative treatments: (1) irradiation of a lesion before it fractures, (2) internal fixation of an impending fracture followed by irradiation, or (3) internal fixation of an established fracture on the assumption that healing is unlikely.

Prophylactic Fixation. The second alternative, prophylactic internal fixation of an impending fracture followed by irradiation, has a poor prognosis for bony union. We therefore recommend fixation of all humeral metastases *before* irradiation unless the lesion is largely extraosseus and the likelihood of subsequent fracture seems remote. It should be recognized that the humeral shaft, in particular, has a relatively small cortical mass and, once lytic changes are apparent therein roentgenographically, the amount of bone destruction often is in excess of half the cortical circumference (see Fig. 11-4). Moreover, the strength of remaining cortical bone will decrease, at least temporarily, after irradiation is begun because of a temporary hyperemic softening of bone and a partial devascularization of the periosteum.

When there is any doubt about the likelihood of a fracture occurring through a humeral lesion, it is advisable to internally splint the bone before irradiation is commenced. As already noted, this can be accomplished by a closed technique of intramedullary fixation so long as the lytic focus is not too extensive. Brumbach et al.[3] have popularized a technique for closed intramedullary fixation of such lesions whereby the extremity is draped freely and suspended by olecranon pin traction (Fig. 10-3, *A*). An image intensifier is used.

For lesions involving the middle and distal thirds of the humerus, a small triceps-splitting approach is made to the posterior humerus just proximal to the olecranon process but well distal to the spiral groove and radial nerve.

A hole is drilled through the posterior cortex of this surface, marking the distal extent of the insertion slot 1.5 cm proximal to the palpable lip of the olecranon fossa.

This hole is enlarged with a high-speed bur until it is approximately 1 cm wide (as wide as the distal humeral canal) and 1.5 cm long. If it is not made sufficiently long, attempts at subsequent rod insertion will require unnecessary force, thereby increasing the risk of a complete iatrogenic fracture.

Usually two Ender or Rush rods of between 23 and 30 cm are required, care being taken not to use rods that are too long lest they penetrate the humeral head. The rods should be prebent in an effort to allow their tips to bounce off the opposite humeral cortex without penetrating the often soft cortical bone at the tumor focus.

The first rod is inserted no deeper than 2 cm from its final intended position so the risk of its being driven into an irretrievable position as the second rod is inserted will be minimized.

After the second rod is inserted to the same depth, an 18-gauge wire is passed through the eye of each rod and the two are twisted together, thereby forcing the devices to work in tandem as a single construct (Fig. 10-3, *B*).

The rod tips and wire are driven beneath the cortical surface and the hole is filled with methylmethacrylate both to ablate the cortical defect as a potential stress riser and to minimize the risk of the rods' subsequently backing out.

No patients have been reported to suffer permanent limitation of elbow motion[3,18] so long as the rod tips have not extended into the olecranon process or impinged on the ole-

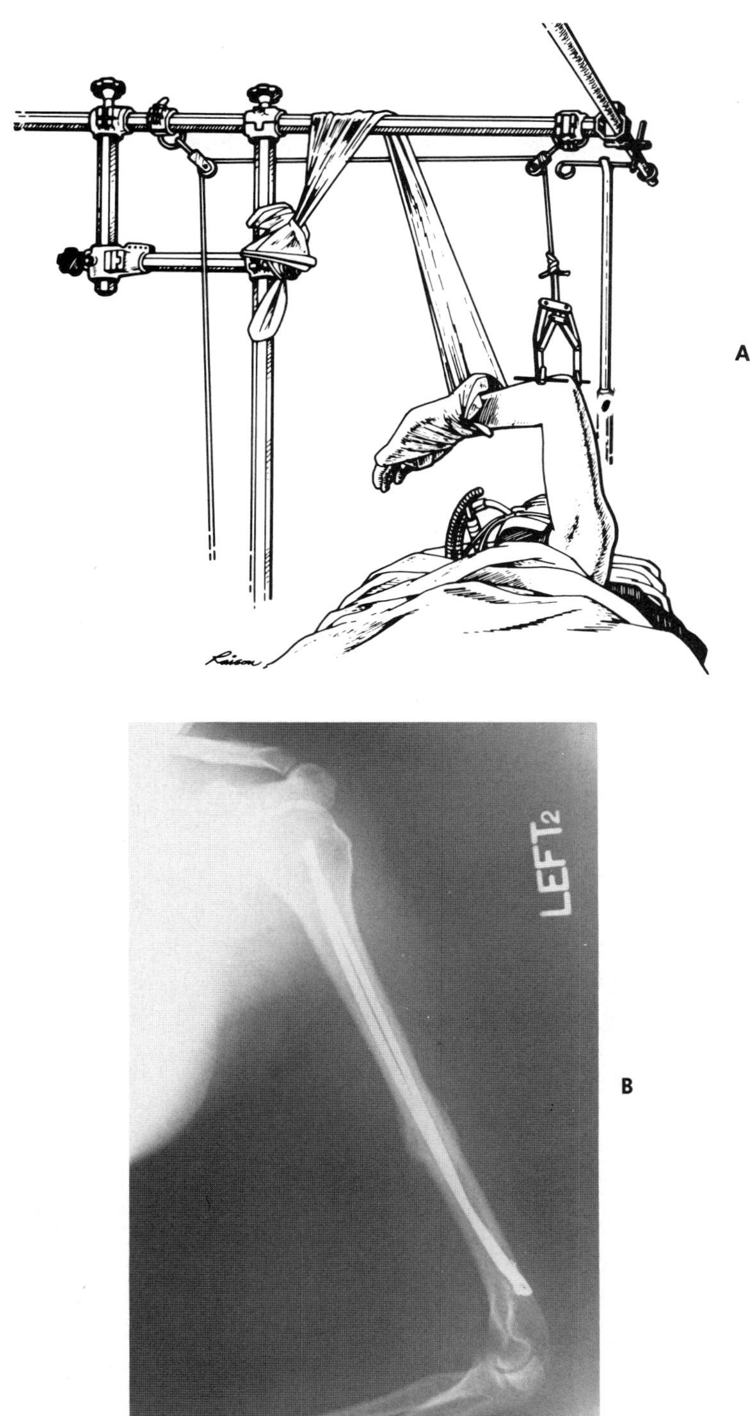

FIGURE 10-3 **A,** Intraoperative suspension apparatus used for "closed" retrograde intramedullary rod fixation of impending humeral shaft fractures. The surgeon stands facing the extensor side of the injured extremity. The image intensifier is parallel to the floor and placed across the patient's torso from the contralateral side. **B,** Lateral roentgenogram of a humerus managed by retrograde Ender nail fixation of a diaphyseal lesion. The nails were inserted proximal to the olecranon groove. The fracture healed, and the patient recovered full shoulder and elbow motion. (Courtesy Robert J. Brumbach, M.D.)

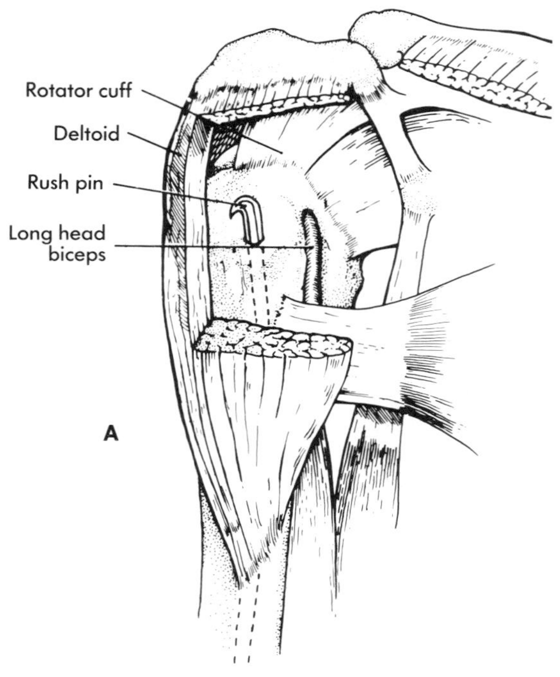

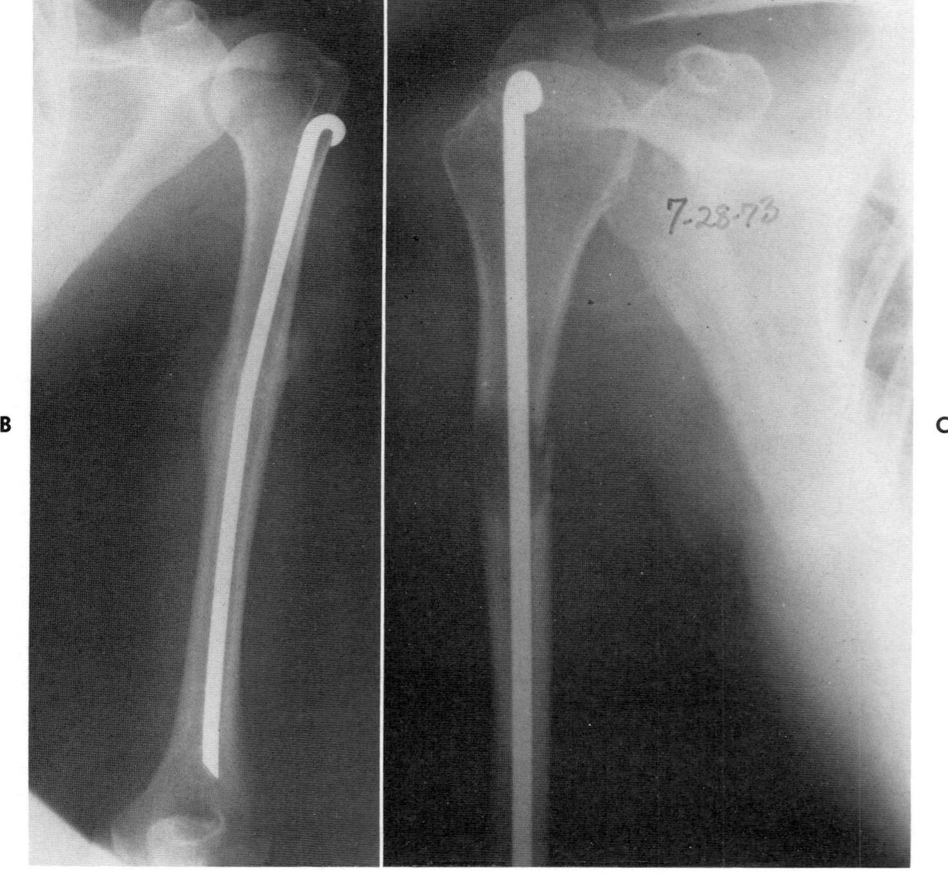

FIGURE 10-4 For legend see opposite page.

FIGURE 10-4 **A,** Diagram of the proximal humerus showing the preferred site for antegrade insertion of a Rush rod, on the superolateral surface of the greater tuberosity. This point is well below the insertion of the supraspinatus muscle and avoids injury to the rotator cuff. **B,** Lytic lesion of the humeral diaphysis, not yet complicated by a fracture, stabilized prophylactically with a Rush rod inserted anterograde. Bony union occurred without difficulty. The entry point of the rod is entirely outside the rotator cuff, and the patient regained full painless shoulder motion. **C,** Similar but larger lytic lesion of the proximal humerus that has progressed to a displaced fracture with the major fragments slightly distracted. In this instance fixation by a Rush rod was inadequate because of the wide separation between the cortices and because the distal shaft fragment had free rotational mobility. The fracture failed to unite. (**A** reprinted with permission from Stern, P.J.: J. Bone Joint Surg. **66A:**644, 1984.)

cranon tip during elbow extension.

More proximal lesions can be prophylactically fixed by Ender or Rush rods inserted anterograde through a cortical hole placed well distal to the prominence of the greater tuberosity (Fig. 10-4, *A*). A similar technique of semiclosed insertion[3] is used under the control of an image intensifier. To avoid impinging on the acromion during shoulder abduction, it is essential that the rod tip protrude from the humeral cortex well distal to the tuberosity (Fig. 10-4, *B*). Stern et al.[18] reported a 56% incidence of adhesive capsulitis of the shoulder when such impingement was allowed to occur because of antegrade fixation by Rush rods inserted in the more conventional manner, through the proximal tip of the greater tuberosity. Sim and Pritchard[16] stated that a Rush rod can be inserted through the proximal tuberosity and its tip can be left extending up to 3 mm above the proximal humeral articular surface without causing an acromial impingement syndrome. In our experience, however, the tolerances for abduction are much closer. Some patients will experience permanent restriction of shoulder abduction, even if the pins do not protrude, because heterotopic ossification or calcification develops above the tuberosity along the track of rod insertion. All these problems are avoided simply by choosing a more distal site for insertion of the rod.

Once prophylactic fixation has been accomplished, irradiation of the metastatic focus can be commenced. Generally a course of between 2000 and 2500 cGy* is sufficient to prevent local recurrence and yet not prevent bone healing of the focus so long as a fracture has not occurred. We favor external splintage of the humerus using a functional sleeve type of brace during the period of radiation and for approximately 3 weeks thereafter. The limb also should be protected for an additional 6 weeks after removal of the splint.

It is to be emphasized again that although the techniques described here are simple, reliable, and therefore ideal for prophylactic fixation of impending humeral fractures, and although the vast majority of such lesions will show bony healing after such fixation and irradiation, these techniques are not appropriate for established pathological fractures. Once an actual fracture has occurred, particularly if the major fragments are at all displaced, such small rods will be inadequate to prevent distraction at the fracture site or to resist rotational forces across the defect. They cannot accomplish lasting humeral stability in the absence of a bony union. The prognosis for union of an established pathological fracture-displacement of the humerus is relatively poor no matter what fixation system is used. Consequently different techniques have been developed for internal stabilization—each involving direct exposure of the fracture site, removal of as much tumor tissue as possible to enhance the efficacy of subsequent irradiation or chemotherapy, and augmentation of conventional internal fixation devices by methylmethacylate injected within the medullary canal. Pugh et al.,[14] using biomechanical strain-gauge analysis, have demonstrated that the most secure means of fixing a fracture model is to insert a large intramedullary nail or two large (⅜ inch or 9.5 mm) Rush rods

*Centigray (cGy) is the currently accepted designation for radiation absorbed dose.

augmented by methylmethacrylate within the medullary canal. It is unfortunate that commercially available Rush rods do not come in sizes larger than 6 mm (¼ inch) and most humeri have an intramedullary canal too small to allow insertion of the 9.5 mm rods, even if they were available. In fact, many women with a humeral fracture have such small canals that it is difficult to force even a single commercially available large (¼-inch) Rush rod down the canal and then augment the fixation by methylmethacrylate (Fig. 10-4, *C*). Moreover, fractures of the most proximal and most distal humerus cannot be stabilized effectively by simple intramedullary fixation techniques.

Because the different areas of the humerus require different techniques for pathological fracture stabilization, it seems most reasonable to approach the discussion by considering the particular requirements of each region of that bone as well as the varieties of challenges that may be encountered in a given region.

Proximal Humerus. As already noted, destructive metastatic lesions of the proximal humerus are different from other metastatic foci in that they not infrequently are the only manifestations of an otherwise occult malignancy (Fig. 10-5, *A*). Moreover, they often are highly vascularized (Fig. 10-5, *B*), representing metastases from retroperitoneal malignancies (particularly hypernephroma) much more commonly than the overall distribution of long bone metastases would suggest. This last peculiarity appears to reflect, at least in part, the anatomical distribution of the paravertebral venous plexuses arising in the retroperitoneal soft tissues, as originally described by Batson.[2]

When such lesions do represent solitary metastases, it may be appropriate to consider wide resection of the proximal humerus as a curative attempt. Before such an operation should be considered, however, it is essential that the surgeon ensure that (1) the primary malignancy has been identified and ablated, (2) there are no other metastases, and (3) wide margins can be achieved around the proximal humeral specimen to be resected. Bone scintigraphy and lung and abdominal computed tomography are essential for ruling out other metastatic disease, as is further more specific evaluation of any questionable site.

To achieve adequate margins around a large solitary metastasis of the proximal humerus, it usually is necessary to perform a resection of the distal clavicle, lateral scapula, and glenoid, as well as of the proximal humerus (the so-called Tikhoff-Lindberg resection). The brachial plexus and brachial artery are spared, but in most cases the radial nerve is removed with the specimen. This procedure usually gives wide margins around the tumor focus and also cleans out the axillary node contents, especially when the neurovascular bundle can be easily cleared from the tumor. The prognosis for separating the neurovascular bundle easily from the tumor can be assessed by preoperative arteriography. The loss of the radial nerve results in a wrist drop deformity, which can be compensated by the use of a cock-up splint.

Much more commonly evidence of metastatic disease elsewhere makes it inappropriate to consider alternatives other than fracture stabilization or palliative prosthetic replacement. Occasionally there will be sufficient bone stock remaining in the humeral head to allow attempts at internal fixation of the fracture (Fig. 10-5, *D*). In such circumstances we have found that a short right-angled blade plate, of the type used for proximal femoral osteotomies in pediatric patients, is the most secure means for stabilizing the short proximal segment. This type of fixation should be augmented by removal of as much gross tumor as possible and by filling the medullary canal with methylmethacrylate. The typical proximal humeral metastasis is managed more appropriately by resection and prosthetic replacement followed by local irradiation. Ideally one can use a custom proximal humeral prosthesis fashioned directly from preoperative roentgenograms (Fig. 10-5, *D*). However, manufacture of such a prosthesis ordinarily requires between 6 and 8 weeks, and many patients with severe post-fracture pain and a limited life expectancy are not best served by such a delay. We have found that with few exceptions the results in terms of restored of function and relief from pain are as good if one simply uses a conventional Neer proximal humeral prosthesis and recreates continuity with the humeral metaphysis using methylmethacrylate (Fig. 10-5, *E*). In situations requiring an extensive resection of the

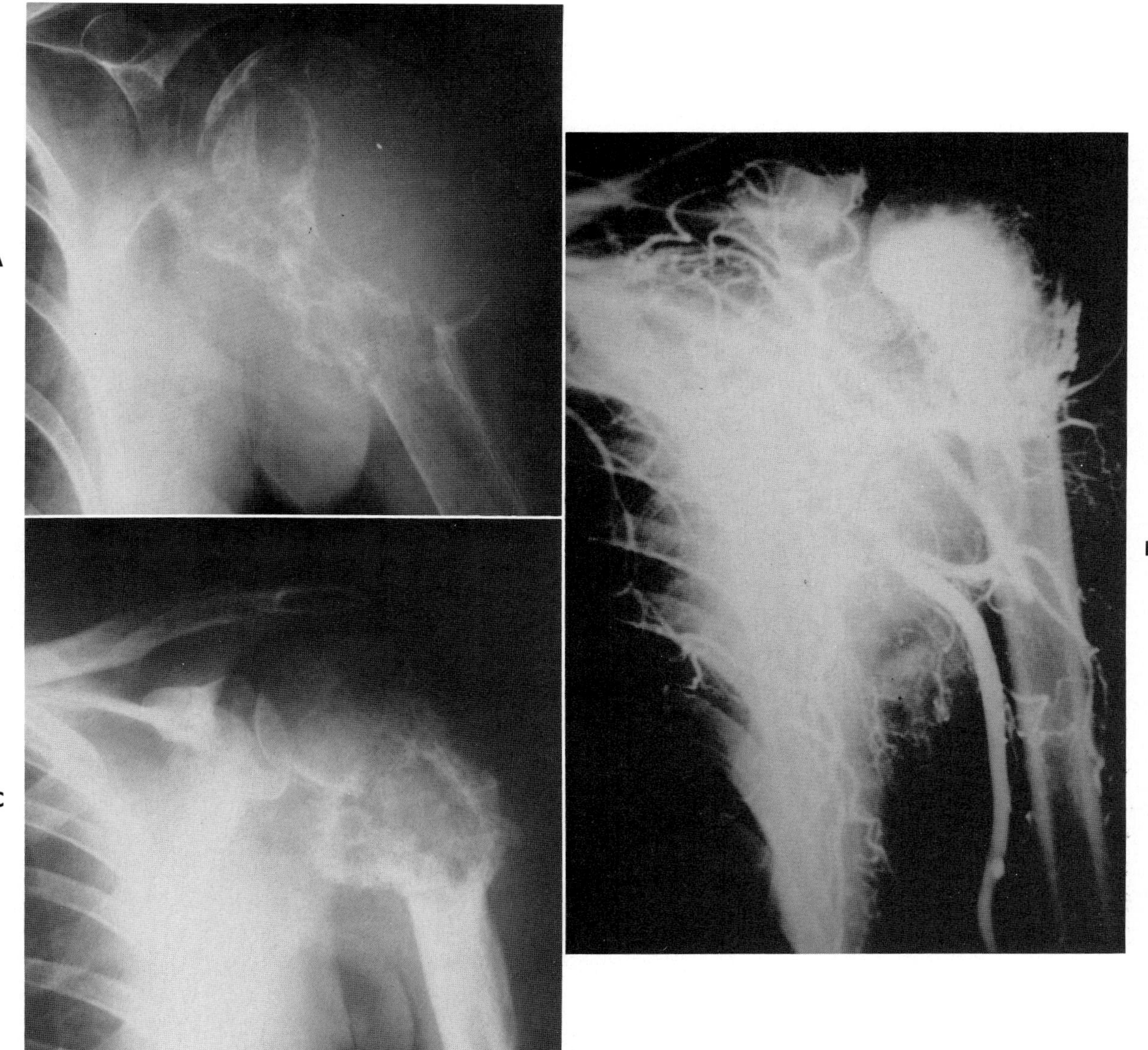

FIGURE 10-5 **A,** Aneurysmal metastatic hypernephroma that has destroyed the proximal humerus in a 52-year-old man with no other demonstrable metastases. A nephrectomy had been performed 3 years before this roentgenogram was obtained. The proximal humerus was resected with wide margins and replaced by a custom prosthesis. The patient enjoyed excellent relief of pain and regained 60 degrees of glenohumeral abduction and 70 degrees of flexion despite the resection of his rotator cuff. **B,** Arteriogram of the left upper extremity in a 45-year-old man with an aggressive metastatic hypernephroma of the proximal humerus. A highly vascularized lesion is apparent. **C,** Proximal humerus of a patient with a metastatic hypernephroma that caused extensive lysis of the humeral metaphysis and a pathological fracture. The humeral head and tuberosities are intact. Such a fracture is best managed by fixation with a pediatric right-angled blade plate augmented by local tumor curettage and packing of the defect with methylmethacrylate. (**B** courtesy Edward T. Habermann, M.D.) *Continued.*

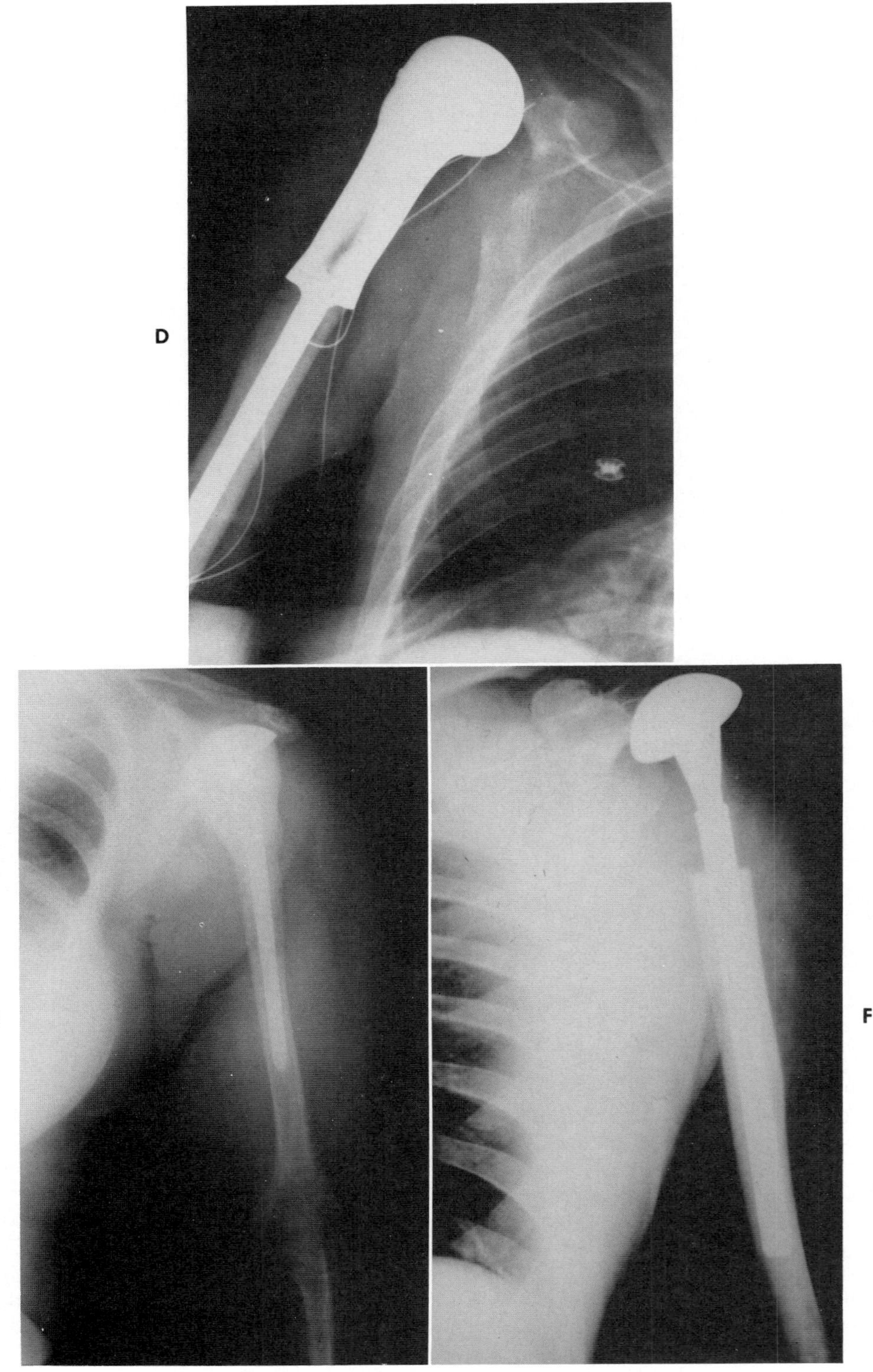

FIGURE 10-5, cont'd. For legend see opposite page.

FIGURE 10-5, cont'd. **D,** An aggressive lytic metastasis in the proximal humerus, again from a primary hypernephroma, has been resected and replaced by a custom fitted prosthesis. Such a prosthesis can be fashioned from properly measured preoperative roentgenographic images. **E,** A similar lesion of the proximal humerus has been resected and replaced by a conventional Neer prosthesis. The junction between the prosthetic articular margin and the remaining humeral metaphyseal shell has been recreated by molded methylmethacrylate. **F,** Postoperative roentgenogram following resection of the lesion in **B.** A Kuntscher nail was inbedded in the humeral diaphysis, the stem of a Neer prosthesis inserted through the nail lumen, and the construct secured with acrylic cement. The patient remained active and engaged in limited athletics until his death 6 years later. (**D** courtesy Franklin H. Sim, M.D.; **F** courtesy Edward T. Habermann, M.D.)

proximal humerus, Habermann has used a technique whereby a Kuntscher nail is inserted into the remaining humeral shaft and the stem of a Neer prosthesis is cemented within that nail (Fig. 10-5, *F*). It must be remembered that all these proximal humeral replacement arthroplasties require resection of the rotator cuff tendons and the prosthesis thus tends to ride high in the subacromial area. Despite this, however, most patients enjoy excellent relief from the pain and approximately one third also are able to demonstrate surprisingly good shoulder abduction and forward flexion. Use of as large a prosthetic head as possible seems to improve the likelihood of the patient's regaining subsequent shoulder motion.

Humeral Diaphysis. A fracture of the humeral shaft must be analyzed carefully before any decision is made about what technique may be employed for fixation. As already demonstrated (Figs. 10-1, *B*, and 10-2, *B*), Rush or Ender rods are not ideal for fixation because they cannot prevent distraction of the major fragments and they are only minimally effective in resisting torque stresses. Alternative techniques for internal stabilization include the use of an intramedullary nail (Kuntscher, A-O, or Sampson) and the use of a compression side plate. Applicability of the former obviously is limited by the diameter of the intramedullary canal. Small women often do not have humeri of sufficient size to allow such fixation. The efficacy of a compression plate may be limited by the extent of tumor destruction of adjacent bone or by the extent of intact bone distal to the fracture (Fig. 10-7, *C* and *E*). Consequently, before undertaking open reduction and fixation of such a fracture, it is essential to evaluate the size of the medullary canal and also carefully consider whether bony cortices on each side of the fracture are sufficiently strong to allow for secure stabilization by a heavy compression plate.

When a fracture occurs through a well-circumscribed metastasis, particularly in the midhumeral diaphysis (Fig. 10-6, *A*), a heavy compression plate is ideal for fixation (Fig. 10-6, *B*). A longitudinal incision paralleling the palpable interval between the biceps and the brachialis is used, and the humeral shaft is approached by blunt dissection through the midportion of the brachialis muscle. According to Henry,[8] who has popularized this approach, the radial nerve will remain protected by the remaining posterior bulk of the brachialis and need not be more specifically identified. In our experience, however, the nerve frequently is displaced from its normal anatomical position either by the tumor mass or by the fracture fragments themselves. On two occasions we have found the radial nerve caught between the fracture fragments (Fig. 10-6, *C*), although in neither instance was there evidence of neurological dysfunction either preoperatively or postoperatively. In one additional instance, in which the patient suffered a pathological fracture at the junction of the middle and distal thirds of her humerus, her oncologist made the decision to manage the fracture himself by external splintage with irradiation. A progressive radial nerve palsy became apparent after 9 months and existed in association with an unstable nonunion of the fracture. At operation the radial nerve was found to be encased in dense scar tissue crossing the pseudoarthrosis site and firmly trapped between the fracture fragments. It recovered within 8 weeks after neurolysis and effective fixation of the fracture, and the fracture healed despite having received 4000 cGy of irradiation.

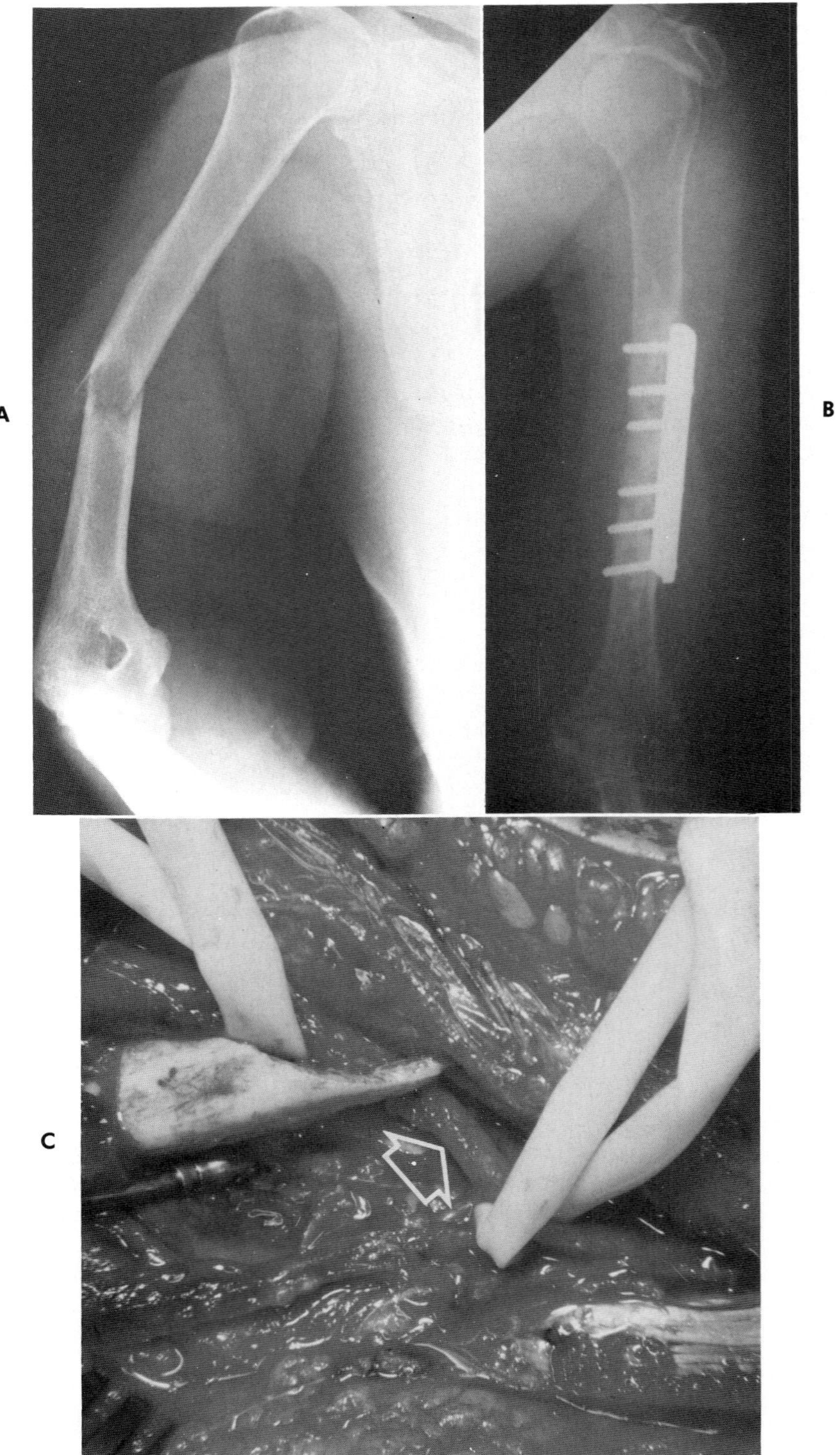

FIGURE 10-6 For legend see opposite page.

FIGURE 10-6 **A,** Well-localized midhumeral lytic lesion from a metastatic breast carcinoma that resulted in a pathological fracture. This fracture is ideal for compression plate fixation augmented by intramedullary methylmethacrylate. **B,** Similar pathological fracture, again from a well-circumscribed lytic breast metastasis, stabilized with a six-hole compression plate augmented by intramedullary cement. At operation the radial nerve was found to be caught between the fracture fragments, although the patient had no neurological deficit. The nerve was freed from the fracture site and gently retracted during stabilization. Postoperatively the fracture progressed to bony union despite 2000 cGy of irradiation. **C,** Intraoperative view of the fracture site showing the radial nerve *(arrow)* caught between the fracture surfaces.

Consequently we recommend identifying the radial nerve deep to the brachialis and well proximal to the fracture site, carefully dissecting it free of tumor and bone debris, and protecting it with two Penrose drains. Using this technique, we have had no radial nerve palsies in 16 open fixations of pathological humeral diaphyseal fractures.

When there is extensive destruction of cortical bone on both sides of the fracture site (Fig. 10-7, *A* and *B*), the conventional technique using screw fixation of six cortices proximal and six distal to the fracture is inadequate (Fig. 10-7, *C* and *E*). Effective alternatives include the use of a large heavy compression plate allowing at least six cortical screws for fixation into good bone on each side of the fracture (Fig. 10-7, *D*) or, in patients with a sufficiently large medullary canal, the use of an intramedullary nail of the Kuntscher type (Fig. 10-7, *F*). When a Kuntscher nail is used, it must be inserted proximally through the point of attachment of the rotator cuff tendons. It is essential that the nail tip be buried beneath the cortical surface and that the rotator cuff insertion be reestablished directly to bone.

With either alternative, methylmethacrylate should be injected and packed within the intramedullary canal to enhance fixation by minimizing varus angulation strains (in the case of the plate) and to increase resistance to torque stress (in the case of the rod). Often it is also necessary to resect some structurally inadequate bone and then bring the intact cortices of the major fragments together by shortening the humerus slightly. Unlike the situation with lower-extremity fractures, significant discrepancy in humeral length is of minimal functional significance.

Supracondylar Fractures. Supracondylar humeral fractures are particularly difficult to stabilize because the marked flattening of the bone at the olecranon fossa precludes both direct intramedullary fixation and the use of an angled blade plate of any sort (Fig. 10-8, *A* and *C*). The most effective means for stabilizing such a fracture is by two Rush rods inserted retrograde, one through the medial and one through the lateral epicondyle (Fig. 10-8, *B*). Some degree of three-point fixation is achieved by each rod (Fig. 10-9, *D*), and the combination of rods effectively prevents varus or valgus malalignment of the fracture fragments. The construct is minimally resistant to torque stresses, however, because the rods usually cross each other right at the level of the fracture-tumor defect (Fig. 10-8, *A* and *C*). Consequently it is essential that the medullary canal be thoroughly debrided of residual tumor tissue and then filled well proximal and well distal to the fracture site with methylmethacrylate. By hollowing out the distal fragment well beyond the metaphyseal flare and, if possible, down along each side of the olecranon fossa (Fig. 10-10, *B* and *C*), one can make the methylmethacrylate filling the defect also diminish the risk of fracture fragment distraction by gravity or lifting-traction stresses. Despite the rather tenuous roentgenographic appearance of these constructs, they function in a remarkably stable manner and almost invariably afford excellent relief from pain. After 19 pathological fractures so managed, we have seen no instances of fixation failure even when, as on three occasions, only a single Rush rod could be used for fixation (Fig. 10-10, *B* and *C*).

The distal humerus is approached via a Henry type of hockey stick incision,[8] the

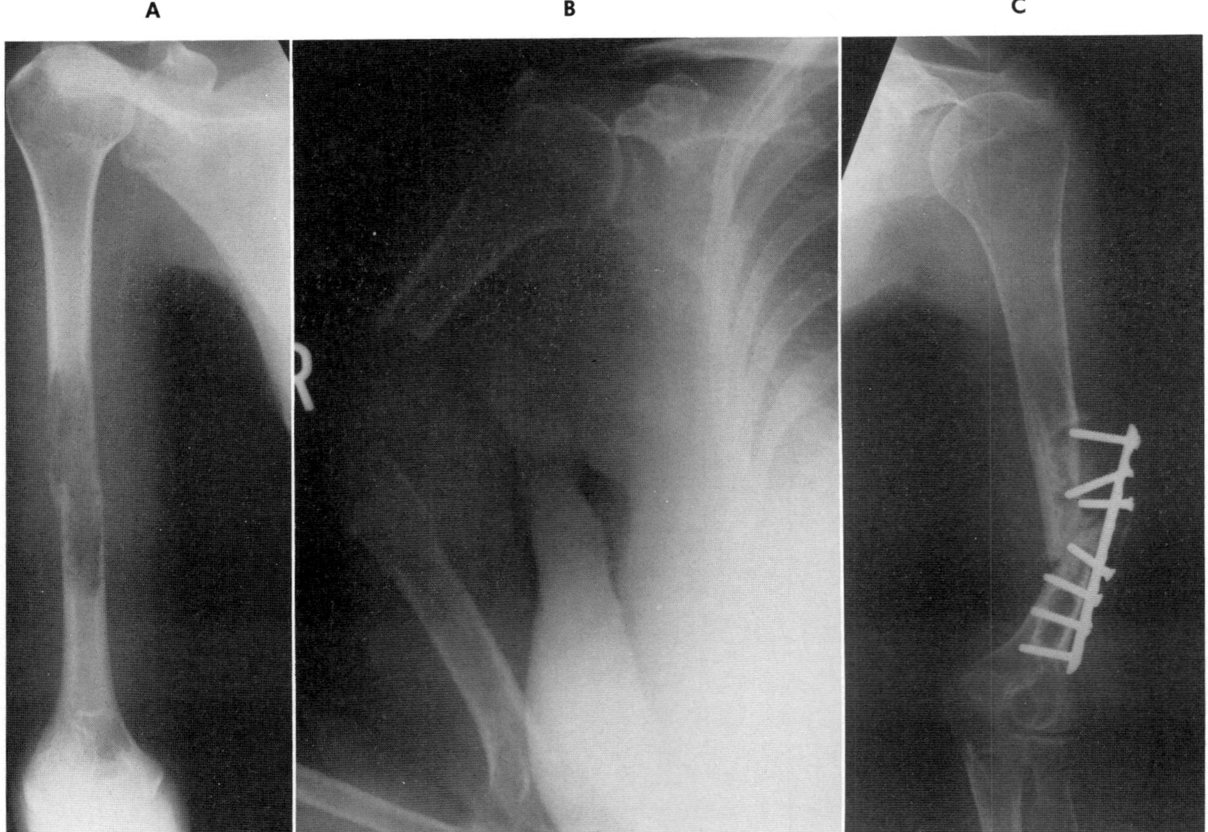

FIGURE 10-7 **A,** Pathological fracture of the humeral shaft through an extensive area of reticulated lysis secondary to breast carcinoma metastases. From a biomechanical viewpoint the entire segment of affected bone must be considered structurally absent. Because the medullary canal is small, stabilization will be best achieved by humeral shortening and plate fixation with 12 screws imbedded in intact cortices, six above and six below the extent of tumor lysis. **B,** Another pathological fracture. Note the more extensive bone loss here than in **A.** However, the requirements for stabilization are virtually identical. **C,** Similar fracture through an extensive lytic lesion. This was managed by attempted plate fixation into structurally inadequate bone. The upper four screws quickly pulled out of the tumor-infiltrated cortex.

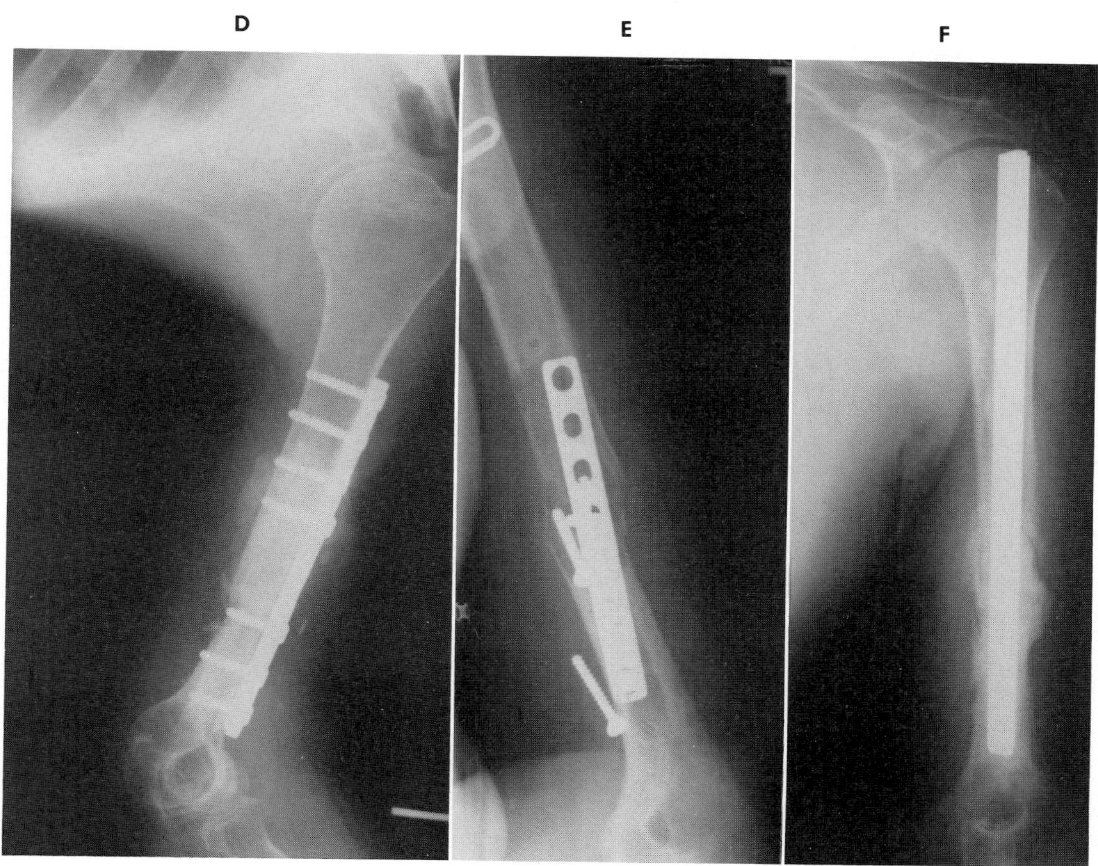

FIGURE 10-7, cont'd. **D,** Shortening of the humerus was then accomplished, with apposition of adequate cortices and fixation by a compression plate augmented with intramedullary cement. Because no further irradiation was contemplated, the fracture was bone grafted. Bony union ensued and the patient regained 15 to 125 degrees of elbow motion. **E,** Extensive lysis from a myeloma in another patient. An attempt at stabilization using a small bone plate with screw fixation into structurally inadequate bone was unsuccessful. Failure ensued promptly. **F,** Because this humerus had a large intramedullary canal, fixation was best accomplished by a slight shortening of the bone and the use of a Kuntscher nail augmented by cement. The nail was inserted through a small incision in the supraspinatus tendon, and its tip was buried beneath the cortical surface.

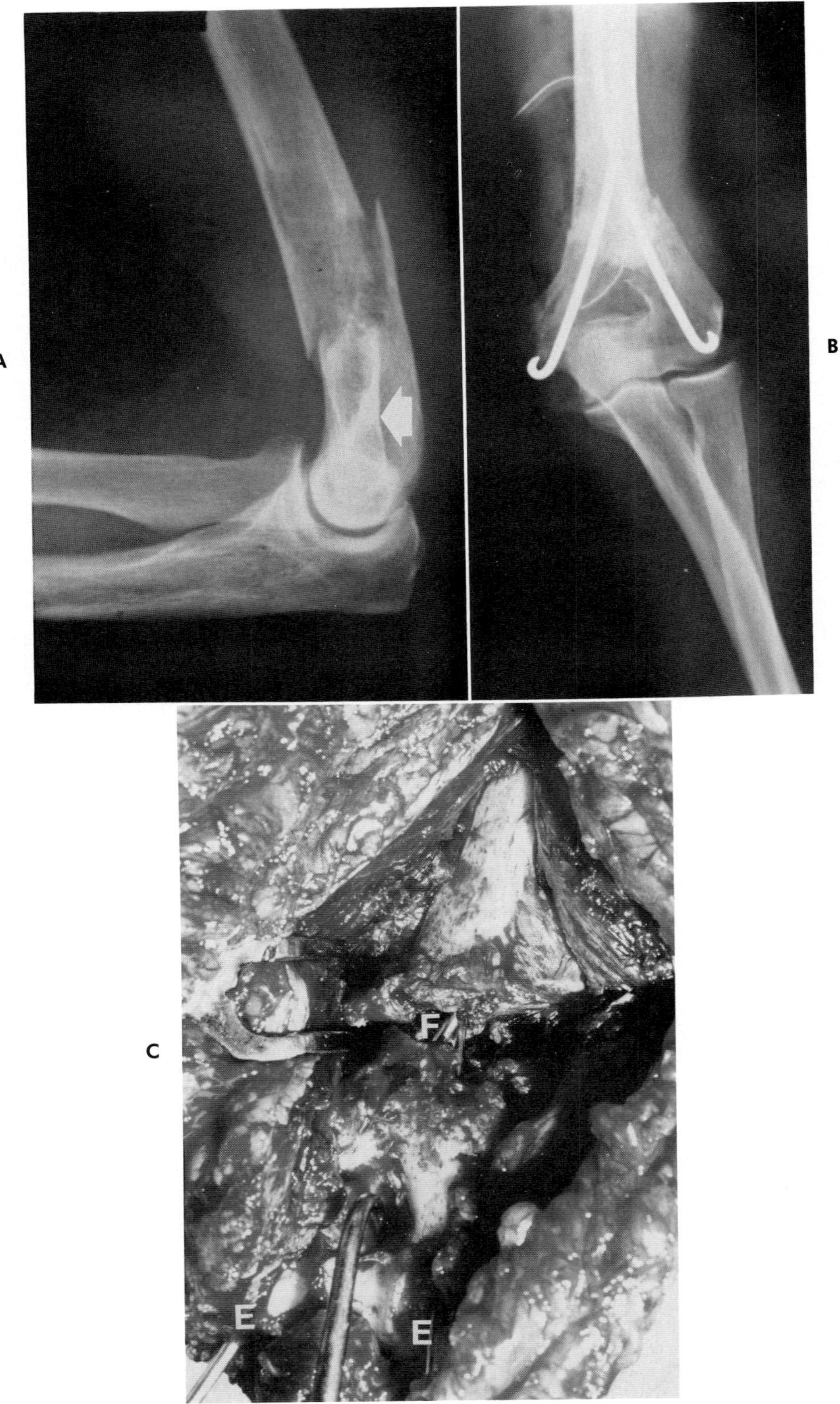

FIGURE 10-8 For legend see opposite page.

FIGURE 10-8 **A,** Destructive lesion of distal humerus secondary to metastatic thyroid cancer. This lateral roentgenogram demonstrates well the anteroposterior narrowness of the humerus at the level of the olecranon fossa *(arrow)*. **B,** The fracture has been internally fixed with two Rush rods inserted retrograde from each epicondyle and reinforced by intramedullary methylmethacrylate. The rods cross one another at the level of the fracture and consequently afford minimum resistance to rotational stresses. It would have been preferable to inject the cement further into the distal fragment for resistance against rotational and distractional forces. **C,** Intraoperative view of a similar pathological fracture exposed from behind by a triceps-splitting incision. Note the bone hook in the olecranon fossa. The two Rush rods have been inserted retrograde from the epicondyles *(E)* across the fracture site *(F)* and they thus intersect right at the fracture, affording little inherent resistance to rotational stress. (**B** reprinted with permission from Sim, F.H., and Pritchard, D.J.: Clin. Orthop. **169:**91, 1982.)

upper end of which parallels the groove between the biceps and the brachialis and then crosses the antecubital fossa obliquely (Fig. 10-9, *A*). As with exposure of the humeral shaft, the brachialis muscle can be split gently by blunt dissection, thereby revealing the radial nerve and allowing it to be retracted out of harm's way. Once the fracture site is exposed, there almost always is evidence of an exophytic tumor mass extending anteriorly or laterally (Fig. 10-10, *A*). The tumor mass is excised and followed through the cortical defect into the medullary canal (Fig. 10-9, *A*). All tumor and debris within the canal are removed by curettage as far proximally and distally as possible.

Via a separate stab incision over the lateral epicondyle, a ¼-inch drill hole is made through the distal cortex of the epicondyle just lateral to the edge of the capitellum (Fig. 10-9, *B*). A similar hole is then made through the distal cortical surface of the medial epicondyle. It is important to make both holes in the *posterior* distal epicondylar cortex, since the distal humerus normally angulates slightly anteriorly and a slightly posterior entrance portal is needed to align the rod with the long axis of the bone.

A Rush rod is inserted into each of the holes and driven proximally across the level of the fracture defect and well into the medullary canal of the humeral shaft above the fracture. Ordinarily two 0.3 cm (⅛ inch) rods are chosen, although in a large patient with a patulous medullary canal it may be possible to use at least one larger (0.6 cm, ¼ inch) Rush rod.

Each rod should be prebent at its tip (to prevent the sharp point from penetrating the cortex above) and in its midportion (to allow the rod to spring against the humeral cortices). An ideal configuration of each rod allows it to contact cortical bone firmly in three places (Fig. 10-1, *D*).

Once both rods are properly positioned and the fracture fragments have been impacted to minimize gaps between the cortices, the medullary canal is filled with methymethacrylate injected under pressure while still quite liquid.

Before polymerization of the cement is complete, any excess exuding out the fracture surfaces or through the cortical defects is removed to minimize interference with bone healing.

When the limb is not to be irradiated postoperatively or has not been irradiated within 4 to 6 months preoperatively, it is worthwhile to pack cancellous bone about the fracture site and across the cortical defect. If such grafting is anticipated, it is well to evaluate the iliac crests preoperatively by roentgenography and/or scintigraphy to ensure that they are not infiltrated as well by metastases. If any question exists, banked allograft bone may be substituted.

Postoperatively no external immobilization is used. Instead, active assisted range-of-motion exercises are begun as soon as comfort

Text continued on p. 278.

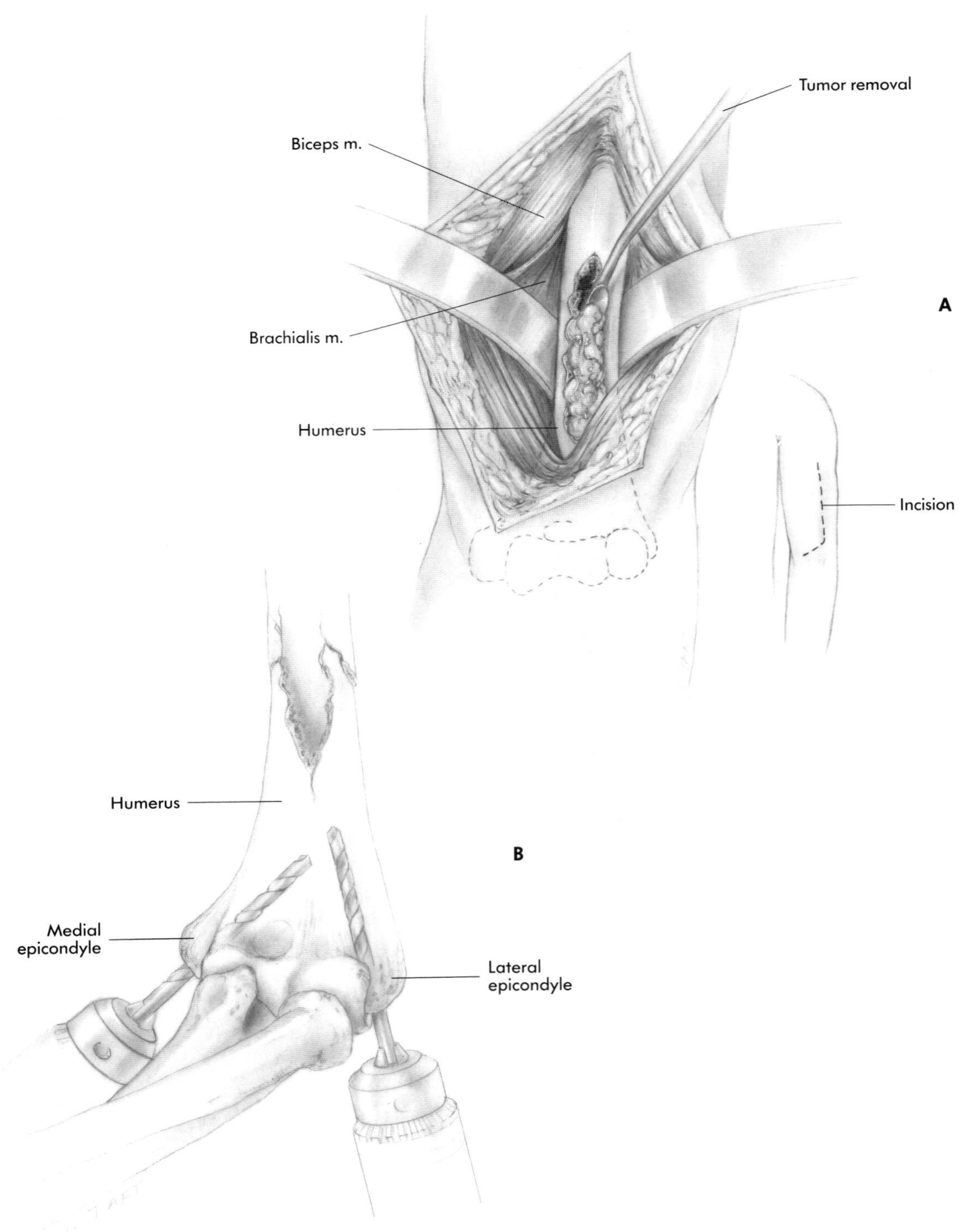

FIGURE 10-9 For legend see opposite page.

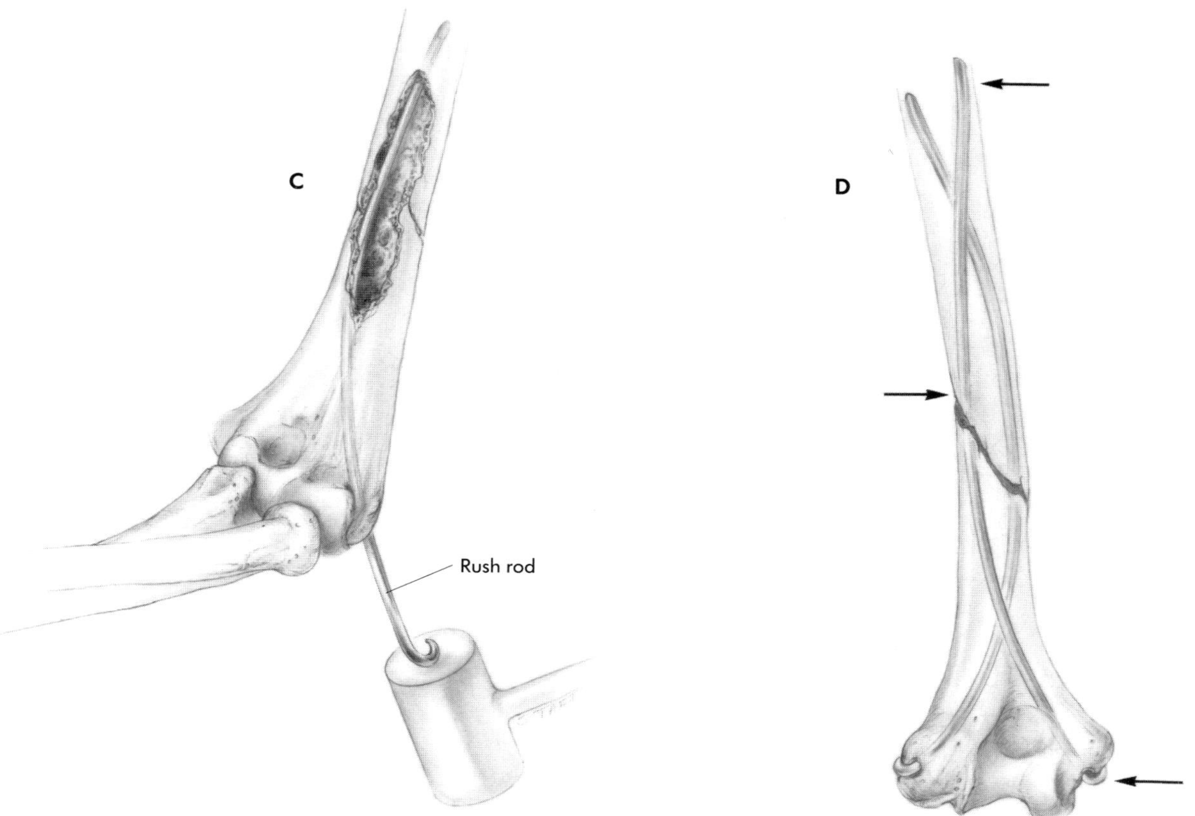

FIGURE 10-9 Pathological fracture of the supracondylar humerus. **A,** The best approach is via the lower half of a Henry[8] extensile incision. The brachialis muscle is split bluntly. Its posterior half and the protected radial nerve are retracted posteriorly. Note: the nerve should be exposed widely when approaching a displaced fracture or when a large tumor mass distorts the normal anatomy. **B,** Through separate stab wounds over each epicondyle, drill holes are made in the distal posterior cortex. It is important to position these holes well behind the midarticular surface so the points of the Rush rod insertions will be aligned with the center of the medullary canal. **C,** Rush rods of the largest possible size that will fit (either ⅛ or ¼ inch) are driven retrograde into the medullary canal and across the fracture site. **D,** Once the rods are seated, there should be solid three-point fixation by each rod *(arrows).*

Continued.

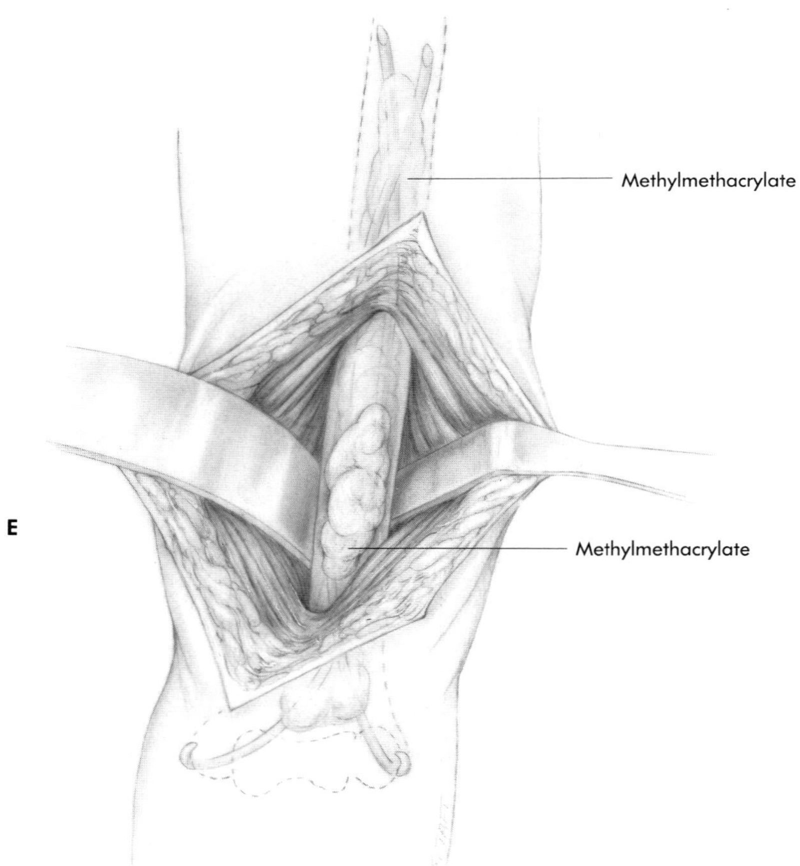

FIGURE 10-9, cont'd. E, Methylmethacrylate is injected into the canal well proximal and well distal to the fracture defect. It is particularly important to inject the cement as far as possible into the distal fragment to minimize the risk of fracture distraction by gravity or lifting activities.

FIGURE 10-10 **A,** Pathological fracture through an expansile lytic breast metastasis in the distal humerus. It was treated by local irradiaton and external splintage but remained painful, unhealed, and unstable 10 months later. **B,** At operation the humeral cortical bone was found to be extremely soft because of disuse osteoporosis. One Rush rod inserted through the medial epicondyle transfixed the fracture fragments, but another, through the lateral epicondyle, penetrated the soft bone of the distal fragment and had to be removed. Effective fixation was afforded primarily by methylmethacrylate injected within the medullary canal and across the fracture. **C,** Sixteen months postoperative. A lateral roentgenogram demonstrates bony union of the fracture without loss of alignment. The methylmethacrylate cement is visible within the medullary canal. **D** and **E,** The patient regained full pronation and supination with 25 to 95 degrees of functional flexion.

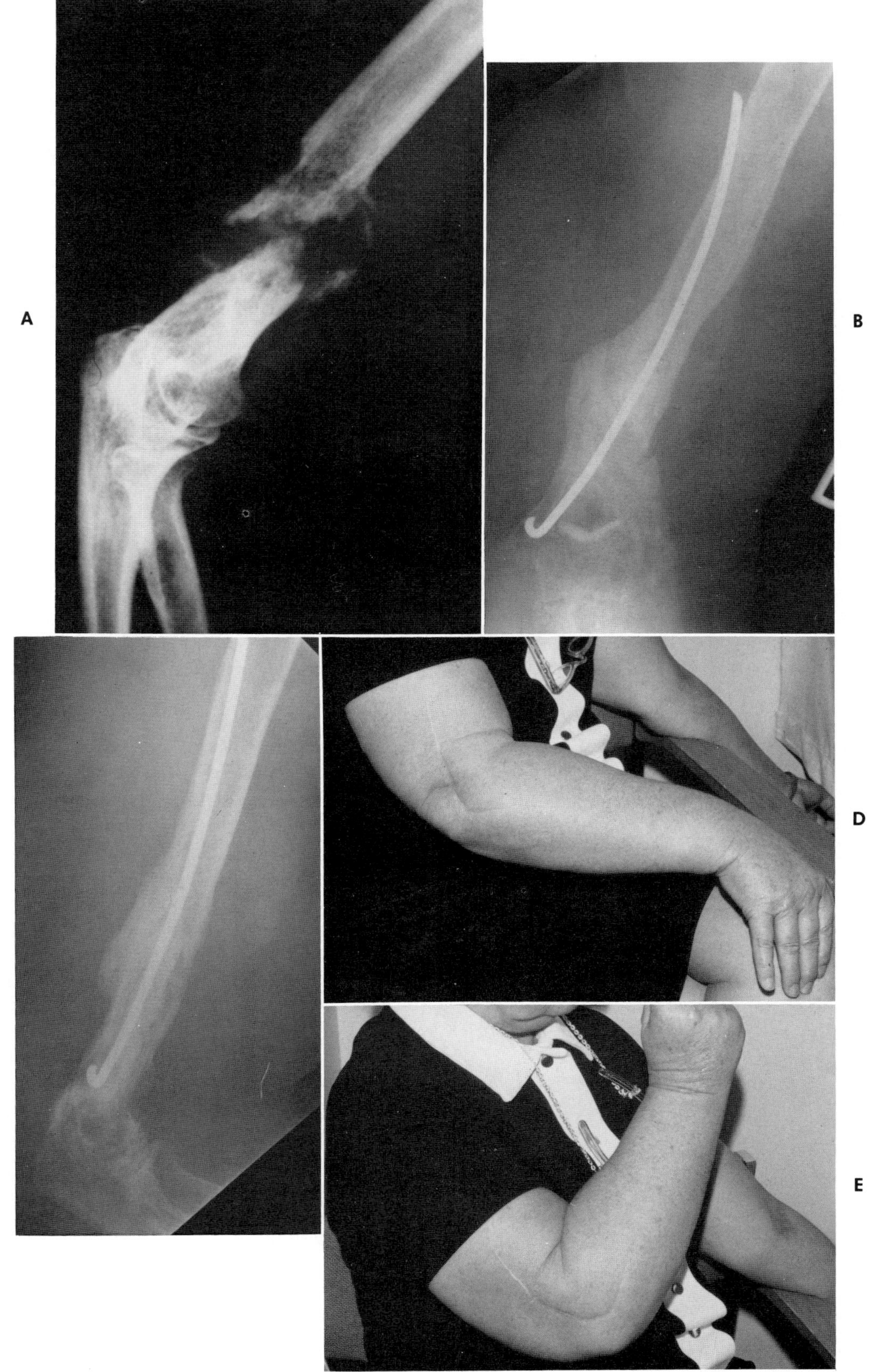

FIGURE 10-10 For legend see opposite page.

allows. In our experience most patients regain all but the final 10 degrees of elbow flexion and all but the final 20 degrees of elbow extension (Fig. 10-10, *D* and *E*). All but one of our 19 patients with a supracondylar fracture regained at least 90 degrees of elbow motion and 120 degrees of pronation and supination.

Intraarticular Fractures of the Elbow

Pathological fractures of the distal humerus extending into the elbow joint are quite uncommon because the articular cartilage acts as an effective avascular barrier to tumor extension. Metastases that do extend into the joint usually are quite aggressive and vascular and typically have broken through the anterior cortex of the humerus intrasynovially. If the articular surfaces of the distal humerus remain intact, the focus is best treated by local irradiation. If the joint surfaces have become disrupted in a patient with sufficient pain to warrant operative intervention and if the life expectancy warrants an attempt at joint arthroplasty, it is best usually to resect the distal humerus and perform a hinge-type total elbow replacement. However, it is our experience that all the currently available prostheses have a high likelihood of loosening in the face of deficient distal humeral bone stock. Consequently, such patients should be counseled carefully preoperatively that stresses to the prosthetic joint must be severely curtailed on a permanent basis.

Fractures of the Scapula and Clavicle

As noted earlier, metastases not uncommonly are demonstrable in both the scapula and the clavicle and, in fact, have been reported in most series to be between 40% and 60% as common as those of the humerus. However, it is exceedingly rare for a lesion or even a secondary fracture of the scapula or clavicle to require operative management. We have performed debulking procedures on a few occasions for patients with aggressive lesions of either bone that were not radiosensitive or had already been irradiated fully. On two occasions we have managed pathological fractures of the distal clavicle by distal clavicular resection, and in each case the patient regained a full range of motion and enjoyed excellent relief of pain.

Fractures of the Radius and Ulna

Pathological fractures of the radius and/or ulna also are uncommon and, when present, usually represent a small segment of widespread bone metastasis in a pre–terminally ill patient. Lung carcinomas not infrequently metastasize to the proximal ulna or distal radius, presumably by direct arterial embolization. Again, the overall prognosis for patients with such lesions generally is poor and rarely is an attempt at operative intervention warranted.

On occasion, however, a pathological fracture of the radius or ulna does occur in a patient with a sufficiently good projected life expectancy to warrant consideration of internal stabilization. For some reason the most commonly affected site under such circumstances seems to be the proximal radius, despite the fact that its blood supply is nowhere near as abundant as is that of the proximal ulna or distal radius.

Pathological fractures of the radial neck, when sufficiently symptomatic to require treatment (Fig. 10-11, *A*) are best treated by radial head excision and a program of early postoperative motion. When internal fixation of the radial neck appears to be warranted (Fig. 10-11, *B*), it can be accomplished relatively easily through a lateral incision paralleling the proximal shaft. The use of two small (⅛-inch) Rush rods augmented by intramedullary cement seems to be an effective means for stabilization (Fig. 10-11, *C*).

We have had experience with only two distal radial fractures requiring internal stabilization. Both were secondary to lung carcinoma metastases and in each instance the resulting lesion was aneurysmal with marked thinning and destruction of the distal radial cortices (Fig. 10-11, *D* and *E*). In the first instance fixation was accomplished with a small Rush rod inserted retrograde through the radial styloid and augmented by cement. Postoperatively the patient complained of persistent pain over the tip of the rod at the styloid, and finally it was removed. The fracture fixation remained stable throughout the last 2 years of the patient's life despite the fact that no true bony healing was observed. In the second instance the distal radius was approached through a dorsal incision with the extensor tendons re-

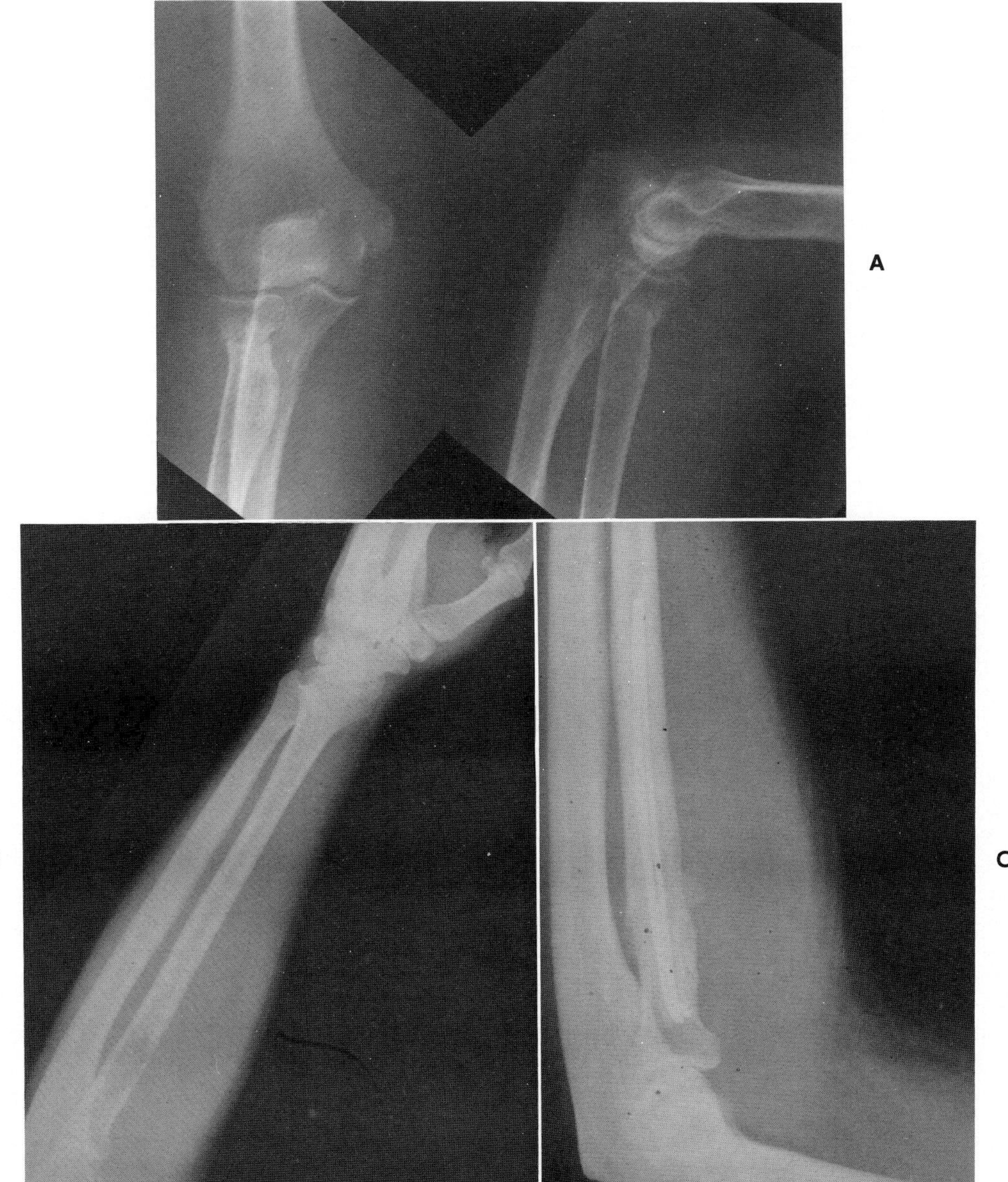

FIGURE 10-11 **A,** Pathological fracture of the radial neck following local irradiation for lymphoma. The patient had been experiencing pain with elbow motion and forearm rotation, but this was relieved completely by radial head resection. **B,** Somewhat more extensive lytic lesion of the proximal radius extending well beyond the level suitable for radial head excision. **C,** Internal fixation was achieved successfully in this patient with two Rush rods augmented by intramedullary cement. *Continued.*

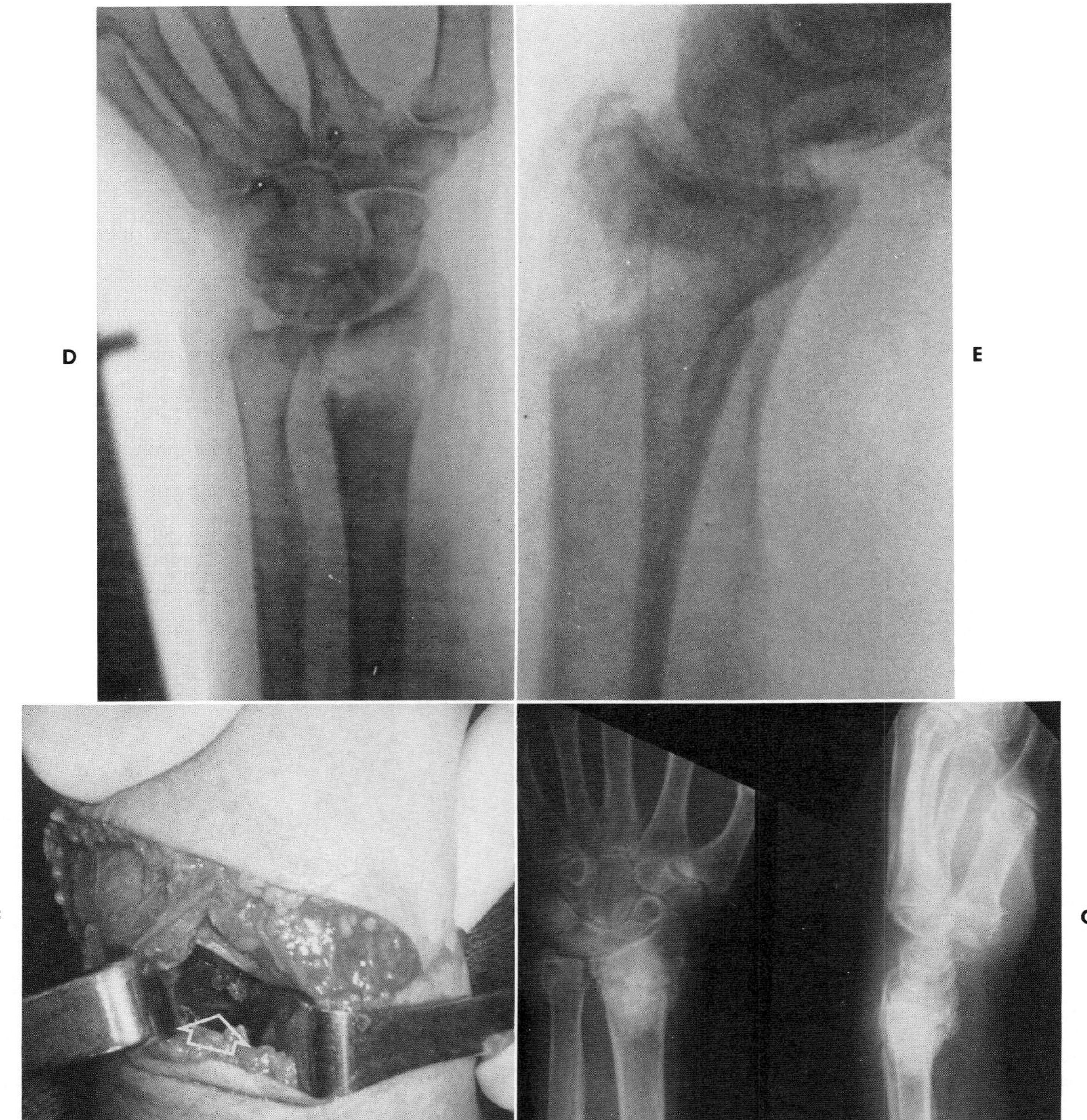

FIGURE 10-11, cont'd. **D** and **E,** AP and lateral roentgenograms of the distal radius in another patient with metastatic lung carcinoma causing extensive bone lysis and a consequent fracture. **F,** Intraoperative view of the dorsal approach used to reduce and stabilize this fracture. Note the large dorsal cortical defect *(arrow)*. **G,** Postoperative roentgenograms 5 months after open reduction and stabilization by intramedullary methylmethacrylate alone. Although it would have been safer to augment fixation with a small Rush rod, this particular patient regained full motion and enjoyed a stable and pain-free wrist until her demise 2 years later.

tracted to expose the cortical defect (Fig. 10-11,*F*). The tumor and destroyed dorsal cortex were resected, the fracture reduced, and the cavity packed with methylmethacrylate extending well into the distal fragment (Fig. 10-11,*G*). Despite the patient's poor overall prognosis because of her lung malignancy, she remains alive and with her disease in remission 2½ years postoperatively. She regained 100 degrees of wrist flexion-extension and has good grip strength without pain. In this instance the fracture progressed eventually to bony union.

COMPLICATIONS

Upper-extremity fractures are subject to the same types of complications that afflict lower-extremity fractures. The surgeon must be wary of approaching a highly vascular lesion operatively without first obtaining an arteriogram and considering arterial embolization (Fig. 10-5,*B*). The risks of wound dehiscence, infection, skin slough, etc. are no less for the upper than for the lower extremity.

The stresses and strains so typically productive of varus angulation at the intertrochanteric area of the femur do not exist in the humerus. The disastrous sequela of a major limb length discrepancy, so important to avoid in managing lower-extremity fractures, is of minimal importance when managing a pathological fracture of the humerus. However, these advantages are more than compensated by the small size of the humeral medullary canal and the consequent difficulty in obtaining strong and rigid fixation. Moreover, the fact that the humerus is alternately loaded and distracted renders intramedullary fixation particularly subject to failure. For these reasons it is important to use the largest and strongest fixation device possible and to augment such fixation with intramedullary cement injected as far proximal and as far distal to the fracture site as one can.

Because early active elbow and shoulder motion is essential in these patients with a limited life expectancy and often with other limb disabilities as well, we do not favor using any operative approaches that detach tendinous origins or insertions and therefore require a period of limb immobilization. The technique of detaching the triceps tendon for exposure of the distal humerus, in particular, should be avoided because of its propensity to result in heterotopic ossification around the elbow and because of the risk of late tendon rupture after irradiation.

REFERENCES

1. Barer, M., et al.: Mastocytosis with osseus lesions resembling metastatic malignant lesions in bone, J. Bone Joint Surg. **50A:**142, 1968.
2. Batson, O.V.: Function of vertebral veins and their role in spread of metastases, Ann. Surg. **112:**138, 1940.
3. Brumback, R.J., et al.: Intramedullary rodding of humeral shaft fractures in polytrauma. Read at the A.A.O.S. meeting, Las Vegas, 1985,
4. Clain, A.: Secondary malignant disease of bone, Br. J. Cancer **19:**15, 1965.
5. Douglass, J.O., Jr., et al.: Treatment of pathological fractures of long bones excluding those due to breast cancer, J. Bone Joint Surg. **58A:**1055, 1976.
6. Habermann, E.T., et al.: The pathology and treatment of metastatic disease of the femur, Clin. Orthop. **169:**70, 1982.
7. Harrington, K.D., et al.: Methylmethacrylate as an adjunct in internal fixation of pathological fractures, J. Bone Joint Surg. **58A:**1047, 1976.
8. Henry, A.K.: Extensile exposure, ed. 2, New York, 1966, Churchill-Livingstone, Inc.
9. Holm, C.L.: Management of humeral shaft fractures. Fundamental nonoperative techniques, Clin. Orthop. **71:**132, 1970.
10. Jaffe, H.L.: Tumors and tumorous conditions of the bones and joints, Philadelphia, 1958, Lea & Febiger.
11. Klenerman, L.: Fractures of the shaft of the humerus, J. Bone Joint Surg. **48B:**105, 1966.
12. Lewallen, R.P., et al.: Treatment of pathologic fractures or impending fractures of the humerus with Rush rods and methylmethacrylate. Experience with 55 cases in 54 patients: 1968-1977, Clin. Orthop. **166:**193, 1982.
13. Mast, J.W., et al.: Fractures of the humeral shaft. A retrospective study of 240 adult fractures, Clin. Orthop. **112:**254, 1975.
14. Pugh, J., et al.: Biomechanics of pathologic fractures, Clin. Orthop. **169:**109, 1982.
15. Sarmiento, A., et al.: Functional bracing of fractures of the shaft of the humerus, J. Bone Joint Surg. **59A:**596, 1977.
16. Sim, F.H., and Pritchard, D.J.: Metastatic disease in the upper extremity, Clin. Orthop. **169:**83, 1982.
17. Sim, F.H., et al.: Postradiation sarcoma of bone, J. Bone Joint Surg. **54A:**1479, 1972.
18. Stern, P.J., et al.: Intramedullary fixation of humeral shaft fractures, J. Bone Joint Surg. **66A:**639, 1984.

CHAPTER 11

PROPHYLACTIC MANAGEMENT OF IMPENDING FRACTURES

It has been estimated that 90% of patients dying of disseminated malignancy will have bone metastases demonstrable by careful postmortem examination. Probably fewer than half of these patients have experienced bone symptoms, and fewer than 10% have suffered a pathological fracture through a tumor focus before their death. Nevertheless, because the development of a fracture is so devastating to a cancer patient, increasing emphasis is being placed on attempts to determine which metastases are likely to produce fractures and how individual lesions can best be managed to avoid this complication.

HISTOMECHANICS

A common misconception is that only lytic metastases are likely to supply sufficient bone to result in a fracture and that the new bone laid down by blastic foci actually may increase cortical strength in many instances or at least make the bone locally harder. There is, in fact, no statistical or histological basis for this belief. A long bone with blastic metastases may seem harder from the viewpoint of the surgeon attempting to attach hardware to it, but it lacks most of the strength and plasticity of normal bone. Approximately 60% of pathological long bone fractures occur through breast carcinoma metastases despite the fact that more than half of these metastases are primarily blastic. Prostatic carcinoma, which almost invariably produces blastic bony metastases, nevertheless ranks high as a cause of long bone pathological fractures.

Experimental evidence suggests that epithelial cells from breast, prostate, bladder, and certain lung carcinomas have the capacity to form bone within metastatic foci.[8] These metastatic tumor cells apparently produce an osteoblast-stimulating factor while forming a fibrous stroma around the developing tumor.[10,14] It seems likely that the two phenomena are synchronous and that the stroma so formed affords a suitable matrix for ossification in the presence of the osteoprogenitor cells produced by the tumor.

Certainly most tumor metastases have the secondary capacity to stimulate endosteal trabecular and even periosteal new bone formation by causing adjacent normal bone to respond to stress while being weakened by tumor lysis (see Fig. 11-2, *A*). The phenomenon is similar only qualitatively to callus repair of a traumatic fracture but differs markedly in a quantitative sense because of the poor strength of the callus. The reactive bone has a haphazard configuration histologically, lacking the parallelism of bone fibers seen in normal stress-responsive lamellar bone. Although often appearing almost normal roentgenographically, these blastic foci are markedly weaker than normal bone and have an only slightly lower predisposition to

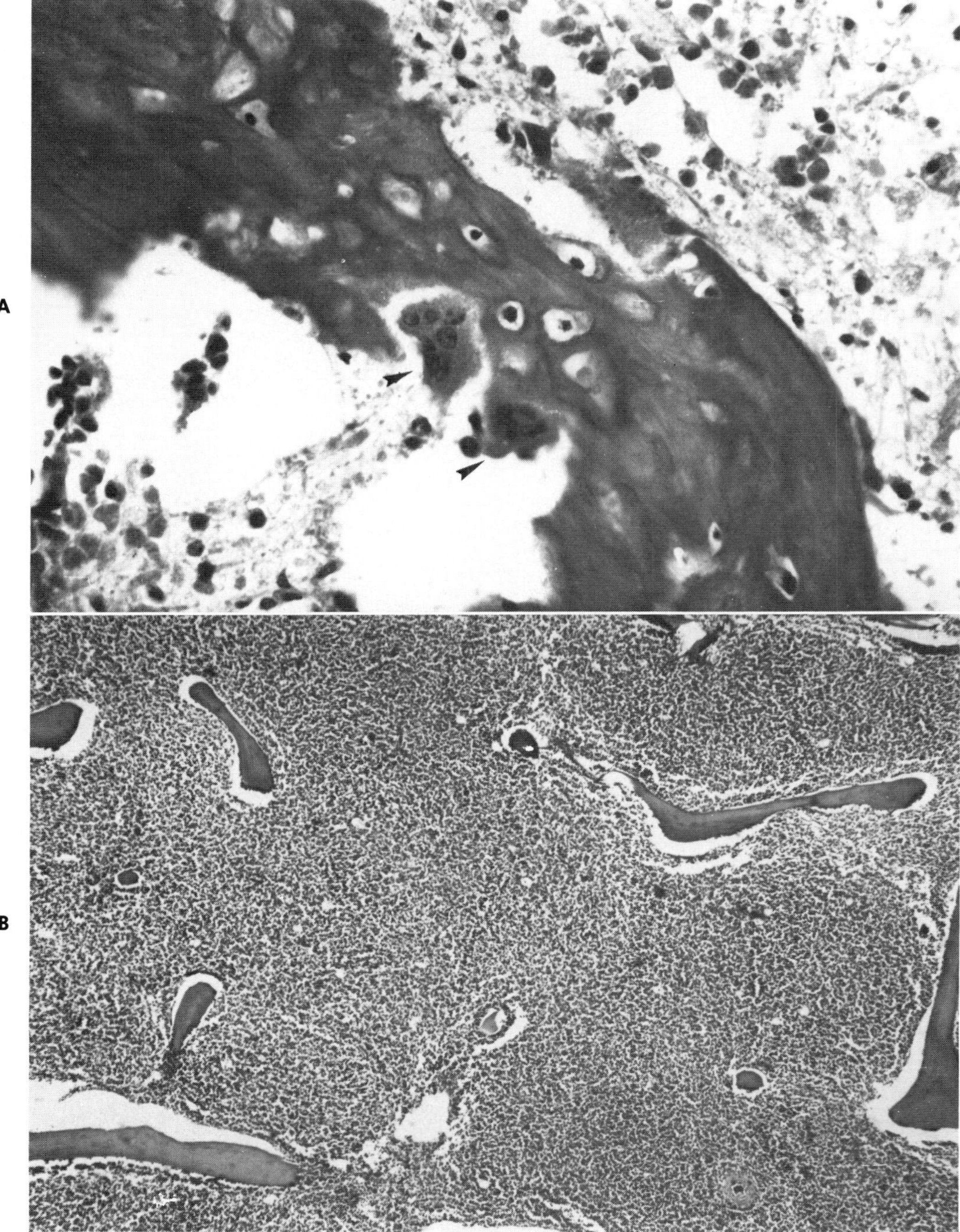

FIGURE 11-1 **A,** High-power photomicrograph of a biopsy taken at the site of a pathological fracture in a patient with metastatic breast carcinoma. Malignant cells are apparent in the soft tissue stroma adjacent to mature trabecular bone. Active resorption of bone is being caused by large multinucleated osteoclasts *(arrows),* which are not malignant. **B,** Low-power photomicrograph of tissue taken from the site of pathological fracture in a patient with malignant lymphoma. No osteoclasts are apparent, but extensive destruction of cortical bone has occurred. The densely packed malignant round cells appear to be causing bone lysis by direct resorption.

pathological fracture than to more obvious lytic foci (Figs. 11-9, *D*, and 11-10, *B*).

Lytic bony metastases appear to weaken bone principally by two mechanisms. The first and quantitatively the most important is mediated by way of osteoclasts. Galasko[10] demonstrated clearly that osteoclast proliferation occurs within 24 hours of innoculation of experimental animals with cancer cell strains. Similar histological changes are seen in the majority of human skeletal metastases and are as pronounced in highly cellular tumors as in relatively acellular sclerotic metastases. The phenomenon is seen in host bone immediately adjacent to tumor foci separated from the tumor cells by the type of reactive fiber stroma already described. The osteoclasts are not malignant cells but rather concentrate in response to some tumor stimulus. Bone resorption occurs in lacunae around each osteoclast. Osteoclastic destruction of the cortex extends to the periosteal surface, the osteoclasts always preceding the tumor itself (Fig. 11-1, *A*).

It appears that such osteoclastic proliferation is mediated by way of an osteoclast-activating factor (OAF) secreted by the tumor.[7,11,12]

Leukocytes concentrating at the tumor-host margin also are capable of producing an OAF.[22] This phenomenon appears to play a particular role in osteoclasis around myelomatous and lymphomatous tumors. A similar phenomenon, however, occurs with many metastatic carcinomas, particularly breast carcinoma, in which the OAF is secreted not directly by leukocytes but rather via prostaglandins (especially PGE_2).

The production of these osteoclastic prostaglandins can be inhibited experimentally by certain nonsteroidal antiinflammatory drugs (e.g., indomethacin[13]) although the drug's efficacy has not been demonstrated consistently in clinical situations in humans. If these agents are to play a role in the control of lytic bony metastases, it will likely need to be before extensive cortical erosion has occurred and while osteoclastic activity is still prominent.

Once cortical bone destruction has extended through from the endosteal to the periosteal surface, the remaining spicules are densely encased by tumor cells and osteoclasts have in fact disappeared. At this point, the tumor cells alone apparently can destroy bone directly via immediate bone resorption[22] or by the secretion of bone-degrading enzymes[14] (Fig. 11-1, *B*).

BIOMECHANICS

From a biomechanical viewpoint it is obvious that cortical defects weaken bone, especially with regard to torsional stress. There are two general categories of cortical defects: those with a dimension less than the diameter of the bone and those with a dimension greater than that diameter.

The smaller defect, termed a *stress riser*, weakens the bone by creating an uneven distribution of stresses in it. Such a stress riser can decrease bone strength by 60% to 70%.[24]

The larger defect, termed an *open-section defect*, has a more profound effect on decreasing shear and torque-loading resistance. In normal bone under torsion loading, the shear stresses are more evenly distributed through the cross section (Fig. 11-2, *H*). The stress distribution in the closed section is radically altered by a large defect. Because the open section does not have a continuous outer surface, only the shear stress developed at the periphery of the section can resist the applied torque (Fig. 11-2, *I*). Consequently, the mass of bone resisting any given load is greatly decreased. Torsional testing of human adult tibiae with open-section defects shows a 90% reduction in load to failure and in energy storage to failure.[24]

INDICATIONS FOR INTERNAL FIXATION

The means for assessing these biomechanical factors in any given patient is the conventional AP and lateral roentgenograms (Fig. 11-3, *A* and *B*). Fidler[9] has demonstrated a technique for estimating the percentage of cortical bone destruction at any level of a long bone using these two views alone (Fig. 11-3, *C* to *E*), and it is my experience that the technique usually is as accurate a prognosticator of impending pathological fracture as is a cross-sectional CT scan. However, when cortical destruction progresses in a patchy or spiral distribution, it may be difficult to assess the circumferential bone loss accurately by this technique and a cross-sectional CT scan of the extremity may be more accurate (Fig. 11-4).

Once tumor lysis has progressed to the point where 50% or more of the cortex is

Text continued on p. 291.

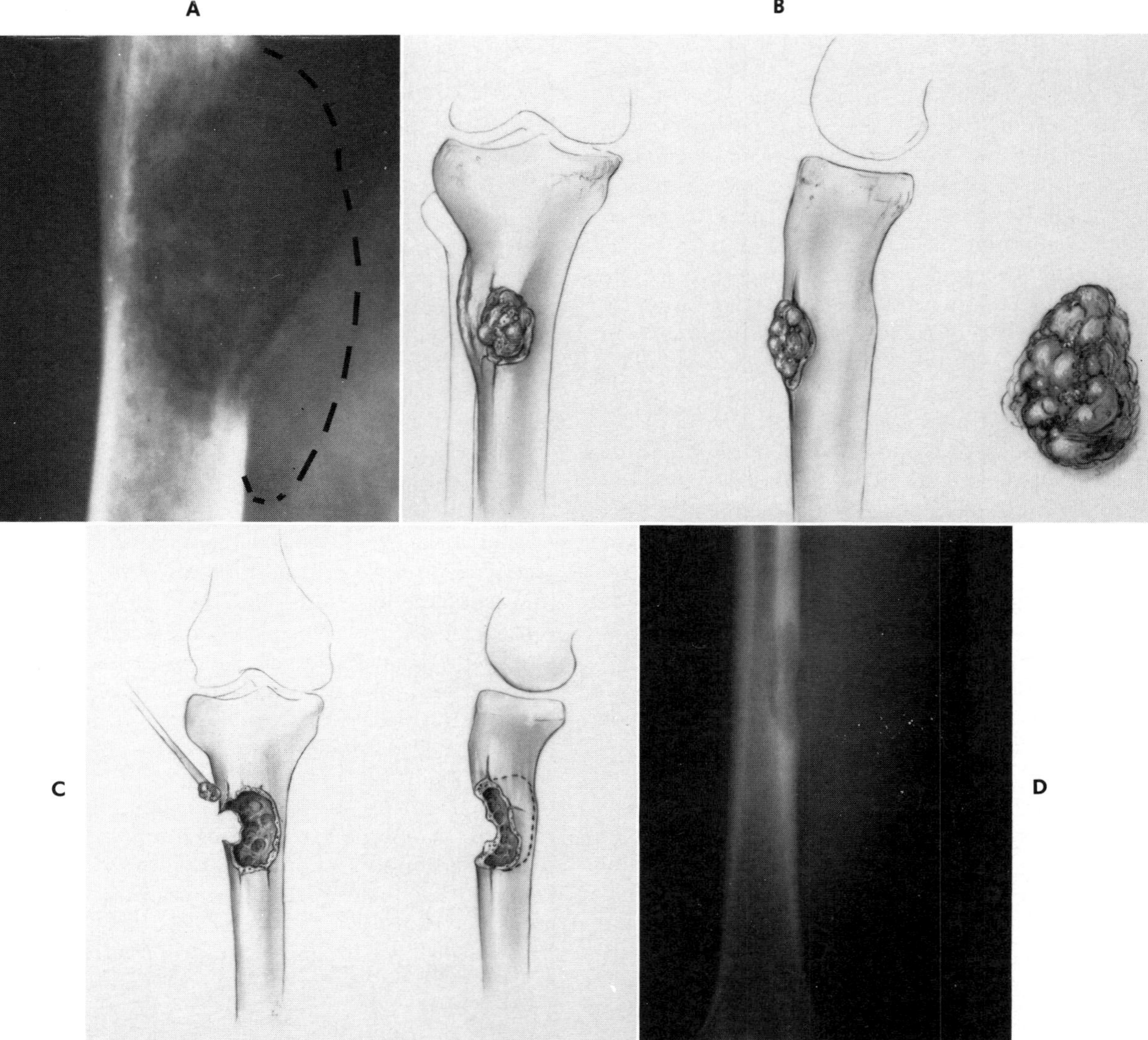

FIGURE 11-2 **A,** Most roentgenographic pictures of metastases show focal destruction and surrounding patchy lysis. This appearance, however, suggests that there is little reactive host bone formation walling the tumor process (unlike that seen in Fig. 11-3, *A* and *B*), although there is evidence of periosteal new bone formed in response to the stress of an impending fracture. Often such lesions will have broken through the cortex by the time they become symptomatic, despite the fact that conventional films usually do not demonstrate the soft tissue mass. This film of the distal femur in a patient with multiple myeloma shows an ill-defined extension of tumor lysis well beyond the confines of the cortical defect. Some reactive bone has formed along the opposite cortex but is of little structural significance. At surgery, a large extracortical soft tissue mass was found *(dotted lines)*, although the mass was not apparent roentgenographically. **B,** Schematic rendering of such a lesion (here in the proximal tibia) as it would be seen at surgery. The tumor tissue typically is soft, multiply lobulated, and moderately vascular. **C,** After curettage of the defect and removal of structurally inadequate bone, the cavity typically is twice the size of the lesion first appreciated on the initial roentgenogram. The extent of cortical destruction is also well in excess of that anticipated preoperatively. **D,** Lesion of the femoral diaphysis in a patient with metastatic breast carcinoma. It appears well circumscribed and involves approximately 60% of the circumferential cortex (when measured by the technique shown in Fig. 11-3, *C* to *E*).

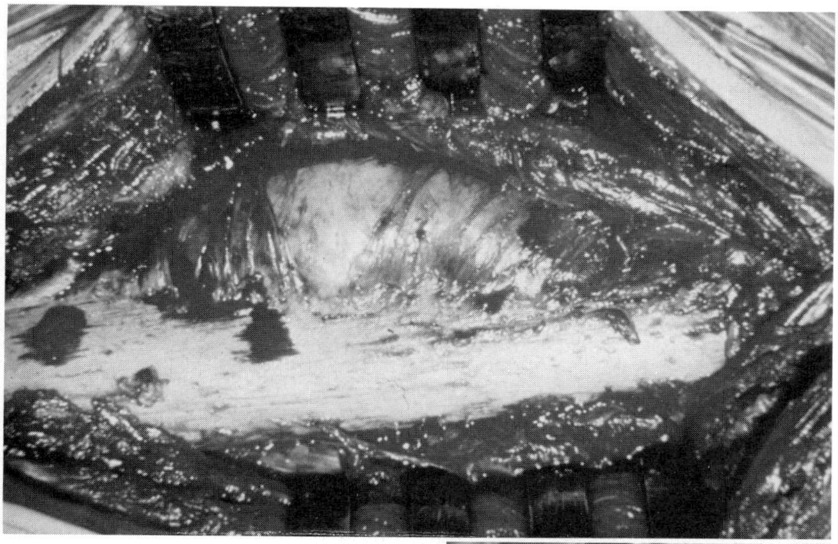

E

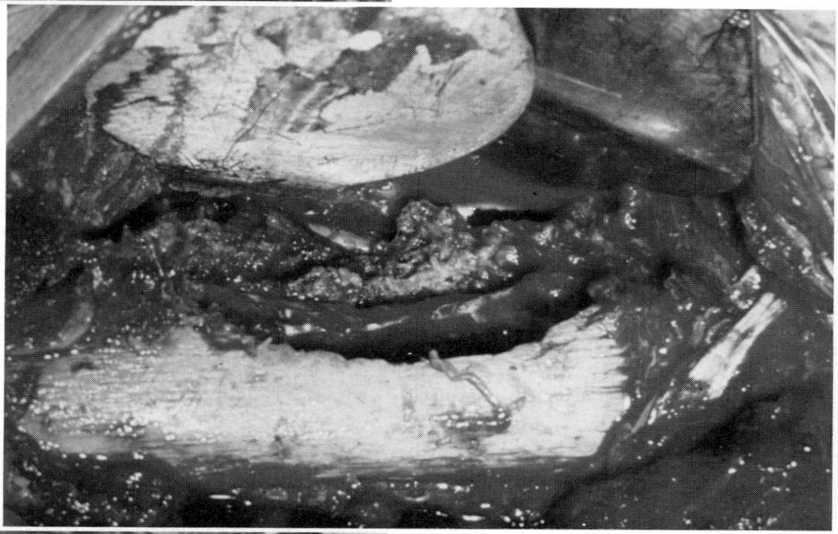

F

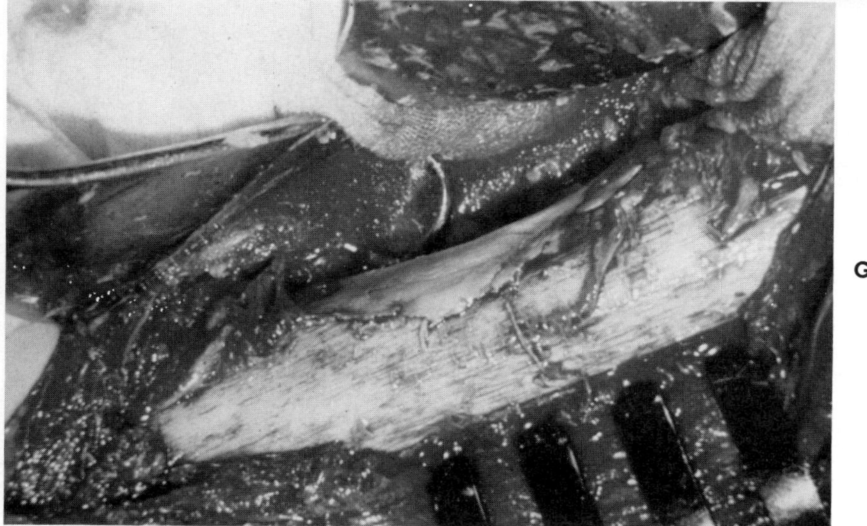

G

FIGURE 11-2, cont'd. For legend see p. 288.

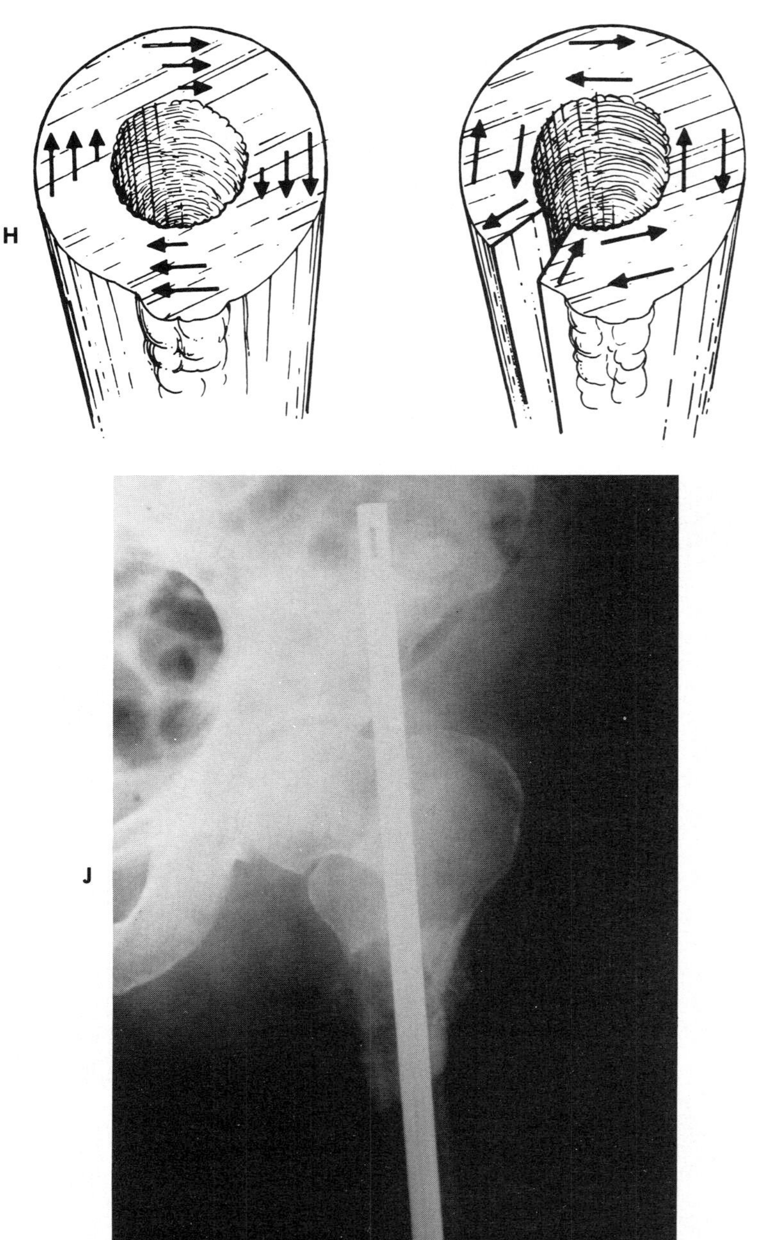

FIGURE 11-2, cont'd. **E,** At surgery an unsuspected large exophytic mass was encountered emerging from the cortical defect. **F,** At curettage of the lesion, the extent of the cortical destruction was apparent. **G,** After closed Kuntscher nail fixation of the femur, the cortical defect and adjacent intramedullary canal were packed with methylmethacrylate in an effort to reduce the localized stress riser created by a large open-section defect in the cortex. **H,** Under torsional loading the distribution of shear stress in a cross section of intact bone is symmetrical and linearly a function of the radius. **I,** An open-section defect causes a redistribution of stresses. Only the stress vectors at the periphery of the cross section are able to resist the tortionally applied load. Thus an open-section defect severely reduces the ability of the bone to carry torsional load. **J,** Another reason for packing large lytic lesions with methylmethacrylate at the time of internal fixation is to avoid the sort of shortening apparent here, which cannot be obviated by fixation with an intramedullary device alone. (**H** and **I** from Pugh, J., et al.: Clin. Orthop. **169:**109, 1982.)

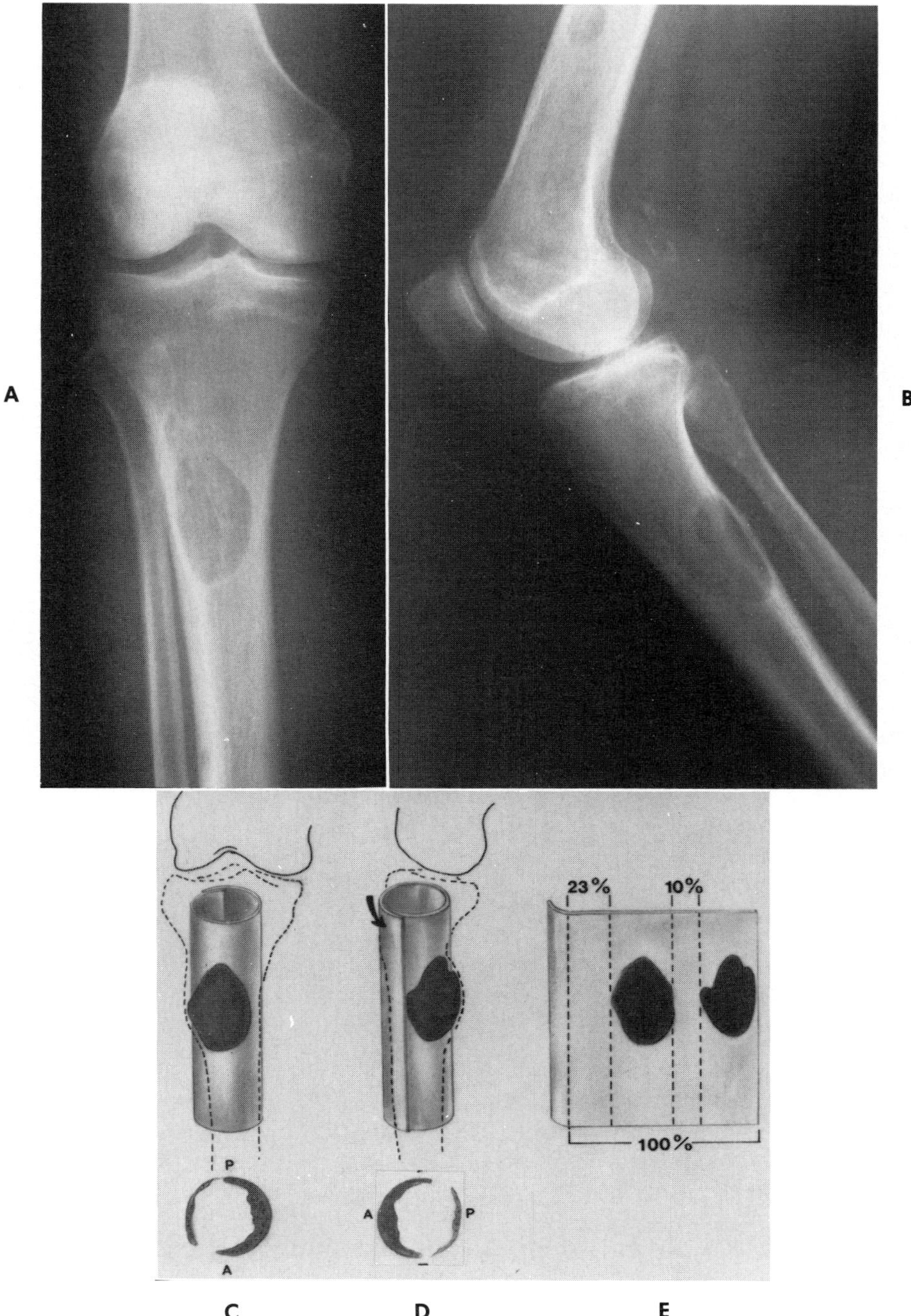

FIGURE 11-3 **A** and **B,** Well-circumscribed lytic myelomatous lesion of the proximal tibia with a similar but smaller focus apparent in the distal femur. Although the lesion's distinct margin and the surrounding reactive bone suggest that it is only slowly progressive, the extent of cortical destruction and persistent pain on weight-bearing indicated a need for prophylactic internal fixation. With such well-circumscribed lesions, the extent of cortical destruction can be surprisingly well estimated from conventional AP and lateral roentgenograms by using the method of Fidler.[9] A sheet of paper is rolled into a tube approximating the shaft of the affected long bone. The lesion outlined is copied from the AP film onto the front of the tube, **C.** The tube is then turned 90 degrees, and the outline from the lateral film is copied, **D.** When the sheet is unfurled, **E,** an accurate assessment can be made of the extent of circumferential cortical destruction. In this instance only 33% of the circumferential cortex remains intact. As noted in the box on p. 297, this patient is at high risk of a spontaneous pathological fracture and should have prophylactic fixation.

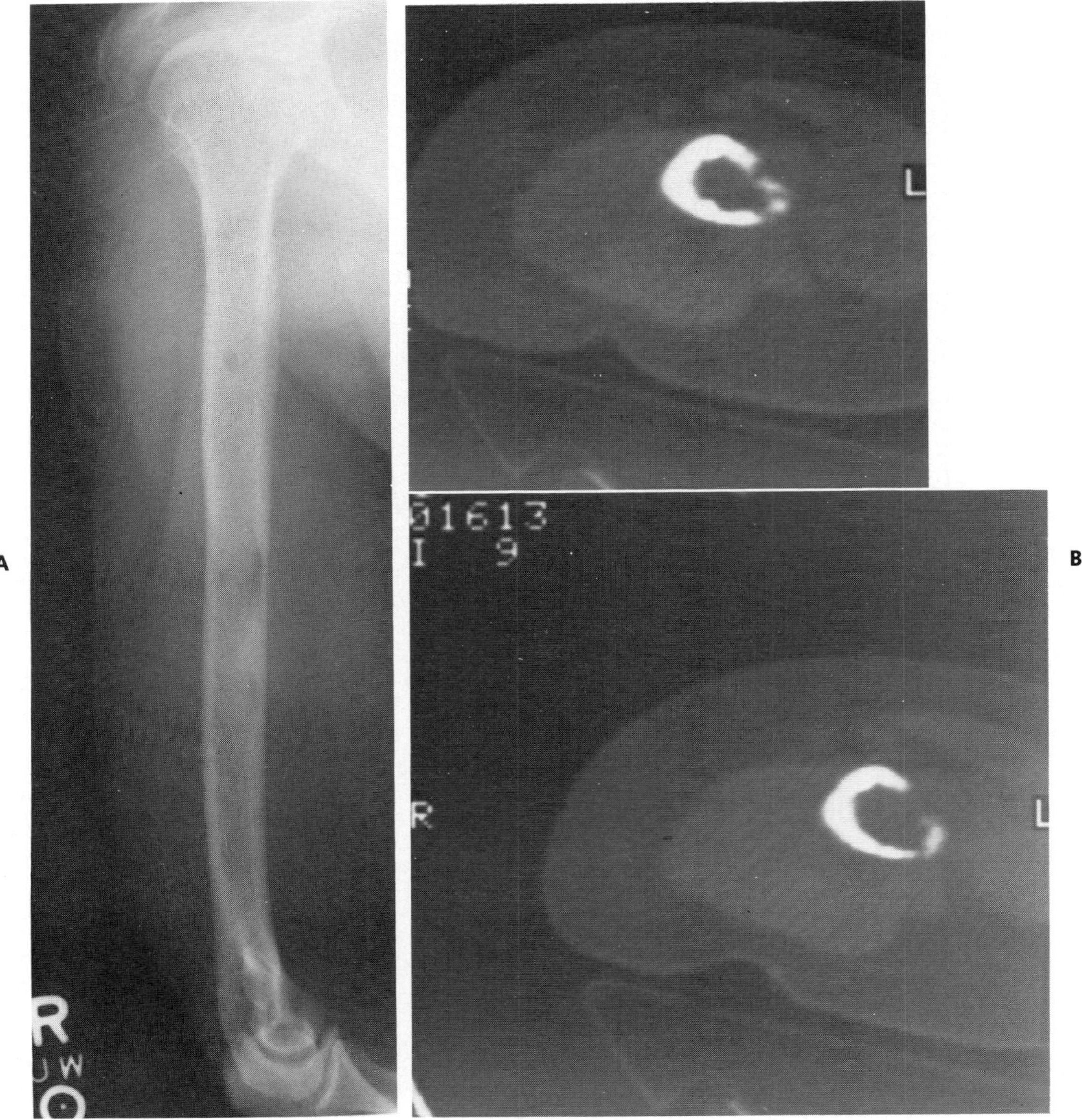

FIGURE 11-4 **A,** Partially circumscribed myelomatous lesion of the midhumeral diaphysis. Although some cortical destruction is apparent, neither an AP nor this lateral roentgenogram suggested that the cortical loss was in excess of 20%. **B,** Because of persistent pain in the area with even the slightest stress on the arm, and because of progressive radial neuralgia, a CT scan was obtained. It revealed at least 50% loss of circumferential cortex and suggested the presence of an exophytic soft tissue mass arising from the cortical defect. At operation, destruction of approximately 50% of the circumferential cortex was apparent and a large soft tissue tumor that had partially encompassed the radial nerve. The tumor was debulked, and prophylactic fixation with an A-O plate reinforced by methylmethacrylate accomplished. The patient, who experienced prompt relief of pain and recovery of neurological function, remains symptom-free 19 months after surgery.

destroyed at any given level, the incidence of spontaneous pathological fracture increases dramatically (Fig. 11-5). In the proximal femur a lytic lesion in excess of 2.5 cm on either the AP or the lateral view almost always can be seen to have an associated cortical disruption in excess of 50%, although demonstrating such cortical destruction by a lateral roentgenogram may be difficult in a patient with a painful hip (Fig. 11-6, *A* and *B*).

A pathological avulsion fracture of the lesser trochanter also suggests that at least 50% of the femoral cortex has been destroyed locally and that there is a significant chance of developing a pathological fracture across the femur at the intertrochanteric or subtrochanteric level[2] (Fig. 11-7).

Based on these observations, it is possible to establish relative criteria for prophylactic internal stabilization of impending pathological fractures.[1,9,14,16,18]

1. A destructive lesion involving more than 50% of the cortical bone circumferentially
2. A lytic lesion of the proximal femur larger than 2.5 cm
3. A lesion of the proximal femur associated with avulsion of the lesser trochanter

It is important to realize that many of these lytic lesions will not be painful before the development of the fracture. Fidler[9] found that less than half of such patients experienced local pain before the fracture occurred.

Unfortunately, all these criteria are based on the assessment of lytic lesions in which the size of the tumor focus or the extent of its destruction can be determined roentgenographically. In fact, the majority of bone metastases ultimately resulting in pathological fractures combine both blastic and lytic changes or show roentgenographic evidence of diffuse or difficult-to-quantify lytic changes; thus it is easy to underestimate the actual extent of tumor lysis (Figs. 11-2, *A* to *G* and 11-8, *A* and *B*). Radionuclide scans using technetium-99 accurately demonstrate the presence of skeletal metastases in over 90% of

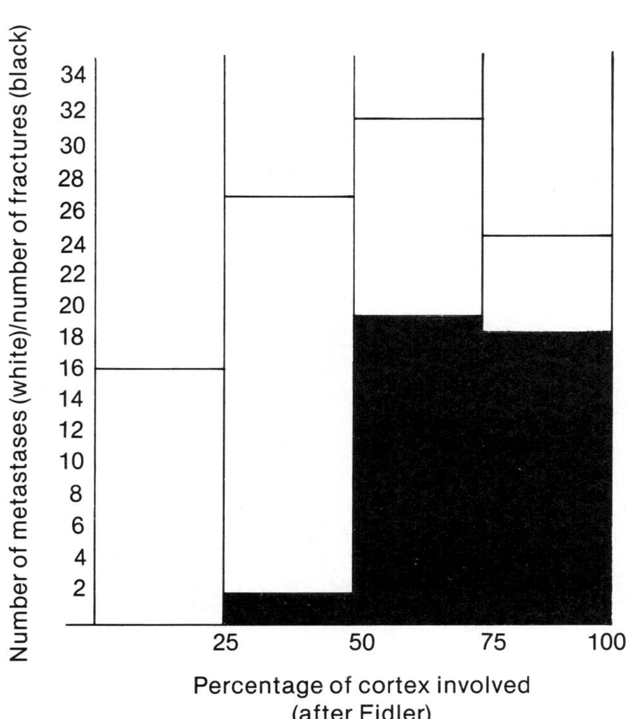

FIGURE 11-5 Incidence of spontaneous pathological fracture in metastatic malignancy.

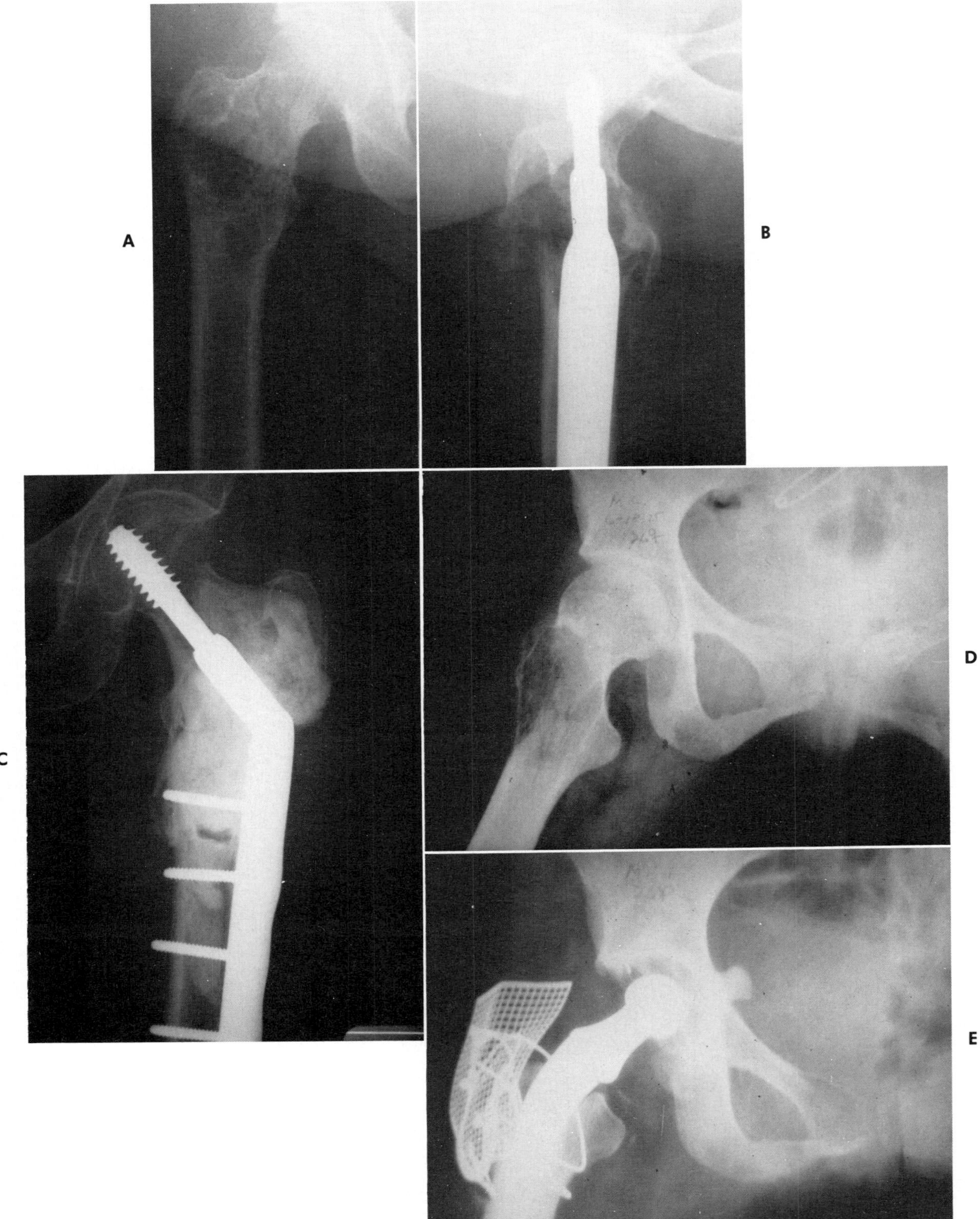

FIGURE 11-6 For legend see opposite page.

FIGURE 11-6 **A,** Extensive lytic metastasis at least 3 cm in diameter involving the proximal femur (carcinoma of the breast). Neither this nor a "frogleg" lateral roentgenogram revealed definite cortical destruction. **B,** Because of the lesion's size, prophylactic fixation was accomplished before the area was irradiated. An intraoperative true lateral roentgenogram after fixation clearly demonstrates extensive destruction of the anterior cortex. The lesion healed after irradiation, and the patient remains alive and pain free 5 years after surgery. **C,** Expansile lytic lesion of the proximal femur associated with expansion of the medullary canal and marked thinning of the cortex. Methylmethacrylate filling the lesion (and the medullary canal proximal and distal to the lesion) greatly enhances prophylactic fixation with a compression hip screw. Ideally the acrylic cement should extend proximally up to the level of the threads of the hip screw and distally to incorporate at least the second screw of the sideplate. An artificial buttress thus is created, effectively resisting compression loads and the tendency for the proximal femur to angulate into varus. Such fixation also complements the resistance to shear and torque forces that are afforded primarily by the hip screw. **D,** A similar expansile lytic lesion of the proximal femur in a 26-year-old woman with metastatic breast cancer. **E,** Rather than attempt prophylactic internal fixation of this femur, the surgeon chose to resect the proximal head and neck and to perform a total hip arthroplasty. Because the greater trochanter had been destroyed by tumor, wire mesh was used to secure the abductor muscles to the shaft. Total hip replacement in preference to internal fixation is favored by many surgeons who believe that the technique obviates further concerns about the permanency of internal fixation in the face of questionable bony union after radiation. (**D** and **E** reprinted from Habermann, E.T., et al.: Clin. Orthop. **169:**70, 1982.)

cases, but such scans are not particularly useful in attempting to quantitate the extent of bone destruction or (more important) the likelihood of a pathological fracture. Because technetium-99 uptake initially is dependent on local blood flow to bone and later on local osteoblastic activity, slowly or rapidly progressive lytic lesions provoking minimal response from adjacent host osteocytes may appear deceptively quiet on bone scan (Fig. 11-9, *A* and *B*). Myeloma, lymphoma, and colon metastases often behave in this way. Galium scanning has offered no improvement in diagnostic accuracy over conventional technetium-99 bone scans.

For patients who experience focal limb pain that is aggravated by weight-bearing and in whom conventional roentgenograms, CT scans, or tomograms do not demonstrate a clear-cut risk of impending fracture, a combination of these studies with radioisotope scanning will better demonstrate the balance between tumor aggressiveness and host response. Such patients are treated typically by local irradiation therapy, and in most instances effective pain control can be achieved. However, the physician must realize that the initial response of bone to irradiation is a focal hyperemia leading to localized osteoporosis, which actually weakens the host bone temporarily. For the first 10 to 18 days after beginning a course of radiotherapy, the patient actually is at higher risk of fracturing through the tumor focus than before the radiation commenced. Patients may frequently incur long-bone fractures while being transferred to or from the radiotherapy table after 2 weeks of a projected 4-week course of treatment.

The vagaries of assessing fracture risk in patients with mixed blastic and lytic lesions and the increased risk of fracture created by the initial response to irradiation have prompted the establishment of another relative indication for prophylactic fixation—the presence of persistent or increasing local pain, particularly when aggravated by weight-bearing, despite the completion of at least 2 weeks of radiotherapy (see box on p. 297). Most such patients probably have microfractures that will progress to displacement even in the face of restricted weight-bearing if the bone is not internally splinted (Fig. 11-9, *C* to *E*).

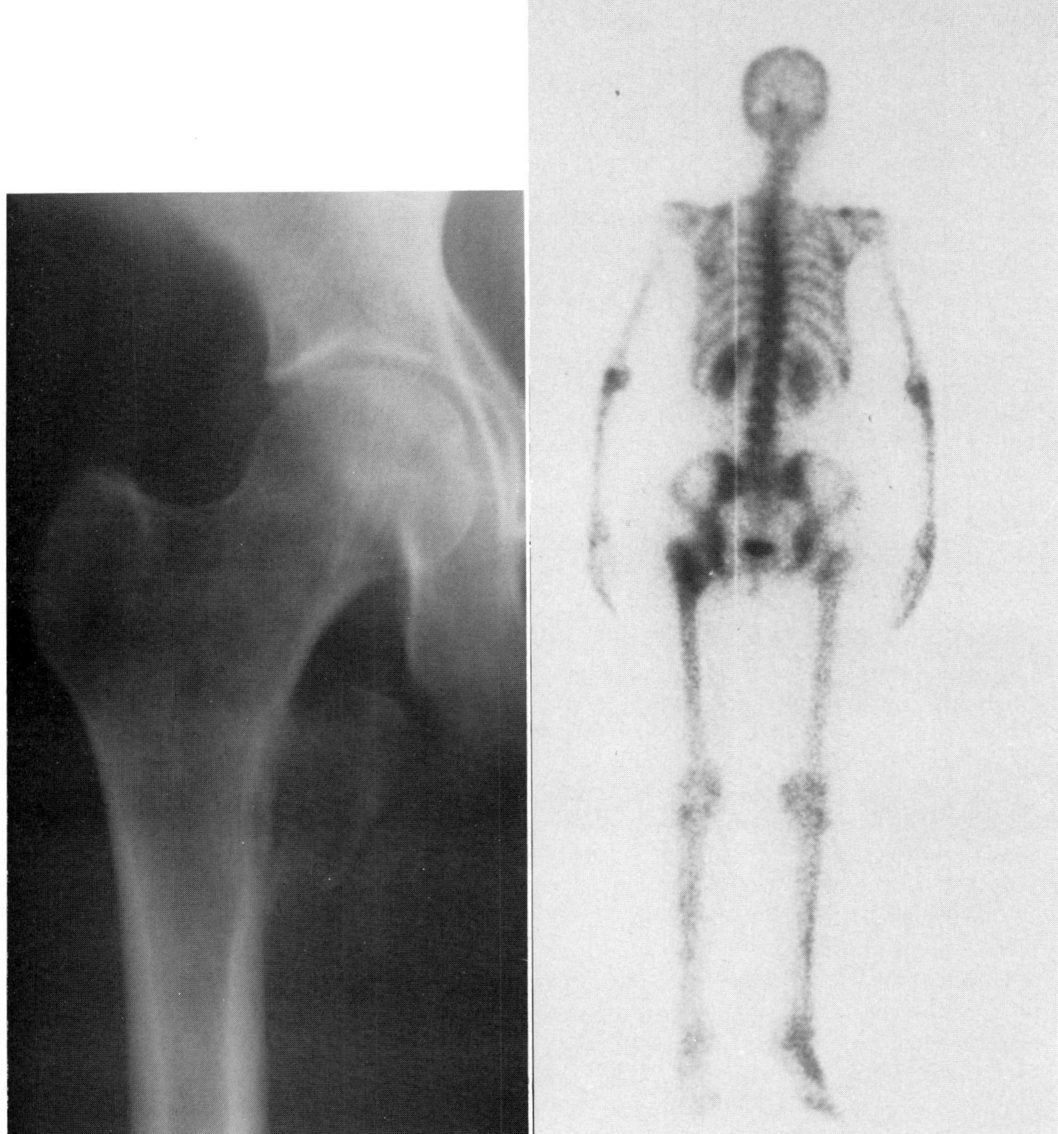

FIGURE 11-7 **A,** Pathological avulsion fracture of the lesser trochanter in a patient with metastatic carcinoma of the breast. Although the femoral neck and subtrochanteric region appeared unaffected by metastases, the lesser trochanter fracture was considered an ominous warning of impending fracture of the proximal femur. **B,** The technetium-99 scan revealed markedly increased uptake in the intertrochanteric femur. The patient refused prophylactic stabilization of the femur and 2 weeks later suffered a spontaneous intertrochanteric fracture when she rolled over in bed.

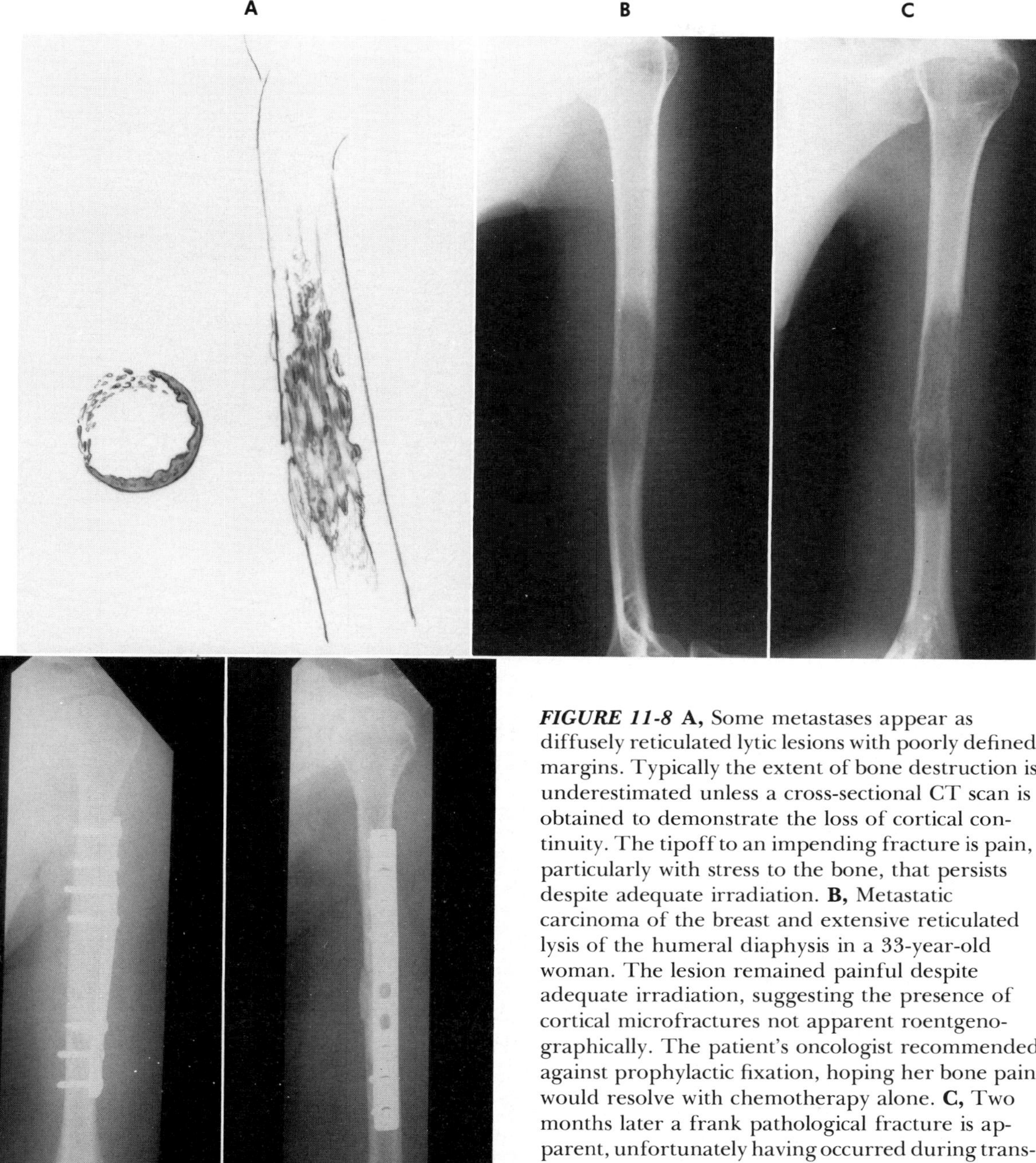

FIGURE 11-8 **A,** Some metastases appear as diffusely reticulated lytic lesions with poorly defined margins. Typically the extent of bone destruction is underestimated unless a cross-sectional CT scan is obtained to demonstrate the loss of cortical continuity. The tipoff to an impending fracture is pain, particularly with stress to the bone, that persists despite adequate irradiation. **B,** Metastatic carcinoma of the breast and extensive reticulated lysis of the humeral diaphysis in a 33-year-old woman. The lesion remained painful despite adequate irradiation, suggesting the presence of cortical microfractures not apparent roentgenographically. The patient's oncologist recommended against prophylactic fixation, hoping her bone pain would resolve with chemotherapy alone. **C,** Two months later a frank pathological fracture is apparent, unfortunately having occurred during transcontinental air travel. The fracture was complicated by a radial nerve palsy persisting 3 months. **D** and **E,** After open fixation and radial neurolysis, the patient was pain free within 10 days. She enjoyed excellent fracture stability, despite the absence of true bone union, until her death 26 months after surgery.

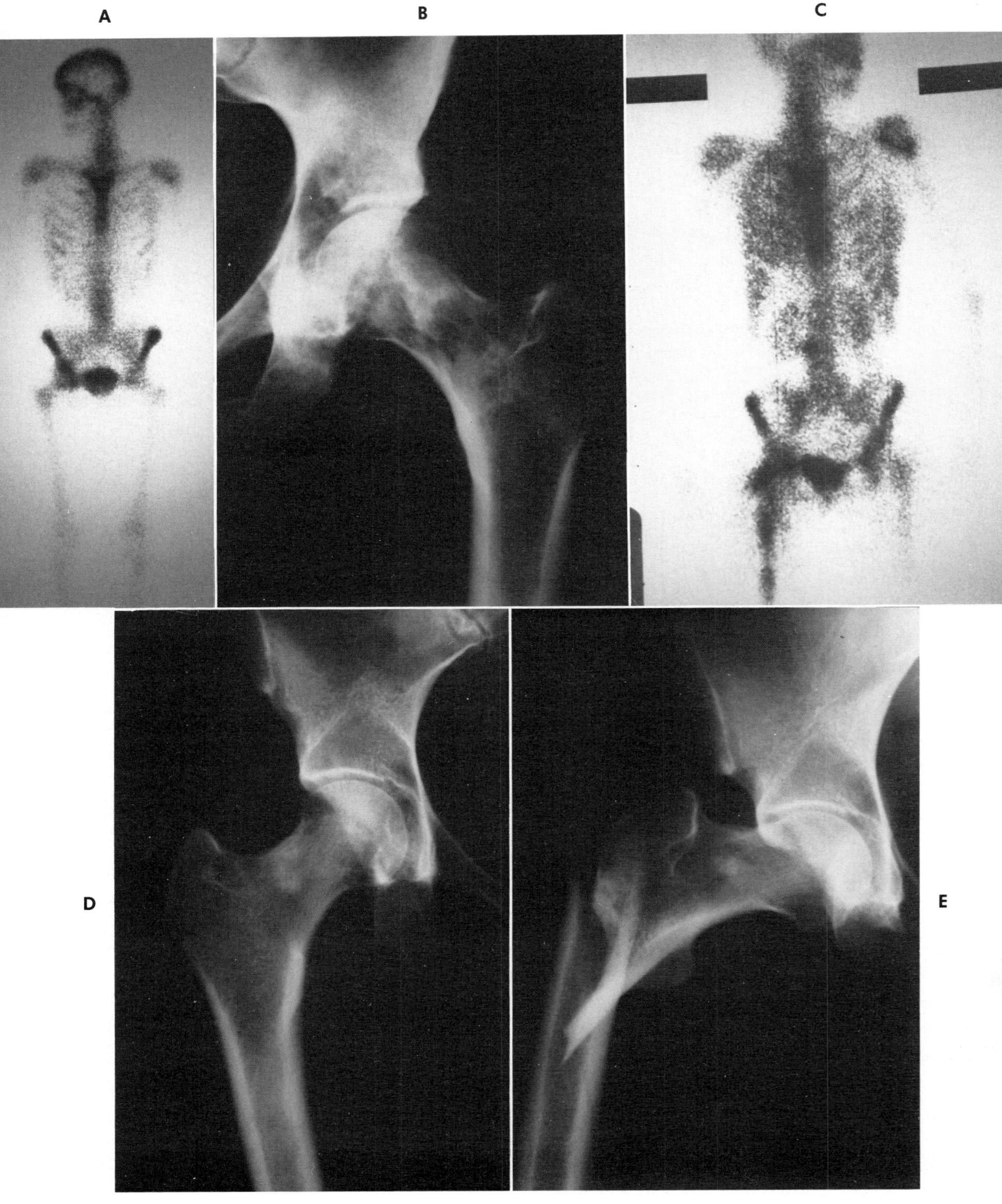

FIGURE 11-9 For legend see opposite page.

FIGURE 11-9 A technetium-99 bone scan reflects blood flow through bone (during the initial vascular phase of the scan) and osteoblastic activity (during the late or secondary phase). Metastatic lesions stimulating minimum increase in blood flow or osteoblastic reaction can appear misleadingly quiet by scan despite aggressive bone destruction apparent roentgenographically. **A,** Technetium-99 scan of a patient with left hip pain. Note the increased uptake in the opposite right supraacetabular region. However, this scan did not suggest the extent of metastatic disease, which was subsequently revealed by a roentgenogram (**B**) of the left proximal femur. **B,** The AP film of the left hip shows extensive lytic destruction of the femoral neck. A spontaneous pathological fracture occurred through this area 3 days after the roentgenogram. **C,** Conversely, intensive hypervascularity and/or osteoblastic activity in bone, suggestive of an aggressive neoplastic process, may not be reflected by discernible changes on conventional films until there is at least 75% destruction of bone locally. This is a technetium-99 scan of a patient with pain in the right hip. Markedly increased uptake is apparent in the proximal half of the right femur. **D,** A roentgenogram of the right hip taken at the same time reveals only a small blastic focus in the femoral neck. The extent of lysis in the subtrochanteric area is not apparent. **E,** A subtrochanteric pathological fracture occurred as the patient was being lifted off the x-ray table. At surgery there was extensive cortical lysis as suggested by the bone scan.

INDICATIONS FOR PROPHYLACTIC FIXATION OF IMPENDING LONG BONE FRACTURES

1. Cortical bone destruction of 50% or more
2. Lesion of 2.5 cm or more in the proximal femur
3. Pathological avulsion fracture of the lesser trochanter
4. Persisting stress pain despite irradiation

HEALING

Tong et al.[25] report that up to 58% of patients with long bone lesions treated by irradiation but without prophylactic fixation suffered late recurrences of pain despite initial complete relief. In addition, 26% of these patients suffered pathological fractures after the completion of a full course (average 4050 cGy*) of radiotherapy. These figures reinforce concern about the existence of unrecognized microfractures that may progress to frank displacement, perhaps after adequate radiotherapy. They also raise concern that, even if the destructive tumor process is ablated by irradiation, the open section defects or stress risers originally created in cortical bone by the tumor may remain and predispose to eventual fracture even in the absence of active tumor lysis.

Various radiotherapists[3,4,25] also have raised the question of how frequently lytic lesions actually reossify following completion of radiation and why there appears to be a large disparity clinically between (1) the high rate of healing and reossification of lytic lesions and (2) the low incidence of bony union if a pathological fracture occurs through that lesion. Although Beals et al.[1] estimated that only 4% of lytic breast metastases reossify, most other workers[6,17,23] have reported an incidence of 65% to 85% reossification under similar circumstances so long as a fracture has not ensued. Some changes roentgenographically interpreted as reossification may actually represent the formation of heterotopic ossification within the lesion (Fig. 11-10); however, in the great majority of instances replacement of the lesion by mature organized bone does occur.

This reparative process following irradiation has been summarized by Matsubayashi[21]: Initially there is evidence of degeneration and necrosis of cancer cells followed by replacement with proliferative fibrous tissue. Col-

*Currently used designation for units of absorbed radiation (centigrays).

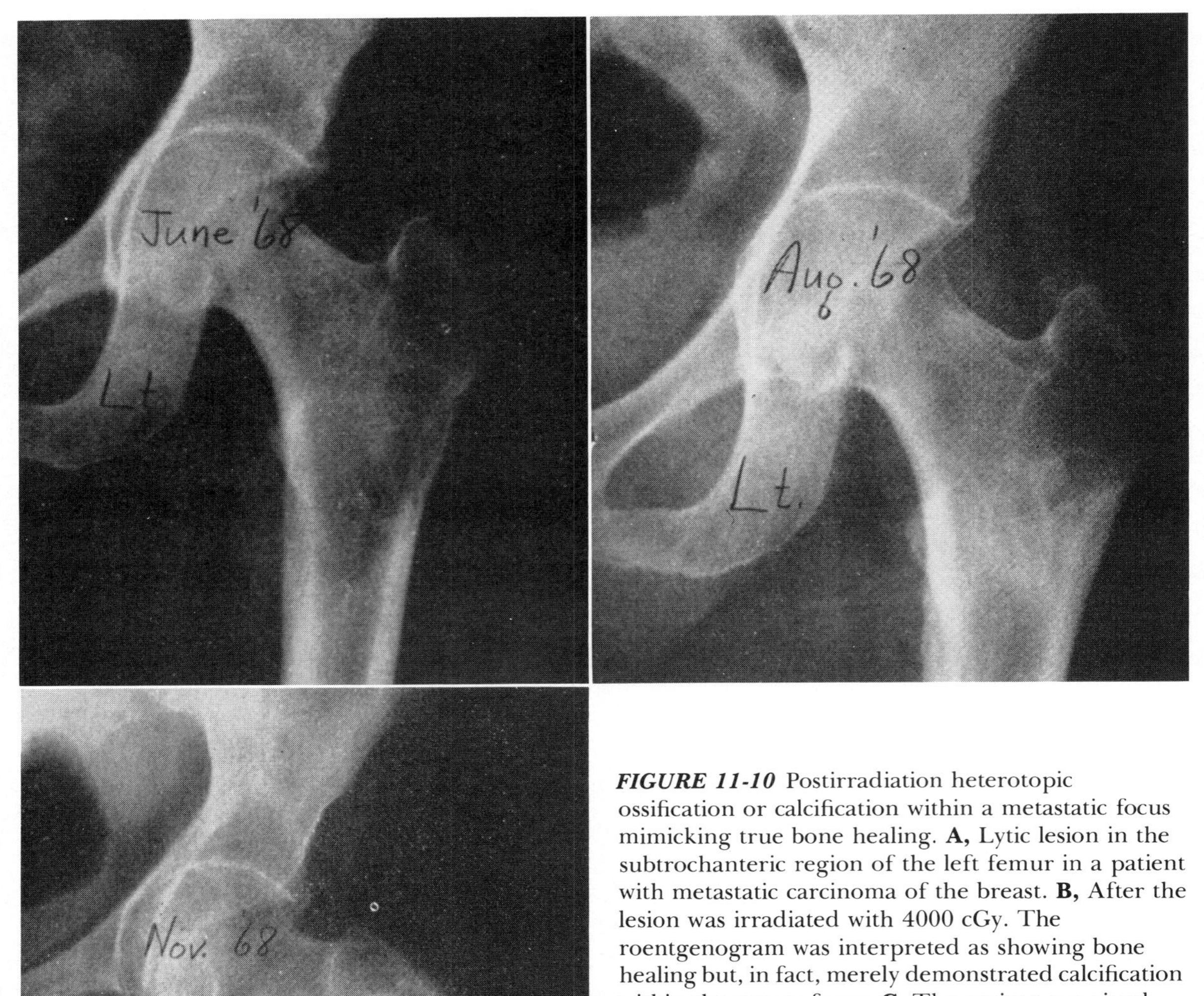

FIGURE 11-10 Postirradiation heterotopic ossification or calcification within a metastatic focus mimicking true bone healing. **A,** Lytic lesion in the subtrochanteric region of the left femur in a patient with metastatic carcinoma of the breast. **B,** After the lesion was irradiated with 4000 cGy. The roentgenogram was interpreted as showing bone healing but, in fact, merely demonstrated calcification within the tumor focus. **C,** The patient remained ambulatory, despite hip pain, and 3 months later suffered a displaced pathological fracture through the original lytic focus. In view of the size and location of the lesion and the fact that it remained painful on weight-bearing after irradiation, prophylactic internal fixation should have been performed. (From Blake, D.D., Clin. Orthop. **73:**89, 1970.)

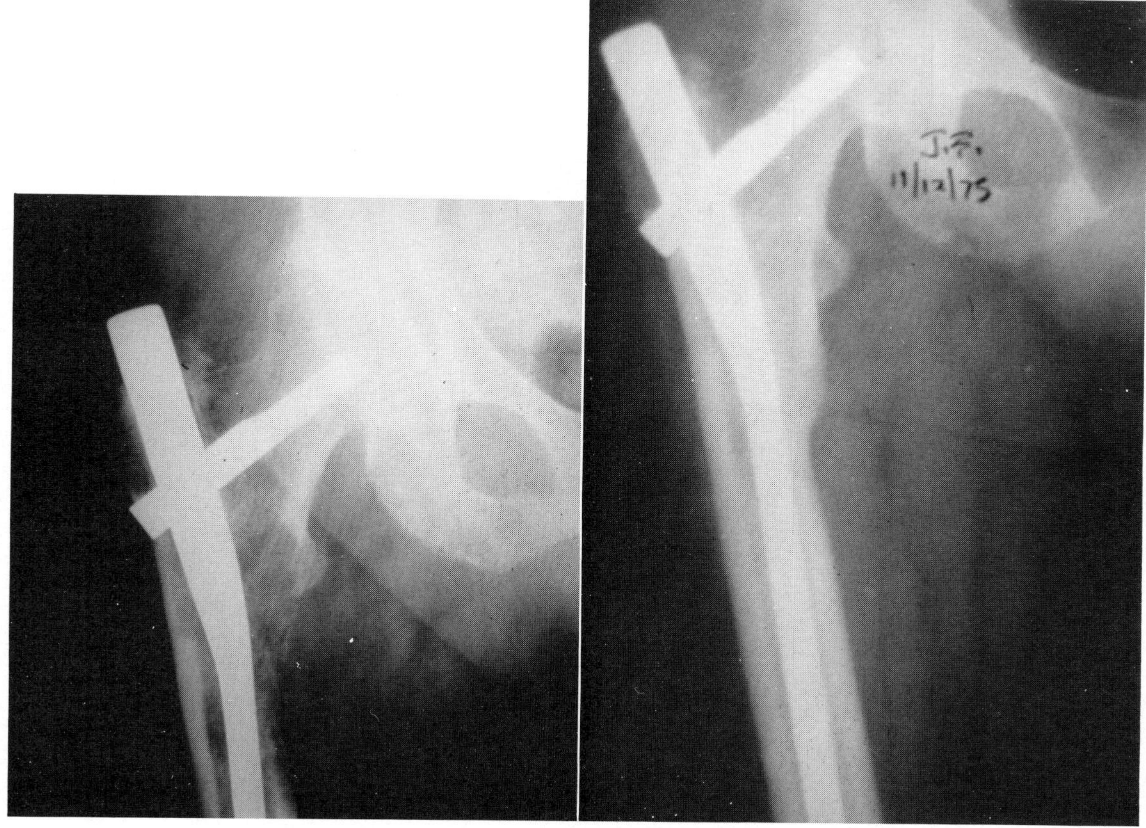

FIGURE 11-11 **A,** Metastatic carcinoma of the breast and large lytic metastases in the subtrochanteric femur of a 63-year-old woman. The impending pathological fracture was prophylactically fixed closed with a Zickel nail and did not need to be exposed. Adjunctive fixation by methylmethacrylate was unnecessary. **B,** Fracture through the lesion was prevented by prophylactic fixation, and 5 months after surgery, despite local irradiation, the lesion had healed completely. *Continued.*

lagen fibers then aggregate within a loose but richly vascularized fibrous stroma. These fluffy strands of aggregated collagen gradually become calcified, and finally woven bone trabeculae appear that eventually mature into lamellar bone.

If a pathological fracture supervenes during this reparative process, a totally different pathway for healing exists. Normally fractures heal by the formation of a bridging callus that develops through the network of organizing hematoma and gradually is differentiated into fibrocartilage and then into hyaline cartilage and eventually is replaced by bone. As noted, this process is in marked contrast to a lytic metastasis, which appears to occur primarily as a result of direct osteogenesis. The chondrogenic phase of healing (formation of fibrocartilage and its evolution into hyaline cartilage) required for a pathological fracture—but not for the filling in of a lytic defect—is extremely sensitive to radiation. Bonarigo and Rubin[4] demonstrated experimentally that radiation in excess of 2500 cGy (rads) seriously interferes with the chondrogenic phase of fracture healing yet causes minimal interference with osteoblastic proliferation. For this reason nonunion of a fracture often occurs after radiation whereas osteogenesis continues healing through a nonfractured lytic area. Here again is a strong argument for prophylactic internal fixation of lytic lesions at high risk of fracture *before* such a fracture occurs (Fig. 11-11, *A* and *B*).

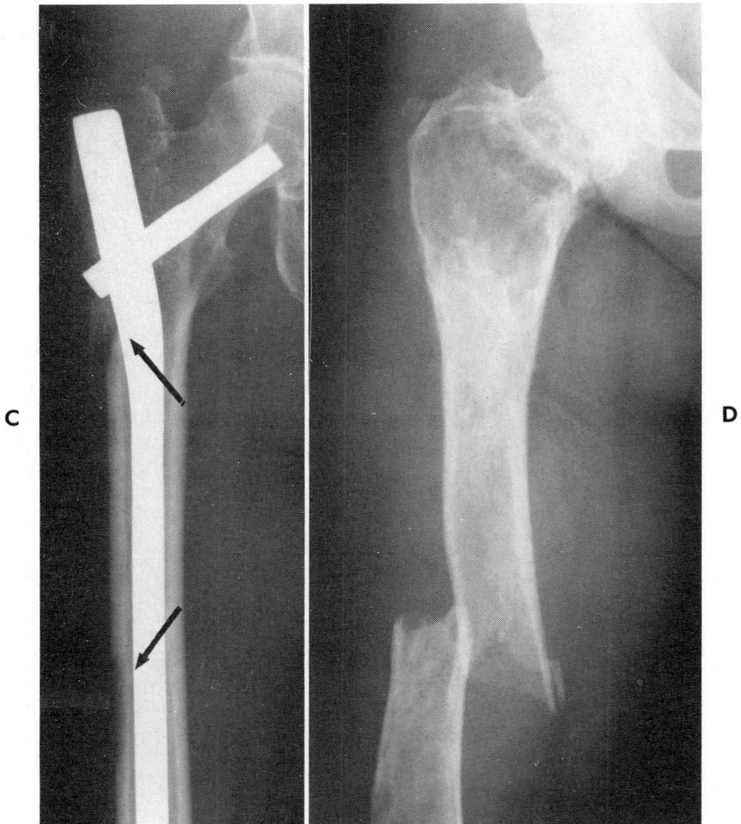

FIGURE 11-11, cont'd. **C,** Another example of an ideal use for the Zickel nail. An extensive lytic focus in the subtrochanteric region *(upper arrow)* has been reinforced prophylactically and, by the same technique, a lesion of the diaphysis with moderate destruction has been stabilized *(lower arrow)*. In this circumstance closed insertion of the Zickel nail components could be accomplished without the necessity of using intramedullary methylmethacrylate. **D,** This is an unusual situation: widespread metastases from a renal carcinoma with cortical destruction and deformity involving almost the entire femur. The patient had been encouraged to undergo prophylactic fixation with a Zickel nail but had refused surgical intervention even after the fracture occurred. Prophylactic fixation by an intramedullary rod before the fracture would not have been appropriate because a major stress riser would have been created at the base of the femoral neck and in the intertrochanteric region and a fracture through this area would have ensued. Once the fracture occurred, a Zickel nail still would have been ideal for fixation but rotational stability of the distal femur could have been achieved only by extensive curettage of the medullary canal and packing the canal with methylmethacrylate around the distal end of the nail. The distal canal would have been filled with cement in a liquid state and the fracture then reduced with the nail inserted the length of the canal before polymerization occurred. (**C** reprinted from Habermann, E.T., et al.: Clin. Orthop. **169:**70, 1982.)

TECHNIQUES OF PROPHYLACTIC INTERNAL FIXATION

Once the decision has been made to fix an impending fracture internally, the surgeon must review several general technical considerations critical to the success of the procedure.

1. To avoid the concomitant higher risk of nonunion, every effort should be made to prevent the occurrence of a fracture during the operative procedure.
2. Soft tissue surrounding the bone should be disturbed as little as possible to preserve the periosteal blood supply. This is particularly important because the endosteal circulation usually has been disrupted locally by the tumor process.
3. When large thin-walled lesions exist or the intramedullary canal varies greatly in size (Fig. 11-11, *D*), closed intramedullary nailing techniques should be augmented by direct reinforcement of the lesion using methylmethacrylate. This will enhance fixation of the distal long bone, particularly with regard to the torsional stability, and will also prevent shortening of the bone. The use of an interlocking intramedullary device (e.g., the Grosse-Kempf nail) that is specifically designed to prevent shortening also may be considered. However, this device is technically more demanding to use than is conventional intramedullary fixation and it is not as secure a method of preventing late shortening of the long bone if bony union does not occur ultimately.
4. When defects extend through the full thickness of cortical bone, they should be plugged by acrylic cement at the time of fixation to minimize the significance of stress risers or open section defects (Fig. 11-2, *H* and *I*).
5. To enhance the efficacy of subsequent irradiation, lesions that have not been irradiated before fixation should be debulked of as much tumor tissue as possible before fixation (Fig. 11-2, *D* to *G*).
6. Lesions appearing likely to be highly vascular should be considered for arteriographic evaluation and possible embolization before open curettage.

Lesions of the femoral neck or the intertrochanteric area of the proximal femur are treated best by fixation with the use of a compression hip screw and side plate. Intramedullary devices such as the Zickel nail, although affording better prophylaxis against subsequent fracture of the subtrochanteric area, do not reinforce the femoral neck adequately if there is tumor lysis extending significantly into that area. I have reviewed the roentgenograms of three patients with such lesions reinforced by a Zickel nail, each of whom suffered a subsequent fracture through the subcapital portion of the femoral neck just proximal to the tip of the cross-fixation pin.

Patients with impending intertrochanteric or femoral neck fracture are positioned on a fracture table, and a guide pin is inserted into the midportion of the femoral head and neck under image intensification. A 2 × 2 cm lateral cortical window is created, and the corkscrew portion of a compression hip screw is inserted over the guide pin under direct vision as proximally as possible so its tip will be in the immediately subchondral bone of the femoral head. As much tumor tissue as possible is removed from the intertrochanteric lesion both proximal and distal to the cortical window. A four- or five-hole side plate is articulated with the corkscrews—care being taken to avoid undue sheer or torque stress across the weakened bone, thereby creating a fracture. Once the surgeon is comfortable that the side plate can be positioned easily over the screws, he removes the side plate and fills the cavity with methylmethacrylate to its fullest extent. Ideally, the cement will fill proximally to the level of the hip screw threads and distally to the level of the first and second side-plate screw (Fig. 11-6, *C*). A side plate should be chosen of sufficient length to allow bicortical fixation by at least three screws below the distal extent of the tumor cavity.

Habermann et al.,[14] Lane et al.,[20] and Sim (Harrington et al.[18]) have advocated resection of the proximal femur where intertrochanteric lesions create a high risk of fracture. The upper femur is thereby replaced by a proximal femoral prosthesis, often necessitating acetabular prosthetic replacement as well (Fig. 11-6, *D* and *E*). Biopsy of the acetabular bone at the time of surgery often reveals evidence of metastases, and Habermann et al.[14] have used this as an indication to replace both sides of the joint.

Such replacement (rather than fixation) of

proximal lesions obviates fears of late local tumor recurrence or fixation-device failure. However, the technique requires the surgeon to maintain a large stock of proximal femoral prostheses. It also subjects the patient to much more operative time and blood loss than does prophylactic fixation, and it introduces the risk of acetabular loosening, hip dislocation, trochanteric avulsion, and nonunion, which are not encountered after internal fixation. For these reasons I still advocate fixation techniques for all but the most severely destroyed. proximal femora.

Subtrochanteric lesions are stabilized best by using a Zickel nail inserted while the patient is in the lateral decubitus position, which allows the affected leg to be freely adducted for insertion of the nail through the tip of the greater trochanter. I have found that attempts to insert the Zickel nail while the patient is supine on the fracture table necessitate forceful adduction and often rotation of the affected limb, thus predisposing to a fracture through weakened subtrochanteric bone where much of that stress is concentrated.

Many subtrochanteric lesions can be effectively fixed prophylactically with the Zickel nail alone, inserted by a closed technique and without augmentation by intramedullary methylmethacrylate (Fig. 11-11, *C*). However, when large cortical defects exist in the subtrochanteric area, I believe that these should be filled with acrylic cement polymerizing in situ in an effort to restore cortical continuity and thereby reduce local stress potentially productive of a subsequent fracture (Fig. 11-2, *H* and *I*). This requires local exposure of the tumor focus, but it offers the additional advantage that extensive debulking of the tumor mass can be established as well, thereby enhancing the efficacy of subsequent radiation therapy. Others[14] have performed such fixation without filling the defect with cement and have reported good results accompanied by a low incidence of late refracture (Fig. 11-11, *A* and *B*).

Lesions of the femoral shaft usually can be fixed internally by closed intramedullary nailing with the patient in the lateral decubitus position. Again, however, when large defects exist, particularly associated with marked cortical thinning or open defects, it may be necessary to expose these areas, remove tissue within the cavity, and fill the resulting defect with acrylic cement. This procedure prevents the all-too-common complication during later weight-bearing that bone about the tumor focus collapses, the proximal shaft fragment slides over the nail to impact on the distal fragment, and femoral shortening with proximal nail protrusion results (Fig. 11-2, *J*). Under these circumstances an alternative method of preventing shortening and maintaining the principles of closed intramedullary fixation is to use an interlocking nail with cross fixation well proximal and distal to the area of tumor lysis. However, a potential disadvantage of this fixation technique is that, if the lytic lesion does not ossify ultimately, the relatively fragile cross-fixation screws eventually will loosen or break.

If a risk does not seem to exist that shortening will occur by telescoping of the major fragments about the intramedullary rod, a conventional closed rodding technique should be accomplished and no attempt made to fill the lytic defect with methylmethacrylate. There is no effective way to augment the fixation by methylmethacrylate unless the lytic focus is approached directly surgically, tumor tissue is removed under direct vision, and the cavity is filled with cement. Low-viscosity acrylic cement can be injected down the full length of the femoral shaft within the intramedullary rod, but in my opinion the cement adds little if any ancillary stability under these circumstances.

Large thin-walled lytic metastases in the distal femur are uncommon, but when present they are especially challenging because of the difficulty of fixing the narrow distal fragment. If sufficient bone of the femoral condyle remains, an angulated condylar plate can be used with augmentation by methylmethacrylate packed into the debrided cavity of the lytic metastasis. Again, care should be taken to use a blade plate of sufficient length to allow at least two and preferably three screws to transfix intact cortices about the confines of the lesion.

Occasionally a metastatic focus will aggressively destroy bone right up to the subchondral bone of the femoral condylar articulate cartilage (Fig. 11-12). Because all cartilage is resistant to tumor invasion,[19] it is extremely unlikely that the malignant process will invade the knee joint unless a pathological fracture has occurred. These lesions are best man-

A 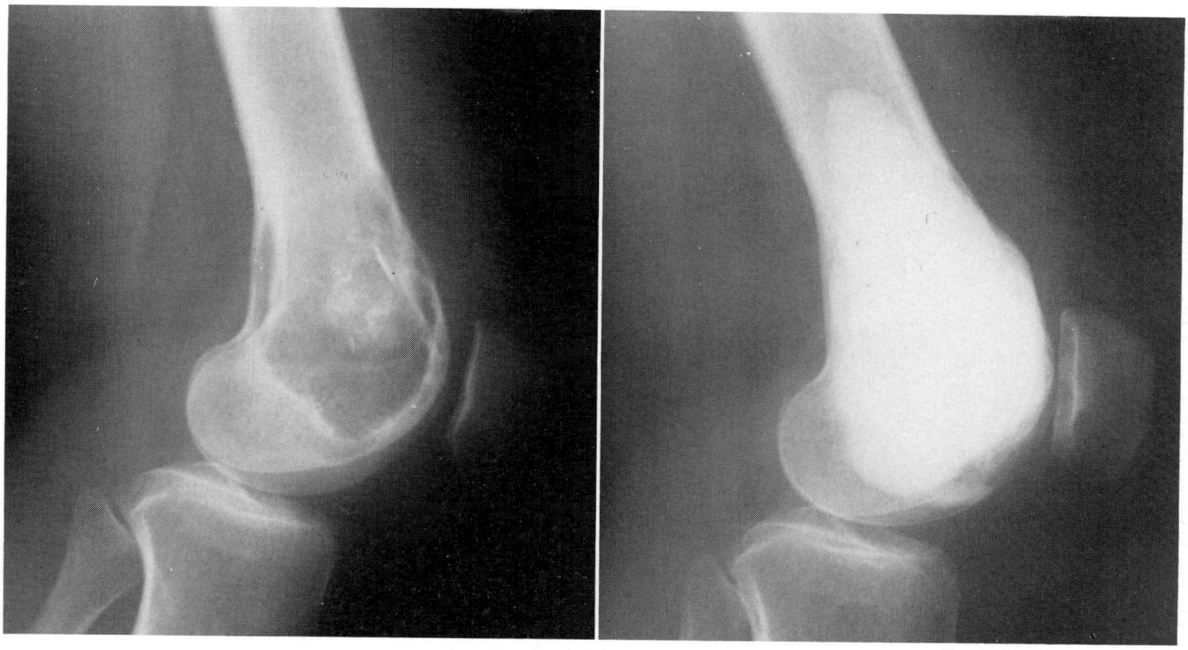 B

FIGURE 11-12 **A,** Occasionally extensive metaphyseal or epiphyseal destructive defects will have insufficient bone proximal or distal to the lesional margins to allow conventional prophylactic fixation. **B,** The technique of intralesional curettage and filling of the defect with methylmethacrylate can be used to prevent subchondral fractures, bone collapse, and disruption of the joint surface. The lesion then can be irradiated with impunity. The presence of methylmethacrylate within the tumor cavity, even if radiopaque, does not interfere with the efficacy of irradiation. Moreover, irradiation does not change the mechanical properties of the cement.

aged by curettage through a cortical window followed by packing of the tumor cavity with cement without attempted reinforcement by any metal fixation device. Care must be taken to prevent extrusion of liquid cement into the knee joint through even a small fracture defect. Intraoperative roentgenograms should be obtained, and if cement is noted in the joint it should be removed through a small arthrotomy.

Large aneurysmal lesions of the distal femur, particularly those from myeloma or retroperitoneal malignancies, often should be studied arteriographically before surgery because of the high likelihood that they will be hypervascular with the consequent risk of intractable intraoperative blood loss. Embolization by free fat or Gelfoam strips soaked in thrombin is indicated for particularly vascular lesions, especially if they have been irradiated. There is some evidence that the effectiveness of radiation administered after such embolization may be lessened by the temporarily diminished oxygen tension in the tumor caused by its embolization.

As already noted, Habermann has taken biopsies of roentgenographically normal–appearing periacetabular bone in many breast carcinoma patients with recognizable proximal femoral lesions and has found a high incidence of metastases. Under these circumstances he often advocates prophylactic acetabular replacement. My experience suggests that the great majority of such metastases can be controlled by focal irradiation and will not progress to fracture or even—in most instances—become symptomatic. However, intractable acetabular pain will develop occasionally and be unresponsive to radiotherapy as well as aggravated by the stress of weight-bearing. These individuals should be considered to have microfractures of the acetabular

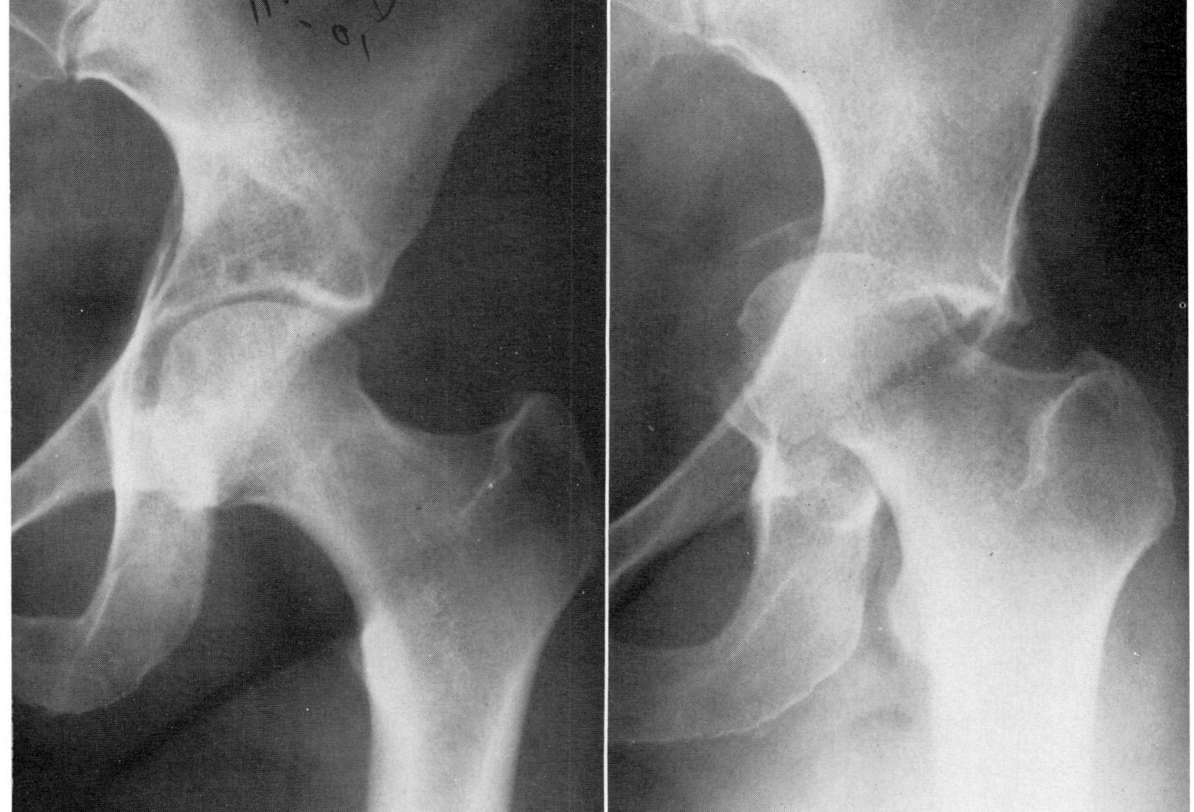

FIGURE 11-13 **A,** Destructive lesion of the supraacetabular bone in a 51-year-old woman 11 years after a mastectomy for breast carcinoma. The patient had no symptoms, and this film was obtained as part of an intravenous pyelographic study for the evaluation of chronic pyelonephritis. No further evaluation of the patient's hip disease was undertaken, but she was given prophylactic irradiation (4500 cGy) because of the changes on her roentgenogram. **B,** Three months later she was running to catch a bus and suddenly suffered a minimally painful superocentral fracture dislocation of the hip. Previously noted changes in the supraacetabular region were minimally apparent after irradiation. This fracture was managed by total hip reconstruction, stabilizing the acetabular component by the use of a protrusio cup with Steinmann pins inserted across the sacroiliac joint.

FIGURE 11-14 **A** and **B,** Another extensive area of reticulated lysis, here involving the distal humerus. A spontaneous fracture occurred as the patient was being transferred from the x-ray table. **C** and **D,** Because of the distal extent of bone destruction, including a portion of the medial epicondyle *(arrow),* fixation was accomplished by using Rush rods inserted retrograde and reinforced with methylmethacrylate packed into the curetted lesion. The fixation, although appearing somewhat tenuous, has remained secure in the absence of bony union for 24 months after surgery.

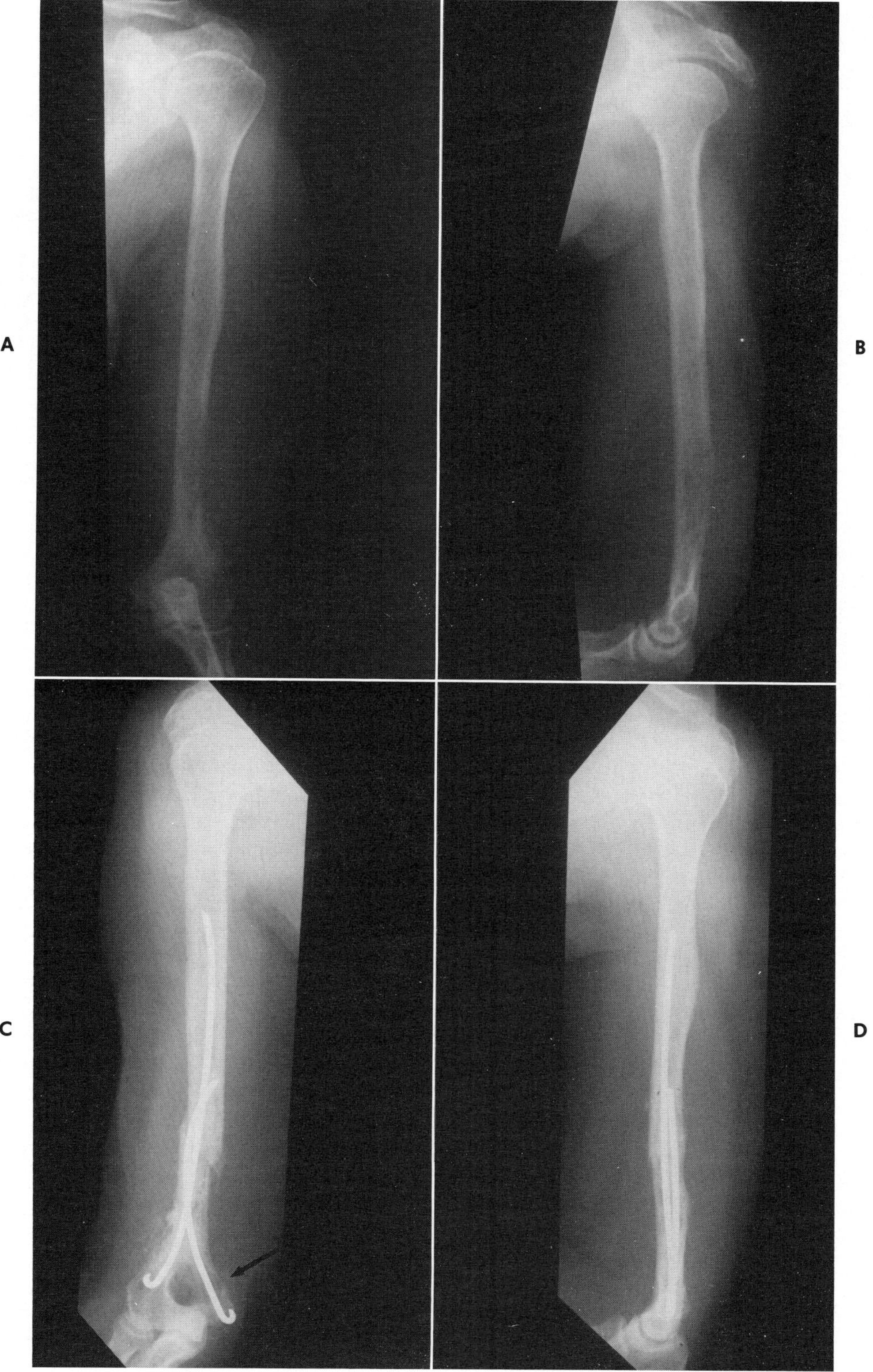

FIGURE 11-14 For legend see opposite page.

bone and be at high risk of central acetabular fracture if a joint replacement and stabilization is not performed (Fig. 11-13). In most instances the extent of bone destruction encountered at surgery and the technical requirements for joint stabilization far exceed what might be anticipated from preoperative roentgenograms.[16] It is the presence of pain on weight-bearing even after the completion of an adequate course of radiation that is the clearest indicator of the need for prophylactic acetabular reconstruction.

Lytic lesions of the humerus generally are considered to have a minimal risk of fracture simply because the humerus is not ordinarily subjected to weight-bearing. However, because patients with widespread metastases often are required to use assistive devices (e.g., canes, crutches, or a walker) necessitated by concomitant metastases of the spine or lower extremities, the humerus may in effect become a weight-bearing bone and require similarly aggressive prophylaxis.

By far, the most common focus for impending humeral fractures is the middiaphysis. Typically lesions that are focal and have minimal risk of shortening are best managed by closed intramedullary fixation with a humeral Kuntscher nail.

When a large lesion with extension and bone destruction exists, fixation by a long compression bone plate is advisable (Figs. 11-4 and 11-8). Although the application of such a plate requires a more difficult anatomical dissection that encompasses some risk to the radial nerve, the advantages of the technique far outweigh its disadvantages: (1) the tumor focus can be entered, debulked, and filled with methylmethacrylate and (2) fixation with a heavy plate augmented by acrylic protects not only against shortening of the humerus but also against subsequent fracture secondary to a distraction force. It must be remembered that the usual stresses on the upper-extremity long bones involve distraction and not compression. I have seen three instances in which such forces caused a distraction through a lytic force despite internal splintage by an intramedullary rod.

Distal humeral lesions are the most difficult to fix prophylactically for several reasons: (1) the thin bone at the olecranon fossa prevents direct axial intramedullary fixation or fixation by a blade plate, (2) one or both epicondyles are frequently involved, thereby obviating adequate fixation by a Y or T plate of the type used for traumatic supracondylar or intracondylar fractures (Fig. 11-14, *A* and *B*), and (3) early elbow motion is essential to minimize upper extremity disability for these patients, who often depend greatly on walking aids. Consequently the most effective method for fixation includes local debridement of the tumor focus and packing of the resulting defect with acrylic cement after first stabilizing the distal humerus by Rush rods inserted percutaneously and retrograde through remaining intact bone of the epicondyles (Fig. 11-14, *C* and *D*).

Whether the prophylactic fixation of spinal metastases ever is indicated is difficult to determine. Spinal metastases are extremely common, particularly from lesions such as breast carcinoma, hypernephroma, colonic carcinoma, prostatic, uterine, and ovarian carcinomas, and myeloma. Pathological compression fractures also are common under such circumstances, but the great majority become inherently stable just as do vertebral compression fractures occurring in women who have osteoporosis without malignant disease. It is not difficult to predict which vertebrae are likely to fracture, particularly if one obtains a cross-sectional CT scan, but the magnitude and risks of the operation required for "prophylactic" stabilization of these lesions generally preclude such a procedure for the spine. However, an exception is the destructive tumor that not only has created a risk of fracture but also has resulted in a progressive neurological compromise necessitating anterior decompression. In such an instance spinal cord or root decompression can be accomplished by resecting much of the remaining bone of the vertebral body, and vertebral replacement and stabilization can be achieved by using methylmethacrylate and distraction rod fixation.[15,17]

SUMMARY

Both lytic and blastic long bone metastases are at risk of producing pathological fractures when more than 50% of the circumferential cortical bone has been destroyed or when pain on weight-bearing stresses persists, increases, or recurs despite adequate local irradiation.

Moreover, the most commonly encountered lesions of the proximal femur are at high risk of fracturing if they are in excess of 2.5 cm in any dimension or are associated with avulsion of the lesser trochanter.

Such lesions should be treated aggressively by prophylactic internal fixation. This will avoid the development of a secondary fracture with its concomitantly high risk that true bony healing will not occur even in the presence of adequate fixation.

When internal fixation is chosen for a large metastasis with extensive cortical destruction, it should be augmented by debulking of the lesion and packing with in situ–polymerizing methylmethacrylate. Such an expedient not only improves the efficacy of subsequent radiotherapy but also prevents shortening of the bone with weight-bearing while enhancing the torque capacity and sheer resistance inherent in the metal fixation device.

REFERENCES

1. Beals, R.K., et al.: Prophylactic internal fixation of the femur in metastatic breast cancer, Cancer, **28:**1350, 1971.
2. Bertin, K.C., et al.: Metastatic malignant disease: isolated fracture of the greater trochanter in adults, J. Bone Joint Surg. **66A:**770, June 1984.
3. Blake, D.D.: Radiation treatment of metastatic bone disease, Clin. Orthop. **73:**89, 1970.
4. Bonarigo, B.C., and Rubin, P.: Nonunion of pathologic fracture after radiation therapy, Radiology **88:**889, 1967.
5. Burstein, A.H., et al: Bone strength: the effect of screw holes, J. Bone Joint Surg. **54A:**1143, 1972.
6. Cheng, D.S., et al.: Nonoperative management of femoral, humeral, and acetabular metastases in patients with breast carcinoma, Cancer **45:**1533, 1980.
7. Cramer, S.F., et al.: The cellular basis of metastatic bone disease in patients with lung cancer, Cancer **48:**2649, 1981.
8. Enneking, W.F.: Metastatic carcinoma. In Musculoskeletal tumor surgery, New York, 1982 Churchill Livingstone, Inc.
9. Fidler, M.: Prophylactic internal fixation of secondary neoplastic deposits in long bones, Br. Med. J. **1:**341, 1973.
10. Galasko, C.S.B.: The pathological basis for skeletal scintigraphy, J. Bone Joint Surg. **57B:**353, 1975.
11. Galasko, C.S.B.: Mechanisms of bone destruction in the development of skeletal metastases, Nature **263:**507, 1976.
12. Galasko, C.S.B.: Mechanisms of lytic and blastic metastastic disease of bone, Clin. Orthop. **169:**20, 1982.
13. Galasko, C.S.B., et al: Prostaglandins, osteoclasts, and bone destruction produced by VX2 carcinoma in rabbits: effects of administering indomethacin at different doses and times, Br. J. Cancer **40:**360, 1979.
14. Habermann, E.T., et al.: The pathology and treatment of metastatic disease of the femur, Clin. Orthop. **169:**70, 1982.
15. Harrington, K.D.: The use of methylmethacrylate or vertebral-body replacement and anterior stabilization of pathological fracture-dislocations of the spine due to metastatic malignant disease, J. Bone Joint Surg. **63A:**36, 1981.
16. Harrington, K.D.: New trends in the management of lower extremity metastases, Clin. Orthop. **169:**53, 1982.
17. Harrington, K.D.: Anterior cord decompression and spine stabilization for patients with metastatic lesions of the spine, J. Neurosurg. **61:**107, 1984.
18. Harrington, K.D., et al: Methylmethacrylate as an adjunct in the internal fixation of pathological fractures, J. Bone Joint Surg. **58A:**1047, 1976.
19. Kuettner, K.E., and Pauli, B.U.: Resistance of cartilage to normal and neoplastic invasion. In Horton, J.E., editor: Mechanisms of localized bone loss, Calcif. Tissue Res. (spec. suppl.), p. 251, 1978.
20. Lane, J.M., et al.: Treatment of pathological fractures of the hip by endoprosthetic replacement, J. Bone Joint Surg. **62A:**954, 1980.
21. Matsubayashi, T.: The reparative process of metastatic bone lesions after radiotherapy, Jap. J. Clin. Oncol. **11**(suppl.):253, 1981.
22. Mundy, G.R., and Raisz, L.G.: Big and little forms of osteoclast activating factor, J. Clin. Invest. **60:**122, 1977.
23. Parrish, F.F., and Murray, J.A.: Surgical treatment for secondary neoplastic fractures: a retrospective study of ninety-six patients, J. Bone Joint Surg. **52A:**665, 1970.
24. Pugh, J., et al.: Biomechanics of pathologic fractures, Clin. Orthop. **169:**109, 1982.
25. Tong, D., et al.: The palliation of symptomatic osseus metastases, Cancer **50:**893, 1982.

CHAPTER 12

METASTATIC DISEASE OF THE SPINE

The spine is the most common site for skeletal metastases, irrespective of the primary tumor involved. Within the spine the vertebral body typically is affected first, although the initial roentgenographic finding often will be destruction of a pedicle. This seeming paradox is explainable by the fact that, in the absence of a blastic or sclerotic reaction from the vertebral cancellous bone, between 30% and 50% of a vertebral body must be destroyed before any changes can be recognized roentgenographically (Fig. 12-1). By contrast, minimal lysis of bone in a pedicle is recognizable because the pedicle cortex tends to be involved earlier and this is easily seen in cross section on AP roentgenograms (Fig. 12-2). Thompson and Keiller[64] demonstrated by postmortem examination of patients who had died of metastatic disease that the posterior vertebral elements were significantly involved only one seventh as often as was the vertebral body. Similar findings were described by Jaffe,[45] who showed that more than 70% of patients dying of cancer had evidence of vertebral metastases at careful postmortem examination. In his series the thoracic spine was the most commonly involved segment of the vertebral column, although other investigators[2,34,75] have found the lumbar spine to be more frequently involved.

In most series, carcinomas of the breast and lung and lymphomas and myelomas are the most common tumors with metastases to the spine. Seventy-five percent of vertebral metastases come from these primaries and from the less frequent carcinomas of the kidney, prostate, and thyroid.[15] Gilbert et al.[37] found that tumors of the breast and lung usually metastasized to the thoracic area, although the entire spine often is involved, and prostatic carcinomas usually affected the lumbar spine, sacrum, and pelvis.

This distribution is not entirely a random phenomenon. As discussed in greater detail in Chapter 2, pp. 25 to 28, the breast drains principally by the azygos veins, communicating with Batson's paravertebral venous plexus initially in the thoracic region. The prostate drains through the pelvic venous plexus,[2] which also communicates with Batson's plexus, initially in the pelvis and lower spine. The lung, by contrast, drains principally via the pulmonary vein into the left heart and showers its tumor cells in a generalized fashion throughout the skeleton. Tumors of the colon and rectum, which drain through the portal system, tend to seed the lung and liver with metastases much earlier and more frequently than they do the bones. Black[4] estimated that for 9% of spinal metastases the primary source of the tumor could not be determined.

PATHOPHYSIOLOGY

Throughout a person's life the vertebral bodies contain active (red) bone marrow, unlike the bones of the peripheral skeleton, which in adulthood contain mostly avascular yellow marrow. As already described in Chapter 2, the vascular sinusoidal system within red marrow is particularly vulnerable

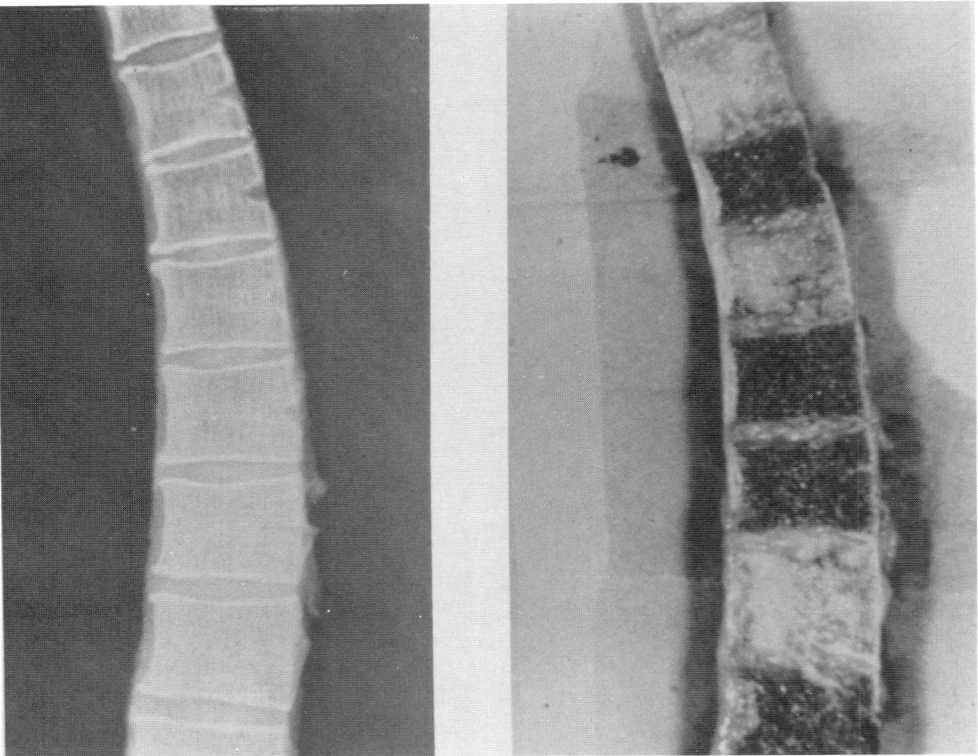

FIGURE 12-1 Postmortem specimen of the spine sectioned sagittally *(right)* and detailed by time-lapse roentgenography *(left)*. Note the extensive metastatic involvement. Four vertebral bodies have been almost completely replaced by tumor, although no abnormalities are appreciable roentgenographically. (Reprinted with permission from Jaffee, H.L.: Tumors and tumorous conditions of the bones and joints, Philadelphia, 1958, Lea & Febiger.)

to cancer cells, allowing them easily to escape the circulation and become established within the cancellous network of bone. The ability of these cells[34,35] to produce a protective fibrin sheath and secrete osteoclast-activating factors and perhaps prostaglandins also appears to be enhanced within the red marrow of vertebrae.

Vertebral metastases per se are often asymptomatic and may be discovered only on routine bone scans or plain roentgenograms. When symptoms do develop, they are the consequence of one or more of the following: (1) an enlarging mass within the vertebral body that may break through the cortex and invade paravertebral soft tissues, (2) compression or invasion of local nerve roots by such a mass, (3) a pathological fracture secondary to vertebral destruction, (4) the development of spinal instability from such a fracture, particularly when associated with lytic destructive changes in the posterior elements, and (5) spinal cord compression.

Spinal cord compression is the most serious sequela of spinal metastases and is reported to occur in 5% to 10% of patients with widespread cancer.[1,16] The causes of cord compression, illustrated in Figs. 12-3 and 12-4 and Plate 1, include direct pressure from tumor, which infiltrates and weakens the vertebral bone, leading to compression and backward bulging of the cord into the spinal canal, direct pressure from an enlarging epidural mass, cord and root compression from a soft tissue mass growing into the spinal canal through a neural foramen, severe spinal angulation secondary to vertebral wedging with posterior extrusion of bone and tumor detritus, direct cord or root pressure by intradural metastases, and carcinomatous meningitis.

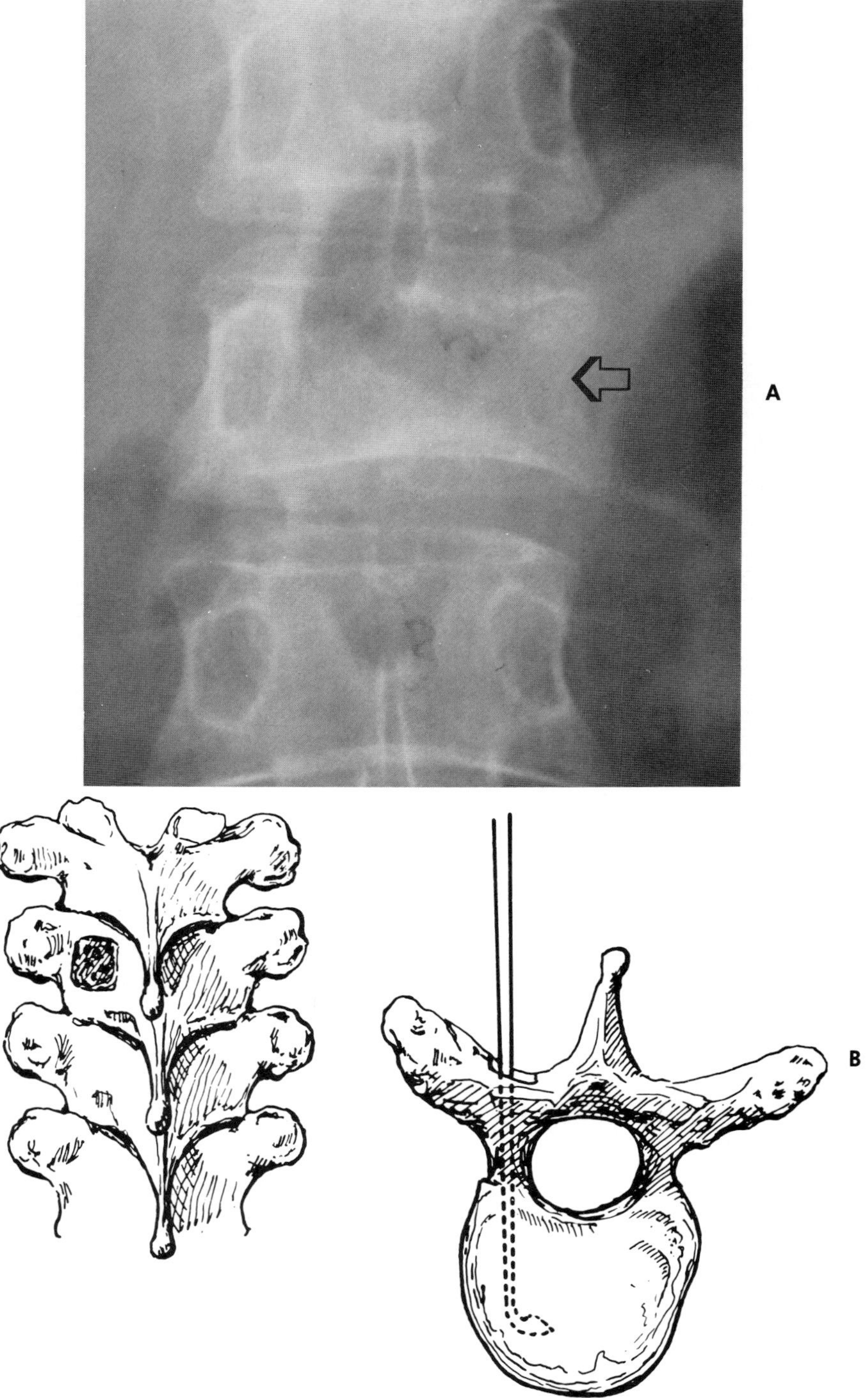

FIGURE 12-2 **A,** An AP roentgenogram of the lumbar spine in a patient with known metastatic breast cancer, low back pain, and a negative bone scan. Destruction of the left pedicle of L2 is apparent *(arrow)*. The patient's pain was completely relieved by irradiation. **B,** Technique of open biopsy of a thoracic vertebra. The paravertebral muscles are split sufficiently to expose the lamina of the involved vertebra. A 5 mm window is made in the lamina immediately behind the superior facet directly overlying the involved pedicle. Abundant biopsy material can be obtained safely by using an angled curet. (Reprinted with permission from Dunn, H.K.: In Evarts, C.M., editor: Surgery of the musculoskeletal system, New York, 1983, Churchill-Livingstone, Inc., chap. 9.)

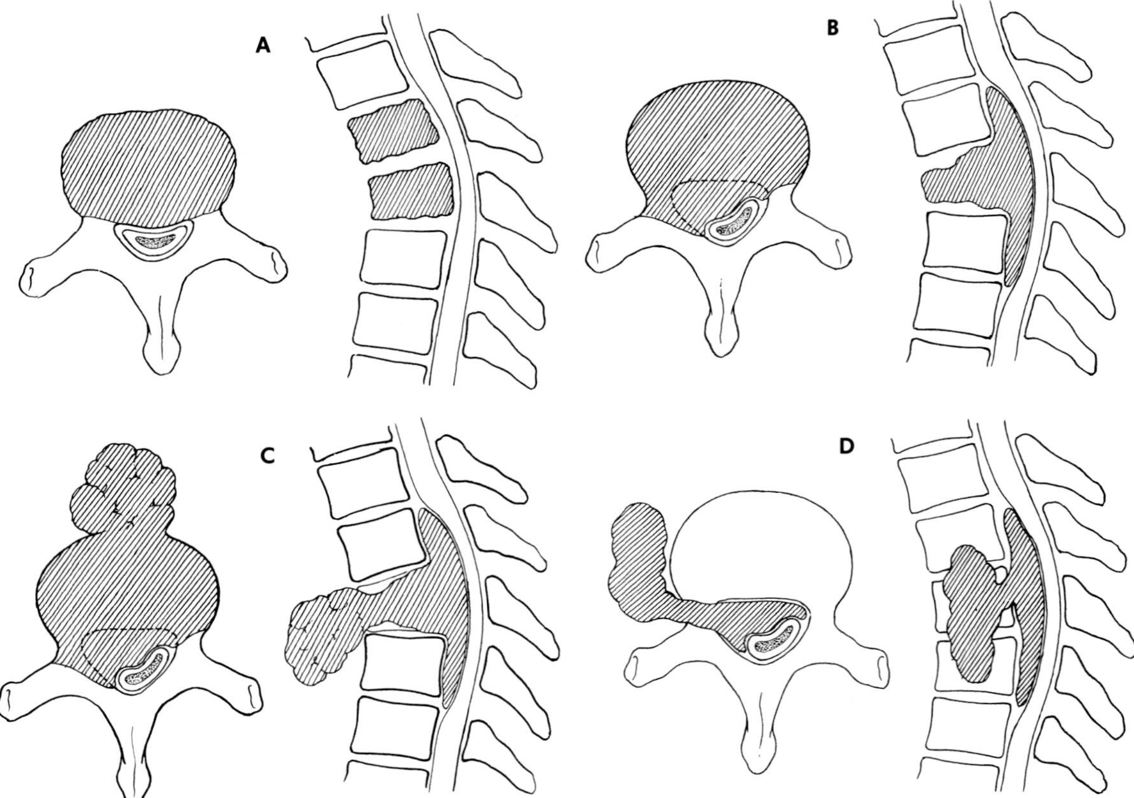

FIGURE 12-3 The mechanisms by which metastases of the vertebrae can cause neurological manifestations. **A,** Partial collapse of one or more vertebral bodies may cause an extrusion of soft bone and tumor tissue into the canal, and cord compression may be accentuated by the gradual development of kyphosis. As the tumor expands further within the canal, **B,** a progressive sleevelike compression of the cord may result. The confines of this process can be demonstrated adequately only by myelography (see Fig. 12-5, *A*). If metastatic tumor tissue breaks out of the vertebral body anteriorly, **C,** a paravertebral mass may develop and hinder the surgeon's attempts to decompress the spine anteriorly. This process can be demonstrated accurately only by computerized tomography (Fig. 12-9, *A*). Rarely a paravertebral metastatic lesion (often from a lymph node) may grow through the neural foramen and create cord compression in the absence of vertebral destruction, **D.** Adequate evaluation of such a process requires both CT and myelography. (**A** to **D** reproduced with permission from Constans, J.P., et al.: J. Neurosurg. **59:**111, 1983.)

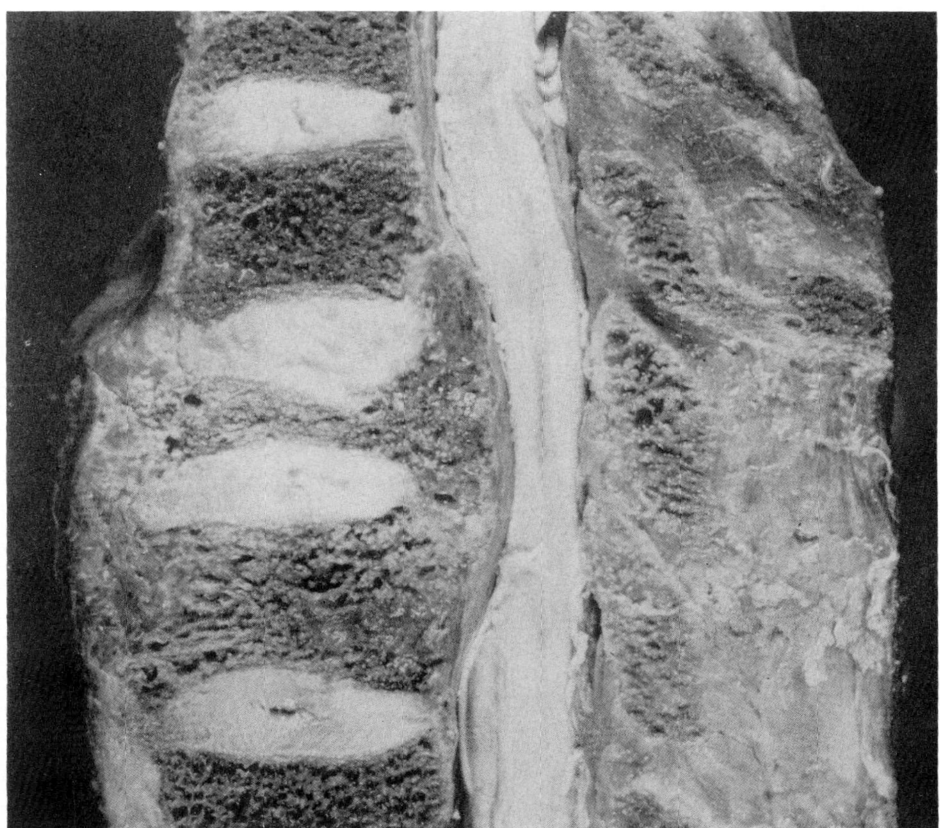

FIGURE 12-4 Metastatic adenocarcinoma of the lung that presented as progressive lower neck pain and paraparesis. The primary bronchogenic lesion was silent. Note the almost total collapse of the body of the seventh cervical vertebra and the partial collapse of the body of the first thoracic vertebra. Bulging of these bodies posteriorly has narrowed the vertebral canal and compressed the cord. (Reprinted with permission from Jaffe, H.L.: Tumors and tumorous conditions of the bones and joints, Philadelphia, 1958, Lea & Febiger.)

Bernat et al.[3] in a retrospective study of 133 patients with metastatic neurological compromise found that 24% suffered from intradural cord compression or carcinomatous meningitis and 21% had primarily root compression without cord involvement. However, comparable studies* have found intradural metastases to be rare, accounting for less than 5% of neurological symptoms. The dura functions as an effective barrier to tumor invasion and, in fact, becomes markedly thickened in response to adjacent tumor tissue. At the time of operative decompression the dura typically is found to have become a firm whitish structure, often as much as 1 mm thick and amazingly resistant to tearing or penetration. In a series of almost 100 such decompressions, we have seen only one dural tear and it was repaired without subsequent evidence of intradural tumor invasion.

Because the metastatic tumor mass invades the canal from the vertebral body or causes cord or root compression by collapse or extrusion of the vertebral body, neurological compromise occurs from in front of the cord in the great majority of instances. Only in unusual situations, when tumor tissue invades the canal from a metastatic focus in the posterior elements or when once within the canal the tumor grows to surround the cord in a

*References 1, 5, 16, 28, 41, 42, 44.

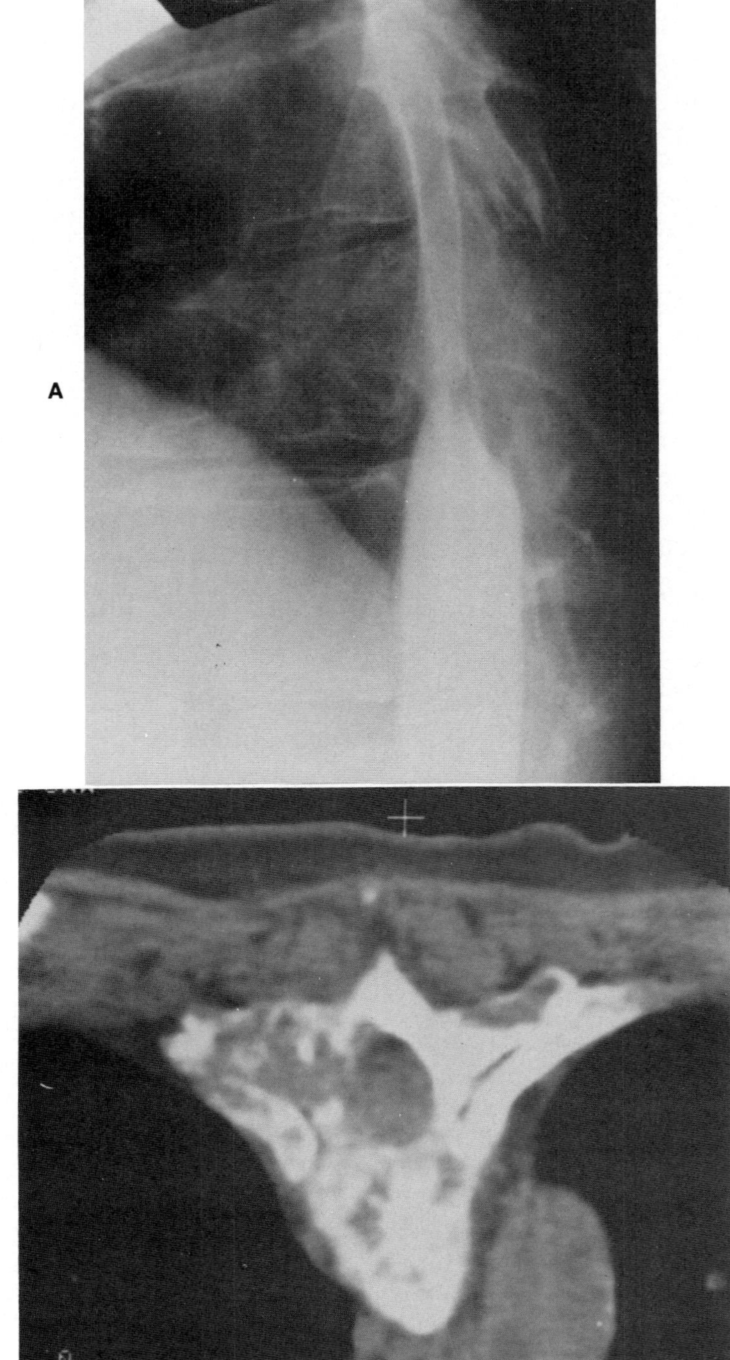

FIGURE 12-5 **A,** Unusual "napkin ring" constriction of the cord caused by a metastatic tumor within the spinal canal growing around the dura to compress the cord circumferentially. **B,** A CT scan of the spine demonstrates anterior and posterior bone destruction and canal compromise. Under such circumstances both anterior and posterior decompression and stabilization probably will be necessary.

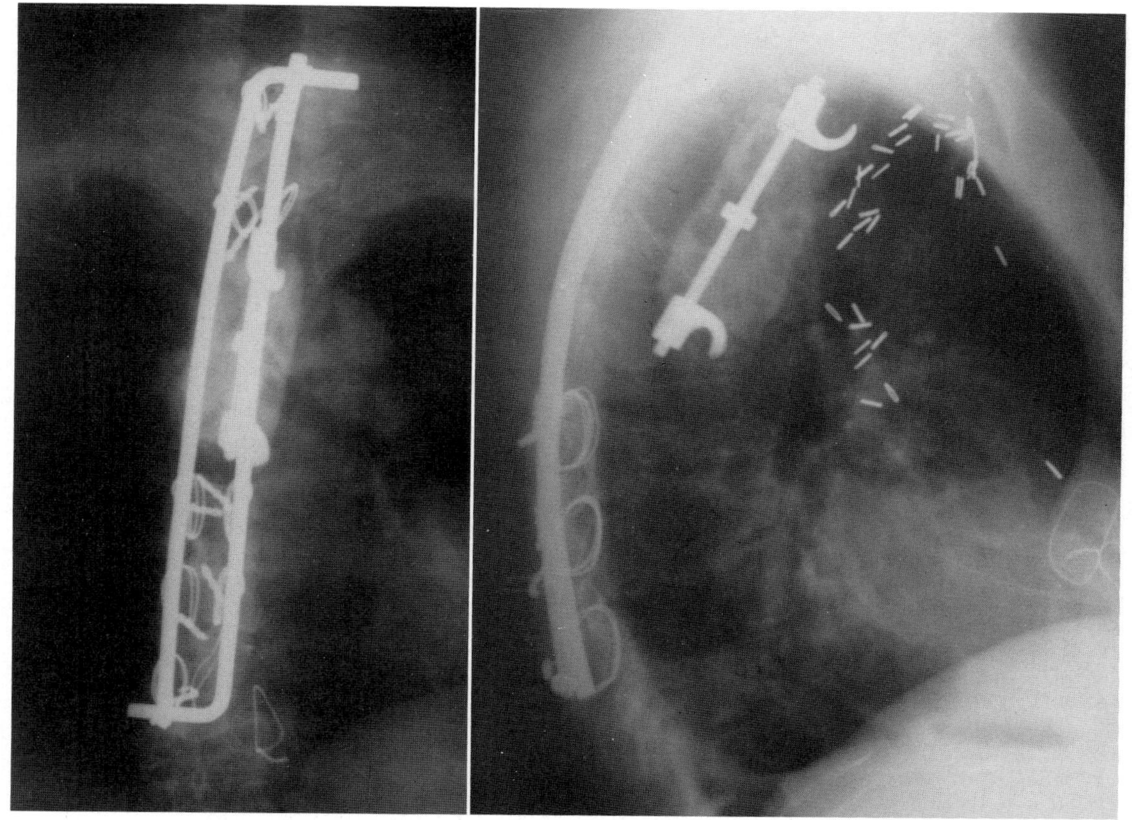

FIGURE 12-5, cont'd. **C** and **D,** AP and lateral roentgenograms taken 1 year after successful decompression and stabilization.

napkin ring constriction (Fig. 12-5), is the posterior aspect of the cord involved. However, there is a contrecoup phenomenon whereby tumor tissue invading the canal from in front will cause the cord to become displaced against the unyielding intact lamina and thus secondarily result in compression of the posterior columns (Fig. 12-3). For this reason most patients in whom cord compression develops will demonstrate more motor than sensory disability, at least in the early stages of their neurological deficit.

Although the lumbar vertebrae are most commonly affected by tumor metastases, it is in the thoracic spine that cord compromise usually occurs. This is because the cord here is largest relative to the diameter of the canal and thus suffers compression earlier from a tumor mass. Extradural tumor may cause compression at more than one level in the same patient. In his series of 52 patients, Smith[60] found that in 27 cases the tumor involved the cord in more than one contiguous segment and that in 4 there were two widely separated foci of significant canal compromise. This incidence of multilevel involvement must always be kept in mind before the physician begins treatment and is one of the strongest arguments for routine preoperative myelography.

Barron et al.[1] reported microscopic cord changes at postmortem examination of patients who had died with clinical evidence of cord compression. There was no consistent histological pattern, however, and in fact the pathological alterations often were minimal despite severe and long-standing clinical disease. Edema and cellular degeneration were noted in the myelenated tissues at the level of compression, but the gray matter was relatively well preserved. The distribution of these changes did not conform to the arterial supply

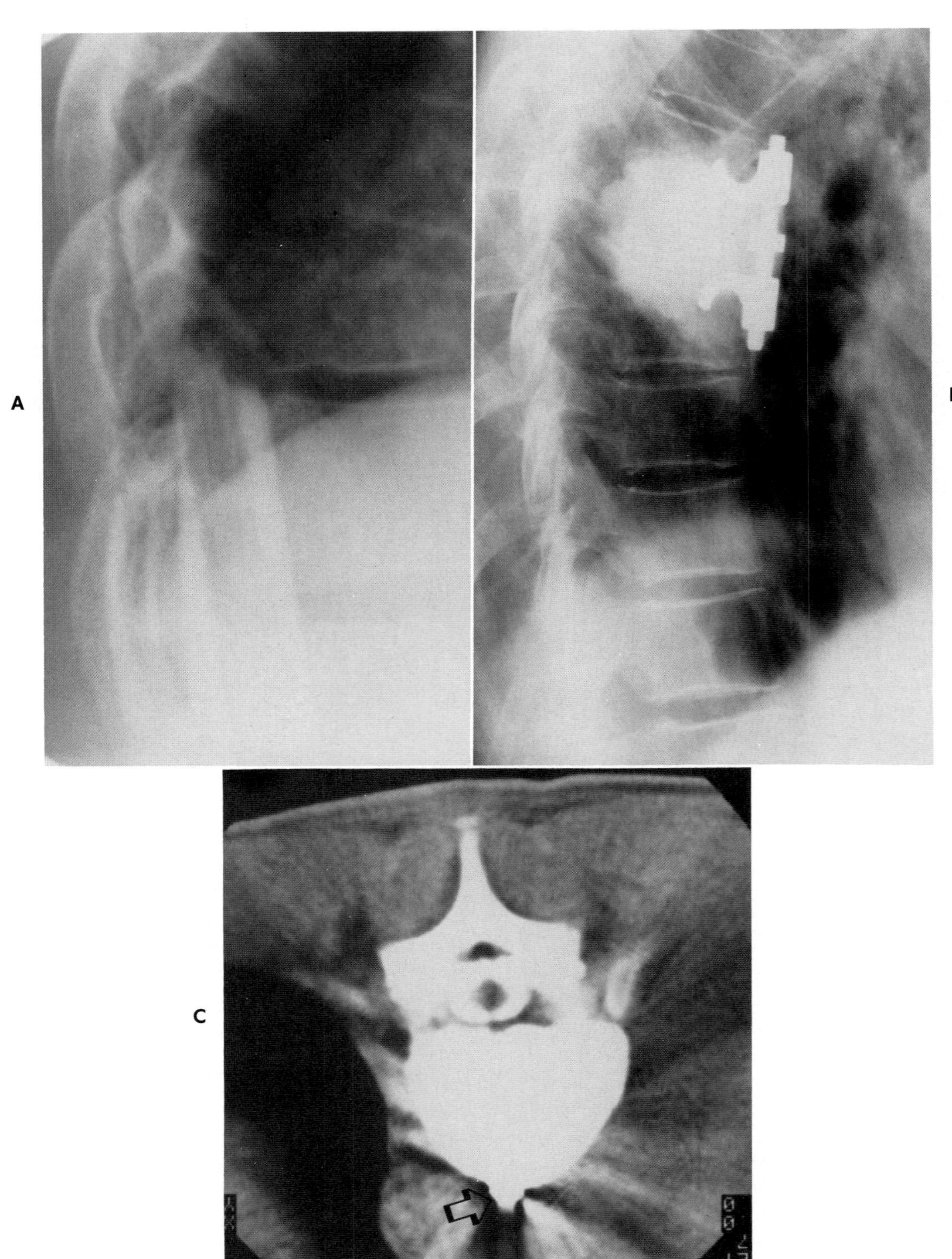

FIGURE 12-6 For legend see opposite page.

or venous drainage, although the authors postulated that venous occlusion might be the most important factor leading to neuronal degeneration.

CLINICAL COURSE

The most frequent manifestation of osseous metastases is pain. Usually it is localized, of gradual onset, relentlessly progressive over weeks or months, tender to percussion, and worse at night. It has been attributed to stretching of the periosteum by direct pressure of the tumor[8] or to microfractures occurring sequentially in the weakened bone. Not infrequently the patient will locate the pain at the level below the actual metastatic lesion, which may lead the unsuspecting physician to attribute initial symptoms to arthritis or disc disease and to continue conservative and ineffective treatment measures in the face of progressive neurological compromise (Fig. 12-6). Until proved otherwise, the onset of back pain in a patient known to have cancer should be attributed to metastases.

Patients in whom progressive cord or root compression ultimately develops usually present initially with the same type of constant and gradually worsening spinal pain without neurological involvement. Radicular pain, when present, may assist the clinician in locating the level of vertebral involvement. Approximately 50% of patients with thoracic cord impingement complain of radicular pain before they manifest symptoms of cord involvement. Such pain often is described as "girdle pain," particularly with lesions at T9 or below, and may not be recognized as reflective of intercostal root irritation.

With more central neural involvement, motor deficits usually precede sensory changes because of the typical anterior location of cord compression. Except in the unusual situation when there is direct compression of the conus medullaris, loss of sphincter control is a late phenomenon and usually occurs only in patients with the most profound cord involvement.[55,74,76] In a series of 600 cases of spinal metastases with neurological compromise, Constans et al.[16] found but 14 cases (2.3%) with isolated sphincter disturbances as a presenting symptom.

The sensory level often is not a reliable indicator of the level of cord compression. In Nather and Bose's[55] series a discrepancy was found in 7 of 31 cases in which sensory changes were recorded. The sensory level also is frequently recorded several segments below the site of cord compression and therefore, unlike radicular symptoms, tends not to be a reliable indicator of the lesion site.

The rapidity of onset of muscle weakness has considerable bearing on the prognosis. Constans et al.[16] reported that 166 of 600 patients (28%) had an acute onset when there was a delay of less than 48 hours between the manifestation of initial symptoms and the appearance of a complete neurological syndrome. These patients had the worst prognosis for recovery, no matter what treatment was rendered: 61% of those with an acute onset and progression of symptoms over 7 to 10 days, 11% of those with an insidious onset and progression continuing up to 1 month. Patients with a slower evolution of neurological compromise (indicating in most instances a slower growth rate of the metastases) had a

FIGURE 12-6 **A,** Lateral myelographic view of the thoracolumbar spine in a 67-year-old woman with progressive paraparesis (Frankel grade B) secondary to multiple myeloma involving the T8 vertebral body. A complete block is apparent at the level of the partially collapsed vertebra. The patient had complained of back pain for 3 months prior to the onset of her neurological compromise, but her symptoms were attributed to "arthritis" even though she was undergoing chemotherapy for multiple myeloma. **B,** Postoperative roentgenogram 18 months after anterior decompression and stabilization with a Knodt rod and methylmethacrylate. The vertebrectomy space was too small to allow the rod to be placed within the vertebrae above and below the decompression. **C,** Postoperative CT scan of the construct demonstrating complete decompression of the spinal cord. The slight prominence of the Knodt hook is apparent anteriorly *(arrow)*. The patient enjoyed a complete recovery neurologically and remains free of symptoms after 2.4 years.

decidedly better prognosis. Tarlov and Herz[63] demonstrated experimentally that even major neurological compromise caused by gradual cord compression was reversible for a longer period than was compromise due to an acute cord lesion. Smith[60] found that less than 10% of patients with symptoms of 8 weeks' duration or less benefited from surgery whereas 33% having symptoms for more than 2 months benefited. His figures are quantitatively misleading, however, in that they show the results of posterior laminectomy decompression only; nevertheless, the implication is correct that the more slowly progressing metastases create neurological disabilities that are increasingly amenable to surgical decompression.

Conversely, a sudden onset of paralysis is almost invariably associated with a poor prognosis.* Such cases most often involve the thoracic spine and in many instances are the result more of vascular compromise than of direct cord compression. Dommisse[22] has shown that the blood supply is least rich from T4 to T9 and describes this as the "critical vascular zone" of the spinal cord.

The upper three segments of the thoracic spine, above the level of borderline cord vascularity, actually are associated with the worst prognosis.[42,44,54] This fact is probably a reflection of several factors, including (1) the tendency for more aggressive tumors (e.g., Pancoast's tumor of the lung apex) to involve this region of the spine by direct extension or local metastasis, (2) the still less than abundant cord vascularity, and (3) the fact that thoracic kyphosis is more acute in this area, thereby encouraging posterior extrusion of bone and tumor debris whenever vertebral collapse ensues (Fig. 12-4, *A*).

When paraplegia has become complete before the onset of treatment, the prognosis for recovery generally is poor.† Similarly a loss of sphincter control, indicating profound cord dysfunction, gives a poor prognosis for recovery no matter what treatment is rendered. In the series of Nather and Bose,[55] when sphincter control was intact 50% of patients enjoyed a "satisfactory" recovery of neurological function after posterior cord decompression but when sphincter control was already lost satisfactory recovery occurred in only 13%. All of their patients who recovered the ability to walk retained or regained sphincter control postoperatively.

*References 5, 9, 40-42, 44, 55.

†References 6, 9, 40, 42, 44, 55.

DIAGNOSIS

Once an individual is suspected of harboring a significant spinal metastasis, studies must be initiated to determine the level(s) of involvement, the likelihood of vertebral collapse or progressive neurological impairment, and the most reasonable approach to treatment.

Laboratory Studies

Laboratory studies are rarely of much value in defining these three parameters but may be critical in preparing a patient for surgical intervention. Anemia must be diagnosed and corrected. The patient receiving chemotherapy must have his or her white cell and platelet counts determined. An uncorrected insufficiency of either blood component argues strongly against immediate operative intervention in all but the most critically compromised patient. The individual who has been forced to bedrest by spinal pain must have serum calcium and phosphorus determinations serially for assessment of the possible development of malignant hypercalcemia. This is particularly true of any person with myeloma, lyphoma, or breast carcinoma.

Roentgenography

As already noted, plain roentgenograms are not particularly sensitive in quantitating the extent of spinal metastatic disease. However, they do assist in determining the extent of host bone reaction to the malignancy as well as the presence and configuration of vertebral collapse. The patient with principally blastic lesions is at much less risk for the development of progressive collapse and neurological compromise and generally can be treated nonoperatively. Even one with evident bone destruction and collapse can be determined to be at little risk of neurological involvement depending on the pattern of collapse and the extent of canal impingement apparent on a lateral plain film (Fig. 12-7).

Bone Scintigraphy

Without question, bone scintigraphy[36] is the most sensitive diagnostic aid available for de-

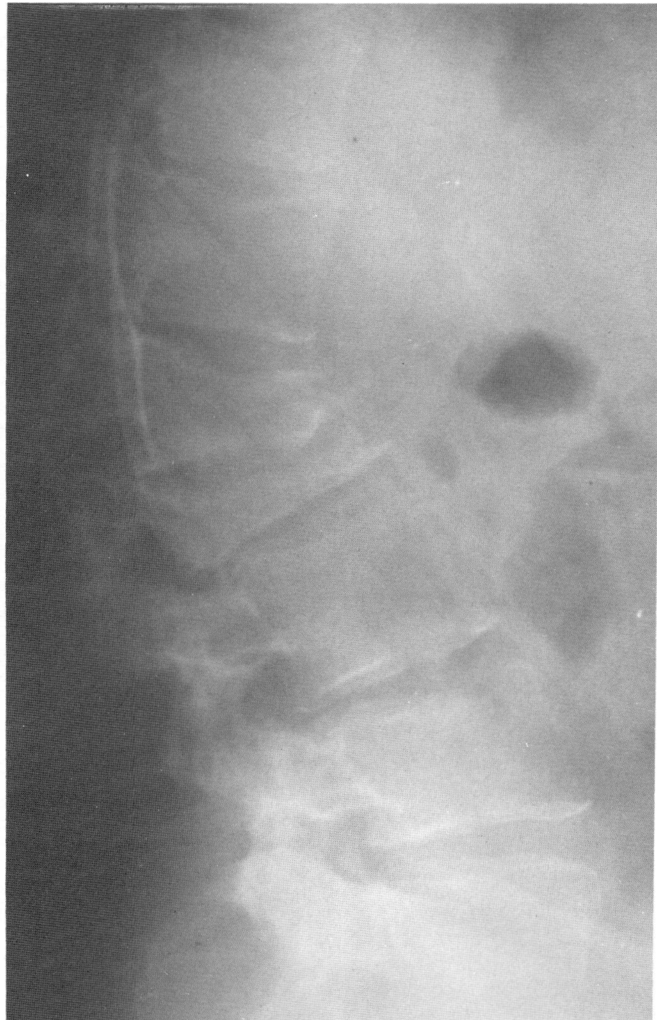

FIGURE 12-7 Roentgenogram of a 66-year-old woman with known breast cancer and scintigraphically demonstrable metastases to T11 and T12. Eventually, despite irradiation, pathological wedge compression fractures occurred in both vertebral bodies but without extrusion of bone into the spinal canal. The patient suffered no neurological compromise, and her pain was relieved by the use of a corset support. There was no indication for operative intervention.

tecting spinal metastases. The development of vertebral metastases is associated with an increase in vascularity surrounding the tumor, caused by dilation of preexisting capillary-arteriolar plexuses, in part secondary to the secretion of angiogenic hormones by the tumor.[18] The initial phase of technetium-99 uptake is a reflection of this locally increased vascularity. The second or delayed phase is a reflection of radioisotopic concentration in the reactive newly woven bone, which usually develops as a response to tumor invasion. In many instances metastatic lesions of the spine will be apparent by bone scan long before they are detectable roentgenographically, and in many instances even before they become symptomatic. However, scintigraphy is not necessarily diagnostic of metastatic disease. The patient with a pathological fracture secondary to osteoporosis but not to malignancy will often show changes on scan that are indistinguishable from the effects of met-

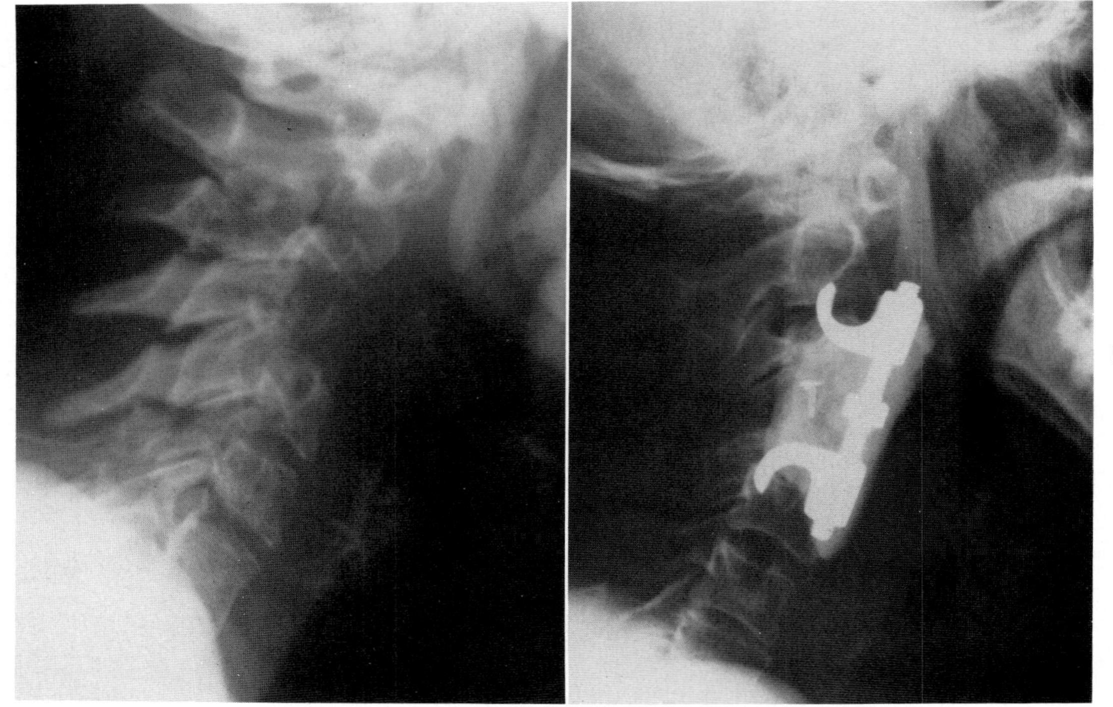

FIGURE 12-8 **A,** Extensive destruction of C3 and C4 from an aggressively metastatic breast carcinoma in a 52-year-old woman. Despite the changes so obvious roentgenographically, the patient's technetium-99 bone scan revealed no abnormalities in the cervical spine. Presumably this false-negative scan reflected minimum if any increase in vascularity of the metastases and an absence of blastic response in the affected bone. **B,** Nine months postoperative. The vertebral reconstruction remained secure, and the patient had no neurological deficit or neck pain. Surprisingly, she also had no complaints of dysphagia.

astatic disease. Occasionally even extensive arthritis will present a picture difficult to differentiate from focal metastatic destruction. Moreover, false-negative scans may occur in lesions where lytic destruction prompts minimal reactive bone formation and where little if any vascular response is elicited (Fig. 12-8).

The most common and serious deficiency of bone scintigraphy is that it often reflects multiple areas of vertebral involvement without clarifying which level is associated with progressive pain, neurological compromise, or vertebral collapse. The extent of isotopic uptake, in either the early or the late phases of the scan, does not correlate well with the extent of vertebral destruction, the prognosis for progressive collapse or cord compromise, or the likelihood of the patient's responding to conservative as opposed to operative intervention.

Computed Tomography

The introduction of spinal CT scans has markedly enhanced the ability to assess spinal metastases. One can see clearly even small areas of destruction within a vertebra, assess the extent of paravertebral soft tissue masses, and (most important) quantify the degree and direction of spinal canal impingement by bone debris and tumor (Fig. 12-9, *A* and *D*). CT has the additional advantage of being noninvasive and rapid, so it can be performed safely even in a patient with progressive spinal instability. Osteoporosis can be differentiated from tumor destruction; with osteoporosis the cortical outline generally is intact and multiple small areas of low density are present whereas with metastatic lesions the cortex frequently is destroyed and the osteolytic areas are larger and more irregular.[5]

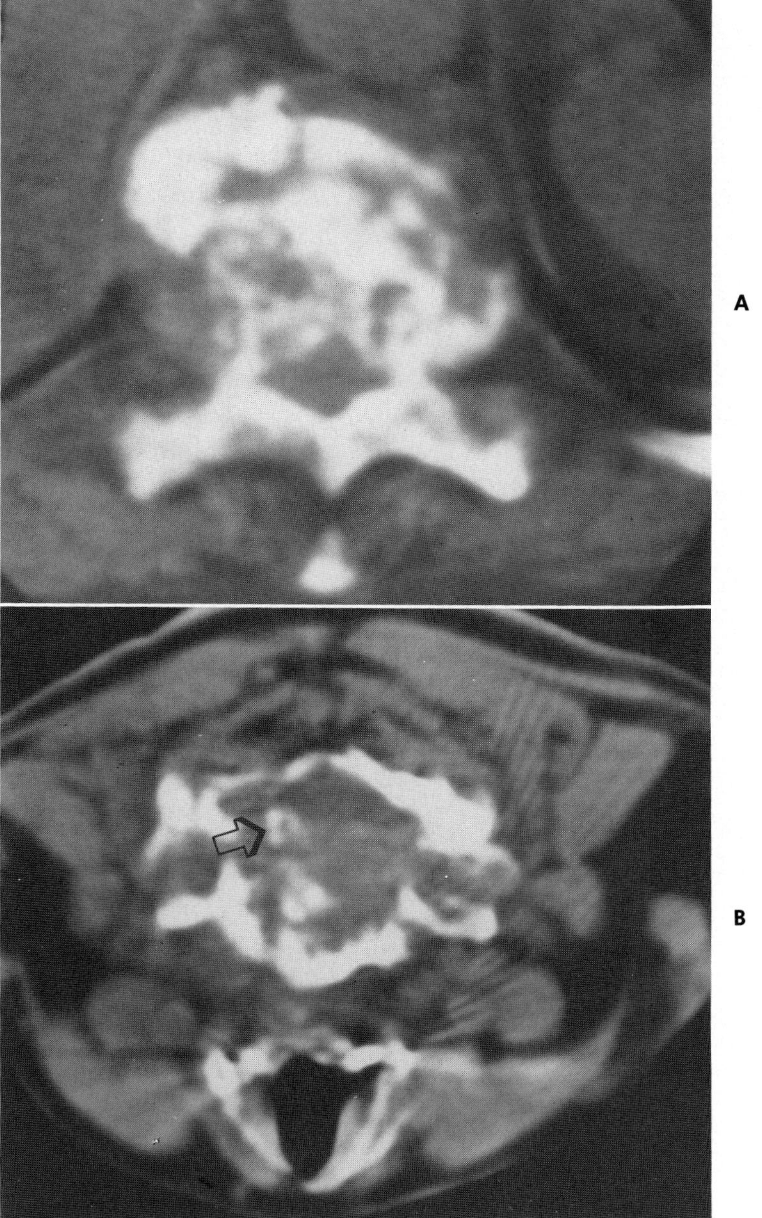

FIGURE 12-9 **A,** CT scan of the L3 vertebral body in a man with a progressive cauda equina syndrome secondary to a metastatic prostate carcinoma. Fragmentation of the vertebral body by tumor can be seen, but on this and other CT cuts the canal did not appear to be severely compromised. A myelogram revealed very localized high-grade narrowing of the canal, apparently just above the level of this cut and thus not demonstrated by the CT scan. This case demonstrates one of the limitations of computerized tomography of the spine, also one of the concomitant indications for myelography when CT does not correlate well with the clinical picute presented. **B,** CT scan of the cervical spine in a woman with metastatic breast carcinoma. She had minimal left-sided C5 root symptoms but no clinical evidence of spinal cord compromise. Because the density (attenuation number) of the tumor was almost identical to that of the spinal cord, this scan was not particularly helpful in quantitating how much if any spinal cord compromise existed. However, one large bone fragment *(arrow)* can be seen to extrude into the area of the C5 nerve root. A myelogram showed minimum canal compromise but displacement of the root by the bone fragment.

Continued.

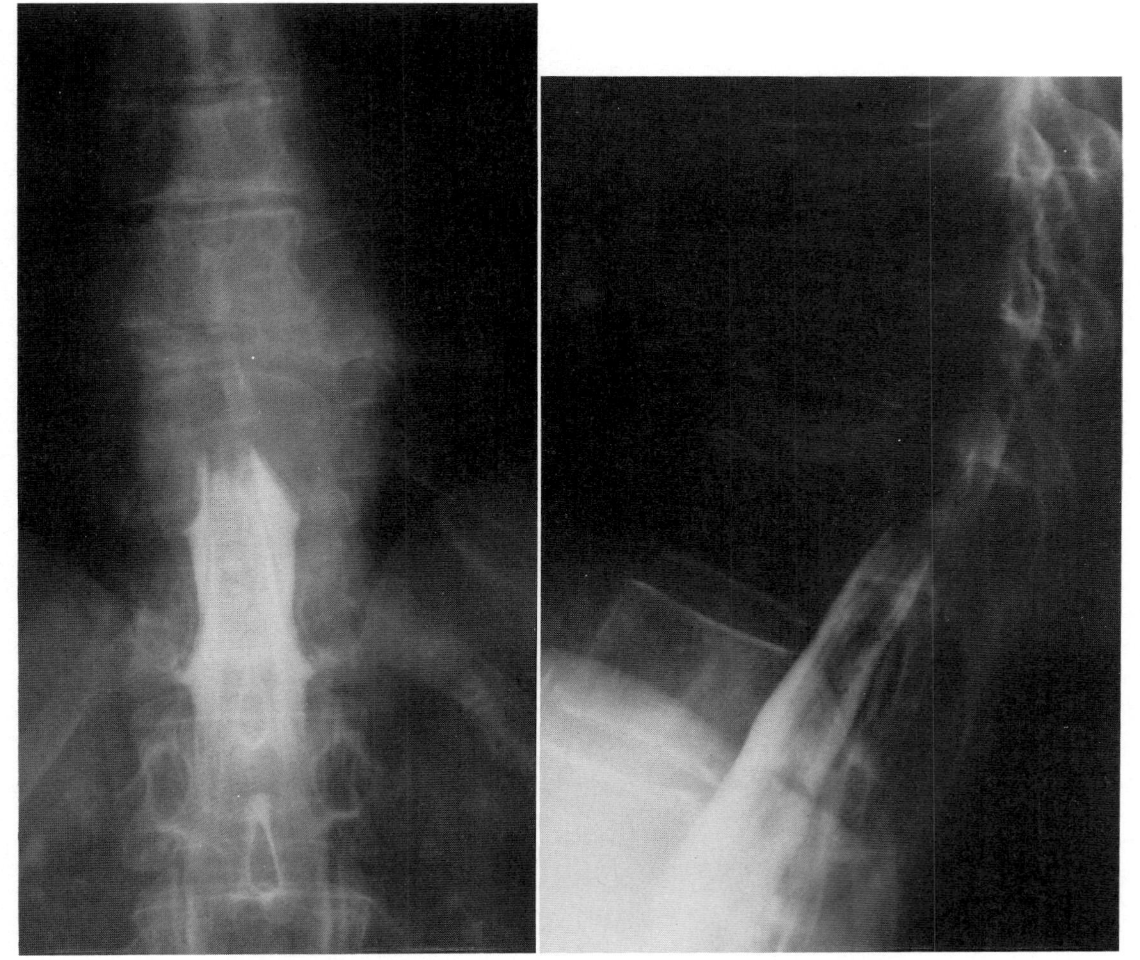

FIGURE 12-9, cont'd. **C** and **D,** AP and lateral metrizamide myelograms of the thoracolumbar spine in another woman with metastatic breast carcinoma. She had a severe (Frankel grade B) paraparesis and a complete myelographic block. The AP shows that the spinal cord is compressed eccentrically from the left, and the lateral confirms that the compression comes from in front at the level of the collapsed vertebral body.

The principal limitation of CT scanning is its potential failure to disclose a second site of cord compression. In the series of Bernat et al.[3] involving 133 patients studied myelographically, multiple sites were discernible in 9% with cord compression, the sites being separated by a mean of 12 vertebral segments.

Another disadvantage of CT is that the cross-section cuts generally are made at 1 cm intervals and the possibility exists for missing the area of maximal canal impingement and thus failing to recognize an indication for anterior decompression (Fig. 12-9, *A* to *C*). The CT scan will on occasion also fail to demonstrate the extent or configuration of spinal cord displacement when the attenuation value (CT number) of the soft tissue tumor mass bulging into the spinal canal happens to approximate that of the spinal cord itself (Fig. 12-9, *D*). However, this problem can be overcome by obtaining a metrizamide-enhanced scan. The use of metrizamide enhancement also has resolved the dilemma of differentiating between intradural and extradural metastases, although myelography is still a better means of making this distinction (Fig. 12-9, *E* and *F*).

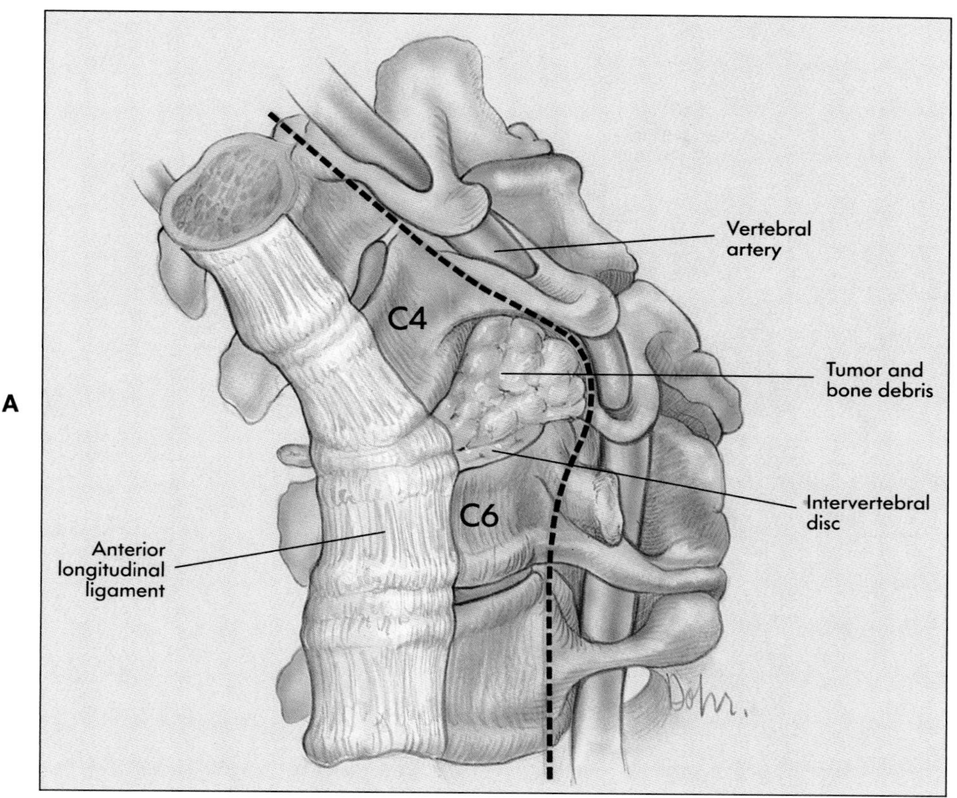

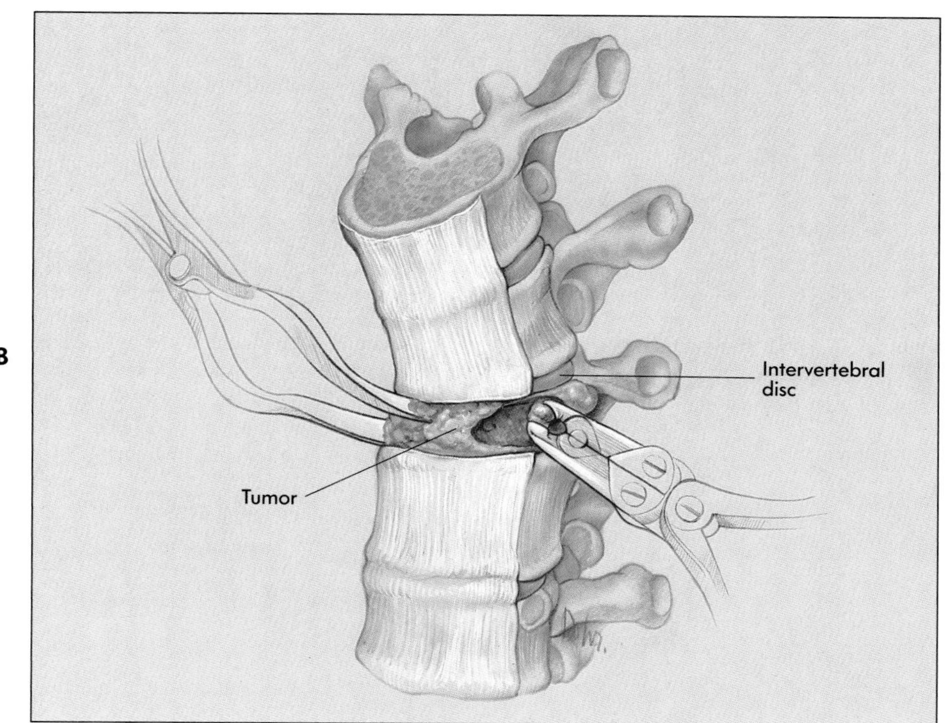

PLATE 1 Technique for anterior vertebrectomy and spinal cord decompression. **A,** Replacement of the vertebral body by tumor results in collapse of the body, increasing kyphosis, and extrusion of the tumor and bone fragments into the epidural space. **B,** By means of a lamina spreader the vertebral space is reconstituted anteriorly. Tumor is resected with a rongeur and curets.

Continued.

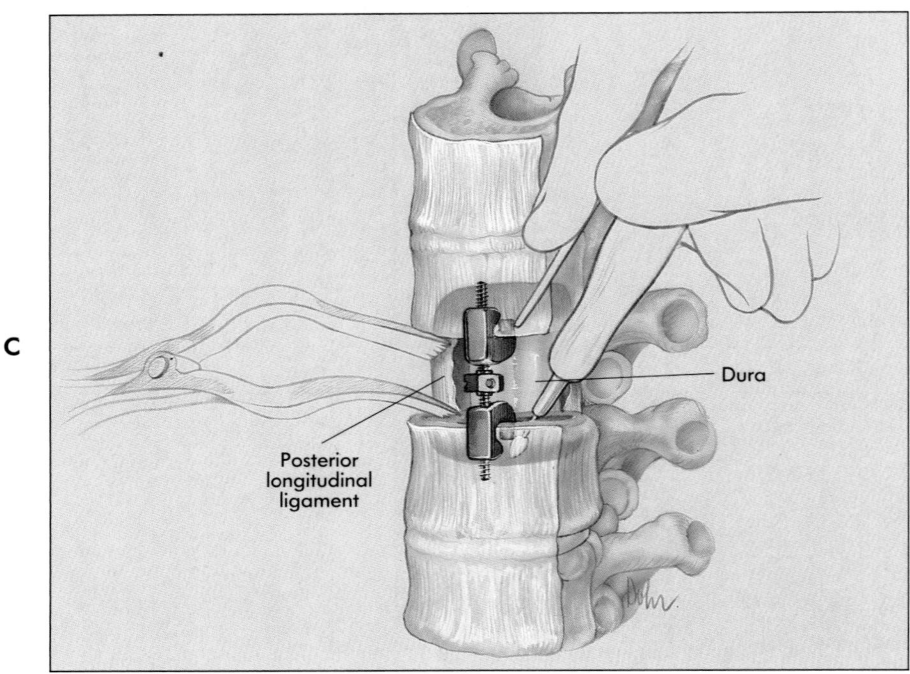

PLATE 1, cont'd **C,** Once the vertebral space has been restored and the neural elements are completely exposed and decompressed, the end plates of the adjacent vertebrae are opened with a power bur and the bone is undercut to enhance fixation of the methylmethacrylate.

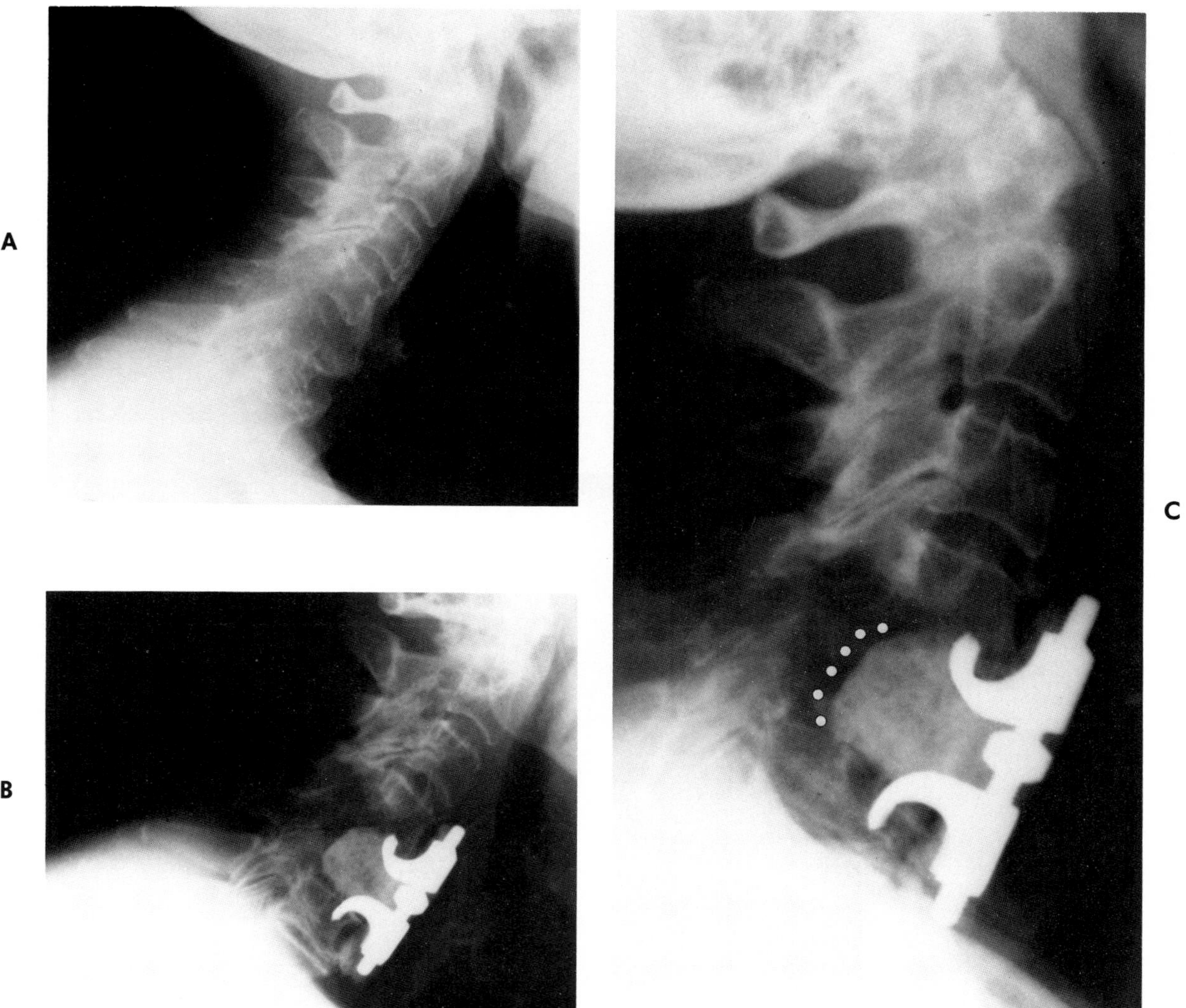

PLATE 2 **A,** Lateral roentgenogram of the cervical spine in a 68-year-old woman with myelomatous destruction of the C5 vertebral body. The neurological deficit was Frankel grade D. **B,** The diseased vertebral body was resected and replaced by methylmethacrylate incorporating a Knodt distraction rod. Fixation within the body of C6, which also had been found to be weakened by tumor, appears tenuous. **C,** Two weeks postoperative. The lower hook and cement have become displaced as the anterior cortex of the diseased bone has given way. The extent of displacement is indicated *(dots)*. The patient's neurological deficit did not recur, but her severe mechanical spinal pain returned. *Continued.*

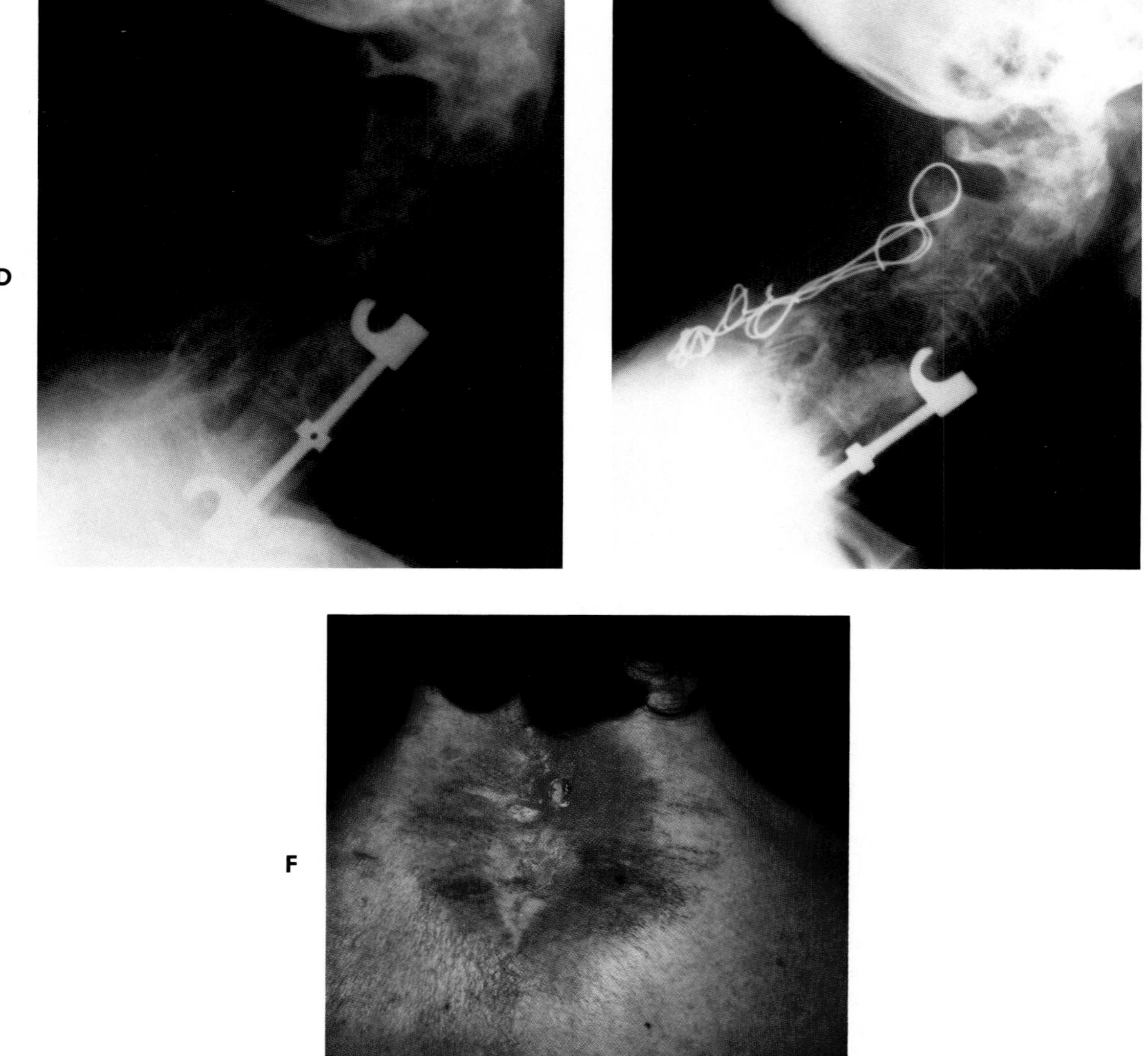

PLATE 2, cont'd **D,** The cervical spine was stabilized again, now with the cement and Knodt rod replacing three diseased vertebrae. The patient enjoyed complete neurological recovery and remained free of symptoms for 47 months postoperatively. She received 4500 cGy of postoperative irradiation. **E,** Forty-seven months after the stabilization her neck pain returned, along with Frankel grade 5 neurological disability. Roentgenograms now revealed extensive lytic destruction of the posterior elements above the previous fusion. The anterior vertebral construct appeared to be secure. A posterior stabilization from C2 to C7 was accomplished through heavily irradiated tissue. **F,** This freed the patient of her neck symptoms and neurological deficit, but a skin breakdown developed and subsequently progressed to a chronic draining sinus posteriorly. Two years postoperative she remains symptom free except for the skin deficit. Bone and a portion of the fixation wire can be seen in the depths of the defect. Because a bone arthrodesis had been achieved posteriorly, it was possible to remove the wire and dead bone and to rotate a vascularized latissimus dorsi musculocutaneous flap to cover the defect.

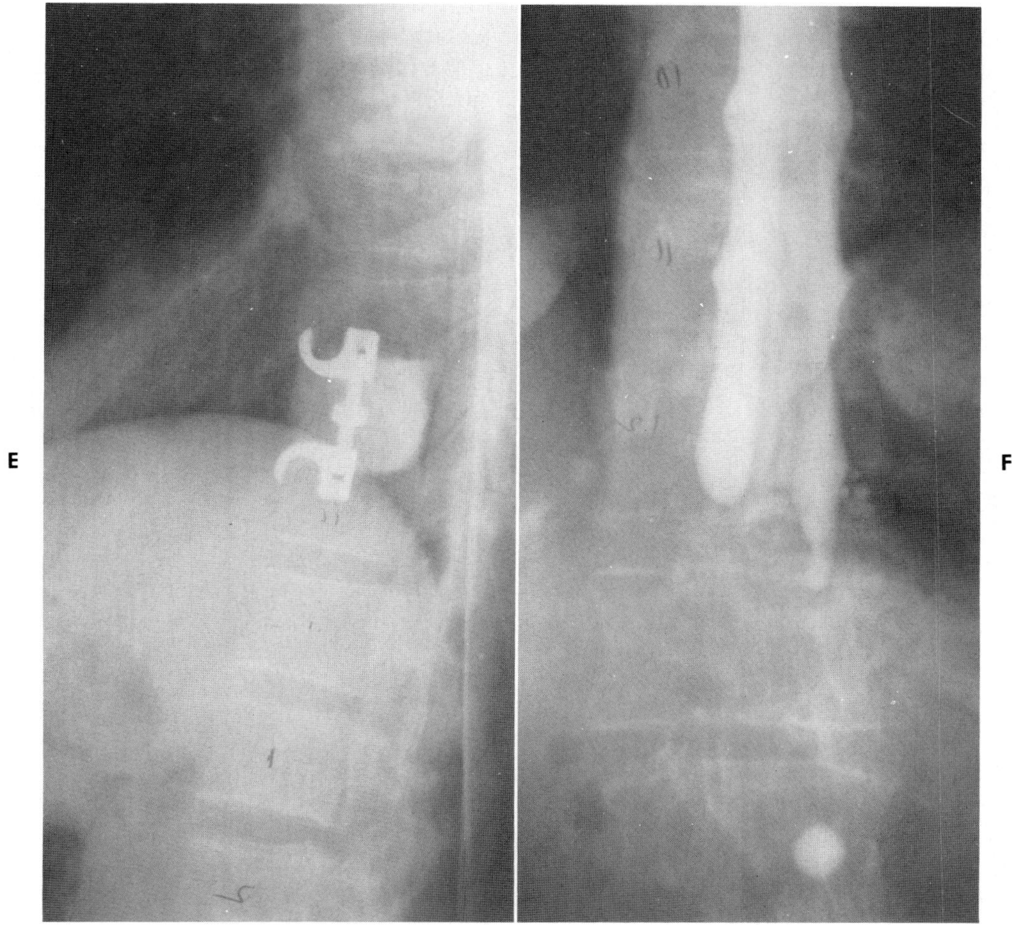

FIGURE 12-9, cont'd. **E,** Follow-up metrizamide myelogram 19 months after anterior vertebrectomy decompression and stabilization with a Knodt rod and methylmethacrylate. There is no evidence of residual canal compromise at the operated level, although a new lesion at C7 was demonstrated on different films. **F,** Non–water soluble myelogram showing a complete block at the T12-L1 level from a rare intradural metastasis (lung carcinoma). At operation it was found that the malignancy had grown through the dura at the L2 area and spread intrathecally to the T9 level.

Myelography

Despite the emergence of enhanced computed tomography as an ideal tool for studying spinal metastases, myelography remains an important if not inevitably necessary means of clarifying the nature of intraspinal disease leading to neurological disabilities. When water-soluable metrizamide is used as the myelographic contrast material, it is usually possible to assess displacement of the cord not only in the lateral projection but in the AP view as well (Fig. 12-9, *E*). The configuration of extradural masses, which tend to grow circumferentially around the dura, can also be appreciated in most instances (Fig. 12-5, *A*), as can the extent and configuration of intrathecal masses (Fig. 12-9, *D*).

Some workers have recommended using only non–water-soluble iophendylate (Pantopaque) as the contrast material so repeated roentgenographic examinations of the spine can be performed after operative decompression without the necessity of reinjecting the dye. In our experience, however, the improved quality of the metrizamide study exceeds the potential disadvantages of not having the dye still present for postoperative evaluation. In addition, we have observed several instances in which Pantopaque used preoperatively and left in place suggested the persistence of a complete extradural block postoperatively despite the fact that adequate dural decompression had been confirmed directly at operation and by the subsequent clinical course (Fig. 12-21). That such a block may persist roentgenograpically but have no significance clinically discourages us from routinely obtaining such postoperative studies.

If a complete block is suspected on the basis of clinical evidence, a myelogram is mandatory. A small amount of dye (usually 3 ml) should be injected in the lumbar area and allowed to run cephalad to define the level and configuration of the block. The upper limit of the block can be defined by installation of an additional 2 ml of dye laterally at the C1-C2 level or by suboccipital puncture, in each instance under fluoroscopic control. We have found this necessary only rarely because dilute metrizamide usually will move cephalad above the block in time and thus reveal the full dimensions of the obstructing mass on one or more delayed follow-up views.

Myelography is not without risk of increasing the patient's disability.[6,9,55,60,66] Removal of even a small amount of CSF may exacerbate the already existing neurological compromise. Moreover, the technical difficulties of performing an invasive study in an already debilitated person may be immense. For this reason, Bernat et al.[3] attempted to establish criteria for determining prospectively which patients with metastatic spinal involvement and neurological symptoms would require myelography and which could be assessed adequately by noninvasive roentgenograms alone. They were unsuccessful in their attempt. Patients with myelographically demonstrable complete blocks presented symptoms that were often indistinguishable from those of patients who had free flow intrathecally. There were no significant differences in regard to primary tumor type, level of cord involvement, extent of vertebral collapse, severity of spinal pain, or any other measurable parameter.

These results may prompt questions to be asked as to whether the presence of an intraspinal block demonstrable at myelography, in fact, has much clinical significance. It has long been a maxim among spinal surgeons that the diagnosis of such a block warrants immediate decompression. However, in reviewing our own experience, it seems clear that clinical evidence of progressive neurological compromise, irrespective of the myelographic picture, should be the proper indication for operative intervention. Like Bernat et al.,[3] we have not found myelography to be universally helpful in reaching this decision.

In the age of CT and MRI, the place of conventional myelography seems to be more limited than it was previously. At present we obtain myelograms in only about one third of our patients with spinal metastases and clinical evidence of neurological compromise. We have found them helpful for excluding multiple foci of cord or root impingement in patients with separate levels of vertebral collapse in whom bone scintigraphy has revealed a particularly high area of vertebral uptake well away from the focus of apparent cord compression. Myelography has been helpful also whenever the overall neurological picture did not seem to be explainable by a single level of disease demonstrable by enhanced computed tomography. Finally, we advocate getting a myelogram in any patient who has undergone seemingly adequate decompression yet failed to respond neurologically or in whom neurological compromise has reappeared after an initially encouraging recovery (Fig. 12-5).

Magnetic Resonance Imaging

MRI is a relatively new technique whose applications to spinal metastases have not yet been explored fully. To date we have found it particularly helpful in studying patients who have already undergone spinal decompression and stabilization with metallic implants and in whom spinal instability or cord compromise has subsequently developed at the same site (Fig. 12-13). Because of the large defraction artifact created by the metal implants, these patients are not ideally restudied by computed tomography. So long as the metal implants are not ferrous material and therefore not adversely affected by a strong magnetic field, MRI is perfectly safe. Occasionally patients in whom metal fixation devices have already been implanted in adjacent bones (e.g., the proximal humerus or pelvis) will be better studied by magnetic resonance imaging than by computed tomography, and for the same reason (Fig. 12-10). MRI also appears to be preferable to CT for delineating certain extraspinal soft tissue masses that have eroded into adjacent vertebral bodies and the spinal canal and are potentially resectable at the time of operative decompression (Fig. 12-11).

Biopsy

Direct microscopic examination of tissues obtained percutaneously will occasionally be helpful in planning a course of treatment when there is some question as to whether a painful or even partially collapsed vertebra is a focus of metastatic disease (Chapter 4). When an obvious metastatic focus cannot be linked to a known primary tumor, open or percutaneous needle biopsy may lead to a definitive histological diagnosis and assist greatly in planning radiotherapy or chemotherapy protocols. Lytic lesions are much more likely to yield positive results than are blastic foci. In fact, it is our opinion that the risks of neurological injury during needle biopsy attempts, particularly in the thoracic spine, probably preclude using the technique on blastic lesions; the reason is that there is only a 25% likelihood of obtaining a definitive histological specimen.[5] This is true even for such biopsies performed with the assistance of CT.

Open biopsy of metastatic lesions, except at the time of operative decompression, rarely is indicated. When appropriate,[2] it can best be performed through a small window in the laminar cortex, directly over the pedicle, through which a small angle curet can be inserted directly into the cancellous bone of the vertebral body. At the time of open decompression and stabilization of the spine in patients with metastatic breast carcinoma, it is extremely important that fresh tumor tissue be sent to the pathology laboratory for estrogen receptor assay. It is our experience that initially estrogen receptor–negative breast

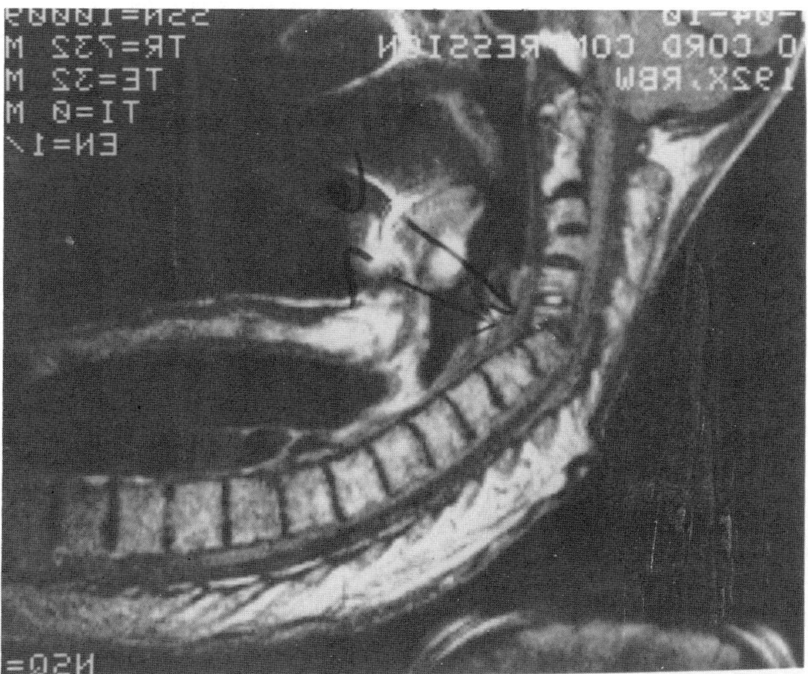

FIGURE 12-10 Lateral MR image of the cervicothoracic spine in a patient with a pathological fracture at C6. The kyphotic deformity, extent of C6 vertebral destruction, involvement of the adjacent C7 vertebra, and spinal canal compromise all are well seen. This patient had a large metal plate in his proximal humerus after treatment for a previous pathological fracture there. Computerized tomography could not be used because of the defraction artifact from that plate.

A

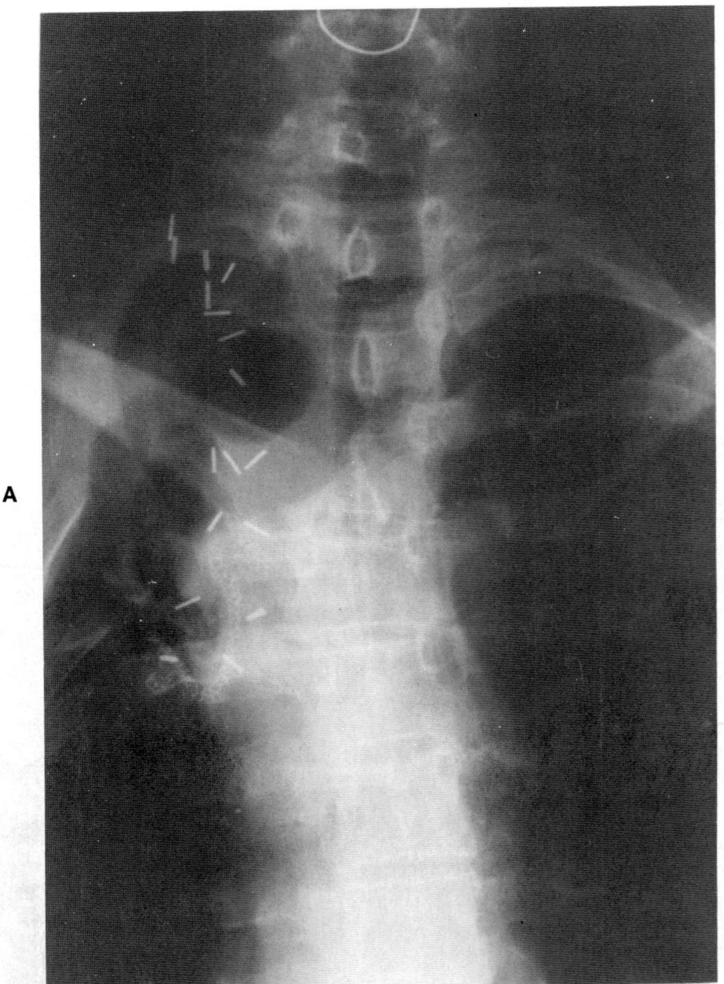

FIGURE 12-11 **A,** An AP roentgenogram of the upper thoracic spine in a 41-year-old woman 4 months after resection of a Pancoast lung carcinoma. Local destruction of the T1-T3 vertebral bodies is apparent. Clinically, the patient evidenced early long tract signs and symptoms.

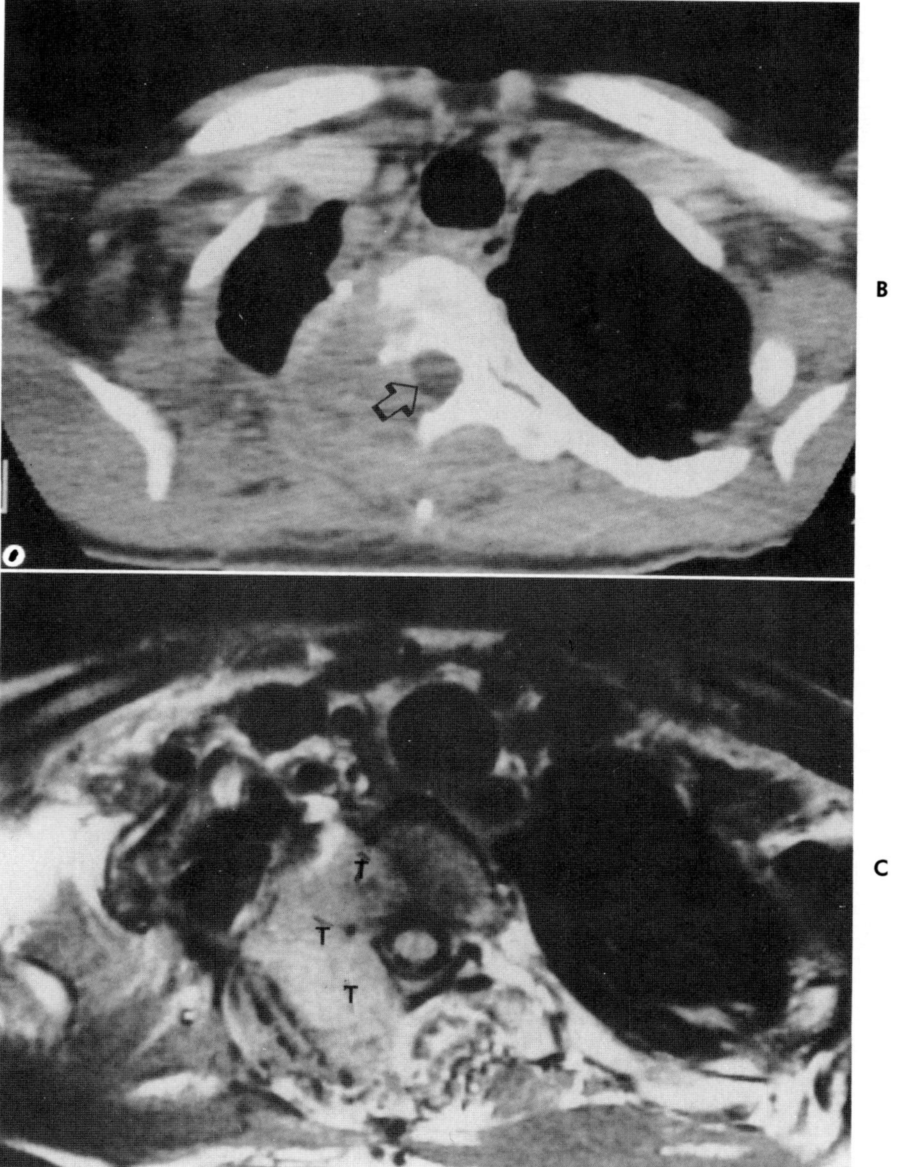

FIGURE 12-11, cont'd. **B,** CT scan at the T4 level. Note the extensive bone lysis both anteriorly and posteriorly, also the concave edge of the soft tissue tumor mass *(arrow)* compromising approximately half the spinal canal. The extraspinal dimensions of the tumor mass are not clearly seen. **C,** Cross-sectional MR scan at the same level obtained at the same time. The extent of the soft tissue tumor extraspinally *(T)* is much more clearly demonstrated, although the extent of canal compromise is less apparent than on the CT scan.

Continued.

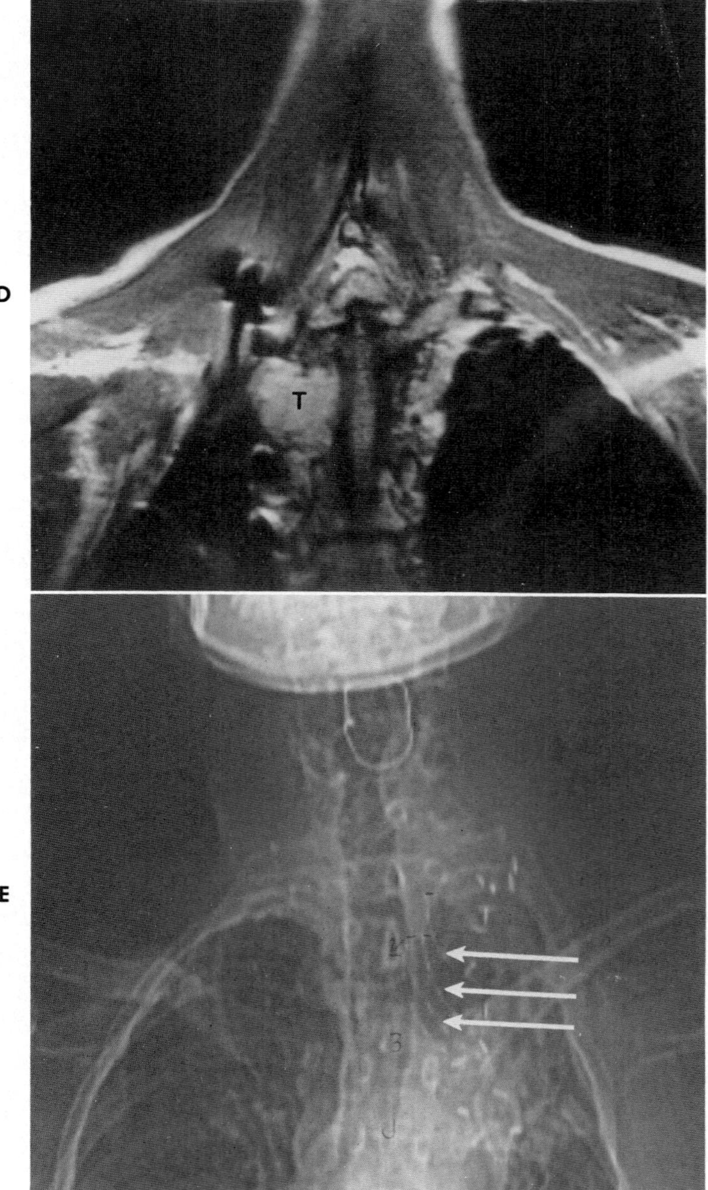

FIGURE 12-11, cont'd. **D,** Anteroposterior MR scan of this patient. The extent of canal compromise and cord displacement by the tumor *(T)* is seen better than on the lateral view but not as clearly as on the CT scan. **E,** Posteroanterior MR image obtained immediately after an anterolateral spinal decompression and placement of four radiopaque plastic radium-bead catheters *(arrows)*. The patient remains alive and well without recurrence of bony or neurological compromise 13 months postoperatively.

tumors may become ER+ as metastases, thus creating an opportunity for effective hormonal manipulation as an adjunct to surgical management.

Cerebrospinal fluid obtained at the time of myelography or enhanced CT also is worthy of histological examination and chemical analysis. Markedly elevated CSF protein, when present, is a strong indicator of either intradural metastases or significant extradural cord compression. Almost all patients with intradural tumors will have somewhat elevated CSF protein; unfortunately, it is relatively uncommon even with profound extradural compression. Nevertheless, occasionally the presence of malignant cells in the CSF will be helpful in defining the primary tumor focus. As already noted, only a few drops of fluid should be removed when there is the likelihood of a complete extradural block.

TREATMENT

The philosophy of treatment of vertebral metastases has undergone considerable change during recent years. With improvement in chemotherapy and hormonal manipulation, many patients survive for long periods with metastases without apparent involvement of vital organs. Progressive bone disease, particularly of the spine, is not uncommon, however, and spinal pain often becomes the principal focus of symptoms. Some spinal surgeons[21] have advocated an aggressive operative approach to vertebral metastases, advocating in essence prophylactic stabilization where there is destruction of 50% or more of a vertebral body. They have supported this approach by stating that prophylactic stabilization of the spine should be considered analogous to prophylactic nailing of a femur with a pathological lesion, because both the femur and the spine are weight-bearing structures. In our opinion, this represents an overly aggressive approach to the problem. Prophylactic stabilization of the femur can be performed with relative ease, often through a closed nailing approach, and with minimal morbidity. Spinal stabilization, whether prophylactic or otherwise, is a major operative proceeding entailing multiple risks and prolonged recovery not encountered with extremity-stabilization procedures. More important, the majority of patients with spinal metastases do not have progressive spinal instability or neurological involvement and can therefore be treated successfully by hormonal manipulation, chemotherapy, local irradiation, or temporary bracing. Even most of those who sustain a pathological compression fracture of one or more vertebral bodies can be treated by temporary bedrest and soft bracing, much like what is used in the osteoporotic patient with a nonmalignant but equally pathological compression fracture of a vertebra (Fig. 12-7). In our experience[41-44] approximately 80% of patients with this disease can be treated effectively with one of these nonoperative modalities.

Chemotherapy and Hormonal Manipulation

If patients who have no symptoms show positive bone scan or roentgenographic evidence of spinal metastases without vertebral collapse, there is little evidence that local radiotherapy is indicated. However, they do warrant chemotherapy or hormonal manipulation in an effort to reverse the process, which otherwise will progress to cause pain and eventual neurological disability. The patient with widespread spinal pain from diffuse metastatic involvement is an appropriate candidate for hormonal manipulation or chemotherapy if there is no evidence of impending vertebral collapse, spinal instability, or neurological compromise.

Hormonal manipulation is the most common form of management, at least initially, for carcinomas of the breast and prostate with spinal metastases. Breast metastases from tumors determined histologically to be ER+ usually will respond for some time to tamoxifen or other hormone-suppression measures. ER− lesions are much less likely to improve, either symptomatically or roentgenographically, with additive hormonal therapy. In the case of breast cancer the response or lack thereof to one form of hormonal manipulation correlates well with the likelihood of responding to further and often quite different hormonal therapy, although exceptions to this rule certainly abound.[67] Prostatic cancer seems to be the most consistently sensitive to hormonal therapy, whether androgen removal or estrogen addition. Spinal metastases respond to either in the majority of instances, at least temporarily.

In contrast to the experience with hormonal manipulation, the response of spinal metastases to chemotherapeutic agents is somewhat more difficult to predict. In breast cancer patients with spinal metastases, for example, the response rate reported even for similar chemotherapy protocols varies from 0% to 84%.[11-13] One reason for this wide range is the variability of response criteria used to evaluate such skeletal disease. The problem has been highlighted by Carter,[11] who examined response criteria for six large breast cancer trials. In two of the trials no mention was made of how bone lesions were assessed for response. In the others, four criteria were used, some requiring the patients to manifest radiographic improvement for at least 3 months before qualifying as partial responders and some not even considering bone lesions in the evaluation. Few patients with breast cancer metastatic to the spine have roentgenographically demonstrable regression of spinal metastases after chemotherapy. It is thus unlikely that chemotherapy has any significant effect in enhancing restoration of cortical or cancellous bone destroyed by metastatic tumor. However, the overall survival time[19] for these patients is significantly better than for those with untreated spinal metastases, even in the absence of pain or neurological compromise. The patient with bone marrow involvement usually will show measurable improvement after chemotherapy. It is this response that is probably the major reason why most patients with spinal metastases improve symptomatically while on chemotherapy even without demonstrable bone healing. Because of the symptomatic improvement and the prolongation of survival, we advocate early intervention with chemotherapy particularly in a patient with breast or prostatic spinal metastases, once hormonal manipulation no longer appears beneficial.

One caveat with regard to chemotherapy needs brief discussion. There appears to be a tendency on the part of some oncologists to employ increasingly aggressive chemotherapy regimens in patients with spinal pain unresponsive to more conventional therapy. Care must be taken to ensure that such uncontrolled pain is not indicative of a microfracture, progressive vertebral collapse, or neurological impairment. All too often, when the mechanical factors finally are established and the patient is recognized as a suitable candidate for surgical intervention, iatrogenic bone marrow depression has become sufficiently severe that the operation must be postponed and the destructive process thus allowed to continue unabated. Similarly there is good evidence that some chemotherapeutic agents, particularly methotrexate and doxorubicin (Adriamycin), interfere with incorporation of the bone grafts that may be indicated at the time of spinal stabilization. This fact should be considered and chemotherapy discontinued as early as possible once the decision has been made to proceed with operative intervention.

Radiotherapy

The most controversial question in the treatment in spinal metastases is whether local irradiation should be used in conjunction with or as an alternative to surgical decompression and stabilization. A decade ago "operative intervention" usually meant laminectomy decompression, and the results of this procedure for the management of advanced spinal metastases were dismal. The majority of patients with neurological compromise did not improve, and in many progressive spinal deformities and instability developed as a result of, rather than in spite of, the decompression (Fig. 12-27).

In a retrospective series published in 1978 and based on a review of 20 years' experience, Gilbert et al.[37] suggested that radiation therapy alone was as effective as decompressive laminectomy (with or without radiotherapy) in the treatment of epidural cord compression. When successful treatment was measured in terms of how many patients regained the ability to walk, both modalities were less than 50% effective. With regard to pain relief, however, radiation alone seemed to be superior to laminectomy and was associated with a much lower incidence of progressive spinal deformity. Both types of treatment had a significant complication rate, although the complications were quite different between the two groups. Similar experiences have been reported by other radiotherapists.[7,50,78]

While advocating laminectomy decompression for patients with neurological compromise, Constans et al.[16] admitted that the overall results of such management were no better than those following radiation alone.

They maintained, nevertheless, that operative decompression before radiation was indicated because it allowed more rapid pain relief and enabled the patient to undergo subsequent irradiation with less risk of a sudden progression of symptoms. We do not agree with these authors' conclusions. There is nothing about laminectomy that ensures rapid alleviation of pain. In our experience the single problem of pain alone can usually be effectively relieved after only 2000 cGy,* far more rapidly than a debilitated cancer patient can expect to find relief after any type of surgery. Moreover, as noted, the likelihood of progressive spinal deformity, worsening spinal pain, and even recurrence of the neurological compromise because of increasing spinal instability is far higher after laminectomy than after irradiation.

What appears to be missing from this comparison is acknowledgment of the fact that not all spinal metastases result in the same complications, not all metastatic tumors are equally radiosensitive, and not all modes of intervention necessarily involve laminectomy.

At one extreme are surgeons who expect spinal metastases from anaplastic breast carcinoma, or other similar undifferentiated primary, to respond favorably to local irradiation. If metastases are causing minimal bone destruction and pain appears to be the result of reaction by the bone to tumor, then radiation may be the ideal means of achieving relief. Even if the metastatic tumor has extended into the extradural space and is causing early neurological compromise, radiation will usually be effective in reversing this so long as there is no evidence of spinal cord or root compression by fragments of bone or disc detritus.

The patient with spinal pain and/or neurological compromise secondary to widespread metastases involving more than one level (Fig. 12-9, *E*) also is an appropriate candidate for irradiation, because multilevel decompression is impractical by any method and is least well tolerated by the patient already debilitated from widely disseminated cancer.

The technique of wide-field or hemibody irradiation (HBI) has found many advocates under these circumstances. Typically such patients, poorly controlled by large doses of analgesics before irradiation, will experience marked improvement by half-body doses of between 700 and 1000 cGy. For example, in Fitzpatrick and Rider's[31] series of patients with widespread breast metastases to the spine in whom pain was the major symptom, 53% who received one HBI treatment obtained complete or partial relief whereas 91% who received radiation to both halves obtained relief. Two thirds of those who responded experienced continuing pain relief for more than half of their remaining life despite inexorable progression of their disease. Radiobiological evidence suggests that a single dose of 300 cGy has a cell lethality of approximately 90% but at 800 cGy has a lethality of about 99.5% or better. Thus, if a tumor has a doubling time of 3 months it might be anticipated to have a remission time of about 30 months following 800 cGy.

A limitation of HBI is sensitivity of the lung, particularly if it has been subjected to previous irradiation or possibly sensitized by cytotoxic agents. Bone marrow suppression is also a limiting factor, reducing the applicability of widespread irradiation. Eight hundred centigrays, for example, is lethal to bone marrow and could not be tolerated as a whole-body dose although it is probably safe as a single HBI dose (800 to the lower half, 500 to the upper half) depending on the extent of previous focal radiation. However, when tumor has destroyed enough bone to result in vertebral collapse and that collapse is causing fragments of bone, ligament, or disc to compress the cord directly (Fig. 12-4), it is illogical to assume that any improvement could result from irradiation no matter how radiosensitive the malignancy might be. Similarly, when vertebral collapse has resulted in progressive spinal deformity and instability, local irradiation cannot be expected to afford any relief from that pain. In fact, because of the hyperemic softening that occurs in bone during the early stages of irradiation, a patient may be at greater risk of progressive deformity then than if no treatment whatsoever had been rendered.

Although irradiation generally is well tolerated, a multiplicity of complications have been described.

---

*Centigrays (cGy) are the currently used designation for amounts of radiation absorbed dose.

The most feared of these is radiation myelopathy, often developing months and occasionally even years after exposure. It causes progressive and at times severe disturbances in spinal cord function for which there is no known effective treatment. As Dorfman et al.[23] have demonstrated, the incidence of this complication exhibits a threshold effect generally related to radiation dose, time, and fractionation and to the length and location of the irradiated spinal segment. Most patients with overt paraparesis or quadriparesis as a manifestation of radiation myelopathy have received second-dose treatments[47] either because of local recurrence or, more commonly, as a complication of double irradiation in overlapping fields from separate treatment courses. However, morphological changes in the spinal cord have also been described in some experimental animal models after only low-dose exposure.[52] Dorfman et al.[23] consistently demonstrated prolongation of the somatosensory conduction velocity (SSCV) in patients receiving cord irradiation doses between 3800 and 4400 cGy, noting, however, that this was infrequent if less than 3000 cGy was administered.

Radiation osteitis, another complication, develops unpredictably but, again, is more common after local irradiation in excess of 3500 cGy. The effect on bone is probably due to damage produced in the fine intraosseous and periosteal vasculature, which may not manifest radiographic changes for many months. Most often these changes take the form of poorly defined patchy sclerosis. The trabecular pattern tends to be maintained, although the trabeculae are thicker and more dense. Such changes may be mistaken for recurrence of an active metastasis, particularly if the osteitis is productive of local spine pain. When a techetium-99 bone scan is performed, the area of osteitis will show increased uptake that is indistinguishable from the pattern typical of recurrent metastases. Tragic results can occur if such sites are given additional irradiation on the assumption that the symptoms and radiographic findings represent metastatic disease (Fig. 12-12, *A* and *B*). Progressive bone necrosis and vertebral collapse may develop[17] with consequent spinal deformity, severe and intractable mechanical spine pain, and even neurological compromise from local cord or root compression.

In patients who have undergone spinal stabilization and bone grafting, the likelihood of graft incorporation and the risk of major wound breakdown are increased by preoperative irradiation in excess of 3500 cGy.* In our own experience (involving over 60 unstable spines managed by operative decompression, stabilization, and postoperative irradiation of 2800 to 3000 cGy) there have been no instances of wound healing problems and 16 patients who underwent bone grafting showed uncomplicated graft incorporation. By contrast, of 30 patients who received preoperative spinal irradiation in excess of 3500 cGy, six suffered wound healing complications and none of the four whose fixation was augmented by corticocancellous grafts showed radiographic evidence of graft incorporation. None of the patients who received low-dose irradiation, even as low as 2200 cGy, had evidence of local tumor recurrence, although two who received no irradiation did have recurrences. Similar results have been described by others.[29,30]

The threshold for radiation complications, including myelopathy, osteitis, wound healing problems, and interference with graft incorporation, consistently appears to be between 3000 and 3500 cGy. Because the control of local tumor recurrence in the spine does not seem to improve with doses in excess of 3000 cGy, we recommend that irradiation be limited to this and if possible be postponed for a minimum of 3 to 4 weeks postoperatively to limit further the risks to wound healing and graft incorporation.

At the other extreme are surgeons who advocate an aggressive philosophy of operative intervention early in the course of spinal metastases and, in many instances, on a prophylactic basis to avoid the complications of instability and neurological compromise. Schaberg and Gainor,[59] for example, have estimated that in 20% of patients with spinal metastases, significant neurological deficits would develop if untreated; however, their estimate derives from a retrospective review of only 179 patients. Based on a similar projection, Constans et al.[16] have advocated decompressive laminectomy for almost all patients with spinal metastases and any neuro-

*References 5, 29, 43, 62, 63.

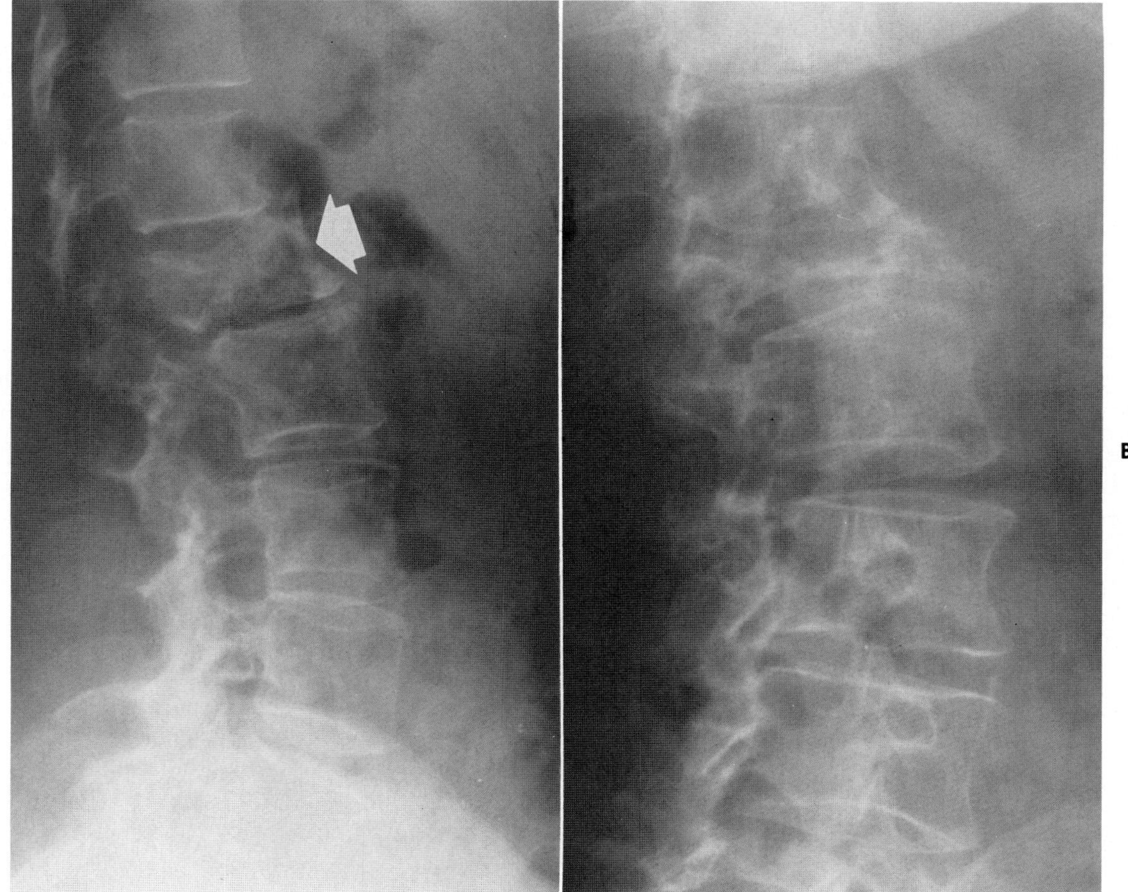

FIGURE 12-12 **A,** Spontaneous fracture of L1 in a 58-year-old woman with breast cancer known to be metastatic to the lower lumbar spine. Two years earlier she had received local irradiation (3500 cGy) because of increasing back pain. The pain had resolved but then returned in conjunction with the fracture apparent here *(arrow)*. An additional 2000 cGy of radiation was given on the presumption that this was a pathological fracture from recurrent cancer. **B,** Within 6 weeks the vertebral body had collapsed completely and a severe cauda equina syndrome had developed with marked segmental instability. At operation, no evidence of tumor was noted but there were histological signs of extensive radiation necrosis. Apparently the vertebra had sustained a so-called "insufficiency fracture" attributable entirely to the irradiation.[17] This case demonstrates the dangers of routinely reirradiating a site after vertebral collapse simply on the assumption that such collapse represents a recurrence of localized malignancy. *Continued.*

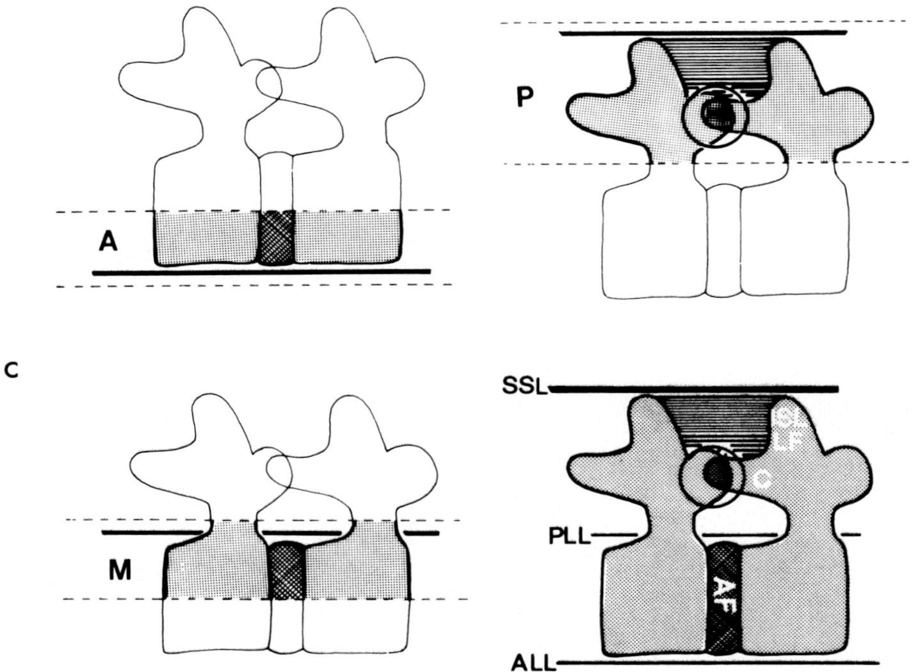

FIGURE 12-12, cont'd. **C,** The three-column biomechanical concept of Denis.[20] The anterior column *(A)* is formed by the anterior longitudinal ligament, anterior annulus fibrosus, and anterior part of the vertebral body. The middle column *(M)* is formed by the posterior longitudinal ligament, posterior annulus fibrosus, and posterior wall of the vertebral body. The posterior column *(P)* is formed by the posterior bony complex (posterior arch) alternating with the posterior ligamentous complex (supraspinous ligament, interspinous ligament, capsule, and ligamentum flavum). There must be disruption of both the anterior and the middle columns for a kyphotic deformity to develop; all three columns must be disrupted for anterior or posterior subluxation to occur (see Fig. 12-11, *B*). (**C** reprinted with permission from Denis, F.: Clin. Orthop. **189:**65, 1984.)

logical symptoms. These authors performed such a decompression in 80% of 600 patients with spinal metastases but noted that overall results were no better than for similar patient groups treated by irradiation alone. DeWald et al.[21] have advocated "prophylactic stabilization" of the spine for all patients with 50% destruction of a vertebral body or with involvement of the pedicles, maintaining that such patients are at high risk of collapse, progressive deformity, or paralysis, whether or not they have symptoms. Such spinal stabilization is likened by them to prophylactic fixation of the femur with a lytic focus because both the spine and the femur are weight-bearing structures.

Just as it seems unreasonable to conclude that all patients with spinal instability or cord compression should be treated nonoperatively, the opposite extreme, advocacy of early surgical intervention espoused by Constans et al.[16] and DeWald et al.,[21] seems overly aggressive. In our experience during the last 15 years, the incidence of significant neurological impairment in patients with spinal metastases has been low, slightly less than 5%. Moreover, many patients who do manifest neurological impairment can be treated effectively with irradiation. Constans' belief that laminectomy decompression before radiation markedly accelerates pain relief has not been supported by our experience. Similarly we have seen many individuals with more than 50% vertebral destruction, or with combined anterior and posterior destruction, who have not required stabilization and yet have not progressed to spinal instability (Fig. 12-11). Prophylactic stabilization of the spine, particularly if performed by both an anterior and a posterior approach (as advocated by DeWald et al.[21]), is a far more extensive, costly, and dangerous operation than is prophylactic fixation of any long bone and in our opinion is not indicated simply on a theoretical basis.

Operative Intervention

Operative intervention is indicated when neurological compromise clearly is related to mechanical cord or root compression by bone or disc detritus, by radioresistent tumor, or by recurrent tumor in an area of the spine already subjected to the maximal safe dosage of irradiation. A separate indication for operation is the necessity for spinal stabilization anteriorly, posteriorly, or both, either in conjunction with or as an alternative to neurological decompression. Controversy abounds concerning whether anterior or posterior decompression is more appropriate, what means and approach should be employed for stabilization, and how aggressive the surgeon should be in recommending operative intervention after the presence of spinal metastases has been detected.

With regard to the last question, it already has been noted that some oncologists and radiotherapists advocate irradiation and chemotherapy as the most appropriate management for every case of spinal metastases even after the development of vertebral collapse, spinal instability, or cord compression. Clearly this philosophy is inappropriate in instances of mechanical disruption, which cannot possibly be improved by irradiation alone.

Biomechanical Considerations

Denis[20] and White and Panjabi[69] have popularized the concept of the three-column spine (Fig. 12-12) and defined from both a biomechanical and a clinical viewpoint the extent of bone or soft tissue disruption necessary to result in true spinal instability. The vertebral bodies and discs function as the fulcrum of weight-bearing and are loaded primarily in compression. Except in the lower lumbar area, the center of gravity falls slightly forward of this fulcrum, tending to bend the spine forward. The posterior elements, particularly their ligamentous connections, resist these forward-bending stresses by exerting tensile forces. Severe destruction of the posterior elements associated with sheer stresses across intact anterior columns could result in a forward flexion deformity, but such a situation rarely occurs with metastatic disease except iatrogenically after wide laminectomy. Lytic destruction of an anterior vertebral body (anterior column) often is the initial manifestation of metastic involvement. The tumor process will break out through the anterior longitudinal ligament, resulting in a paraspinous mass. In such a situation, because the middle and posterior columns have not been weakened significantly, spinal instability does not ensue. Only when the entire vertebral body (both the anterior and the middle columns) is involved by tumor lysis does the risk of progressive deformity and neurological compromise become a major concern. As the vertebral body is destroyed and begins to collapse, its ability to function as a weight-bearing fulcrum decreases, the bending moment of the spine shifts posteriorly, and the compression load on the remaining vertebral body increases geometrically. With progressing kyphosis a vector of this compression load encourages the extrusion of tumor tissue, disc, and bone detritus posteriorly into the spinal canal, often resulting in cord or root compression (Fig. 12-4). If the posterior elements are minimally involved and tensile stability remains intact, the stability of the spine can be restored entirely through the anterior approach. The diseased anterior structures can be resected, the spinal cord decompressed, and the anterior and middle column stability restored by a variety of means (see Fig. 12-13). This is the circumstance usually encountered. However, if tumor destruction of the posterior elements (particularly the pedicles) is advanced, the greatly enhanced tensile loads posteriorly cannot be resisted. Typically a forward-shearing deformity will develop, further compromising the spinal canal and necessitating both anterior and posterior decompression and stabilization (Plate 2).

In summary, the indications for surgical intervention include (1) progressive spinal

Text continued on p. 340.

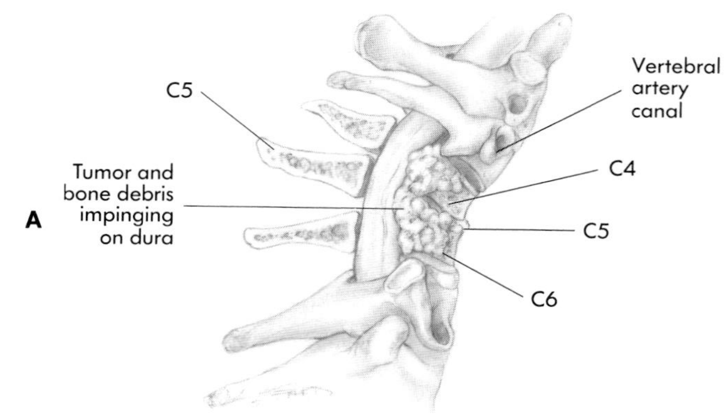

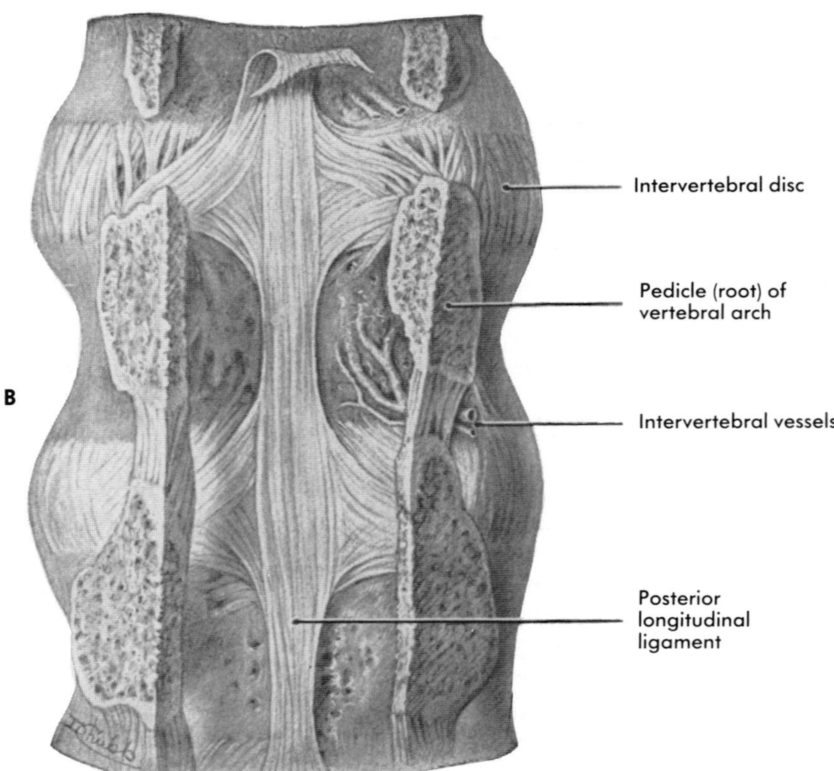

FIGURE 12-13 Technique for anterior decompression and stabilization of the cervical spine. **A,** Lateral presentation, with metastatic tumor destruction of C5 and partial destruction of C4 and C6. Typically a kyphotic deformity has developed, resulting in extrusion of tumor, disc, and bone detritus into the spinal canal. **B,** The posterior longitudinal ligament from behind. Note that it is thin directly behind the vertebral bodies and offers little resistance to posterior extrusion of tumor or bone debris. This is in constant to the thick and diamond-shaped expansion of the ligament behind the intervertebral discs. (**B** reprinted with permission from Grant, J.C.B.: An atlas of anatomy, Baltimore, 1956, The Williams & Wilkins Co., Plate 366.)

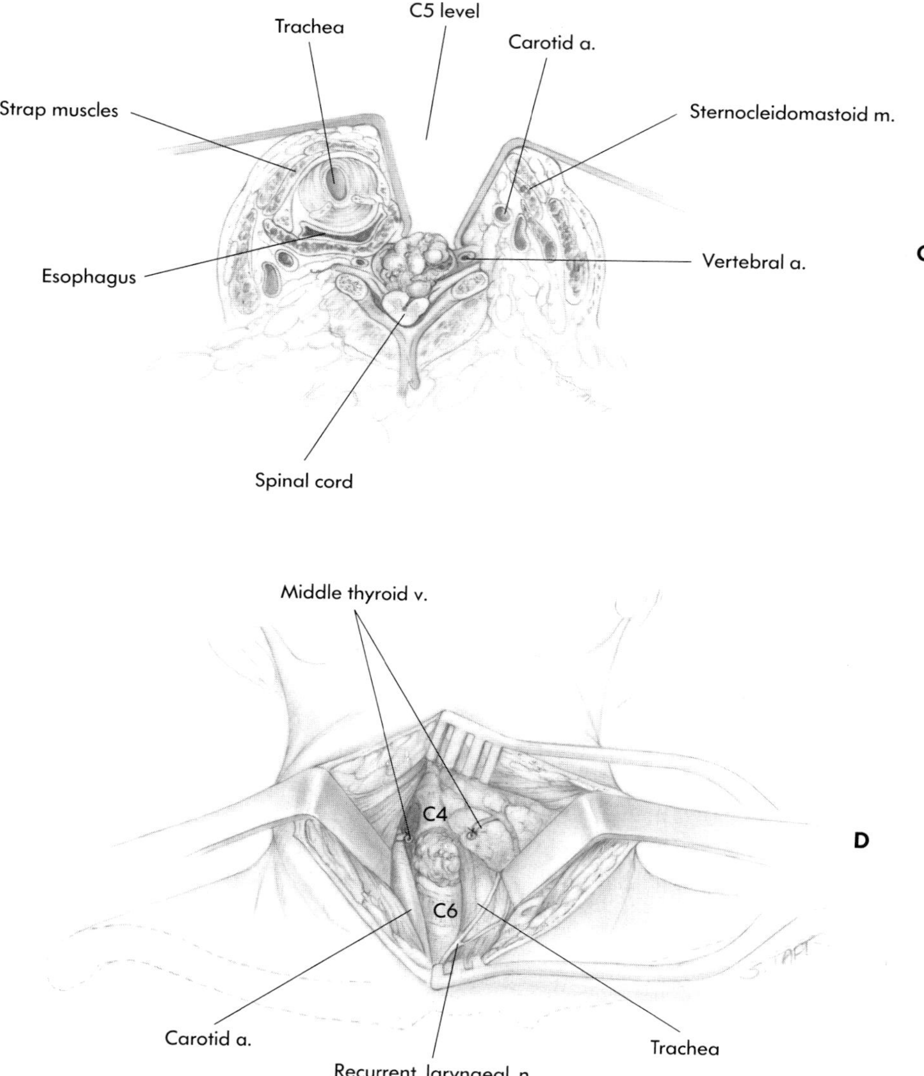

FIGURE 12-13, cont'd. **C,** Cross-sectional view of the neck demonstrating displacement and compression of the spinal cord by an expanding tumor mass. The anterior approach is shown with the trachea, esophagus, and paratracheal muscles retracted medially and the sternocleidomastoid and carotid sheath retracted laterally. **D,** Anterior view of the operative approach demonstrating the level of vertebral involvement (C5). The retracted thyroid gland and its ligated and transected middle thyroid vein are shown. The location of the recurrent laryngeal nerve is also indicated, although this is not invariably visualized.

Continued.

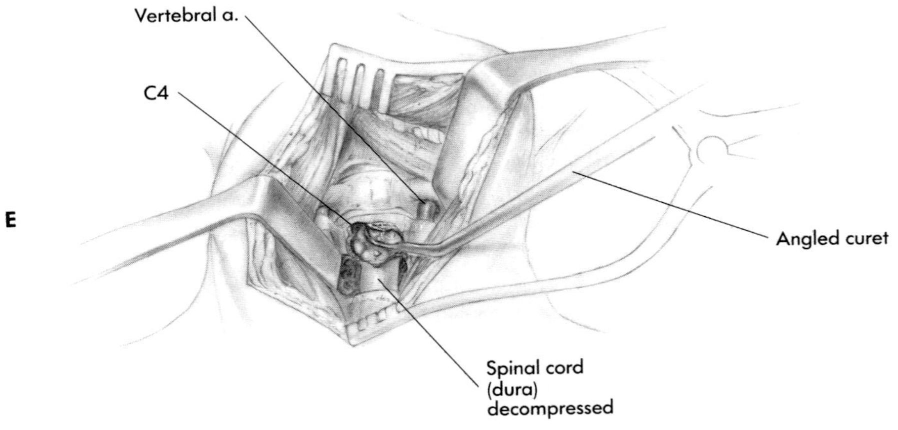

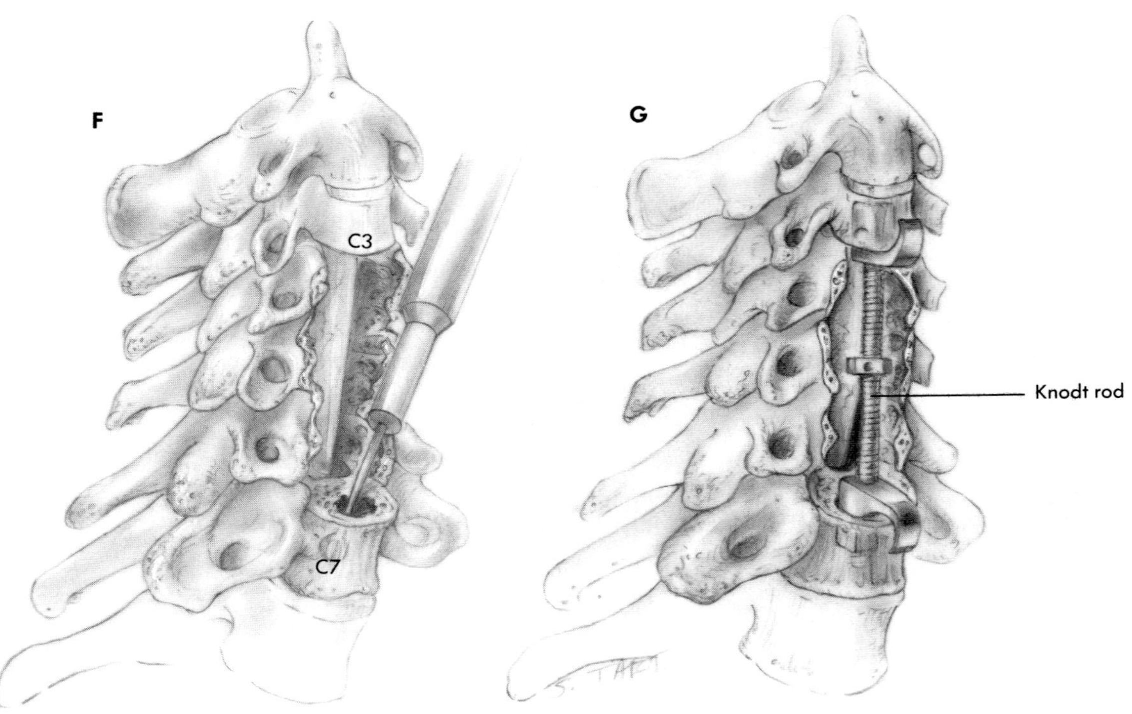

***FIGURE 12-13, cont'd.* E,** The spinal cord has been decompressed anteriorly by resection of the C5 vertebral body, and the C4 vertebra is being removed piecemeal by an angled curet. **F,** Once the spinal canal has been decompressed completely, the end plates of the adjacent intact vertebral bodies are perforated with a high-speed dental bur and a cavity is created just large enough to accommodate the Knodt rod and its hook. **G,** The Knodt rod has been positioned, its hooks imbedded in the adjacent vertebral bodies by twisting the rod.

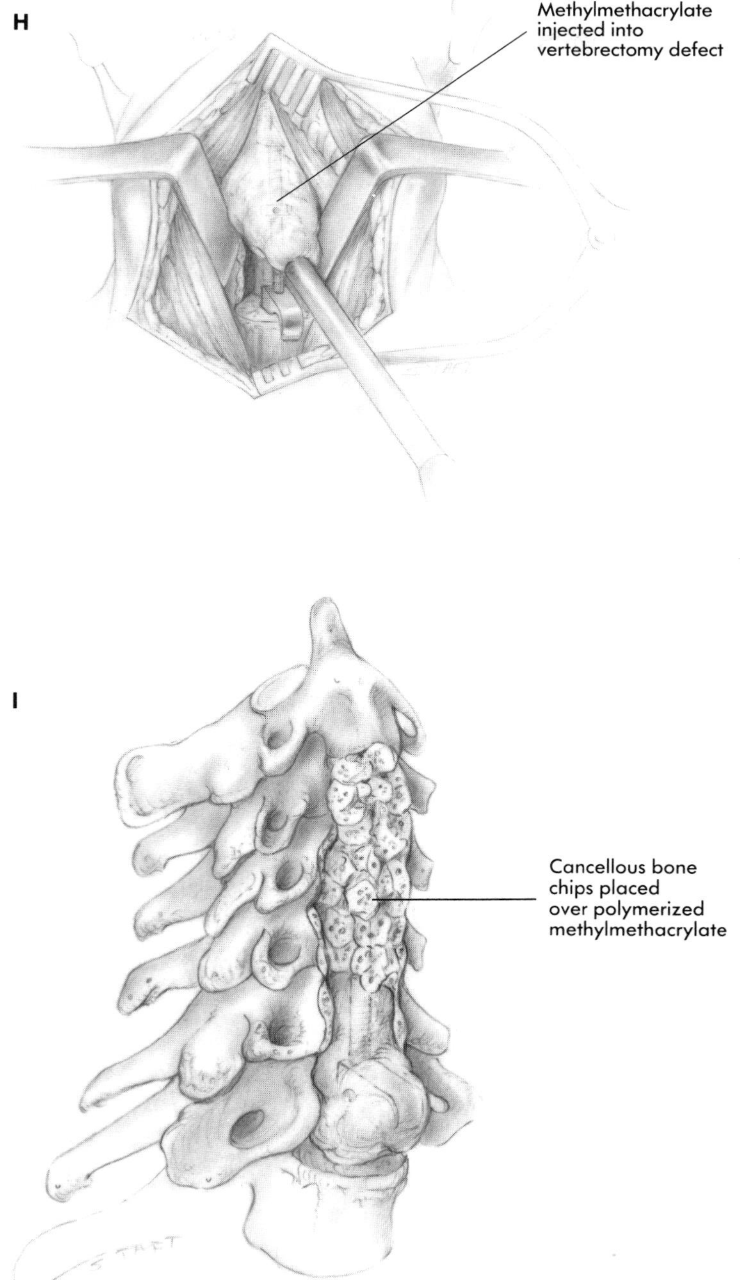

FIGURE 12-13, cont'd. **H,** The defect is filled with methylmethacrylate that polymerizes in situ, incorporating the rod and hooks. Care has been taken to prevent expansion of the acrylic into the spinal canal by placing a malleable retractor between the cement construct and the canal. **I,** In patients who have not been irradiated within 3 months preoperatively and who will not be irradiated within 3 months postoperatively, cancellous bone chips are packed anterior to the cement and metal construct in an effort to achieve a permanent bony arthrodesis.

canal impingement and cord compression by radioresistent tumor, by recurrent tumor in an area already subjected to maximal irradiation, or by bone or soft tissue detritus extruded into the canal as a result of progressive spinal deformity (decompression anteriorly, anterolaterally, or posteriorly, with or without spinal stabilization), (2) progressive spinal deformity (anterior decompression and spinal stabilization), and (3) progressive kyphotic deformity associated with posterior element disruption and shear deformity (anterior and posterior decompression and stabilization).

Preoperative Preparation

Before embarking on a discussion of the techniques of spinal decompression and stabilization, it is necessary to consider at least briefly the immediate preoperative preparation for such undertakings:

1. Because most patients have been given chemotherapeutic agents for variable periods before the necessity for operative intervention was recognized, it is exceedingly important to obtain a complete hemogram, including a coagulation panel, immediately preoperatively. Except under emergency circumstances, the operation should be postponed until the WBC count has returned to a level above 1200. This is necessary because of the obvious immunological restrictions of severe leukocytopenia.
2. Patients should be in positive nitrogen balance, if possible. On occasion a brief period of hyperalimentation preoperatively will improve the rapidity of wound healing and reduce the risk of sepsis dramatically.
3. All patients requiring anterior thoracic and upper lumbar decompressions and stabilizations should have at least bedside pulmonary studies preoperatively because of the necessity of approaching the spine via a thoracotomy. In patients with borderline pulmonary function, consideration also should be given to continuing intubation during the first 18 to 24 hours postoperatively. Most well-sedated patients tolerate overnight intubation and benefit greatly from the improved ventilation and pulmonary toilet that this measure affords during the critical period immediately postoperative.
4. The extent of intraoperative bleeding is difficult to predict accurately preoperatively. Generally patients who are in the midst of a course of radiation when surgery becomes necessary can be expected to bleed actively because of the hyperemia induced by irradiation. Expansile lytic lesions and those without clearly defined margins roentgenographically are the most likely to be highly vascular and, on occasion, consideration must be given to selective arterial embolization preoperatively if severe hemorrhage is anticipated. However, the technique is infrequently used before spinal decompression or stabilization because of the risks of inadvertent embolic occlusion of the anterior spinal artery. This is particularly true for middle and upper thoracic lesions, where cord vascularization is tenuous and unpredictable under any circumstances.

   Ordinarily, to be prepared for the occasional instance of rapid blood loss from a vascular bony bed that cannot be controlled by local pressure or electrocoagulation, we type and cross-match all patients for 50% more blood than we anticipate losing. It is unwise to assume that the blood bank will be able to provide additional blood rapidly in an emergency, since many cancer patients subjected to previous chemotherapy regimens and intermittent transfusions have blood cell antibodies that can cause extensive delays in cross-matching.
5. Patients who have been maintained on corticosteroids as part of their chemotherapy will be adrenally suppressed and require steroid augmentation perioperatively. Although there are many regimens used for such replacement, we have found that, except for the most severely depleted patients, it is sufficient to administer 100 mg of hydrocortisone intravenously at the beginning of the operation, 100 mg IV in the recovery room, and 50 mg IV on the

following morning. We have recognized no instances of clinical renal insufficiency using this simple regimen.

6. The questions of whether steroids are effective in the acute management of cases with incipient cord compression is somewhat more controversial. Sundaresan (Boland et al.[5]) and Sundaresan et al.[61] have advocated the use of high-dose steroids immediately preoperatively, believing them to be effective in reducing the ultimate neurological deficit after adequate decompression. Their recommendation is to use dexamethasone 10 mg IV as a loading dose and then to continue 4 mg intravenously every 6 hours during the perioperative period.

   No controlled studies have been performed to document the effectiveness of this regimen, but there have been prospective studies on the use of steroids in patients with acute cord trauma and these have shown no convincing benefit. We have not found steroids perioperatively to be of any benefit in improving cord function and have therefore, after an initial trial, discontinued their use.

TECHNIQUES OF DECOMPRESSION AND STABILIZATION

As already noted, cord or root decompression can be performed via a posterior, posterolateral, or anterior route or occasionally by a combined anterior and posterior route. The indications for one of these approaches in preference to another are based solely on the direction from which the metastatic tumor is compressing the cord. This information can be obtained most accurately from a computerized tomographic scan or from a myelogram or occasionally from a magnetic resonance study (Figs. 12-9 and 12-10).

With few exceptions, decompression must be followed by spinal stabilization, although the route for such stabilization may not coincide with the decompression approach. Thus a patient requiring anterior decompression and consequent stabilization may also require posterior stabilization when sufficient posterior element destruction has occurred and there exists a predisposition for forward slippage or rotation of the vertebral elements even after anterior stability has been achieved (Fig. 12-13).

I have chosen to discuss the techniques of spinal decompression and stabilization together because they are performed at the same operation. For ease of presentation they will be considered under the following, somewhat artificial, categories:

Anterior decompression and stabilization
Posterior decompression and stabilization
Anterolateral decompression
Combined anterior and posterior stabilization

Anterior Decompression and Stabilization

In most instances compression of the cord and roots occurs from in front as a result of bone detritus extruded from the vertebral body into the spinal canal (Fig. 12-13, *A*). The vertebral body has a network of thin-walled sinusoids where pooling of blood occurs and whence metastatic tumor cells can escape with relative ease. As a consequence it is in the vertebral body itself, anterior to the spinal canal, that metastatic tumor foci are likely to colonize and thence to invade the neural canal.

The normal anatomy of the posterior longitudinal ligament is such that immediately behind the intervertebral disc the ligament not only is thickest but also is widened into a diamond-shaped barrier that encourages disc herniation to occur posterolaterally rather than centrally against the cord. In contrast, immediately behind the vertebral body itself, the ligament is thin and narrow and therefore offers little resistance to central extrusion of tumor tissue and bone fragments directly against the cord (Fig. 12-13, *B*). Consequently, when an anterior decompression of the cord is necessary, the dissection must extend well across the midline and the posterior half of the vertebral body, at least from pedicle to pedicle, must be resected.

Cervical Spine. For lesions of the cervical spine an anterior approach is employed through the avascular interval between the sternocleidomastoid and carotid sheath laterally and the strap muscles, trachea, and esophagus medially (Fig. 12-13, *C*). When resection of one or two vertebrae is contemplated, a transverse thyroidectomy incision centered over the level of involvement and paralleling the normal skin folds (Langer's lines) of the neck is used.

Technique. If the skin and subcutaneous tissue are infiltrated by a combination of 1% lidocaine and epinephrine (1:50), bleeding is markedly reduced.

The platysma is incised in line with the skin incision, care being taken to avoid damage to the superficial jugular veins. By undermining these layers proximally and distally, exposure of at least four vertebral levels is facilitated.

The medial edge of the sternocleidomastoid is identified and mobilized by blunt disection. Beneath it the carotid pulse can be palpated easily. The middle thyroid vein is the only structure ordinarily encountered, traversing the space thus created, and this vessel can be ligated and transected with impunity (Fig. 12-13, *D*). Dissections high in the neck may necessitate transection-ligation of the superior thyroid artery and vein.

Using longitudinal blunt disection, one exposes the anterior longitudinal ligament and gently reflects the longus coli to either side. This reveals the transverse processes and the canal for the vertebral artery.

As the medial structures are freed and retracted, care must be taken to avoid injury to the recurrent laryngeal nerve and the esophagus (Fig. 12-13, *D*).

The nerve may not always be identifiable; but if only blunt dissection is used in this area, there will be little risk of damage. When the patient has received local ir-

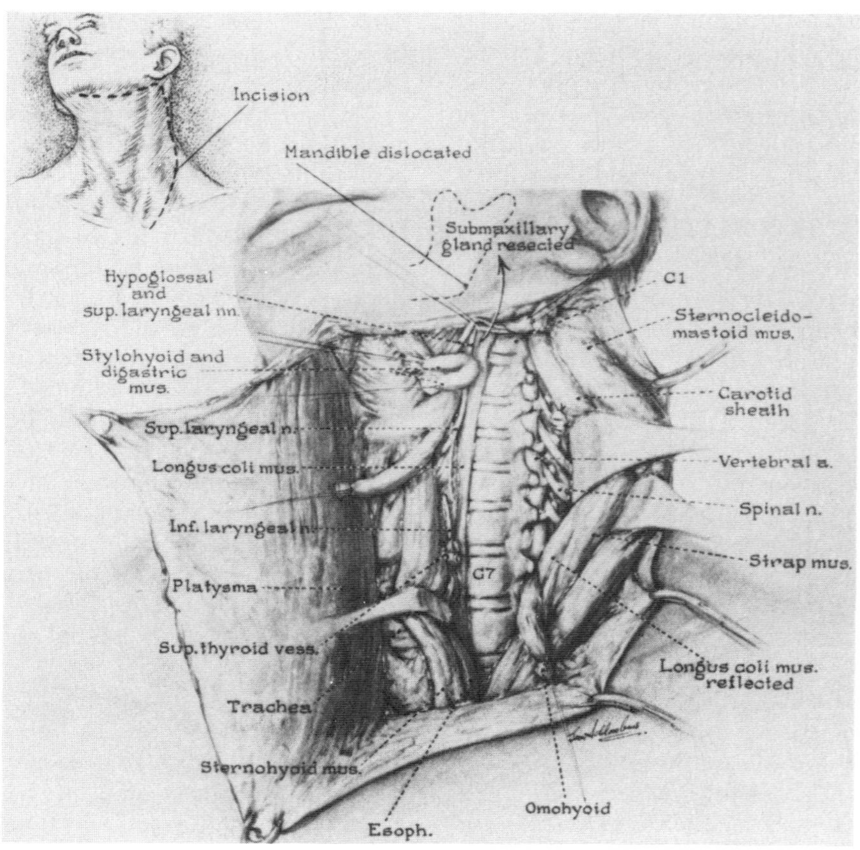

FIGURE 12-14 Exposure of the entire anterior surface of the cervical spine, the base of the skull, and C1 and C2 can be facilitated by excision of the submaxillary gland and even by dislocation of the temporomandibular joint. (Reprinted with permission from Riley, L.: Clin. Orthop. **91:**16, 1973.)

radiation preoperatively, particular care must be taken in retracting the esophagus, which is friable and prone to perforation. Even in the absence of such a major complication, however, most patients experience mild and temporary dysphagia postoperatively; nevertheless, this can be minimized by careful handling of the periesophageal tissues.

When exposure of more than three vertebral levels is anticipated a longitudinal incision paralleling the anterior border of the sternocleidomastoid may be required. In extreme circumstances, when exposure from C1 to T1 is required, the inverted L approach (popularized by Riley[58]) may be employed (Fig. 12-14).

The narrowed vertebral height and forward bulge of tumor tissue (Fig. 12-13, *A*) will usually be apparent and is helpful in identifying the level or levels of vertebral collapse. Occasionally intraoperative roentgenographic confirmation of the level is advisable before cord decompression commences. On occasion the collapsed vertebral space can be opened with assistance of a lamina spreader, which will allow correction of the kyphosis as tumor resection proceeds (Plate 1, *B*).

Initial removal of tumor and destroyed bone can be expedited by using a rongeur, care being taken to avoid damage to the intact vertebral bodies above and below the level(s) to be resected.

When approximately two thirds of the body has been resected, it is safer to proceed with an angled curet, whose smooth rounded back surface is not so likely to penetrate the spinal canal (Fig. 12-13, *E*). The angled curet also is an effective instrument for undercutting the vertebral end plates proximal and distal to the vertebrae resected to ensure that no tumor tissue is left within the spinal canal anteriorly.

The posterior longitudinal ligament may remain intact and prevent tumor tissue and bone from actually entering the spinal canal. More commonly, however, the ligament will be disrupted and its remnants must be removed so the tumor and bone fragments can be eliminated from the cord. Under these circumstances, and particularly if the patient has been irradiated preoperatively, the dura will be a gray-white and markedly thickened with tissue firmly adherent to its anterior surface. By careful dissection using a small angled curet, it is possible to remove the tumor with-

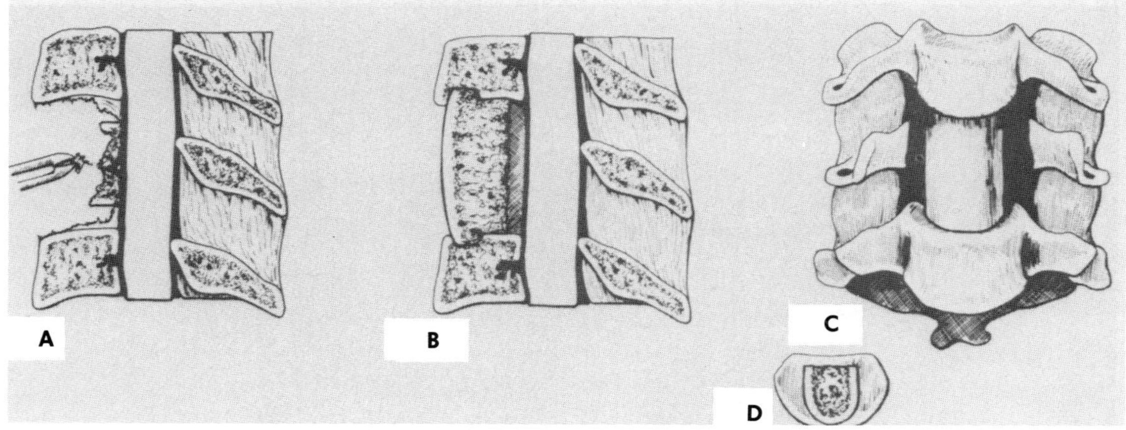

FIGURE 12-15 White's technique for anterior decompression and stabilization of the cervical spine using a corticocancellous graft. **A,** Excision of the destroyed bone and tumor to anteriorly decompress the spinal cord. **B,** Iliac bone used as a spacer. This construct is clinically unstable in the immediate postoperative period. **C,** The bone graft is notched in place to prevent extrusion or posterior displacement into the spinal cord. This construct is relatively stable postoperatively during flexion if the posterior elements are intact but is clinically unstable in both flexion and extension if they are not. **D,** Cortical bone purchase of the intact portion of the end plate offers resistance to vertical compression loading. (**A** to **D** reprinted with permission from White, A.A., and Panjabi, M.M.: Spine **9:**512, 1984.)

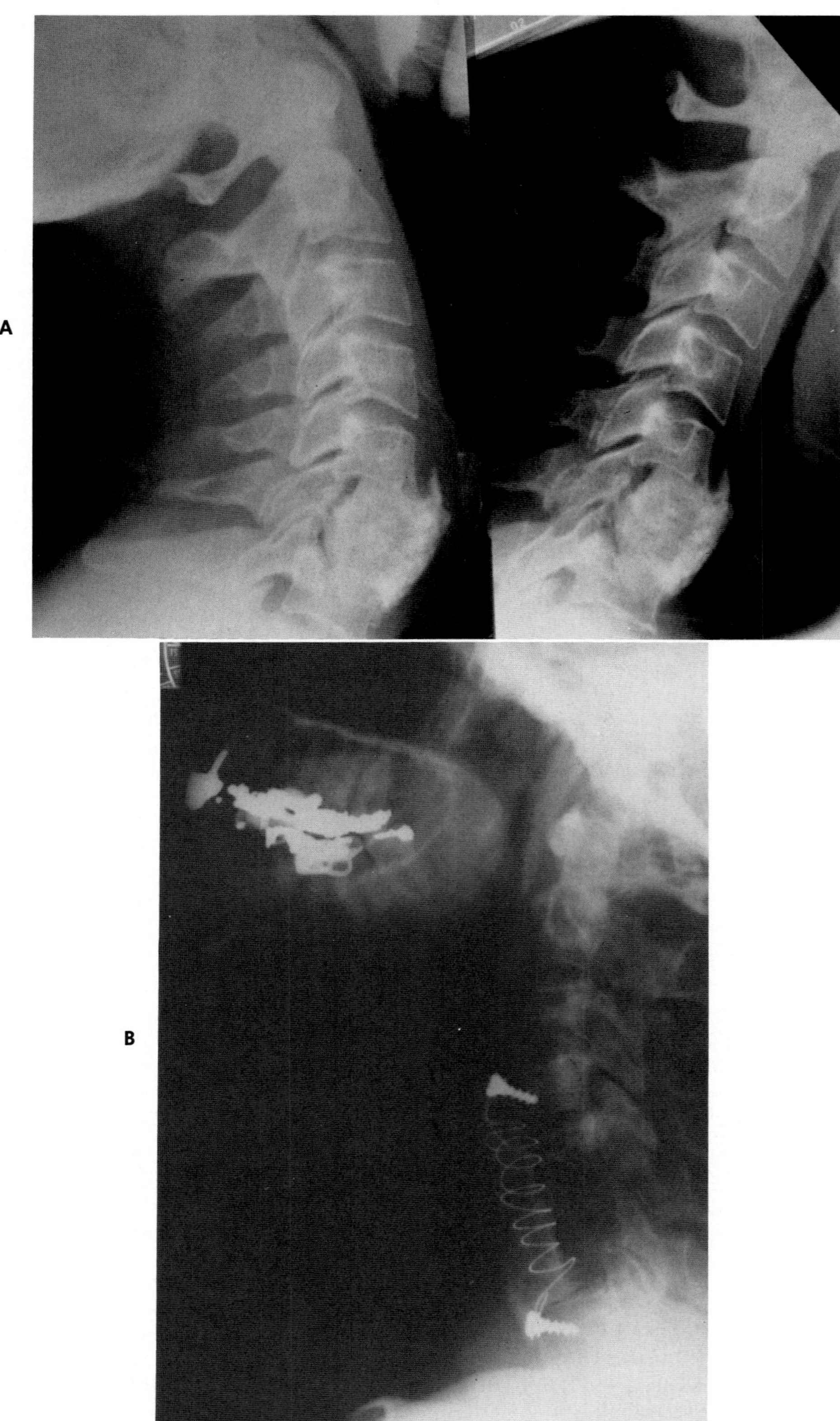

FIGURE 12-16 For legend see opposite page.

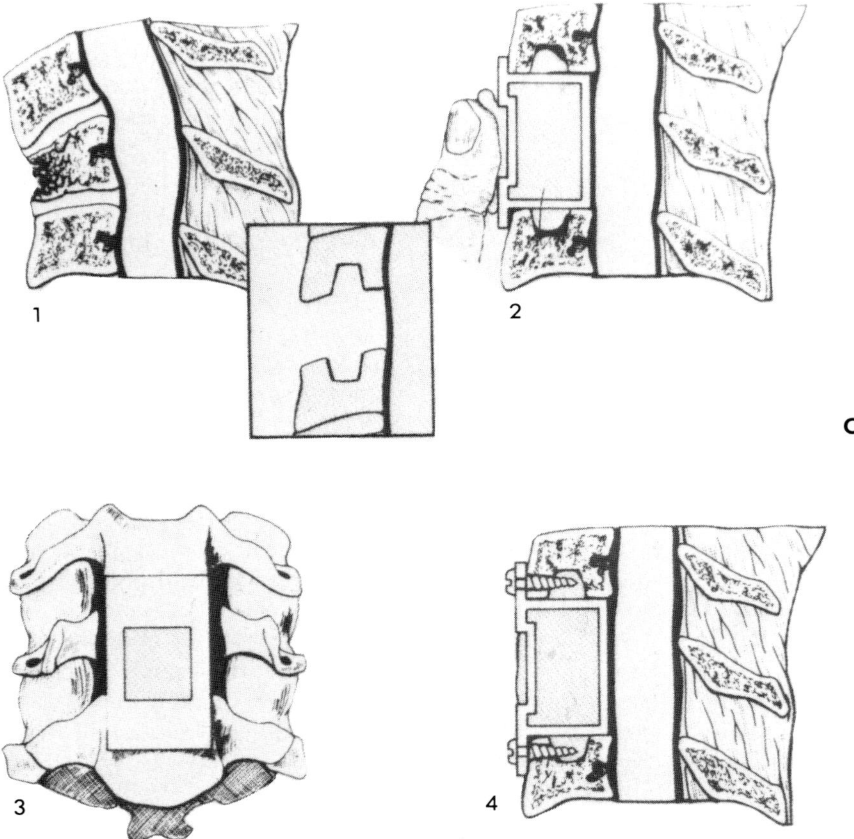

FIGURE 12-16 **A,** Postoperative flexion-extension roentgenograms 9 months after replacement-stabilization at the sixth cervical vertebra in a patient with metastatic gastric carcinoma. Little if any motion is demonstrable at the "fusion" site despite the fact that methylmethacrylate alone was used for stabilization. The patient had no neck symptoms. **B,** Anterior dislodgment of a wire-screw-methylmethacrylate construct after 4 days in a 42-year-old woman with metastatic breast carcinoma to C5 through C7. The construct was removed and the spine restabilized by a posterior wiring and iliac graft fusion from C4 to T1. **C,** The Ono device, one of several designed for vertebral replacement and stabilization after anterior decompression. It has two major disadvantages: inflexibility of size and the fact that its stability depends in great part on screw fixation to adjacent, often weakened, vertebral bodies. *1,* The diseased vertebra (inset, resected and a rectangular tunnel made in the two adjacent vertebrae); *2,* the device in place, and methylmethacrylate packed into it; *3,* anterior view of the construct with the cement in place (neural structures are protected from the cement, which is thoroughly packed into the cavity); bone is wedged between the methylmethacrylate and the outside rim of the shell; the locking of this little segment of bone tends to resist extension and makes the construct more stable; *4,* White and Panjabi's[68] suggested modification of this construct for additional immediate postoperative stability against extension: the rectangular steel device is altered so a screw can be placed into the anterior portion of each adjacent vertebral body and into the methylmethacrylate. (**B** reprinted with permission from McAfee, P.C., et al.: J. Bone Joint Surgery. **68A:**1145, 1986. **C** reprinted with permission from White, A.A., and Panjabi, M.M.: Clinical biomechanics of the spine, Philadelphia, 1978, J.B. Lippincott Co.)

out perforating the surprisingly tough dura.

When the cord and roots have been decompressed completely, preparations are made for spinal stabilization. However, there is lack of agreement among spinal surgeons as to the most effective way to accomplish this.

1. Some[46] advocate using an anterior interbody *corticocancellous bone graft* keyed into the adjacent vertebral end plates and stabilized until a natural bony fusion occurs by the use of external halo-vest immobilization (Fig. 12-15, *A*). The rationale for this is that once graft incorporation is complete there need be no further concern for spinal instability. However, in these patients, who are chronically debilitated and facing a limited life expectancy, the requirement for prolonged external immobilization must be viewed as a major drawback. Free bone grafts undergo vascular invasion and significant resorption before they become incorporated into the fusion mass, and these processes markedly weaken the stabilization construct in the absence of external immobilization. Thus some type of halo-vest support would be needed for at least 10 weeks postoperatively. Moreover, in patients who have undergone local irradiation within the preceding 6 months or who are receiving certain chemotherapeutic agents perioperatively, the likelihood that the graft will be incorporated at any point is markedly reduced.[10,29,42,44] It is difficult to achieve effective internal stability with conventional techniques of bone graft interposition, because no room is left for the placement of rigid fixation devices.

2. In an effort to achieve instant internal stability not dependent on graft incorporation and not necessitating external immobilization, many surgeons have begun using *methylmethacrylate* as an artificial vertebral construct. This can be effective (Fig. 12-15, *B*) because, once polymerized, the cement has excellent resistance to compressive loads and therefore prevents recurrence of the local kyphotic deformity. However, it is difficult to correct the original deformity with methylmethacrylate alone, and there are no means of affixing the cement mass effectively to the adjacent vertebral bodies. Attempts to secure the acrylic by screws or wire rarely are effective. Methylmethacrylate is a brittle material, and the screws usually break out with repeated stresses (Fig. 12-16, *A* and *B*). The use of anterior semitubular plates or intervertebral threaded pins to augment cement stabilization has been advocated by some[14,49,56,68] (Fig. 12-16, *B*), but again these devices do not enhance restoration of normal vertebral body height before filling of the defect with cement.

3. We have found the most adjustable and effective technique for spinal stabilization to be the use of a *Knodt distraction rod* and hooks, which jack open the collapsed vertebral space to its appropriate height and then are incorporated into the acrylic vertebral replacement (Fig. 12-13, *F* to *H*). Knodt rods come in lengths from 4 to 10 cm and can be used to span up to five vertebral spaces without difficulty.[42,44] The end plates of the intact vertebral bodies above and below the area of decompression are penetrated with a high-speed power bur (Fig. 12-13, *F*), and the cavity thus created is enlarged to accept both the rod and the bodies of the hooks (Fig. 12-13, *G*), leaving the tips of the hooks as the only portion of the device extending in front of the spine. By turning the rod, we progressively separate the hooks and thus open the space to the desired height. On occasion the cervical vertebrae will not be sufficiently large to allow the hooks and rod to be buried within the intact vertebrae above and below the defect. In these instances we position the rod anterior to the vertebral column and leave only the hook tips buried in bone (Plate 2 and Figs. 12-17 and 12-18). The vertebral end plates must then be undercut to allow more effective keying of the acrylic cement within the vertebral space (Fig. 12-4, *C*). The internal fixation thus achieved is significantly less, however, than with the rod and hooks buried in the vertebral bodies and the loss in stability is concomitantly higher (Plate 2, *C*). Moreover, with the rod extending anterior to the vertebral column a theoretical risk exists that dysphagia or even esophageal erosion will occur from local pressure. Nevertheless, in a series of 62 cervical spine stabilizations we have encountered persistent dysphagia only once although its possibility remains a concern.

When the Knodt rod is properly positioned and distracted, further cord and root decompression can be performed as needed.

After the spinal canal is completely decompressed, methylmethacrylate is injected into vertebrectomy defect in a liquid consistency, incorporating the Knodt rod (Fig. 12-13, *H*).

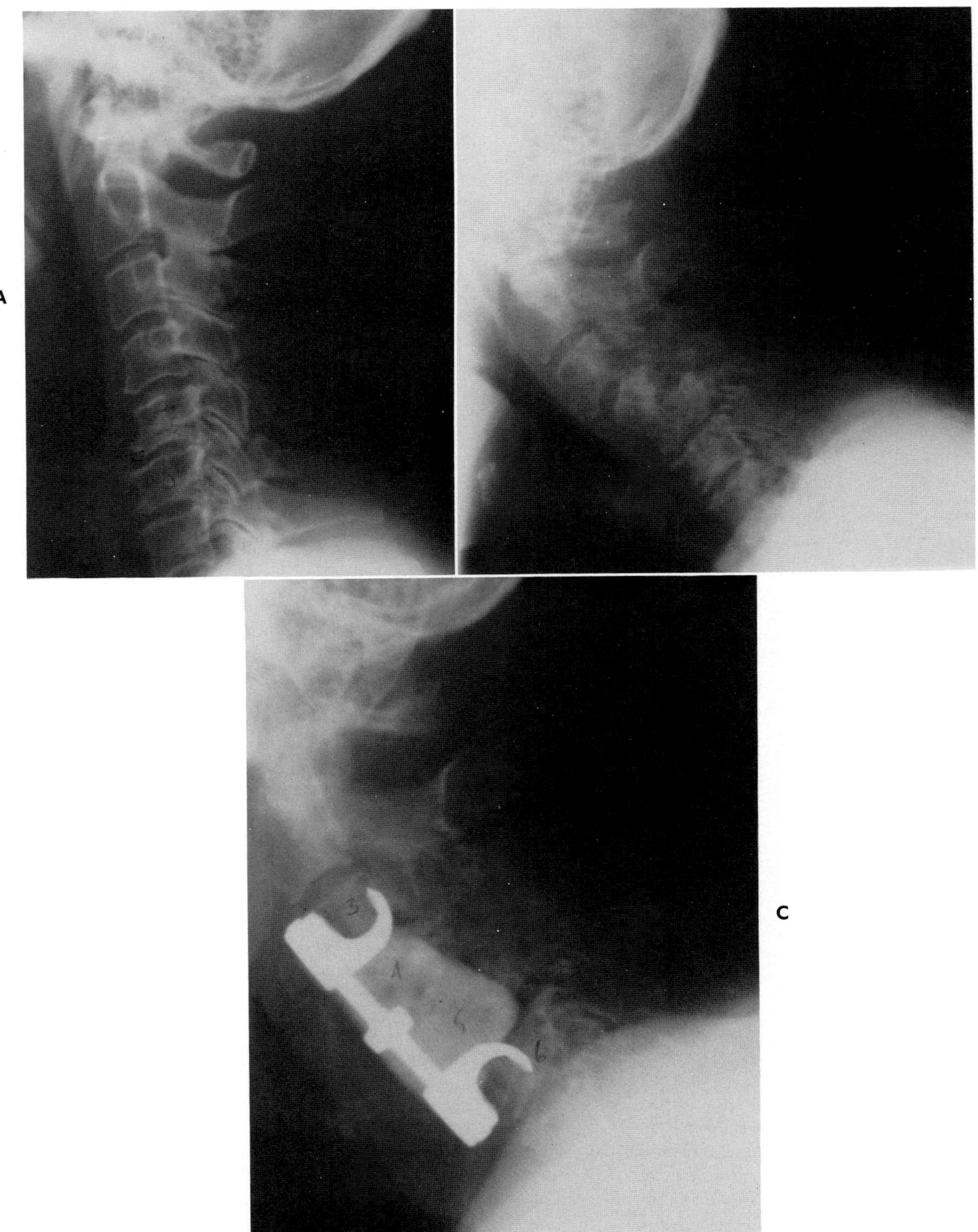

FIGURE 12-17 **A,** Lateral roentgenogram of the cervical spine following an automobile accident in a woman with metastatic breast carcinoma. Some degenerative changes are evident at the C5-C6 level, as is some reversal of the lordotic curve. **B,** Five months later there are pathological fractures of C4 and C5 as well as lytic changes of the posterior elements and an acute kyphosis at C4-C5. Surprisingly there was minimum neurological dysfunction, with evidence only of unilateral C5 root loss. However, the patient had severe mechanical pain in her neck. A CT scan revealed marked displacement of the root by a bone fragment (see Fig. 12-9, *B*). **C,** Eleven months after anterior decompression and stabilization with methylmethacrylate and a Knodt rod. The patient was essentially free of symptoms.

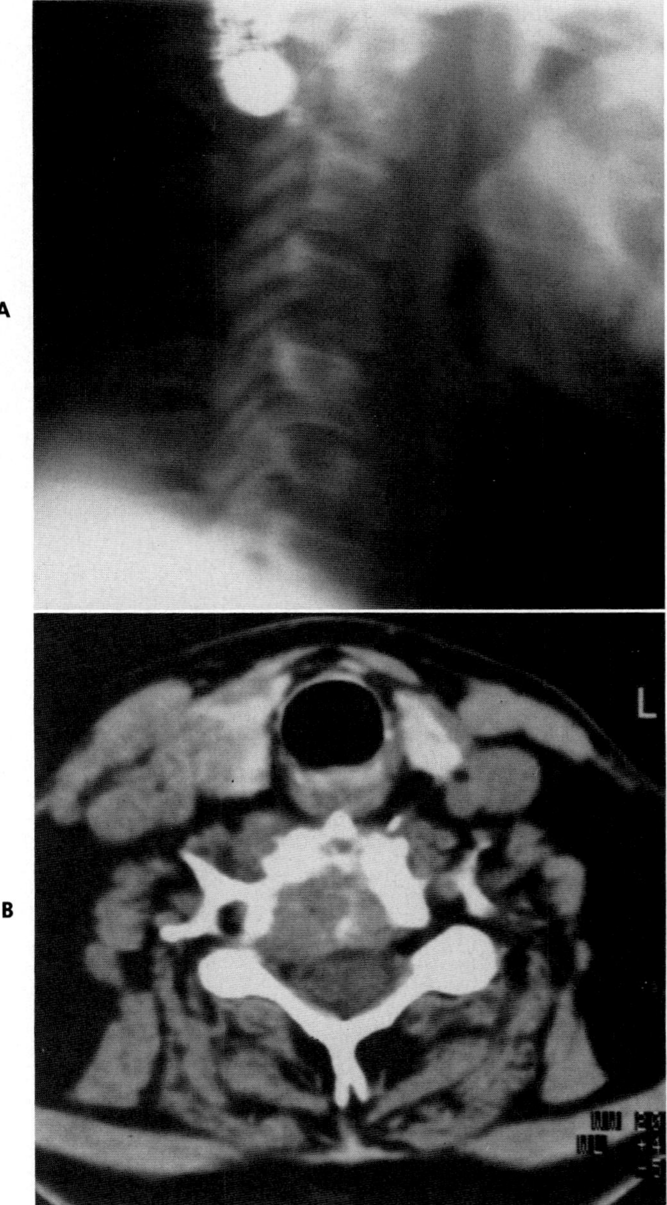

FIGURE 12-18 **A,** Lateral roentgenogram (tomogram) of the cervical spine in a 31-year-old woman with metastatic breast carcinoma and a severe neurological deficit (Frankel B). There are extensive lytic disruptive changes involving the C6 vertebral body. **B,** CT scan of this vertebra demonstrating the destructive changes of bone and the posterior extrusion of tumor tissue into the spinal canal. **C,** The diseased vertebra has been resected and replaced by methylmethacrylate incorporating a Knodt distraction rod. The patient had complete neurological recovery within a period of 2 weeks. **D,** Five months postoperative. Although there was no antecedent history of trauma, she again presented with severe neck pain. The lateral roentgenogram revealed extensive lytic changes with collapse of C4, one vertebra above the previous stabilization. There was no neurological deficit. **E,** Cervical spine restabilized, now with the cement and Knodt rod spanning C2 to C7. For 19 months postoperatively, she has had no further evidence of spinal instability or neurological compromise and has remained essentially symptom free. She returned to work as a secretary.

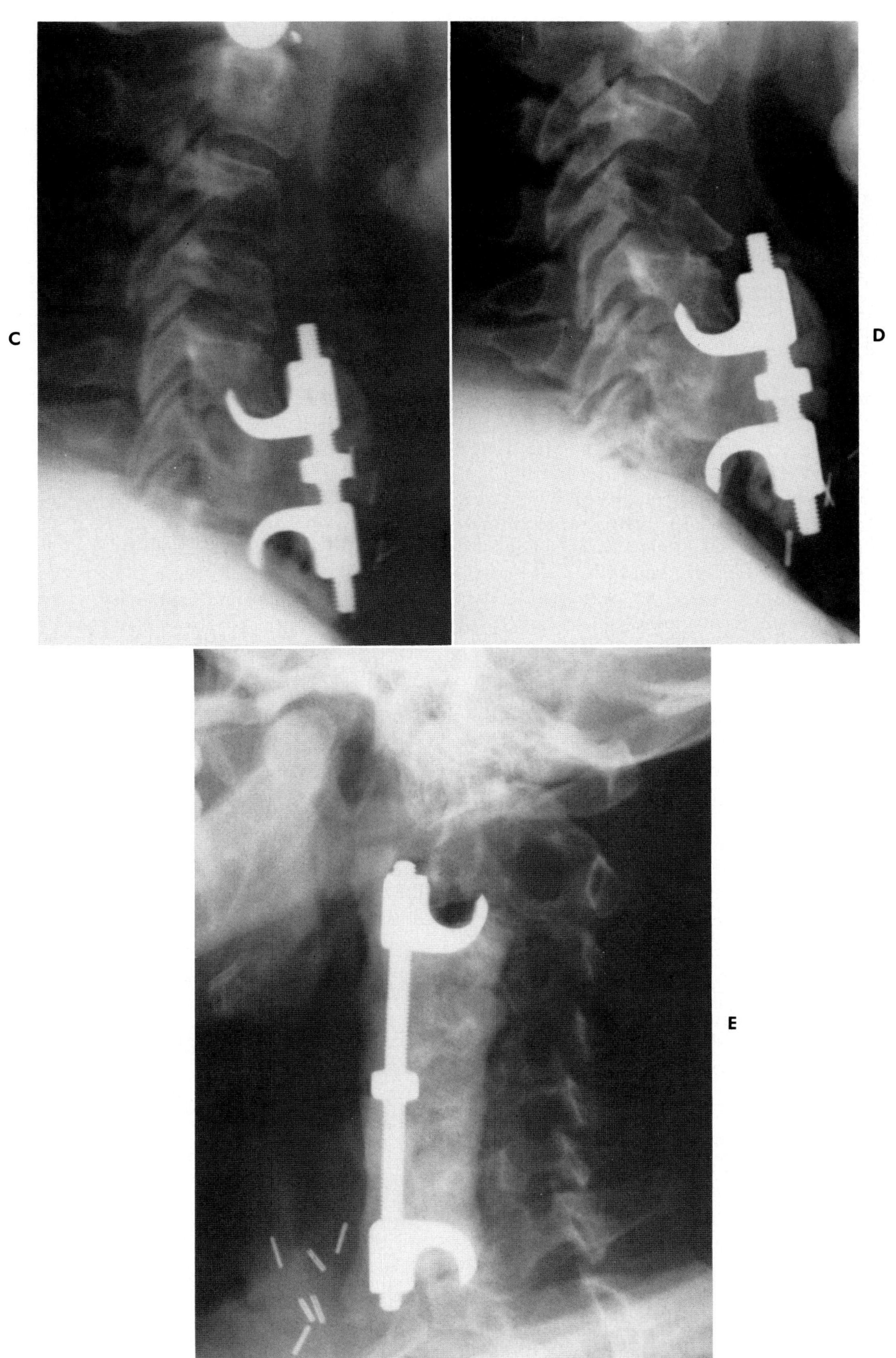

FIGURE 12-18, cont'd. For legend see opposite page.

As polymerization takes place, the cement is packed firmly into the space and trimmed to minimize extension outside the normal cylindrical confines of the vertebral column.

A malleable retractor is placed posterolaterally between the dura and the expanding acrylic mass to keep the cement from impinging on the neural structures and thereby recreating the original cord or root compromise (Fig. 12-13, *H*).

Barium-impregnated radiopaque cement is used so the position of the cement can be monitored postoperatively by serial roentgenograms (Plate 2). There is experimental evidence[41,42,44,67] that the polymerizing cement has no adverse thermal or chemical effect on the underlying dura or neural elements. The cerebrospinal fluid acts as a heat sink, preventing the temperature in the subdural space from rising more than 1° C even during the major exothermic phase of polymerization.[67]

Blood loss from cervical decompressions and stabilizations never exceeds 250 ml, even in the presence of a vascular tumor, so we do not advocate placing Gelfoam or similar hemostatic materials against the dura before injecting the methylmethacrylate. Their presence would interfere with the effective use of a malleable retractor to protect the cord from the expanding cement.

Postoperatively no external immobilization of any kind is required. A Penrose drain is placed deep in the wound and removed the morning after surgery. Patients are encouraged not to attempt the extremes of neck motion, which would place undue stress on the cement-bone construct, but no other limitations are imposed.

The question of long-term stability of this type of spinal stabilization, in the absence of a bony arthrodesis, must be considered. Although many patients in our series have survived 3 or 4 years following stabilization, without evidence of deterioration of their reconstruction, it is at least theoretically likely that many of these constructs, not reinforced by a bone arthrodesis, will ultimately fail. For this reason, in patients with a projected survival exceeding 2 years we ordinarily reinforce the cement–Knodt rod stabilization by surrounding it with cancellous bone graft. The graft is packed over the remaining lateral elements of the resected vertebrae and proximally and distally over the exposed cortices of the remaining vertebral bodies above and below the resection (Fig. 12-13, *I*).

Local irradiation can be initiated, if necessary, beginning between 2 and 3 weeks postoperatively. In these patients, however, it is unlikely that the cancellous graft will become incorporated. Conversely, in patients in whom irradiation to the operative site has been completed more than 6 months preoperatively, there is a high likelihood that the graft will become incorporated and a strong permanent bone arthrodesis will ensue.

Thoracic Spine. Anterior stabilization of the thoracic spine obviously requires a thoracotomy, with exposure of the heart, one lung, and the great vessels. A chest tube is required postoperatively for pleural drainage and lung reexpansion, usually for a period of between 48 and 72 hours. Occasionally overnight intubation will be expedient, particularly in the patient who is moderately debilitated, has chest wall or pleural metastases that interfere with ideal ventilation, or shows evidence of pulmonary metastases.

Although these factors represent disadvantages of the anterior approach compared to the posterior approach, there are definite advantages. Blood loss with anterior stabilization is always less than with posterior stabilization, in part because direct control of tumor bleeding is much easier but also because periosteal stripping and bone decortication are less extensive. Decompression and stabilization of a single-level lesion by the posterior approach ordinarily requires a three-level laminectomy followed by stabilization three levels above and three levels below the extent of the laminectomy defect (Fig. 12-28). Thus the posterior elements of nine vertebrae must be exposed to decompress and stabilize a spinal cord impingement emanating from a single vertebral body. If the same decompression and stabilization is accomplished by the anterior approach, only three vertebral bodies need be exposed and only a single vertebral body excised.

The incidence of wound healing problems also is much lower after the anterior than after the posterior approach. This is attributable to the fact that soft tissue coverage of the spinal elements is minimal posteriorly, particularly after irradiation, when the posterior skin, subcutaneous tissue, and muscle become inelastic and often woody hard. After more than 90 spinal decompressions and stabilizations from the anterior approach, we have encountered not a single incidence of wound dehiscence or deep infection. By contrast, in 12 of 26 patients previously irradiated in whom posterior decompression and stabilization was achieved there were complications of either wound healing or deep infection.

The major advantage of the anterior over the posterior approach, however, is the surgeon's ability to reach the tumor focus directly, decompress the neural structures from the side of their compromise, and jack open the collapsed vertebral spaces, thereby correcting the kyphus at its source. The patient undergoing anterior transthoracic decompression is placed in the lateral decubitus position for a standard thoracotomy with the table flexed (Fig. 12-19, *A*). It makes little difference whether a right- or left-sided approach is used. The major determining factors are the predominant side of tumor involvement and the possible presence of unilateral lung pathology. The thoracotomy is performed through the bed of the numbered rib corresponding to the level of vertebral involvement. This allows exposure of at least one vertebra above and several vertebrae below the affected segments.

Technique. In patients who have received extensive chest wall irradiation it is often preferable to make the incision a rib or two higher than the center of the tumor focus, because with a stiff chest wall it is easier to work downward along the slopes of the ribs than upward. The vertebral bodies are easily visualized through the thin overlying parietal pleura. Often the level of involvement is immediately apparent because of the presence of an exophytic tumor mass bulging beneath the pleura (Fig. 12-19, *B*). For lesions of the lower thoracic spine, however, it will be necessary to take down the corner of the diaphragm and reflect it anteriorly to expose the vertebral bodies. By this technique the anterior decompression or stabilization can be extended to L2 via the thoracotomy approach.

The parietal pleura is incised, elevated, and reflected to expose the segmental vessels (Fig. 12-19, *D*).

These are ligated with heavy silk sutures and transected as close to the aorta as possible, thus minimizing disturbance of the paravertebral anastomoses.

Despite theoretical concerns about the fragile arterial supply to the cord at the midthoracic level and the inconsistent but oft-considered artery of Adamkiewicz, we have found no evidence that division of any number of vessels on one side impairs the blood supply to the spinal cord.

Typically, to obtain adequate exposure for decompression and stabilization, division of five vessels is necessary. We have divided as many as nine vessels (Figs. 12-9, *E*, and 12-21) without untoward effects. During the division it is possible to see the hemiazygos (on the left side) and the intercostal veins. The latter require division as well.

After division of these vessels the aorta can be carefully retracted anteriorly, facilitating exposure of the entire anterior aspect of the vertebral bodies involved (Fig. 12-19, *C*).

Careful blunt dissection is continued subperiosteally to expose the lateral aspect of the affected vertebrae on the opposite side.

The process of removing the entire affected vertebral bodies then commences. We believe all remnants of the affected vertebrae should be removed, together with all tumor tissue, whenever an acute kyphus has developed. Only by performing a complete vertebrectomy can the surgeon be sure of removing every bit of debris forced into the spinal canal by that angulation. It is also possible to be more effective in correcting the kyphotic deformity if all the diseased tissue has been resected. When a kyphus does not exist and sufficient unaffected bone remains that such deformity is unlikely, an anterolateral decompression is preferable without the need for stabilization. This will be discussed separately (see Fig. 12-11).

Just as in cervical decompression, the anterior two thirds of the affected thoracic vertebrae are removed rapidly with a gouge and rongeur (Fig. 12-19, *D*).

When only a thin shell of bone and tumor remains in front of the spinal canal, an angled curet is used. This will help avoid inadvertent penetration of the dura or damage to the cord or nerve roots.

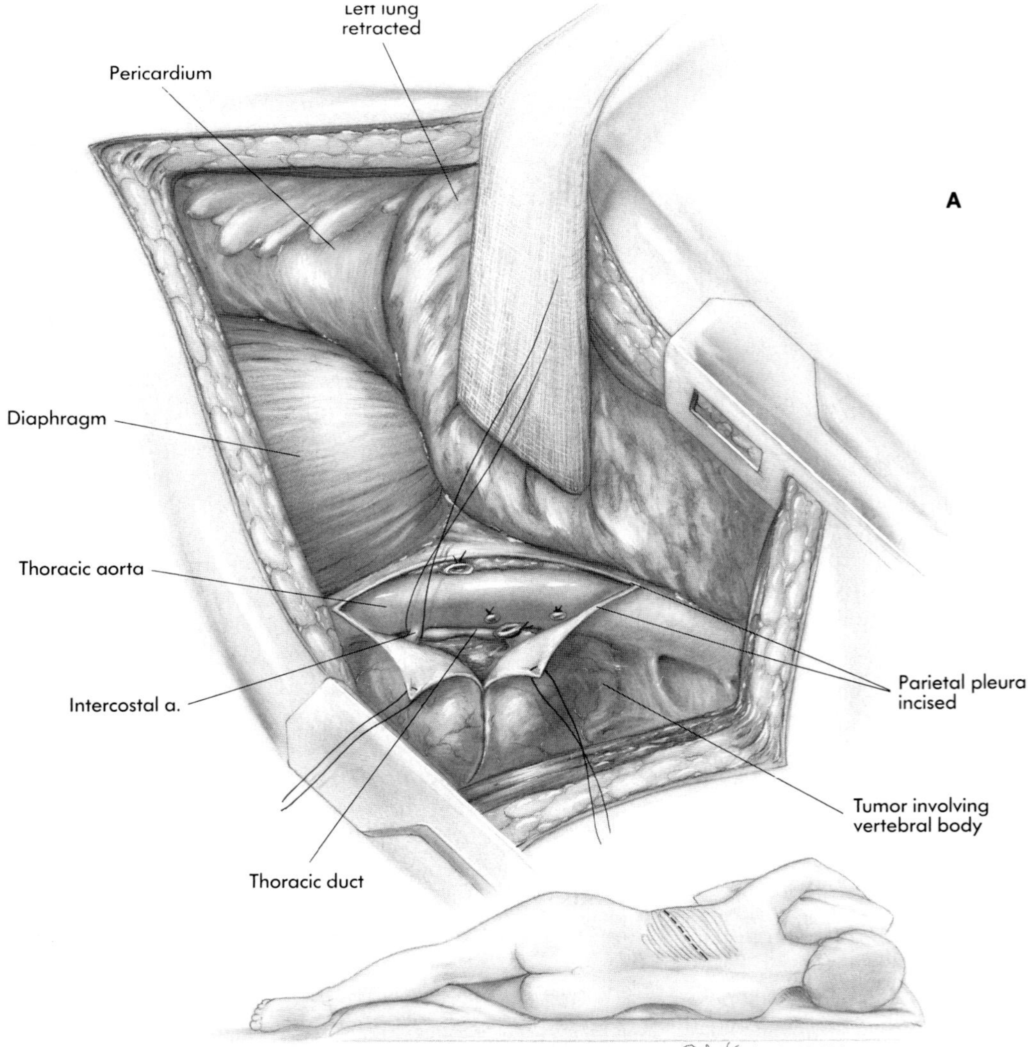

FIGURE 12-19 Technique for anterior decompression and stabilization of the thoracic spine. **A,** Decompression is accomplished via a thoractomy with the patient in the lateral decubitus position. The aorta can be retracted gently, the segmental vessels can be ligated and transected, and the affected vertebral body is easily approached. Often a prominent paravertebral extrapleural tumor mass will assist in locating the focus of destruction.

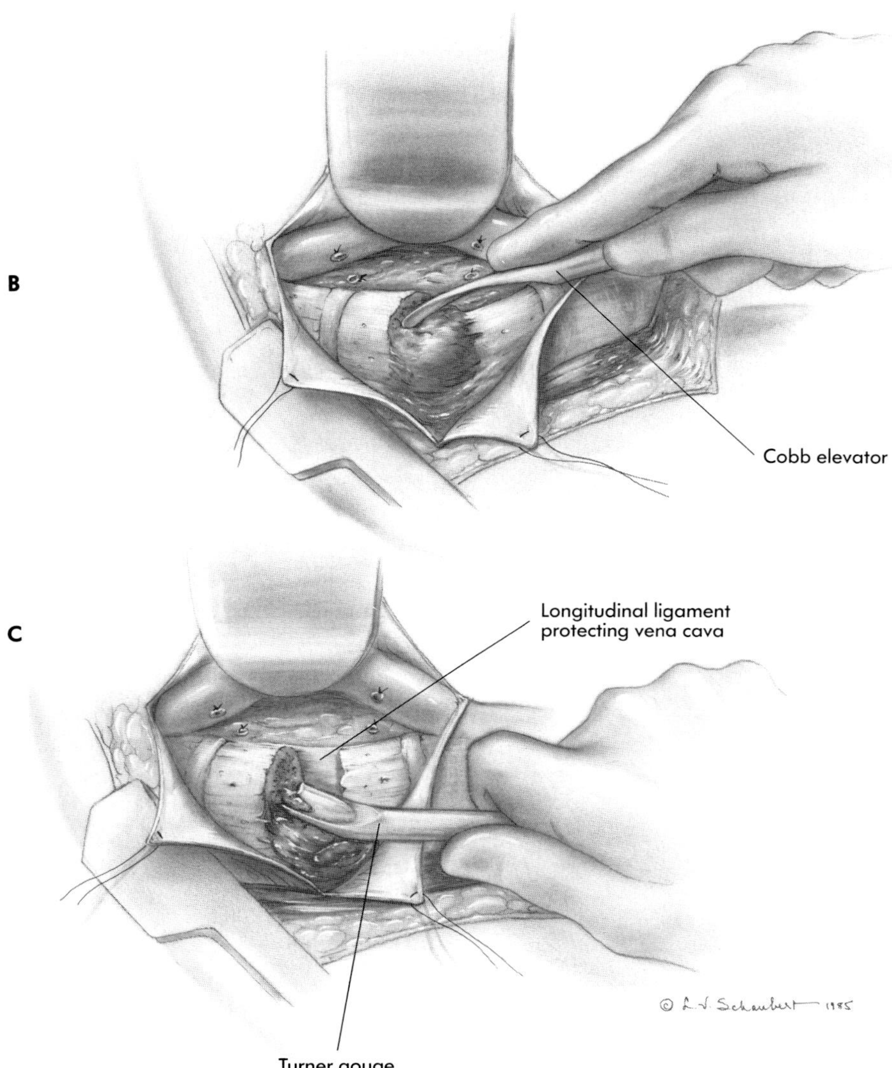

FIGURE 12-19, cont'd. **B,** Most of the tumor and bone-disc debris can be removed with a small periosteal elevator. **C,** As the level of the posterior cortical margin is approached, further decompression should be achieved with an angled gouge or curet. All the material adherent to the adjacent vertebral body is removed. *Continued.*

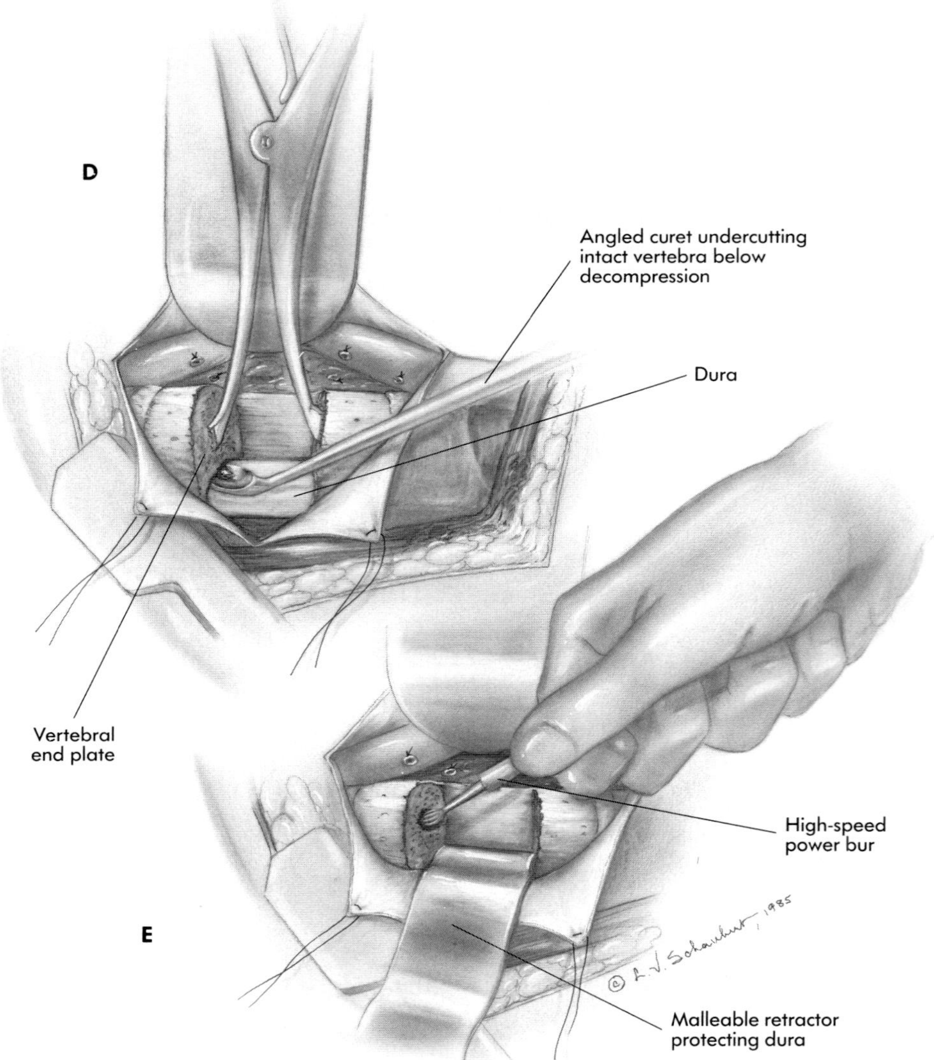

FIGURE 12-19, cont'd. **D,** The vertebral space is recreated with a lamina spreader, and a small angled curet is used to complete decompression of the spinal canal and to round off the edges of the posterior cortices of adjacent vertebrae. **E,** The end plates of the adjacent vertebrae are undercut with a high-speed bur to allow the ends of the Knodt rod and the bodies of its hooks to be buried within the vertebral bone.

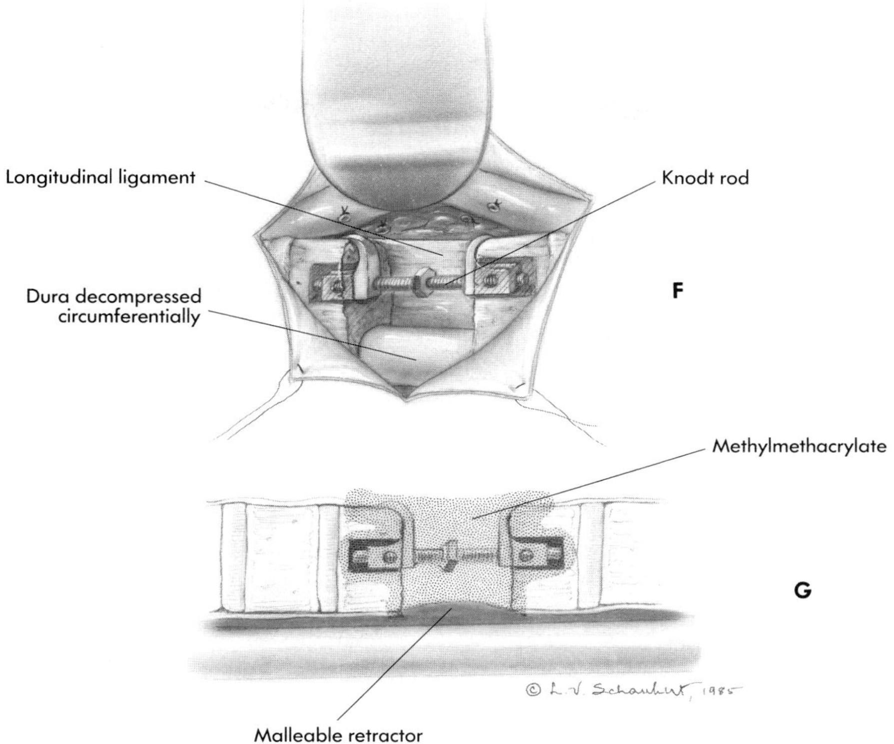

FIGURE 12-19, cont'd. **F,** The Knodt rod has been positioned within the resected space. Twisting distracts its hooks and their bodies become firmly impacted within the adjacent vertebral bone. Only the tips of the hooks extend anterior to the vertebral cortex. **G,** The defect is filled with methylmethacrylate that polymerizes in situ incorporating the rod and hooks. To avoid compression of the cord, a malleable retractor is placed between the expanding mass and the spinal canal.

Great care is taken to decompress the canal completely, using the angled curet to undercut the posterior corners of the intact vertebrae above and below the level of resection. There must be nothing to impinge on the neural structures (Fig. 12-19, *E*). The decompression can be facilitated by using a lamina spreader to open the vertebrectomy space completely and correct the kyphotic deformity. All remnants of disc and annulus attached to intact vertebrae above and below the defect must also be removed.

When the decompression has been completed, stabilization of the thoracic spine is accomplished in a manner similar to that used in the cervical spine.

With a high-speed bur a well is cut into the intact vertebral end plates of sufficient width and depth to seat the Knodt rod and hooks as shown in Fig. 12-19, *E*. When the rod is twisted, the hooks will seat firmly into the vertebrae and the kyphotic angulation will be corrected.

A malleable retractor is placed across the back of the defect to protect the cord from impingement by the expanding cement (Fig. 12-19, *F*). Methylmethacrylate is then injected in liquid form into the vertebrectomy space.

As the polymer reaches a doughy consistency, it is packed firmly about the rod and hooks and into the defects in the vertebral end plates (Fig. 12-19, *G*).

Before polymerization is complete, all excess cement is removed from outside the confines of the vertebral bodies. A computed tomographic scan of the vertebral

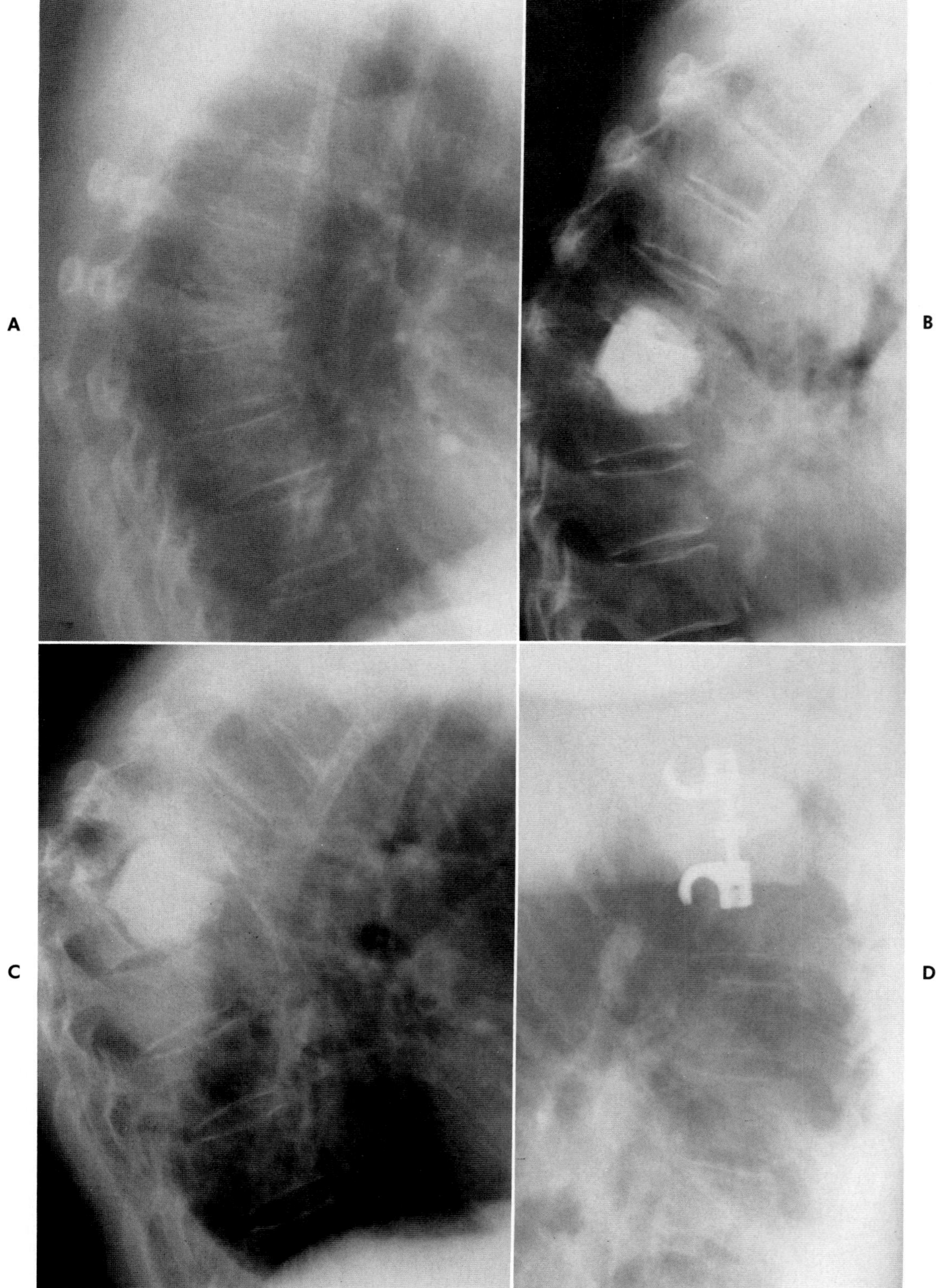

FIGURE 12-20 For legend see opposite page.

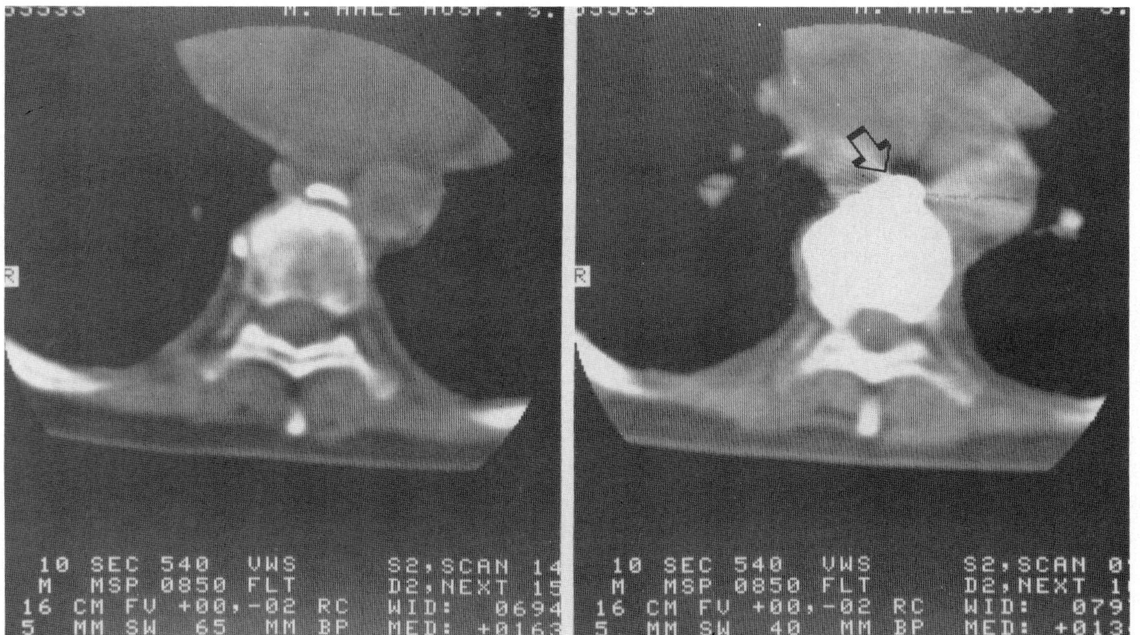

FIGURE 12-20 **A,** Progressive but minimally painful collapse of the T7 vertebral body in a 51-year-old woman with metastatic breast cancer. Deformity occurred over a 2-year period. Shortly after this roentgenogram was obtained, she abruptly became completely paraplegic (Frankel A) during a span of 3 days. **B,** An anterior decompression was performed and the resected vertebra replaced with acrylic cement alone. Because a Knodt rod was not used initially to jack open the vertebral space, it was not possible to reconstitute the normal vertebral height. Nevertheless, the patient enjoyed a complete neurological recovery. **C,** Six years postoperative. She has suffered a progressive kyphosis as the hard cement eroded into the adjacent vertebral bodies. Despite this deformity, she remains essentially without symptoms and without neurological deficit 11 years postoperatively. **D,** Lateral roentgenogram of a midthoracic vertebral construct in another patient 5½ years postoperative. Note that the height of the vertebral space has been reconstituted fully and remains so without evidence of migration of the construct. **E,** CT scans of this patient. On the left is a cut through the vertebral body just above the cement construct. Note that the tip of the Knodt rod hook *(arrow)* protrudes slightly in front of the anterior longitudinal ligament. On the right is a cut through the methylmethacrylate reconstruction. Despite the defraction artifact from the metal rod, the normal dimensions of the spinal canal can be appreciated.

construct obtained postoperatively should show that the cross-sectional diameter of acrylic and metal is nearly identical to that of the normal vertebra, with no encroachment of cement into the spinal canal (Figs. 12-6, *C,* and 12-20, *E*).

Cancellous bone may be packed around the vertebral construct in patients who have a prognosis for longer survival and do not require further irradiation.

Fixation devices other than the Knodt distraction rod have been used with success in the thoracic vertebrae. Early in our experience with vertebral body resection and replacement, we used methylmethacrylate alone to reconstruct the vertebral space (Fig. 12-20), but this was never ideal because the normal height of the vertebral space could not be reconstituted with a lamina spreader and the space simultaneously filled with methylmethacrylate polymerizing in situ. Moreover, unlike the situation in which a Knodt rod is used for partial transmission of weight-bearing loads (Fig. 12-20, *D*), when cement

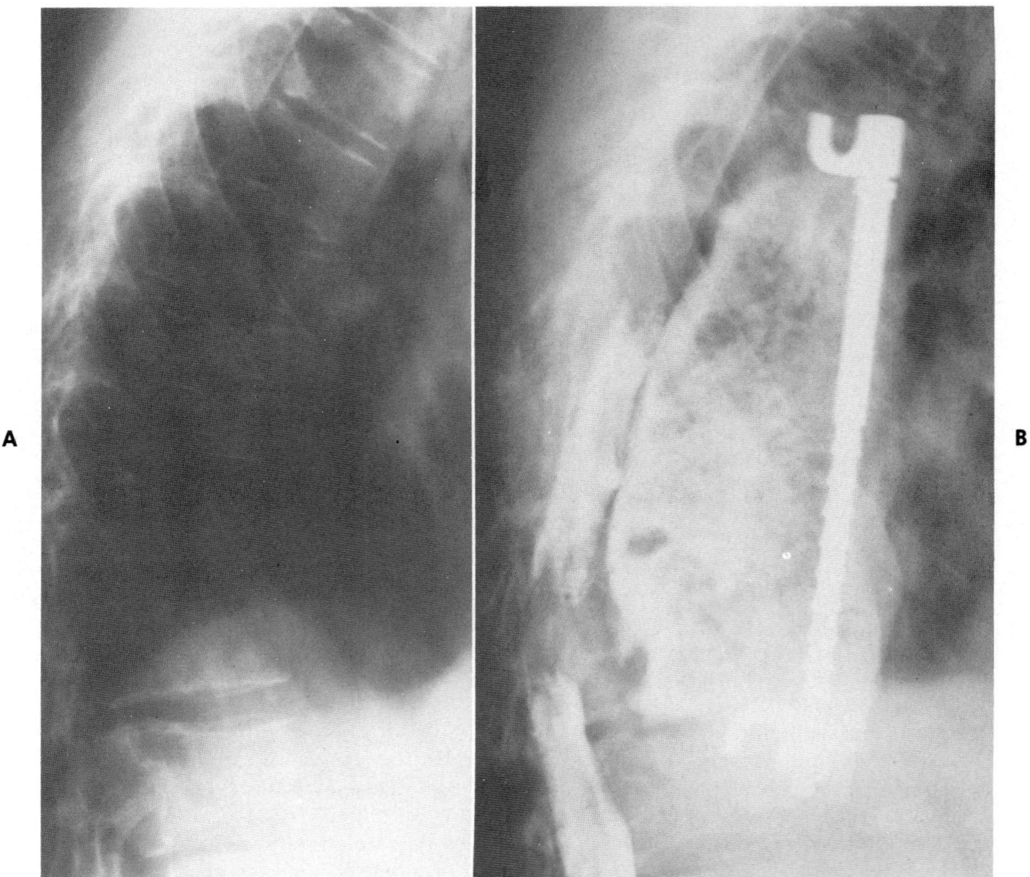

FIGURE 12-21 Partial collapse of four thoracic vertebrae in a 44-year-old woman with breast cancer metastatic to the spine and causing progressive paraparesis (Frankel B). A myelogram, **A,** revealed a complete block extending from T4 to T10. This patient had undergone full irradiation to the spine 16 months earlier. Spinal decompression might well have been accomplished by a multilevel laminectomy and stabilization. As an alternative, a transthoracic anterior decompression was performed from T5 through T9 and the spine was stabilized by a combination of methylmethacrylate and Harrington rod distraction. Although the intraoperative myelogram, **B,** showed a persistent defect at the T9 level, on direct inspection the canal was seen to be decompressed completely and the patient improved to a Frankel grade D. She died of her disease 5 months later.

alone was used it tended to erode into the adjacent vertebral bodies over time and to allow a gradual return of the kyphotic deformity (Fig. 12-20, *C*).

When resection of numerous vertebrae is required and many vertebral spaces must be spanned for stabilization, we have used a Harrington rod with success (Figs. 12-6 and 12-21). Distraction adjustments are much less precise with the Harrington rod, however, and care must be taken not to overdistract the vertebrectomy space and thereby place the cord and roots under excessive tension. Kostuik[49] and Dunn[27] have developed several devices that combine distraction with fixation using a large cancellous screw in the vertebral body (Fig. 12-20). Although we have not had much experience with them, they appear to have three disadvantages as compared to the Knodt distraction rod:

1. They are large and thus cannot be buried within the vertebrectomy space as can the Knodt rod. Therefore a sizable volume of metal is left to displace the adjacent soft tissue

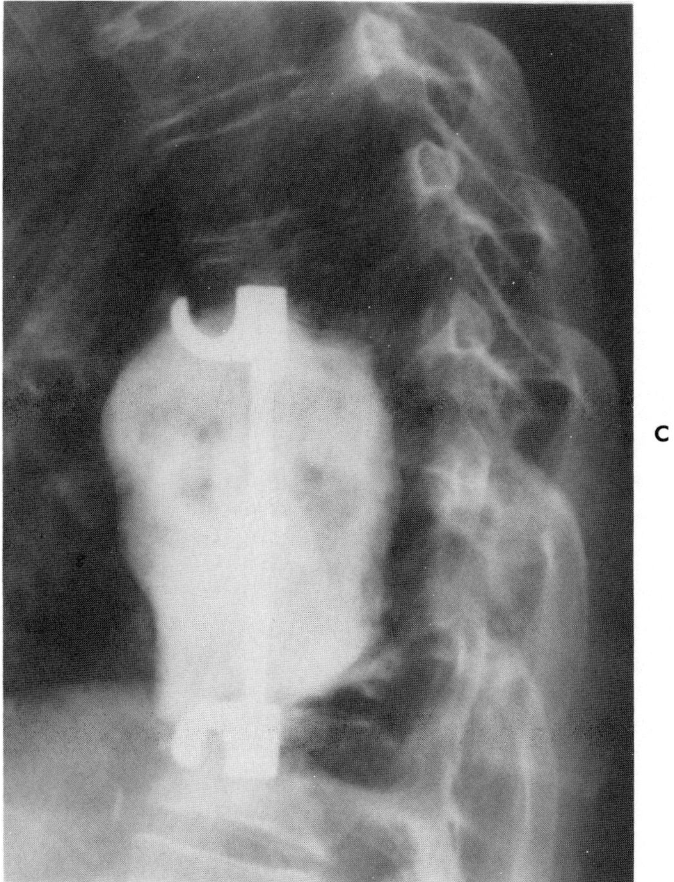

FIGURE 12-21, cont'd. In another patient, **C,** a multilevel anterior decompression-stabilization with methylmethacrylate and a Harrington rod has allowed the patient to carry on without residual spinal pain or neurological dysfunction 4½ years postoperatively.

structures (including the aorta, azygos vein, and vena cava), with the potential for catastrophic erosion into these major vessels over time.

2. Whereas distraction of the positioned Knodt rod enhances seating of its hooks and thus the security of its fixation and, similarly, whereas compression forces across the vertebral construct are exerted parallel to (and thus in concert with) the Knodt rod axis, the same compression forces in the Kostuik (and Dunn) devices act at right angles to the plane of fixation screws and thus encourage gradual loosening within the vertebral body (Fig. 12-26, *C* and *D*).
3. The major theoretical advantage of the Kostuik and the Dunn fixation systems over the Knodt rod is their resistance to torque loads exerted across the vertebral reconstruction. However, although such torque loads do exist in the lumbar spine, they are insignificant in the thoracic spine because the rib cage effectively frustrates them.

For these reasons we have returned to using the Knodt rod and methylmethacrylate fixation system in the thoracic spine, after several trials with the Kostuik and Dunn devices.

Postoperatively, once the chest tube has been removed and the pain has subsided, patients are encouraged to resume full activities as tolerated. No external bracing is necessary, and radiation or chemotherapy may commence 2 weeks postoperatively if needed.

When exposure of the first four vertebral

bodies is called for (Fig. 12-11), a right-sided thoracoplasty approach is used.

The scapular attachments are separated posteriorly, and the scapula is displaced upward and forward.

A thoracotomy is then performed through the fourth rib, and the vertebral bodies are readily exposed. The lowest part of the brachial plexus may be seen in this approach, but it does not interfere with exosure of the spine.

Fixation is accomplished in the same manner as for the cervical or lower thoracic spine. In unusual circumstances the upper thoracic spine can be approached anteriorly through the sternum.

By means of a vertical midline incision the sternum is divided, from the suprasternal notch to the xyphoid. The thymus is retracted, the innominate vein dissected to the left and divided, and the trachea and esophagus displaced to the left.

These structures are not widely exposed by this approach, however, and tend to appear at the bottom of a dark cavity in which blood collects. The vertebral bodies also tend to collapse together and are difficult to separate. Excision of bone with a rongeur and curet must be accomplished extremely carefully since it is necessary to push posteriorly directly toward the spinal canal, thereby transmitting forces anteriorly against the cord. Finally, spinal stabilization is more difficult through this approach because of the poorer exposure than through the thoracotomy approach. For all of these reasons we do not advocate the sternal splitting method except in the unusual circumstance when poor condition of skin overlying the lateral chest wall, perhaps because of irradiation, makes it inadvisable to use the more traditional thoracotomy technique.

Lumbar Spine. The lumbar spine is the least common location for metastatic lesions to develop that ultimately require anterior decompression. This is fortunate, insofar as it is also the area where anterior exposure is most difficult, at least for the L4-L5 and S1 vertebral bodies, and anterior stabilization most problematical.

Exposure is best accomplished through a flank incision paralleling the inferior costal margin (Fig. 12-22, *A*). Dissection then is done retroperitoneally, with the transversalis fascia and abdominal contents displaced medially (Fig. 12-22, *B*). After ligation of the adjacent segmental vessels, the uppermost lumbar vertebra is relatively easy to expose. Distal to it, however, exposure becomes more difficult. The psoas muscles overlie the anterolateral aspect of the vertebral bodies and tend to obscure the segmental vessels (Fig. 12-22, *C*). Brisk bleeding can be a problem unless these vessels are carefully identified and ligated. The sympathetic chain should be preserved if feasible, but again it may be difficult to identify. In most instances the chain can be retracted posteriorly toward the base of the transverse processes. As one proceeds distally, the iliac vessels overlying the L4 and L5 vertebral bodies are often adherent to the soft tissues in front of the spine either because of scarring from previous irradiation or because there is inflammatory reaction coincident with local tumor invasion. The large venous channels are easily torn under such circumstances. For these reasons it is usually better to approach the lower lumbar spine and sacrum transperitoneally.

The patient is placed in the Trendelenburg

FIGURE 12-22 Retroperitoneal anterior decompression and stabilization of the lumbar spine. **A,** Left lateral decubitus position. In the lumbar region a left-sided approach is preferred because the aorta is retracted more easily than the thin-walled inferior vena cava. Note the inflatable mattress and the full flexion of the table, both of which increase the distance between the iliac crest and the costal margin. **B,** Retroperitoneal flank approach to the spine by medial displacement of the transversalis fascia and abdominal contents. Note that the approach is anterior to the psoas muscle. **C,** Vertebral bodies *(V)* exposed immediately behind the aorta. Some branches can be sacrificed, but care must be taken to protect the ureter and the testicular artery and vein. (**A** to **F** courtesy Narayan Sundaresan, M.D.)

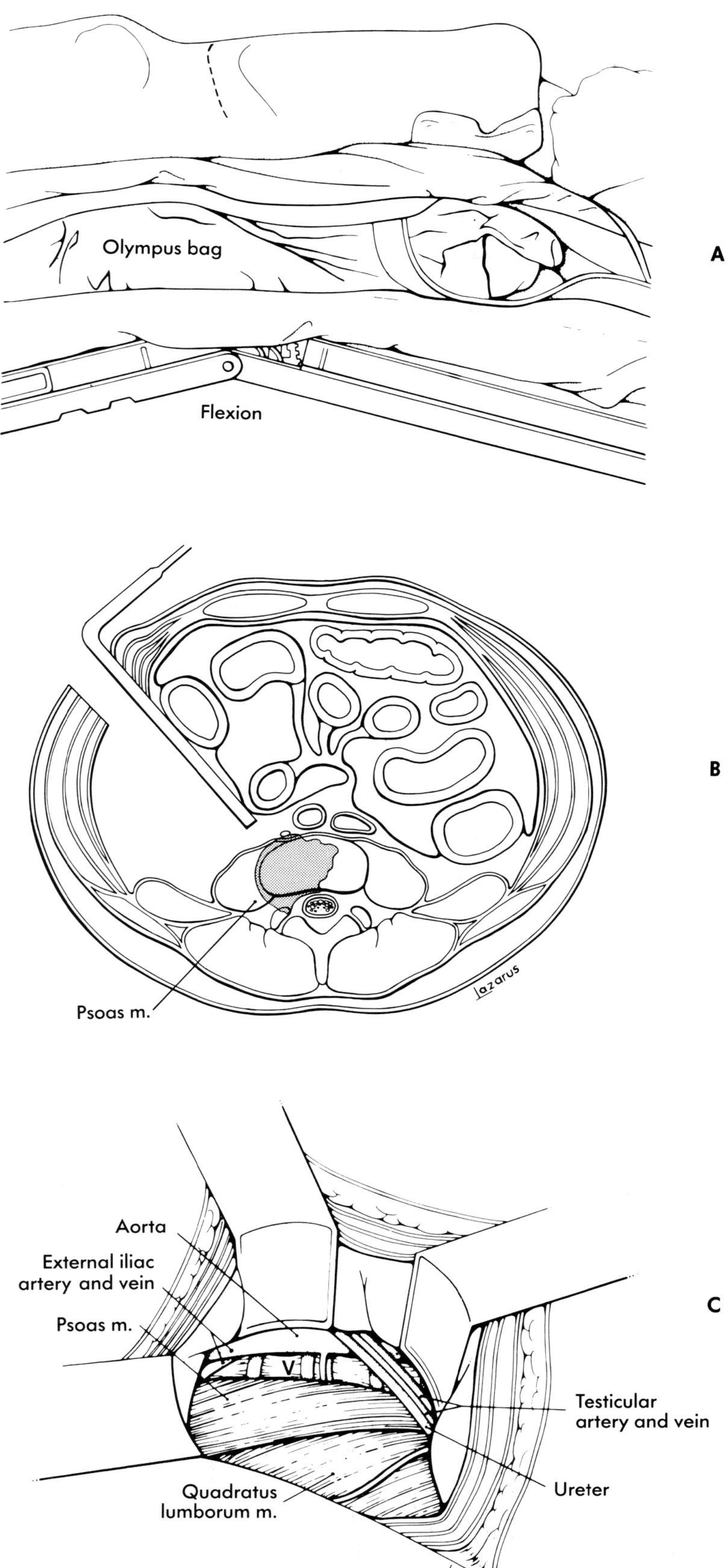

FIGURE 12-22 For legend see opposite page.

Continued.

D

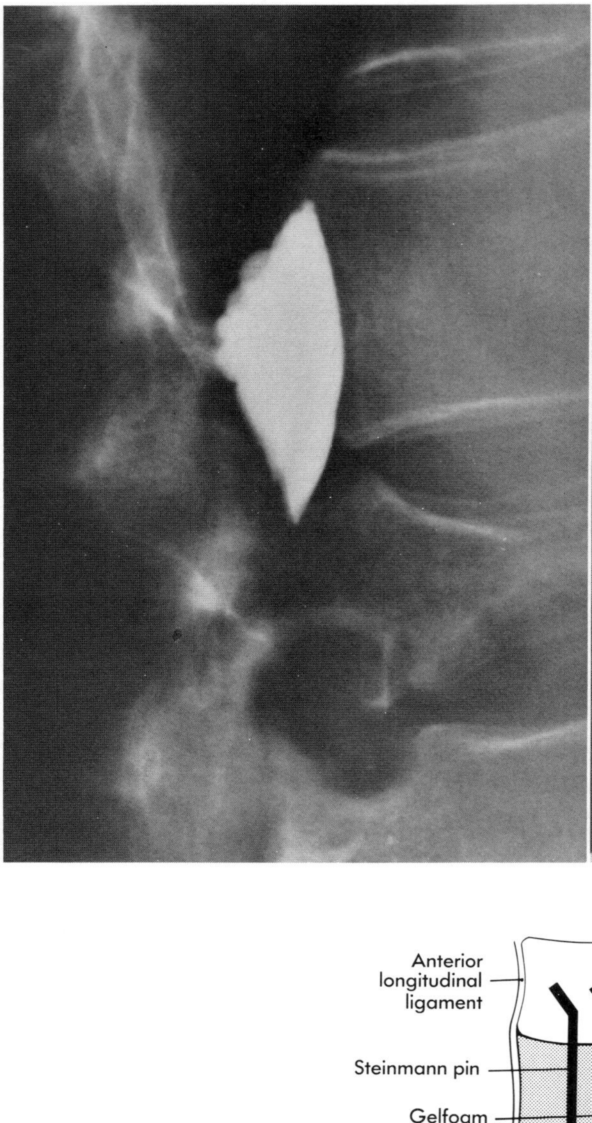

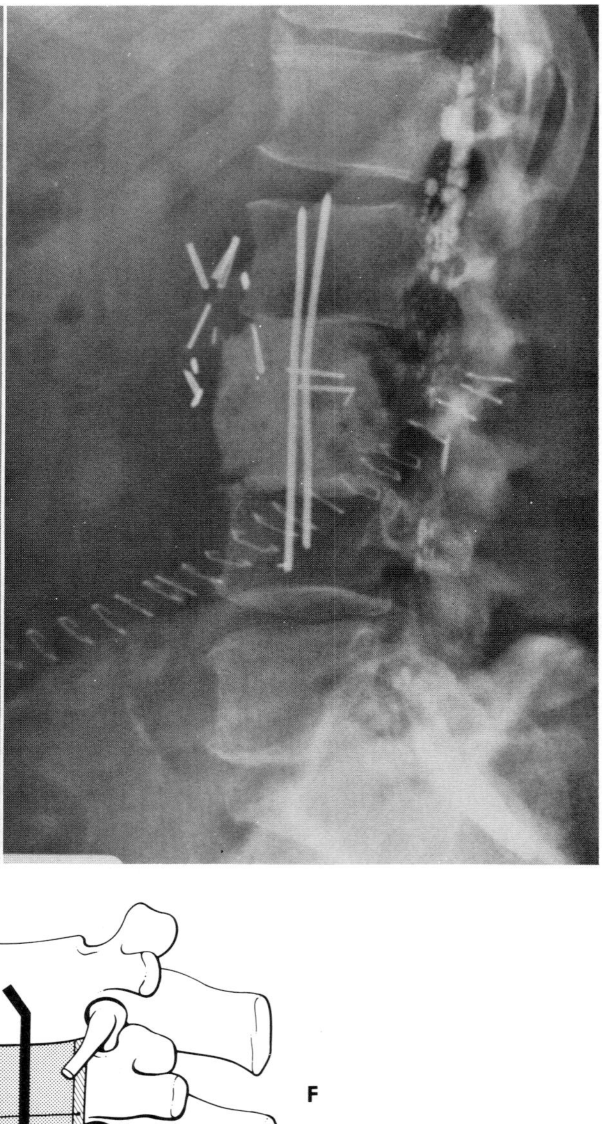

E

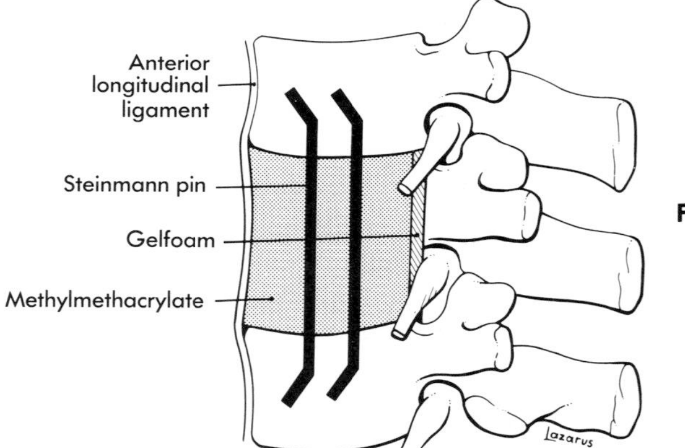

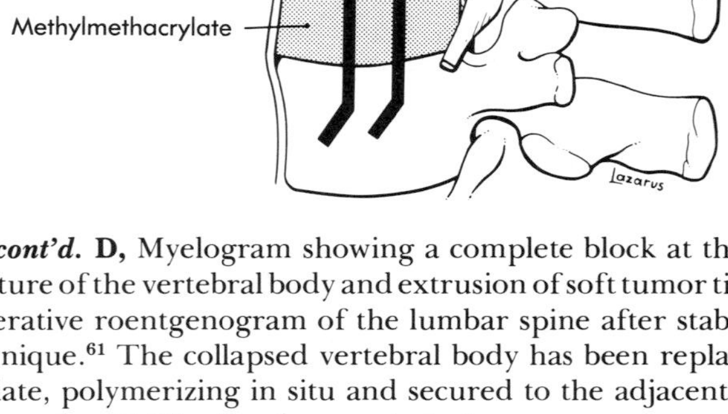

FIGURE 12-22, cont'd. **D,** Myelogram showing a complete block at the L3 level from a pathological fracture of the vertebral body and extrusion of soft tumor tissue into the spinal canal. **E,** Postoperative roentgenogram of the lumbar spine after stabilization by the Sundaresan technique.[61] The collapsed vertebral body has been replaced by a mass of methylmethacrylate, polymerizing in situ and secured to the adjacent vertebrae by two smooth Steinmann pins. **F,** The Sundaresan technique.

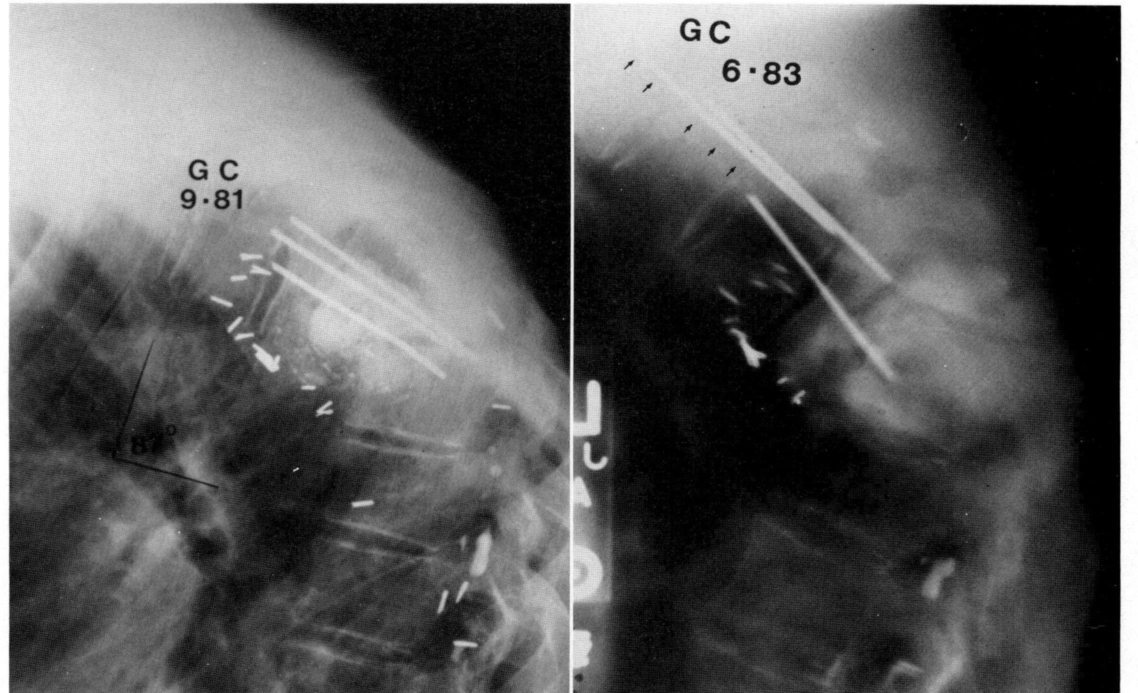

FIGURE 12-22, cont'd. **G,** Lateral roentgenogram of a 27-year-old woman "stabilized" by the Sundaresan technique with three longitudinal Kirschner wires and methylmethacrylate after transthoracic resection of T7. Preoperatively she had a mild T6 paraparesis, but 4 months following this stabilization she was left with an 87-degree gibbus deformity. **H,** Within the next 9 months her wire-cement construct further disrupted; two of the three wires migrated superiorly into the spinal canal. Her neurological function deteriorated, having ascended to become a complete T3 paraplegia (Frankel A). She became wheelchair dependent and required narcotics for the relief of severe mechanical thoracic pain. Note the T6 level fragmentation of cement. At surgical reconstruction one of the Kirschner wires was found to have migrated into the spinal canal and a second had completely become imbedded within the substance of the spinal cord. (**G** and **H** from McAfee, P.C., et al.: J. Bone Joint Surg. **68A:**1145, 1986.)

position, and the abdomen is opened through a lower midline incision. The viscera are retracted into the upper abdomen, the peritoneum is incised below the aortic bifurcation, and the vertebral body and tumor are approached directly through this interval. Care must be taken to avoid injury to the left iliac vein, which crosses the upper part of the fifth lumbar vertebra. Also, as with the transsternal approach to the upper thoracic spine, care must be taken to avoid displacing fragments of bone backward and into the canal, thereby injuring the cauda equina. (This is unlikely, however, since the exposure is quite wide and visualization is much better than with the transsternal approach.)

If a vertebrectomy is necessary to decompress the lumbar spine, stabilization must follow. To date, no consistently effective device for spinal stabilization has been developed. We have employed the technique of Knodt rod fixation augmented by methylmethacrylate effectively on numerous occasions at the T12 to L3 levels without problems. Sundaresan and different groups of coworkers[5,61] have used a combination of Steinmann pins and methylmethacrylate for upper lumbar vertebral replacement (Fig. 12-22, *D* to *F*) and reported consistently good results; others,[53] however, report a significant failure rate compounded by disastrous migration of the pins (Fig. 12-22, *G* and *H*).

Unlike the Knodt rod, whose fixation within the vertebral bodies above and below the defect is secured by the firm impaction of hooks, Steinmann pins must simply be placed within the vertebrae in an effort to reinforce the cement construct. Should that construct fail, there is danger that the rods might migrate, even penetrating the adjacent viscera or vascular structures or entering the spinal canal and damaging the cord or root (Fig. 12-22, *G* and *H*).

Kostuik[49] has advocated extravertebral fixation using a device that attaches to the vertebral bodies above and below the decompression site by large cancellous bone screws. These screws are affixed to each other by laterally placed distraction rods, which not only afford stability but also allow some correction of the kyphotic deformity (Fig. 12-23). Dunn[27] has developed two fixation devices for the lumbar spine based on similar principles. Both the type I (Fig. 12-24) and the type II (Fig. 12-26) devices are similar in concept to the Kostuik fixation system, relying on a large cancellous screw inserted into the vertebral body laterally and at right angles to the longitudinal axis of the spine. Fixation between vertebral bodies is accomplished through the use of vertical distraction rods. The vertebrectomy defect is filled with methylmethacrylate or occasionally with corticocancellous bone graft if prolonged surviv-

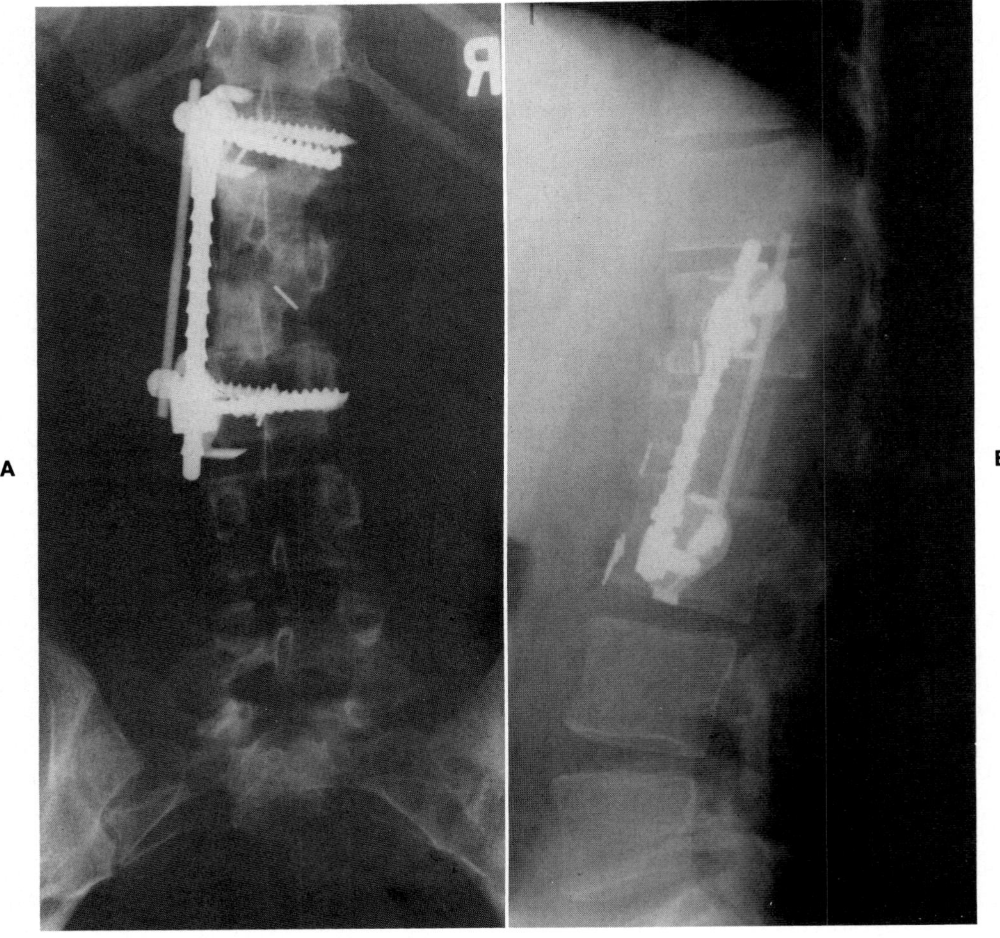

FIGURE 12-23 Kostuik anterior lumbar fixation system. The L2 vertebral body has been resected, and the spinal cord decompressed. Stabilization was performed by an iliac graft with combined anterolateral distraction and compression fixation. (Reprinted with permission from Kostuik, J.P.: Clin. Orthop. **189:**103. 1984.)

al is anticipated and local irradiation is not planned. When a bone graft is used, however, external immobilization of the spine is necessary for an average of 3 months postoperatively or until consolidation of the graft is complete.

In our experience the disadvantages of the Kostuik[49] and Dunn[27] systems are significant:

1. Both leave a large amount of metal outside the vertebral column that can lead to erosion of adjacent soft tissues, particularly an adjacent major vessel.
2. Neither is particularly effective in accomplishing correction of the kyphotic deformity, because the axis of distraction is lateral rather than anterior (Fig. 12-23, *B*). If attempts at distraction are too vigorous, a lateral curvature can be created (Fig. 12-23, *A*).
3. Vertebral fixation is aligned at right angles to both the distraction forces and the weight-bearing axis of the spine, a situation that is biomechanically unsound over the long term unless bony fusion ensues.
4. The devices, placed well outside the rotation of the spine, are subjected to large torque stresses during even modest rotation of the lumbar spine.

At the L4 and S1 levels, the problems of fixation are even more acute. The marked lordosis here adds forward-shearing stresses to the already major torque stresses described. The acute angulation between the L5 vertebral body and the sacrum frustrates anterior fixation attempts by any technique yet devised. In our opinion there simply are no means for anterior stabilization at the lumbosacral junction. If vertebrectomy and dural decompression is necessary at this level (Fig.

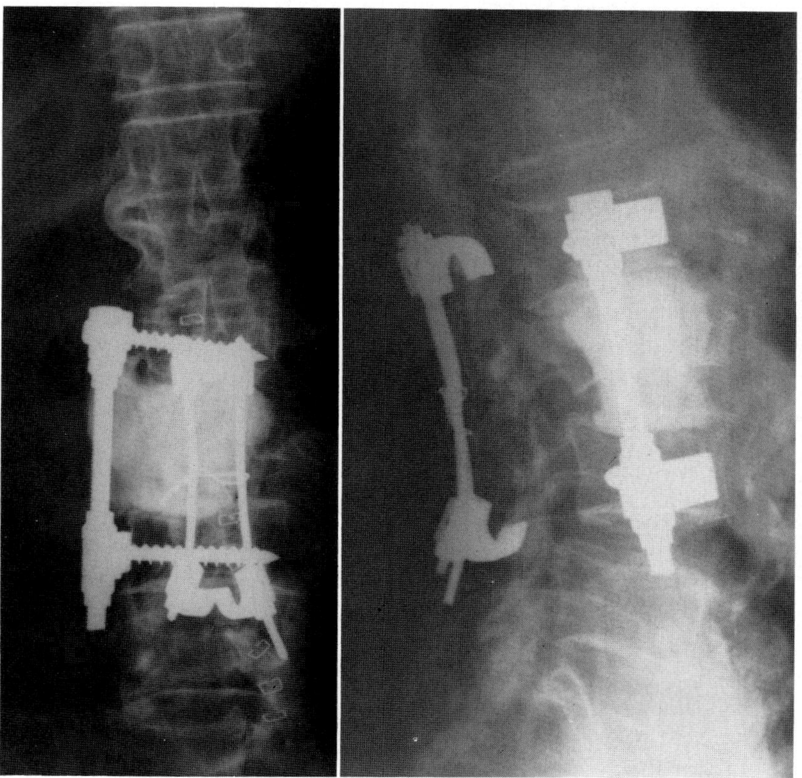

FIGURE 12-24 The L3 vertebral body has been resected, the spinal cord decompressed, and the spine reconstructed with the Dunn type I device anteriorly and Harrington compression rods posteriorly. Only through the use of Harrington compression rods could the kyphosis be corrected completely and a tendency for right lateral angulation of the construct be avoided.

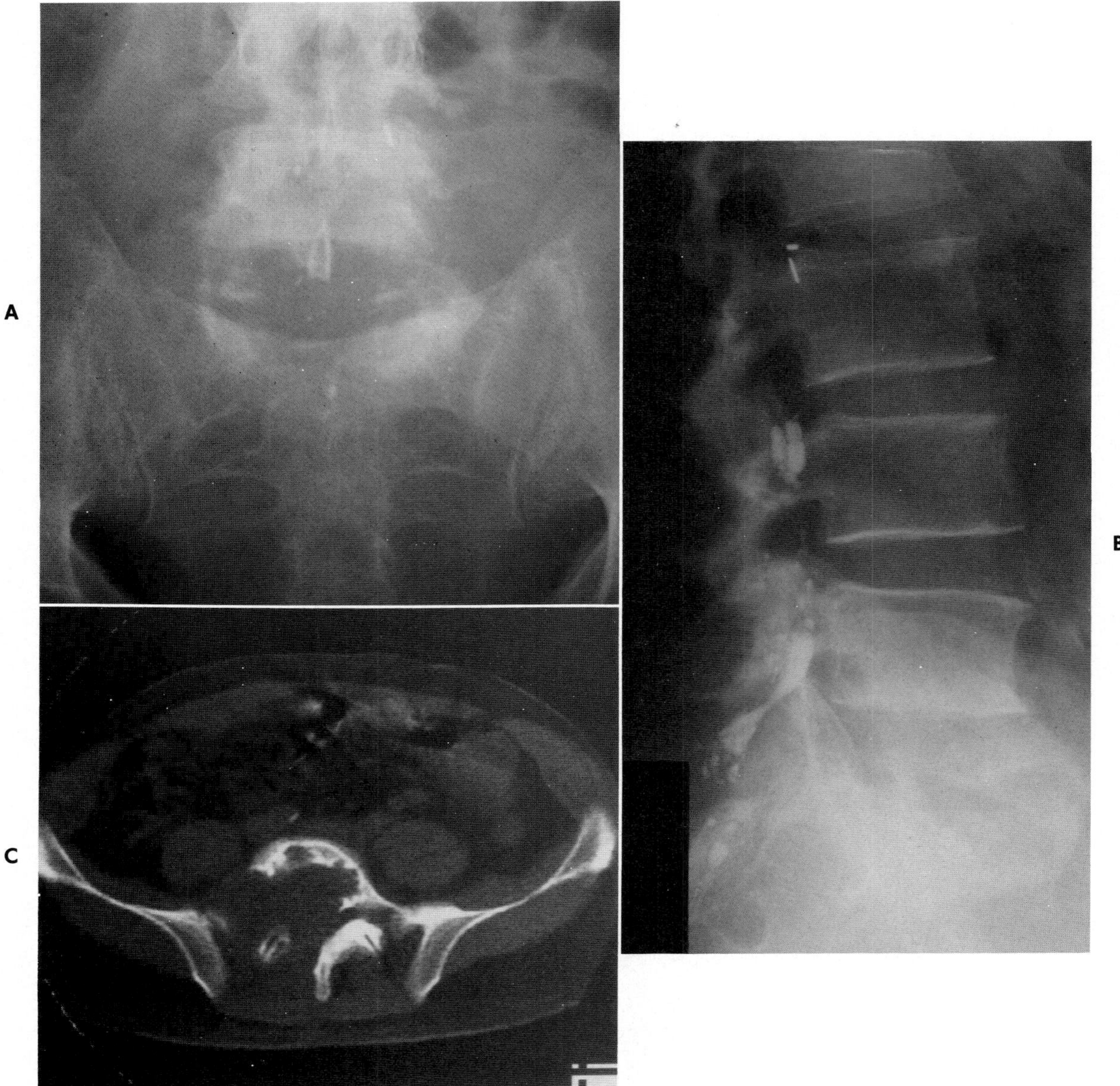

FIGURE 12-25 **A** and **B,** Metastatic carcinoma of the kidney with almost complete dissolution of the L5 vertebral body and posterior elements. **C,** A CT scan reveals only a shell of the anterior L5 vertebra remaining and almost complete dissolution of the facet joints. A progressive forward subluxation of L4 on the sacrum developed. An attempt at combined anterior and posterior stabilization was unsuccessful because of the extensive bone loss.

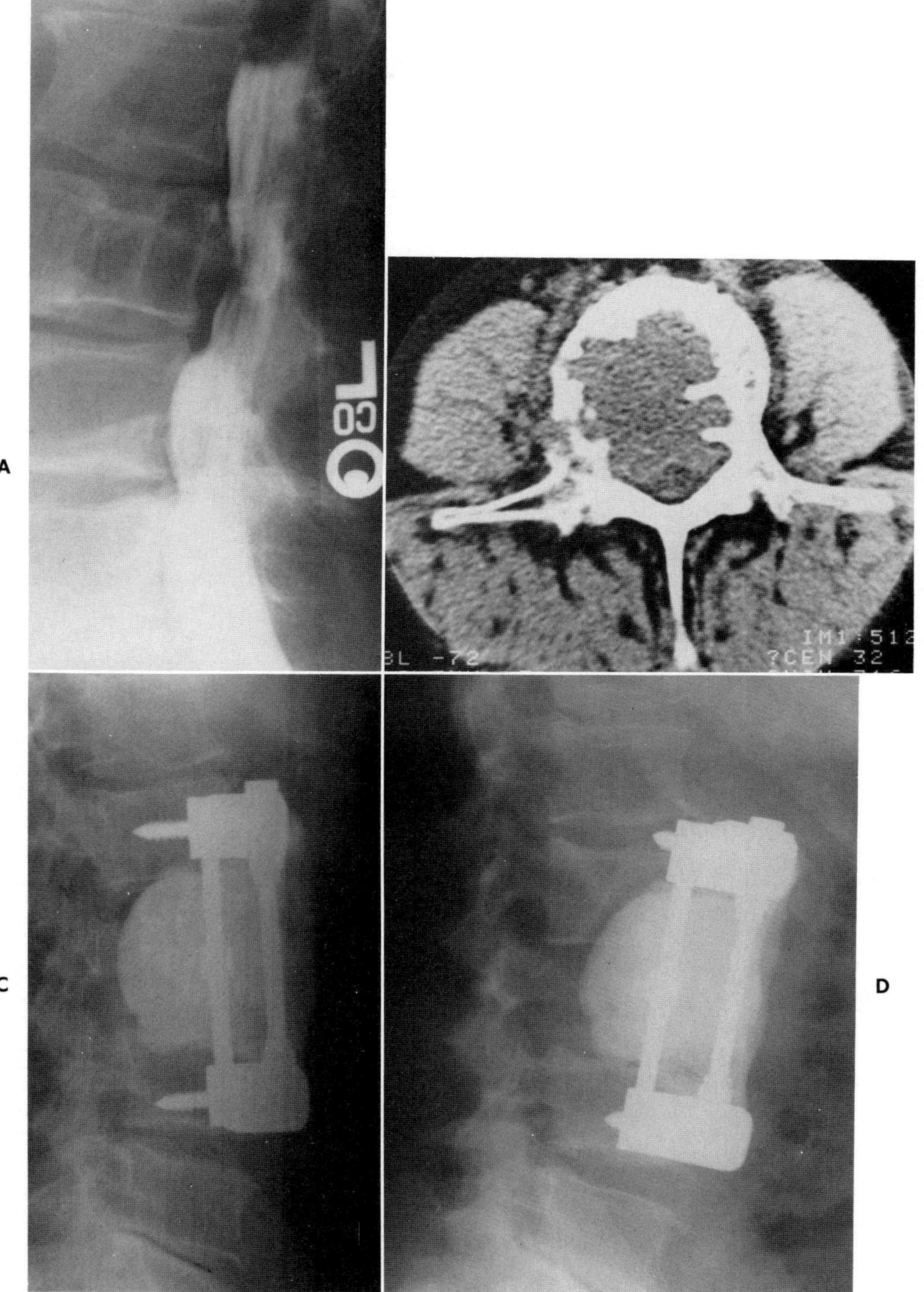

FIGURE 12-26 **A,** Exophytic lytic lesion of the L3 vertebral body from a myeloma. Despite local irradiation, the patient suffered progressive spinal canal impingement and interference with bowel and bladder function. **B,** A CT scan of the affected vertebra shows invasion of the spinal canal by the tumor, which originated within the vertebral body. **C,** Anterior decompression and stabilization was accomplished with the Dunn III fixation system augmented by intervertebral methylmethacrylate. Because of irradiation skin changes posteriorly, no attempt was made to augment this by compression rod fixation. **D,** Within 3 months the fixation screw and staple had pulled out of the L2 vertebral body and the patient was beset with severe back pain. His neurological compromise, however, did not recur.

12-25), stabilization should be accomplished posteriorly. Even with a posterior approach, however, stabilization is difficult and requires the use of a transsacral bar and segmental stabilization with Harrington rods.

The Dunn type III device[27] (Fig. 12-26) allows somewhat rigid fixation of the larger lumbar vertebrae. It is applied more anteriorly than the Kostuik or Dunn II apparatuses, and the rigid two-bar and curved-plate construct is more resistant to torque stresses. However, the curved plates applied to the vertebral bodies are quite large and in smaller patients tend to overlap the vertebral end plates, thereby reducing the solidarity of fixation. The bone staple used to secure the anterior part of the plate to the vertebral body is sufficiently wide that its prongs often enter the disc spaces rather than the vertebral bone itself, obviously minimizing fixation. We have used the Dunn III device for stabilization in eight patients with lower lumbar instability secondary to metastatic malignancy. Six enjoyed lasting stability for up to 2 years postoperatively, but in two the device pulled out of the bone and fixation was lost (Fig. 12-26, *D*).

Posterior Decompression and Stabilization

During the discussion of the indications for radiotherapy it was noted that a retrospective analysis[37] of the use of laminectomy decompression to relieve cord or root compromise from metastases had revealed the technique to be minimally effective and no better than irradiation alone. In fact, our experience[42,44] indicates that most patients subjected to laminectomy decompression for metastatic spinal disease are actually worsened by the procedure, because it leads to progressive instability and a progressive kyphotic deformity (Fig. 12-27). Destruction of the vertebral body by tumor leads to a progressive kyphotic deformity and this can only be accentuated by the type of posterior element resection inherent in a laminectomy decompression. Our experience with 12 patients subjected to wide posterior laminectomy decompression showed that only one improved even temporarily neurologically while nine deteriorated because of progressive spinal deformity. Six of the nine patients, including the one who improved initially, later deteriorated neurologically as the deformity worsened and cord compression increased at the apex of the kyphosis. Other authors* have reported similar results. Dunn, alone[24] and with various co-workers,[25-26] has emphasized the high incidence of spinal instability following posterior laminectomy decompression of as few as two levels.

The concept of laminectomy as more of a destabilization than a decompression is further supported by the fact that it is also impossible to decompress the anterior cord, where tumor invasion usually originates, from a posterior approach. In the cervical and thoracic spines, in particular, the spinal canal is small relative to the size of the cord and there is no way to dissect around to the front safely and remove tumor tissue and bone. The best that can be accomplished from a posterior approach is to remove enough bone (ordinarily three laminae at a minimum) to allow the cord to bulge posteriorly and thereby escape the effects of the tumor mass. Thus the idea that a posterior decompression often is preferable to an anterior decompression in the cancer patient because "the procedure is less extensive"[55] has little validity.

On occasion a posterior spinal decompression will be indicated for the patient with cord or root compression originating from a tumor focus in the laminae or pedicles, or when a circumferential "napkin ring" constriction by tumor and inflammatory tissue cannot be relieved entirely from an anterior approach (Figs. 12-5, *A*, and 12-28, *A* to *C*). A wide complete laminectomy is performed, exposing the roots well laterally and extending at least one level above and one level below the extent of cord constriction (Figs. 12-28, *C*, and 12-29). Ordinarily the tumor and reactive inflammatory tissue can be peeled carefully off the dura, leaving it soft and pulsatile and clearly free of constricting bands.

After decompression has been completed, stabilization is essential. Wide laminectomy decompression is never indicated without concominant stabilization, even if there is no evidence as yet of anterior vertebral collapse.† Posterior stabilization also is indicated when tumor lysis of the posterior ele-

Text continued on p. 374.

*References 16, 21, 24, 25, 32, 76.
†References 14, 21, 32, 42, 44.

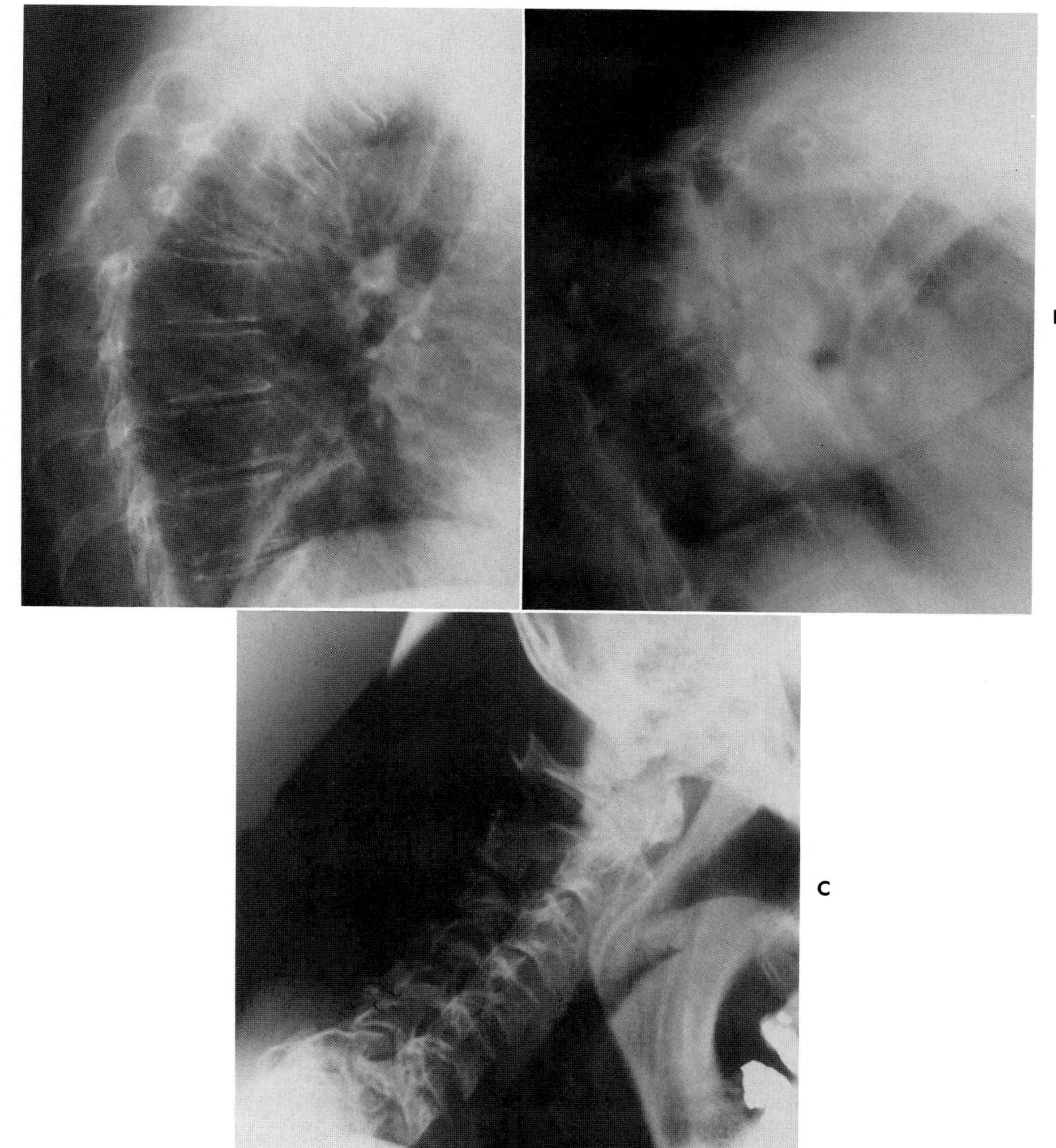

FIGURE 12-27 **A,** Acute pathological compression fracture at T6 with forward subluxation of T5 on T7. The patient had a Frankel grade C neurological deficit. **B,** A two-level laminectomy decompression was performed without stabilization. Within 2 months a 98-degree kyphus developed and the patient deteriorated to a Frankel grade A paraplegia. **C,** Similar disaster following a laminectomy at C6 without stabilization.

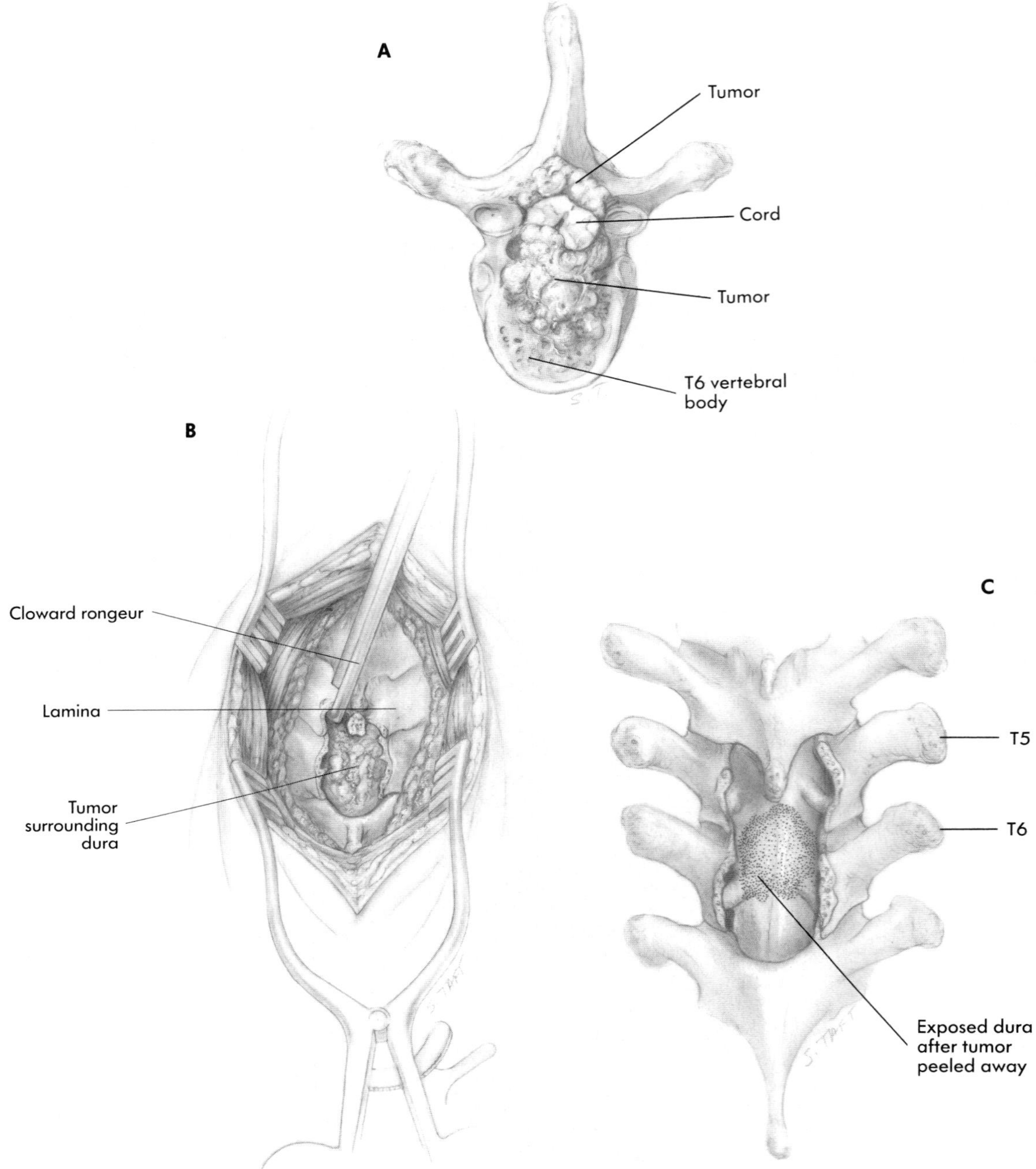

FIGURE 12-28 Technique for posterior decompression and stabilization where significant compression of the cord from behind requires a multilevel laminectomy (see Figs. 12-5 and 12-30). **A,** Type of situation shown in Fig. 12-5. The spinal cord is compressed by tumor circumferentially (so-called "napkin ring") and is displaced posteriorly against the unyielding laminae. **B,** With a variety of curets and rongeurs a complete laminectomy is performed over at least two, and usually three, levels. Epidural bleeding generally is minimal because the thick plaque of tumor has ablated many epidural vessels locally. However, great care must be taken to avoid penetrating the dura where it is plastered against the anterior surface. **C,** After the spinal canal has been decompressed completely, as much tumor tissue as possible is peeled off the dural surface in an effort to relieve the napkin ring constriction.

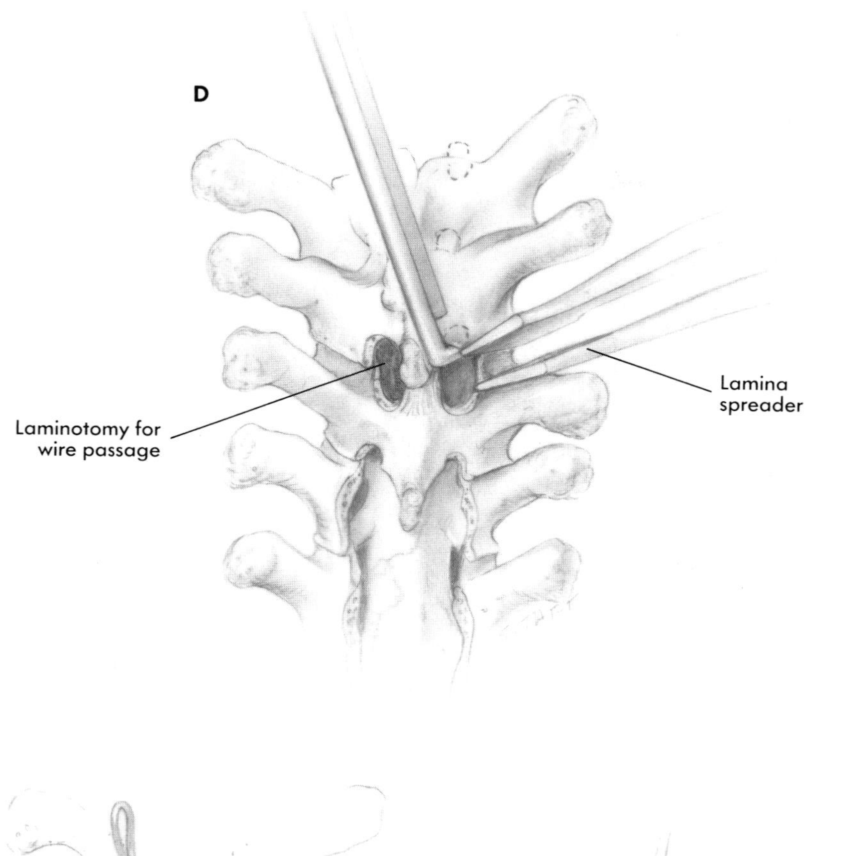

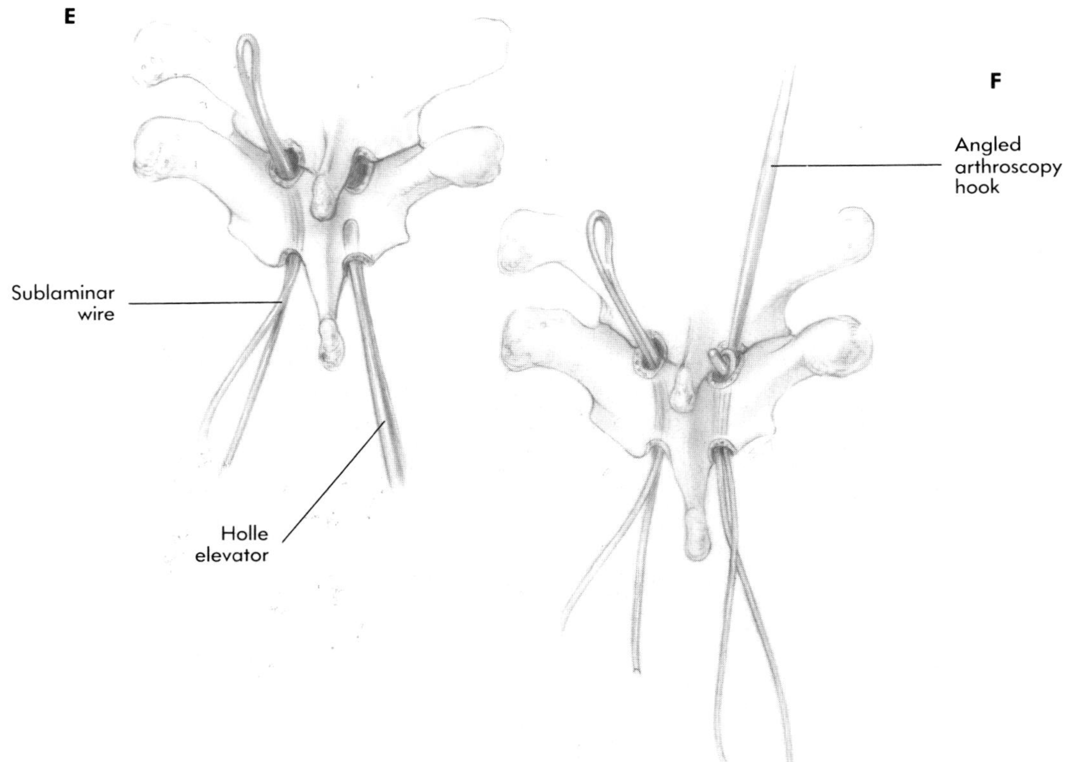

FIGURE 12-28, cont'd. **D,** Following decompression and dural release, preparations are made for stabilization with Luque rods and sublaminar wire fixation. The interlaminar space is widened at each of three levels above and below the extent of the decompression. Notches are cut in the inferior and superior laminar edges with a Lempert or similar rongeur. **E,** A small Holle elevator is passed beneath the lamina to create a space for passage of a doubled 16-gauge wire. **F,** Retrieval of the wire loop may be facilitated by using a small meniscal hook.

Continued.

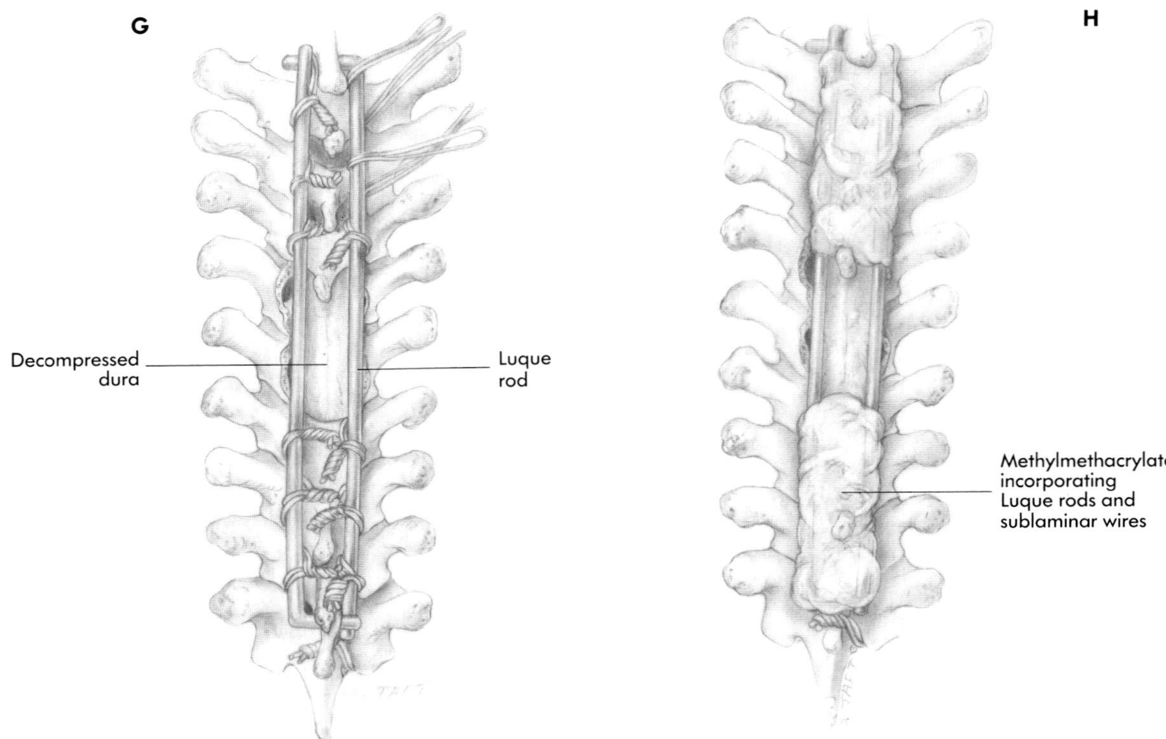

FIGURE 12-28, cont'd. **G,** The Luque rods are cut to appropriate lengths, interdigitated along the laminar sulcus, and secured by the doubled 16-gauge wires at each level. **H,** Stability of the rod and wire fixation above and below the laminectomy is enhanced by packing methylmethacrylate into the areas of wire-rod fixation. This forms a rigid construct which allows sublaminar wire fixation at any single level to reinforce every other level.

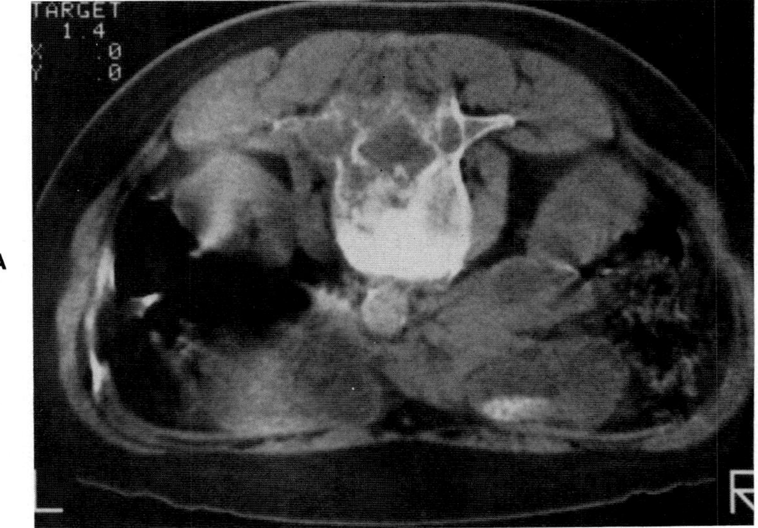

FIGURE 12-29 **A,** CT scan of a typical pattern for metastatic laminar infiltration and spinal canal compromise. Although it is not demonstrated well on this scan, the cord and adjacent nerve roots were found to be compressed from behind over two levels.

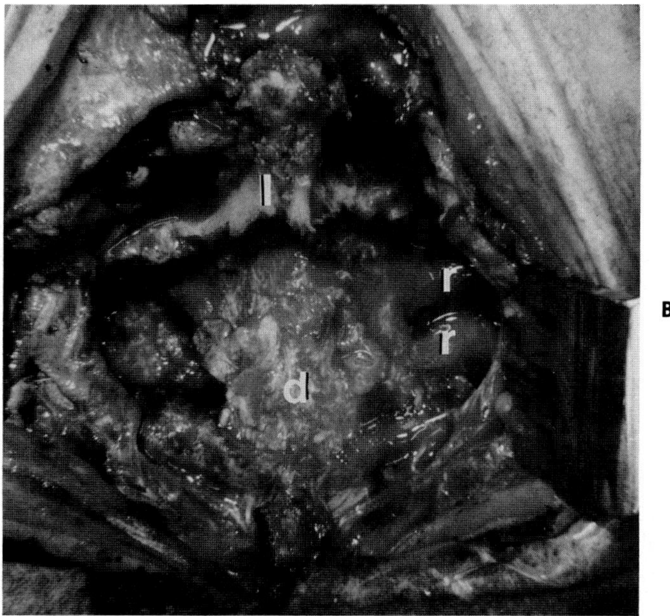

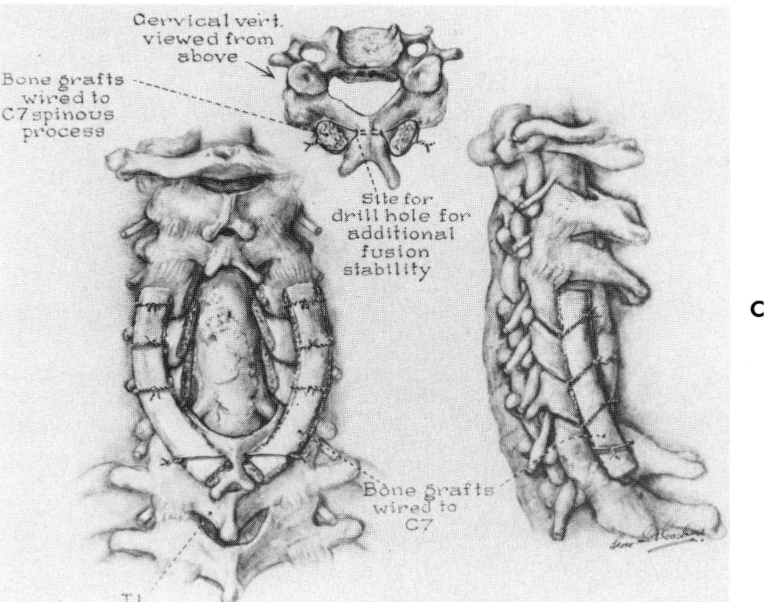

FIGURE 12-29, cont'd. **B,** Intraoperative view of the spine. Note the wide extent of cord and root decompression necessary. The two right roots are clearly seen *(r),* as are the dura *(d)* and first intact lamina *(l)* above the decompression. **C,** After wide multilevel decompression of the cervical spine, it is quite difficult but essential to obtain secondary stability. The technique of Robinson and Southwick is demonstrated. If the site requires irradiation, stability may be achieved by a combination of segmental wiring and methylmethacrylate. (**C** from Riley, L.: Clin Orthop. **91**:16, 1973.)

ments and supporting ligamentous structures has resulted in facet joint instability and a progressive forward slippage of the upper on the lower spine (Plate 2, *E*). Finally, the posterior approach should always be considered when stabilization of the C1-C2 level is necessary either because of anterior or posterior disease or because it is difficult to approach the upper two cervical vertebrae from the front (Fig. 12-30).

Posterior stabilization in the *cervical* spine can be accomplished by sublaminar or spinous process fixation with 16- or 18-gauge wire if no more than a three-level laminectomy decompression has been performed and there is reasonable expectation that cancellous bone graft placed across the stabilized segments will be incorporated (Plate 2, *E*). Such an expectation would exist only if the patient is not to be irradiated postoperatively or has not been irradiated within 4 months preceding the proposed operation. Postoperatively, external immobilization (usually in the form of a halo-vest) is essential for 10 to 12 weeks following bone grafting or until there is evidence of graft incorporation. In most instances this type of stabilization is not possible. The patient may require irradiation postoperatively or may have undergone irradiation recently, and in either case the likelihood of bone graft incorporation is minimal. The patient may require too many levels of posterior decompression to make wire fixation possible or may have a contraindication to external halo-vest immobilization (e.g., skull metastases). When one of these contraindications exists, an attempt must be made to achieve instantaneous stability that will not deteriorate in the absence of bony fusion or require even temporary external reinforcement.

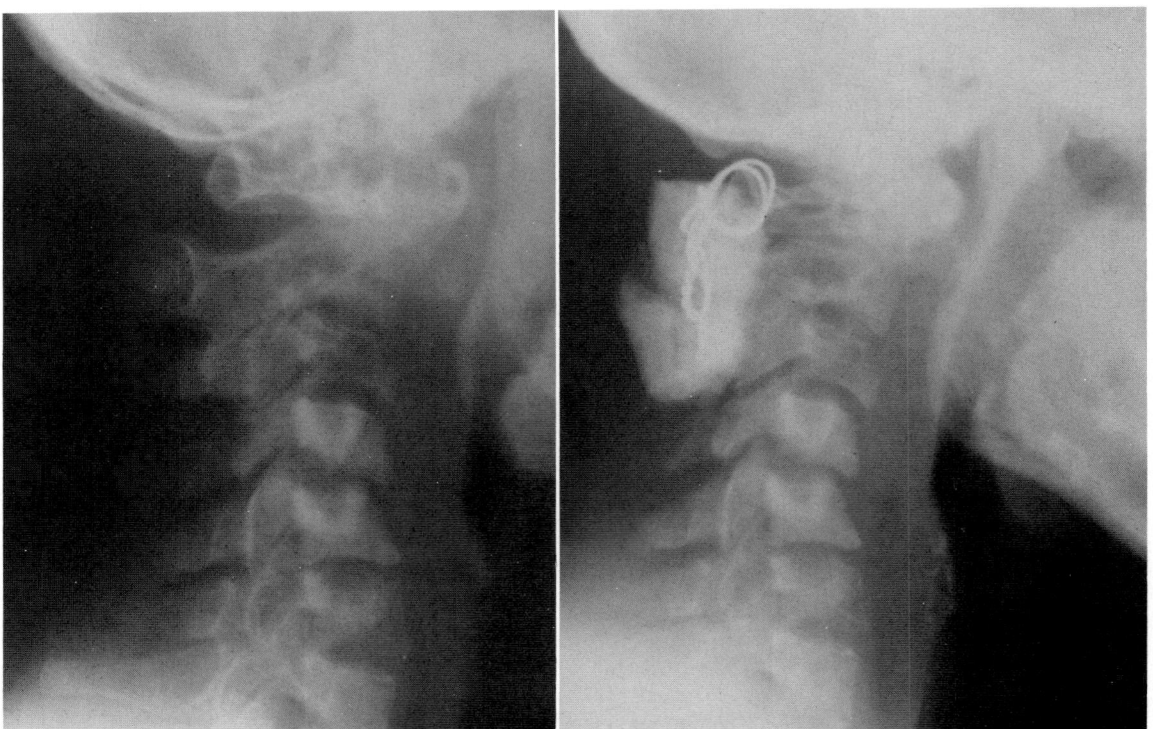

FIGURE 12-30 Indications for posterior stabilization of the upper cervical spine. **A,** Pathological undisplaced odontoid fracture in a 38-year-old woman with metastatic breast cancer. There were no neurological symptoms. **B,** The posterior elements of C1 to C3 were stabilized by wire and methylmethacrylate. The obvious lytic changes in the C3 vertebral body prompted the surgeon to consider extending the stabilization to C4. However, because the posterior elements of C4 were mostly destroyed, it was decided to limit the wiring as shown. The patient survived for 8 months postoperatively and had no further neck symptoms.

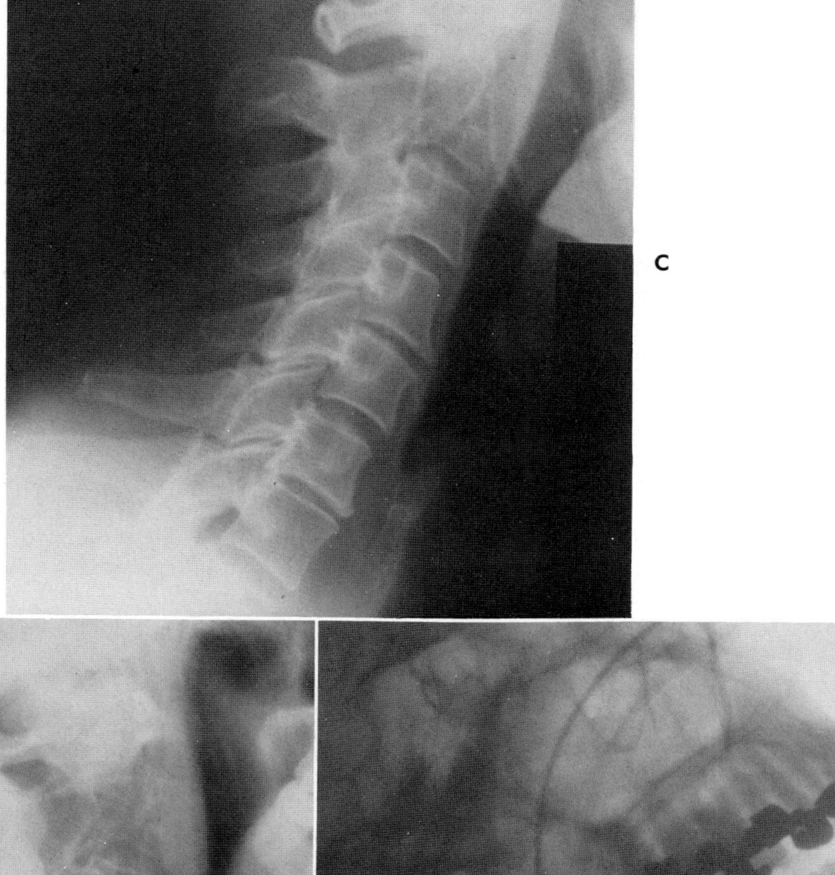

FIGURE 12-30, cont'd. **C,** Roentgenogram of a patient with neck pain, lytic changes in the body of C2, and on tomography a pathological fracture of the basilar odontoid. The primary source of this tumor was unknown. **D,** The upper three vertebrae were stabilized from behind. **E,** Trocar biopsy of the C2 vertebral body and odontoid then was performed. The patient was found to have metastases from an unrecognized esophageal carcinoma.

Occasionally such secure stabilization can be accomplished in the lower cervical spine or for cervicothoracic instability by using Luque rods and multilevel sublaminar wiring (Fig. 12-5, *C* and *D*). However, it is difficult to achieve fixation above the C5 level by this technique because the laminae in the upper cervical spine are thin and fragile and not enough intact laminae exist above the highest level of the posterior decompression to allow for secure fixation of the rods. Fidler[29] has attempted to solve this dilemma by designing a plate shaped like a tuning fork. The short limb can be affixed to the occiput through screw holes; the long parallel limbs are secured to four cervical laminae by sublaminar wiring. We have had no experience with this device and note that Fidler himself reports on its use in only three cases. However, it would seem that the occipital stabilization achieved is tenuous at best, particularly in patients with skull metastases.

The most common technique employed for cervical spine stabilization under these circumstances is as follows: 18- or 16-gauge wires are passed through the spinous processes or beneath the laminae at the appropriate levels and the ends are twisted together to form a rigid wire construct; the wires and the spinous processes are then incorporated together with methylmethacrylate (Figs. 12-28, *H,* and 12-30, *A* and *B*); the acrylic cement thereby forms a continuum between bone and wires, helping to dissipate the highly concentrated stresses of the wire directly on bone that would otherwise exist. Clark et al.[14] reported an extensive experience with this technique, noting good overall results. We have also found it to be effective, particularly in achieving lasting stability in the upper three cervical levels, where the laminae are rather thin and the anterior approach is more difficult. The risk that the wires will cut out of the bone remains moderately high, however Some authors[14,24,26] augment the fixation by packing methylmethacrylate on one side across the laminae and bone-grafting along the opposite side in an attempt to achieve both temporary and permanent stability.

The major difficulty in using posteriorly placed methylmethacrylate to enhance stabilization, particularly in the mobile cervical spine, is that the stresses imposed on this construct attack its greatest weaknesses. Methylmethacrylate has excellent resistance to compressive loads and thus is ideal for anterior vertebral reconstruction. It is minimally able to withstand torque and shear loads, however, and these are the exact stresses to which it is subjected when used for posterior stabilization. Panjabi et al.[57] confirmed this by Instron biomechanical testing on a postmortem C4-T2 posterior methylmethacrylate-wire fixation construct. They showed that failure in flexion occurred at only 70 newtons, the torque exterted by gentle flexion of the neck. Similarly Whitehill and various others[70-72] using canine and in vivo models showed that the posterior methylmethacrylate-wire constructs lose mechanical stability usually within the first month and exhibit radiographic evidence of failure before the second month. The authors also demonstrated a fibrous tissue interface that invariably formed between the posterior laminar surface and the cement mass, indicating that the apparently solid construct created at operation had degenerated quickly into separately moving segments shortly after spinal motion resumed (Fig. 12-31). A similar fibrous interface between bone and methylmethacrylate has been found to contain cells capable of secreting prostaglandins and collagenases that cause progressive lysis of the adjacent bone and may actually further weaken bone already involved by metastases.[38] McAfee et al.[53] collected 22 failures of cement spinal stabilizations, all but three involving posterior approaches and all but two in the cervical spine. The average time to failure for the posterior cement-wire reconstructions was about 7 months, and in almost every instance failure occurred as the acrylic initially loosened its tenuous attachment to bone and the fixation wires pulled out of the laminae.

Despite these problems with posterior *cervical* fixation augmented by methylmethacrylate, there are situations in which the technique is useful and appropriate. Unless irradiation is planned for the immediate postoperative period, such stabilization should be augmented by cancellous bone grafts extending over any portions of the posterior elements that remain exposed. To minimize the transmission of torque or flexion stresses to the cement-bone interface, the wires used for fixation should be doubled 16-gauge stainless steel.

A B

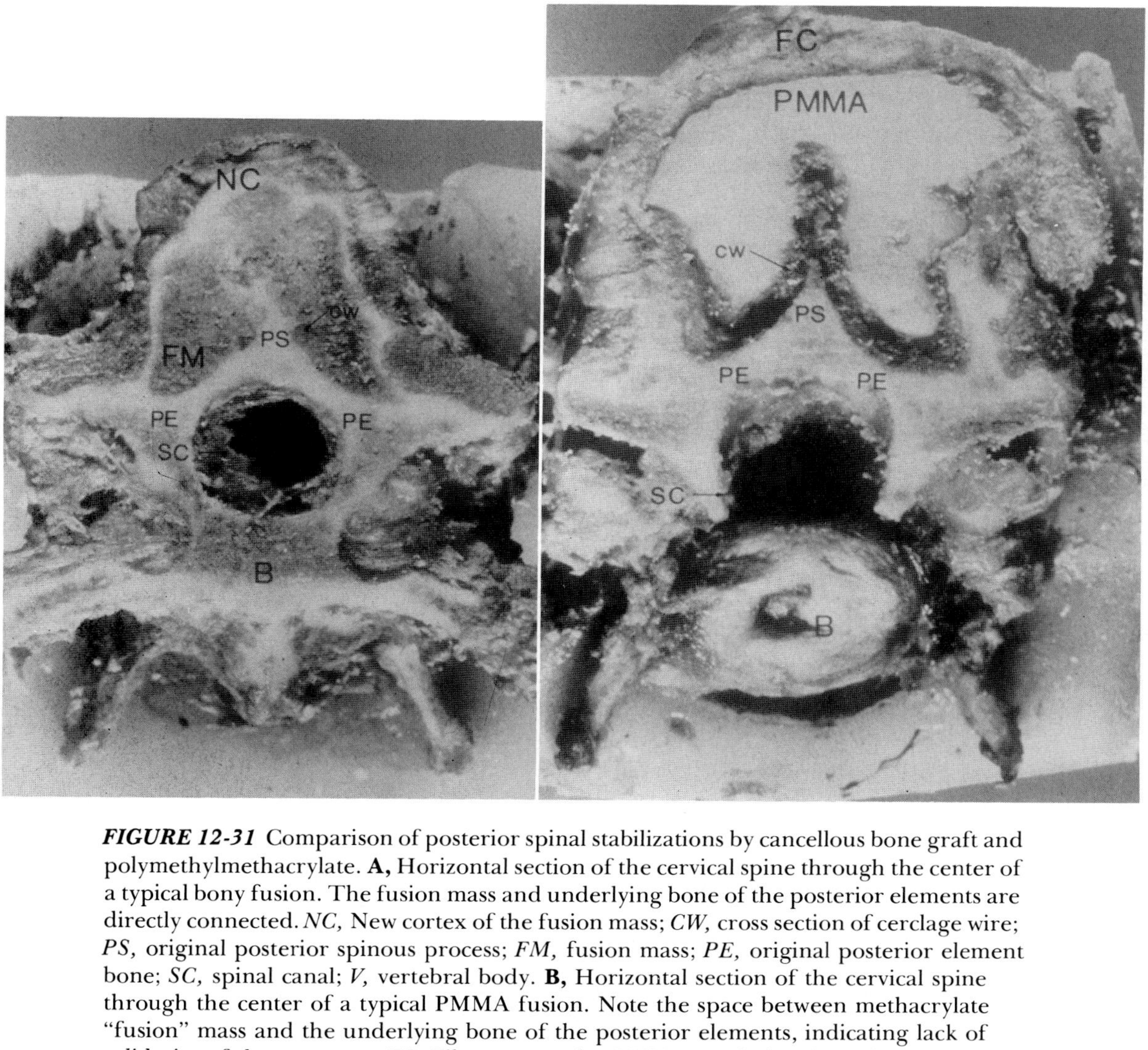

FIGURE 12-31 Comparison of posterior spinal stabilizations by cancellous bone graft and polymethylmethacrylate. **A,** Horizontal section of the cervical spine through the center of a typical bony fusion. The fusion mass and underlying bone of the posterior elements are directly connected. *NC,* New cortex of the fusion mass; *CW,* cross section of cerclage wire; *PS,* original posterior spinous process; *FM,* fusion mass; *PE,* original posterior element bone; *SC,* spinal canal; *V,* vertebral body. **B,** Horizontal section of the cervical spine through the center of a typical PMMA fusion. Note the space between methacrylate "fusion" mass and the underlying bone of the posterior elements, indicating lack of solidarity of the construct. *FC,* Fibrous capsule; *PMMA,* methylmethacrylate mass; *CW,* cross section of cerclage wire; *PS,* original posterior spinous process; *PE,* original posterior element bone; *SC,* spinal canal; *V,* vertebral body. (**A** and **B** reprinted with permission from Whitehill, R., et al.: Spine **9:**246, 1984.)

Posterior stabilization in the *thoracic* and *lumbar* spines can be accomplished much more effectively, because there is room above and below the laminectomy levels to achieve secure rod fixation and augment that fixation by sublaminar wiring. In our opinion Harrington distraction rods alone should not be used for stabilization in metastatic spine disease. They tend to accentuate the kyphotic deformity and there is also a high incidence of the hooks' cutting out of the laminae with even minimal increases in forward angulation (Fig. 12-32). In contrast, Luque rods are ideal for such fixation and are employed with increasing frequency for stabilization of all varieties of traumatic flexion deformities whether or not a laminectomy is required (Fig. 12-33). Luque rods are much more rigid than Harrington rods and are more amenable to sublaminar wire fixations. We ordinarily reinforce Luque rod stabilization above and below a laminectomy defect by incorporating the rods, sublaminar wires, and spinous processes in methylmethacrylate. This minimizes the risks that the wires will cut out through tumor-weakened laminar bone (Fig. 12-28, *H*).

The passage of heavy wires sublaminarly can be accomplished without difficulty so long as certain measures are taken to minimize the risk of dural penetration or injury to the root sleeves. The interlaminar space is spread open, and notches are cut into the adjacent superior and inferior laminal margins to enhance wire placement (Fig. 12-28, *D*). Gently, with a Holle dissector, a tract is created, special care being taken to avoid penetrating the dura or damaging the underlying neural structures (Fig. 12-28, *E*). Doubled 16-gauge wire then is passed sublaminarly. Its looped end can be retrieved easily by using a small right-angle hook probe (Fig. 12-28, *F*). A pair of Luque rods is cut to length and bent to recreate the

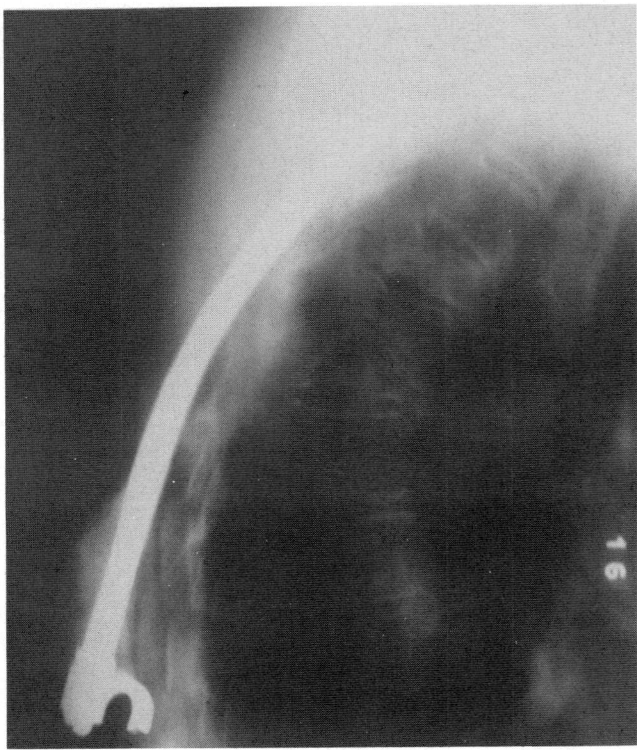

FIGURE 12-32 Example of the ineffectiveness of Harrington distraction rods for stabilizing the spine after vertebral collapse anteriorly and facet instability following wide laminectomy posteriorly. Neither progressive anterior subluxation nor increasing kyphosis is prevented. Moreover, as both worsen, the lower hooks eventually cut out from beneath the laminae.

normal lordotic or kyphotic curves of the spine (Fig. 12-5, *C*). The rods are then secured as shown in Fig. 12-29, *G*, by sublaminar wires three levels above and three levels below the laminectomy defect. External bracing is not required following such stabilization.

Anterolateral Decompression

On rare occasions, tumor growth causing compression of the spinal cord or nerve roots will initially occur laterally and later extend both anteriorly and posteriorly. The tumor may grow in through a neural foramen from a focus in the paraspinal musculature (Fig. 12-3, *D*), or it may break into the spinal canal from the vertebral body early before there has been much destruction of bone (Fig. 12-11, *C*). In either instance it rarely is necessary to attempt any type of stabilization procedure, because sufficient unaffected bone remains that there is little risk of vertebral collapse or spinal instability.

In the thoracic spine it is simplest to use a costotransversectomy approach, beginning posteriorly and removing the medial 3 cm of rib at the level to be decompressed. In the lumbar spine a conventional laminectomy approach is used; but the decompression extends well laterally, usually necessitating resection of the facet joint and a portion of the pedicle on the affected side. The most difficult area in which to perform a wide lateral decompression is the cervical spine because of the presence of the vertebral artery lateral-

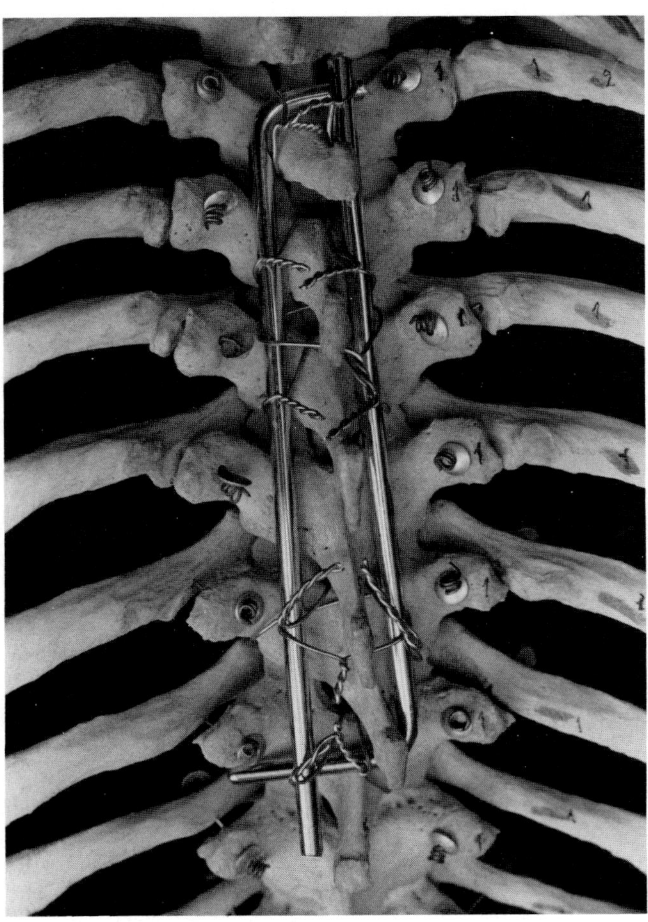

FIGURE 12-33 Segmental posterior stabilization with Luque rods and sublaminar wiring. The strength of the resulting construct is further enhanced by wiring the rods to each other. (Reprinted with the permission from Sullivan, J.A.: Clin. Orthop. **189:**178, 1984.)

ly in its canal. The decompression usually is best accomplished by a wide laminectomy and resection of one or more facet joints on one side as demonstrated in Fig. 12-29, *B*. Needless to say, posterior stabilization is required after such decompression. We have also performed wide anterolateral cervical decompressions on two occasions by sacrificing one of the vertebral arteries, and no complications have been recognized in either case.

Combined Anterior and Posterior Stabilization

In the cervical and thoracic spine we have rarely found it necessary to perform both anterior and posterior stabilizations following an anterior decompression. So long as the posterior column of the spine, as described by Denis,[20] remains intact, anterior distraction stabilization with a Knodt rod and methylmethacrylate is sufficient provided secure fixation of the construct to the adjacent normal vertebral bodies can be achieved (Fig. 12-12). However, if the posterior elements have been destroyed by tumor or by a previous operative decompression, posterior stabilization should be considered. Under these circumstances the anterior decompression and stabilization should be accomplished first and the spine protected by a halo brace until posterior fixation can be completed. For lesions of the lower lumbar spine, where secure anterior fixation is difficult to achieve, we advocate both anterior and posterior stabilization in almost all instances when instability is apparent. Posterior stability is best achieved by using either one of the new transpedicular fixation systems or the short (Harrington or Knodt) compression rods. The compression rods are more effective than distraction rods in maintaining the normal lower lumbar lordosis once anterior stability has been achieved.

RESULTS

It is essential to discuss, at least briefly, our overall results for the treatment of patients with spinal instability and neurological compromise from metastatic malignancy. Only by such an assessment can the reader determine for himself whether the aggressive techniques described here for cord and root decompression and for spinal stabilization seem justified.

As already noted, radiotherapy alone is rarely effective in relieving a well-established neural deficit in the face of a collapsed vertebral body. The combination of radiation and systemic steroids offers little advantage over radiation alone. Neither laminectomy alone nor laminectomy followed by irradiation is more efficacious than radiation alone. By each of these methods, approximately one third of the patients with a major neurological compromise will improve during or after their treatment course, one quarter will become worse, and the remainder will not change.*

For the purpose of accurate comparison, however, it is imperative that the severity of neurological compromise be more specifically quantitated than can be achieved with terms such as "slight" or "major." Frankel et al.[33] established a classification system for quantitating neurological compromise whereby the extent of sensory and motor dysfunction can be conveniently discussed and by which the results of various treatment regimens can be compared.

Grade A: Complete motor and sensory loss
Grade B: Complete motor loss and incomplete sensory loss
Grade C: Some motor function below the level of involvement but no practical use; incomplete sensory loss
Grade D: Useful motor function below the level of involvement; incomplete sensory loss
Grade E: Normal motor and sensory function

Using this system, Nather and Bose[55] reported that fewer than 5% of patients with Frankel grade A, B, or C lesions recovered normal (grade E) or near normal (grade D) function after laminectomy decompression. By comparison, in our series of 78 patients treated by the techniques of anterior decompression described in this chapter, 62% improved to either grade D or grade E levels. More impressively, of 14 patients with complete paraplegia or quadriplegia (Frankel grade A), 8 improved at least two grades and 6 regained the ability to walk and have normal bowel and bladder function. The average

*References 26, 39, 51, 75, 78.

postoperative survival in this group has been 17 months. Twenty-five of the seventy-eight died less than 1 year postoperatively, and the remainder have survived between 1 and 11 years following spinal decompression and stabilization. Twenty-four are still alive more than 1 year postoperative.

Based on these results, we believe that all patients with major neurological compromise (grades A, B, or C) or with intractable mechanical spine pain from vertebral collapse and instability should be considered for decompression and stabilization. We also recommend that in the vast majority of instances this be performed from an anterior approach. Our enthusiasm, however, must not be construed as an advocacy for surgical management of all spinal metastases. Most such patients do not have this degree of localized pain after an initial period of rest and a course of radiotherapy. Most do not experience any great degree of neurological compromise. And many with spinal involvement, even when associated with severe local pain or neurological compromise, do not enjoy a sufficiently long life expectancy to warrant an operative intervention of this magnitude.

REFERENCES

1. Barron, K.D., et al.: Experience with metastatic neoplasms involving the spinal cord, Neurology **9:**91, 1959.
2. Batson, O.V.: The role of the vertebral veins in metastatic processes, Ann. Intern. Med. **16:**38, 1942.
3. Bernat, J.L., et al.: Suspected epidural compression of the spinal cord and cauda equina by metastatic carcinoma. Clinical diagnosis and survival, Cancer **51:**1953, 1983.
4. Black, P.: Metastatic tumors of the central nervous system. In Abelof, M.D., editor: Spinal metastases in complications of cancer, Baltimore, 1979, Johns Hopkins University Press.
5. Boland, P.J., et al.: Metastatic disease of the spine, Clin. Orthop. **169:**95, 1982.
6. Botterell, E.H., and Fitzgerald, G.W.: Spinal cord compression produced by extradural malignant tumours: early recognition, treatment, and results, Can. Med. Assoc. J. **80:**791, 1959.
7. Brady, L.W., et al.: The treatment of metastatic disease of the nervous system by radiation therapy. In Seydel, H.H., editor: Tumors of the nervous system, New York, 1975, John Wiley & Sons, Inc.
8. Bredt, A.: Chemotherapy of bone metastases. In Weiss, L., and Gilbert, H.A., editors: Bone metastases, Boston, 1981, G.K. Hall & Co.
9. Brice, J., and McKissock, W.: Surgical treatment of malignant extradural spinal tumours, Br. Med. J. **1:**1341, 1965.
10. Burchardt, H., et al.: The effect of Adriamycin and methotrexate on the repair of segmental cortical autografts in dogs, J. Bone Joint Surg. **65A:**103, 1983.
11. Carter, S.K.: Methodology of data reporting in advanced breast cancer trials, Cancer Chemother. Pharmacol. **3:**1, 1979.
12. Chlebowski, R.T., et al.: Combination vs sequential single-agent chemotherapy in advanced breast cancer: relationship between survival and metastatic site, Proc. Am. Assoc. Cancer Res. **20:**603, 1979.
13. Chlebowski, R.T., et al.: Survival of patients with metastatic breast cancer treated with either combination or sequential chemotherapy, Cancer Res. **39:**4503, 1979.
14. Clark, C.R., et al.: Methylmethacrylate stabilization of the cervical spine, J. Bone Joint Surg. **66A:**40, 1984.
15. Cohen, D., et al.: Apparently solitary tumors of the vertebral column, Proc. Mayo Clin. **39:**508, 1964.
16. Constans, J.P., et al.: Spinal metastases with neurological manifestations, J. Neurosurg. **59:**111, 1983.
17. Cooper, K.J., et al.: Insufficiency fractures of the sacrum, Radiology **156:**15, 1985.
18. Davies, D.R., et al.: Transcapillary exchange of strontium and sucrose in canine tibia, J. Appl. Physiol. **40:**17, 1976.
19. Decker, D.A., et al.: Characterization and analysis of complete regression to chemotherapy in metastatic breast cancer, Proc. Am. Assoc. Cancer Res. **20:**241, 1979.
20. Denis, F.: Spinal instability as defined by the three-column spine concept in acute spinal trauma, Clin. Orthop. **189:**65, 1984.
21. DeWald, R.L., et al.: Reconstructive spinal surgery as palliation for metastatic malignancies of the spine, Spine **10:**21, 1985.
22. Dommisse, G.F.: The blood supply of the spinal cord: a critical vascular zone in spinal surgery, J. Bone Joint Surg. **56B:**225, 1974.
23. Dorfman, L.J., et al.: Electrophysiological evidence of subclinical injury to the posterior columns of the human spinal cord after therapeutic radiation, Cancer **50:**2815, 1982.
24. Dunn, E.J.: The role of methylmethacrylate in the stabilization and replacement of tumors of the cervical spine: a project of the Cervical Spine Research Society, Spine **2:**15, 1977.
25. Dunn, E.J., and Anas, P.O.: The management of tumors of the upper cervical spine, Orthop. Clin. North Am. **9:**1065, 1978.
26. Dunn, E.J., et al.: Tumors involving the cervical spine: diagnosis and management. In Bailey, R.W., et al., editors: The cervical spine, Philadelphia, 1983, J.B. Lippincott Co.
27. Dunn, H.K.: Anterior stabilization of thoracolumbar injuries, Clin. Orthop. **189:**116, 1984.
28. Edelson, R.N., et al.: Intramedullary spinal cord metastases: clinical and radiographic findings in nine cases, Neurology **22:**1222, 1972.
29. Fidler, M.W.: Pathological fractures of the cervical spine: palliative surgical treatment, J. Bone Joint Surg. **67B:**352, 1985.
30. Fielding, J.W., et al.: Anterior cervical vertebral body

resection and bone-grafting for benign and malignant tumors: a survey under the auspices of the Cervical Spine Research Society, J. Bone Joint Surg. **61A:**251, 1979.

31. Fitzpatrick, P.J., and Rider, W.D.: Half-body radiotherapy, Int. J. Radiat. Oncol. Biol. Phys. **1:**197, 1976.
32. Flatley, T.J., et al.: Spinal instability due to malignant disease, J. Bone Joint Surg. **66A:**47, 1984.
33. Frankel, H.L., et al.: The value of postural reduction in the initial management of closed injuries of the spine paraplegia and tetraplegia. I, Paraplegia **7:** 179, 1969.
34. Galasko, C.S.B.: Mechanisms of bone destruction in the development of skeletal metastases, Nature **263:** 507, 1976.
35. Galasko, C.S.B., and Bennett, A.: Relationship of bone destruction in skeletal metastases to osteoclast activation and prostaglandins, Nature **263:**508, 1976.
36. Galasko, C.S.B., and Doyle, F.H. The detection of skeletal metastases from mammary cancer. A regional comparison between radiology and scintigraphy, Clin. Radiol. **23:**295, 1972.
37. Gilbert, R.N., et al.: Epidural spinal cord compression from metastatic tumors: diagnosis and treatment, Ann. Neurol. **3:**40, 1978.
38. Goldring, S.R., et al.: The synovial-like membrane at the bone-cement interface in loose total hip replacements and its proposed role in bone lysis, J. Bone Joint Surg. **65A:**575, 1983.
39. Greenberg, H.S., et al.: Epidural spinal cord compression from metastatic tumor: results with a new treatment protocol, Ann. Neurol. **8:**361, 1980.
40. Hall, A.J., and MacKay, N.S.: The results of laminectomy for compression of the cord or cauda equina by extradural malignant tumour, J. Bone Joint Surg. **55B:**497, 1973.
41. Harrington, K.D.: Management of unstable pathologic fracture-dislocations of the spine and acetabulum secondary to metastic malignancy. In American Academy of Orthopaedic Surgeons: Instructional course lectures. Vol. 29, St. Louis 1980, The C.V. Mosby Co.
42. Harrington, K.D.: The use of methylmethacrylate for vertebral body replacement anterior stabilization of pathological fracture dislocations of the spine due to metastatic disease, J. Bone Joint Surg. **63A:**36, 1981.
43. Harrington, K.D.: The management of metastatic disease of the lower extremity, Clin. Orthop. **169:**34, 1982.
44. Harrington, K.D.: Anterior cord decompression and spine stabilization for patients with metastatic lesions of the spine, J. Neurosurg. **61:**107, 1984.
45. Jaffe, W.L.: Tumors and tumorous conditions of the bones and joints, Philadelphia, 1958, Lea & Febiger.
46. Johnson, J.R., et al.: Anterior decompression of the spinal cord for neurological deficit, Spine **8:**396, 1983.
47. Kagan, A.R., et al.: Comparisons of tolerance of the brain and spinal cord to injury by radiations. In Gilbert, H.A., and Kagan, A.R., editors: Radiation damage to the nervous system, a delayed therapeutic hazard, New York, 1980, Raven Press.
48. Kennealey, G.T., et al.: Combination chemotherapy for advanced breast cancer. Two regimens containing Adriamycin, Cancer **42:**27, 1978.
49. Kostuik, J.P.: Anterior spinal cord decompression for lesions of the thoracic and lumbar spine. Techniques, new methods of internal fixation, results, Spine **8:**512, 1983.
50. Livingston, K.E., and Perrin, R.G.: The neurosurgical management of spinal metastases causing cord and cauda equina compression, J. Neurosurg. **49:** 839, 1978.
51. Martin, N.S., and Williamson, J.: The role of surgery in the treatment of malignant tumors of the spine, J. Bone Joint Surg. **52B:**227, 1970.
52. Mastaglia, F.L., et al.: Effects of x-radiation on the spinal cord: an experimental study of the morphological changes in central nerve fibers, Brain **99:**101, 1976.
53. McAfee, P.C., et al.: Failure of stabilization of the spine with methylmethacrylate. A retrospective analysis of twenty-four cases, J. Bone Joint Surg. **68A:**1145, 1986.
54. McAlhany, H.J., and Netsky, M.G.: Compression of the spinal cord by extramedullary neoplasms: a clinical and pathologic study, J. Neuropathol. Exp. Neurol. **14:**276. 1955.
55. Nather, A., and Bose, K.: The results of decompression of cord or cauda equina compression from metastatic extradural tumors, Clin. Orthop. **169:**103, 1982.
56. Ono, K., and Tada, K.: Metal prosthesis of the cervical vertebra, J. Neurosurg. **42:**562, 1975.
57. Panjabi, M.M., et al.: Posterior stabilization with methylmethacrylate. Biomechanical testing of a surgical specimen, Spine **2:**241, 1977.
58. Riley, L.: Surgical approaches to the anterior structures of the cervical spine, Clin. Orthop. **91:**16, 1973.
59. Schaberg, J., and Gainor, B.J.: A profile of metastatic carcinoma of the spine, Spine **10:**19, 1985.
60. Smith, R.: An evaluation of surgical treatment for spinal cord compression due to metastatic carcinoma, J. Neurol. Neurosurg. Psychiatry **28:**152, 1965.
61. Sundaresan, N., et al.: Harrington rod stabilization for pathological fractures of the spine, J. Neurosurg. **60:**282, 1984.
62. Tarlov, I.M.: Spinal cord compression studies. III, Time limits for recovery after gradual compression in dogs, Arch. Neurol. Psychiatry **71:**588, 1954.
63. Tarlov, I.M., and Herz, E.: Spinal cord compression studies. IV, Outlook with complete paralysis in man, Arch. Neurol. Psychiatry **72:**43, 1954.
64. Thompson, J.E., and Keiller, V.M.: Multiple skeletal metastases from cancer of the breast, Surg. Gynecol. Obstet. **38:**369, 1924.

65. Torma, T.: Malignant tumours of the spine and the spinal extradural space: a study based on 250 histologically verified cases, Acta Chir. Scand. (suppl.) **225:**157, 1957.
66. Van Scoy-Mosher, M.B.: Hormonal therapy of metastatic bone disease in bone metastases. In Weiss, L., and Gilbert, H.A., editors: Bone metastasis, Boston, 1981, G.K. Hall & Co.
67. Wang, G.J., et al.: Safety of cement fixation in cervical spine (studies of a rabbit model). Unpublished data, 1978.
68. Ward, E.F., and Kapp, J.P.: Reconstruction of the cervical vertebrae using the ASIF cervical plate. Unpublished data, 1985.
69. White, A.A., III, and Panjabi, M.M.: Clinical biomechanics of the spine, Philadelphia, 1978, J.B. Lippincott Co.
70. Whitehill, R., and Barry, J.C.: The evolution of stability in cervical spinal constructs using either autogenous bone graft or methylmethacrylate cement. A follow-up report on a canine *in vivo* model, Spine **10:**32, 1985.
71. Whitehill, R., et al.: A biomechanical analysis of posterior cervical fusions using polymethylmethacrylate as an instantaneous fusion mass, Spine **8:**368, 1983.
72. Whitehill, R., et al.: The use of methylmethacrylate cement as an instantaneous fusion mass in posterior cervical fusions: a canine in vivo experimental model, Spine **9:**246, 1984.
73. Wild, O., and Porter, R.W.: Metastatic epidural tumour of the spine, Arch. Surg. **87:**137, 1963.
74. Willis, R.A.: The spread of tumours in the human body, ed. 3, London, 1973, Butterworth & Co. (Publishers), Ltd.
75. Wright, R.L.: Malignant tumours of the spinal extradural space: Results of surgical treatment, Ann. Surg. **157:**227, 1963.
76. Yablon, I.G.: The effect of methylmethacrylate on fracture healing, Clin. Orthop. **114:**358, 1976.
77. Yasuoka, S., et al.: Incidence of spinal column deformity after multilevel laminectomy in children and adults, J. Neurosurg. **57:**441, 1982.
78. Young, R.F., et al.: Treatment of spinal epidural metastases. Randomized prospective comparison of laminectomy and radiotherapy, J. Neurosurg. **53:** 741, 1980.

INDEX